Tropical Veterinary Toxicology

Tropical Veterinary Toxicology

Mohd Hezmee Mohd Noor

Department of Veterinary Preclinical Sciences
Faculty of Veterinary Medicine
Universiti Putra Malaysia
Serdang, Selangor Darul Ehsan, Malaysia

WILEY

This edition first published 2026

Registered Offices
John Wiley & Sons, Inc., 111 River Street, Hoboken, NJ 07030, USA
John Wiley & Sons Ltd, New Era House, 8 Oldlands Way, Bognor Regis, West Sussex, PO22 9NQ, UK

For details of our global editorial offices, customer services, and more information about Wiley products visit us at www.wiley.com.

The manufacturer's authorized representative according to the EU General Product Safety Regulation is Wiley-VCH GmbH, Boschstr. 12, 69469 Weinheim, Germany, e-mail: Product_Safety@wiley.com.

Wiley also publishes its books in a variety of electronic formats and by print-on-demand. Some content that appears in standard print versions of this book may not be available in other formats.

Library of Congress Cataloging-in-Publication Data Applied for:

Paperback ISBN: 9781394365524

Cover Design: Wiley
Cover Image: © Mohd Hezmee Mohd Noor

Set in 9.5/12.5pt STIXTwoText by Straive, Pondicherry, India

Printed in Singapore
M136345260626

Dedication

To the veterinarians, livestock producers, wildlife officers, and animal health professionals working under the tropical sun: this book is dedicated to you. Your daily efforts to diagnose, treat, and prevent poisonings in challenging environments make a vital difference in animal and human lives. May this book serve as a helpful companion on the front lines of tropical veterinary medicine, and may your work continue to advance the health of animals and people across the tropics.

Contents

About the Author

Professor Dr. Mohd Hezmee Mohd Noor (born 10 January 1981) is a Malaysian veterinary pharmacologist and toxicologist based at Universiti Putra Malaysia (UPM). He earned his Doctor of Veterinary Medicine (DVM) degree from UPM in 2005 and completed a PhD in Veterinary Pharmacology at the University of Queensland, Australia, in 2011. These qualifications established the foundation of his expertise in animal health and pharmacology. His research career focuses on the impact of chemical and natural toxins on animals in tropical environments. Reflecting this focus, he authored the book *Tropical Veterinary Toxicology* (2026), which draws on his experience in tropical veterinary medicine.

Dr. Hezmee serves in the Department of Veterinary Preclinical Sciences, Faculty of Veterinary Medicine at UPM. He joined UPM's faculty in 2011 and was promoted to Associate Professor in 2017, evidencing his advancement in academia. In this role, he teaches core courses such as veterinary pharmacology and toxicology to undergraduate students and leads postgraduate modules on advanced toxicology topics. He also supervises graduate research projects in pharmacology and toxicology, helping to train new veterinarians and scientists. Through his teaching and mentorship, he ensures that students appreciate both the scientific principles and the real-world relevance of toxicology in tropical animal practice.

Dr. Hezmee's research spans a wide range of toxicology topics relevant to tropical animal health. He has made notable contributions on environmental toxicants – for example, he co-authored a *Veterinary World* review of lead poisoning in animals and humans, addressing a critical contaminant issue in developing countries. He has also investigated natural toxins: One recent study he co-authored examined the chemical constituents and subacute toxicity of *Morus alba* (white mulberry) leaf extract in mice. These projects link veterinary pharmacology to regional challenges, from heavy metal contamination to the safety of traditional plant remedies. By focusing on problems encountered in Southeast Asia, his work advances the understanding of toxicology under tropical conditions.

Beyond pure toxicology, Dr. Hezmee is active in One Health and interdisciplinary programs. He co-authored a guide for in situ, problem-based One Health learning as part of Malaysia's university network, and has organized workshops that bring together veterinary, medical, and environmental professionals. These activities reflect his commitment to the One Health perspective, recognizing the interconnectedness of animal, human, and environmental health – an approach especially important in tropical ecosystems. By linking toxicology to broader health and ecological contexts, he helps prepare the next generation of scientists to address emerging challenges.

In summary, Professor Dr. Mohd Hezmee Mohd Noor combines deep academic training with a regional focus to advance veterinary toxicology in Southeast Asia. Based in Malaysia, he applies pharmacological principles to practical problems such as toxin exposure in livestock and wildlife, agricultural chemical risks, and safety of local remedies. His career – spanning field and laboratory research as well as innovative teaching – illustrates a dedication to tropical veterinary science. He brings this breadth of experience to his roles as author and educator, shaping *Tropical Veterinary Toxicology* with both rigorous scholarship and an understanding of local needs.

Foreword

I began writing *Tropical Veterinary Toxicology* to fill a critical gap for veterinary practitioners who work in equatorial and tropical climates. Animal health challenges in the tropics are very different from those in temperate regions, and solutions must be designed specifically for these environments. As one recent editorial notes, "given the striking differences between temperate and tropical realities, it is of the utmost importance to design specific solutions to animal production and health in the tropics." In other words, simply importing veterinary practices and toxicology knowledge from temperate countries often proves "inadequate, irrelevant and creates additional problems" in tropical contexts. This book therefore focuses on the toxins and poisonings unique to tropical ecosystems – from poisonous plants and fungi to venomous animals and tropical contaminants – and on how to diagnose and manage them effectively in tropical veterinary practice.

Veterinary toxicology is by nature a complex, interdisciplinary field. As one expert source emphasizes, "veterinary toxicology is an important branch and interdisciplinary field of veterinary medicine and toxicology." In the tropics especially, animal exposures are closely linked to human and environmental health – a classic "One Health" situation. For example, tropical animals may ingest pesticide residues or mycotoxins that also threaten human food supplies, and venomous snakes in rural areas can endanger both livestock and people. This book therefore integrates knowledge from animal physiology, pharmacology, ecology, and One Health public health. Throughout, I have highlighted how understanding the interplay of animals, people, and environment is critical to preventing and treating toxicological problems in the tropics.

The scope of this volume is broad – because veterinary toxicology itself encompasses thousands of potential toxins. Livestock and companion animals living outdoors in tropical climates are exposed to myriad natural toxins (in plants, molds, animals) and human-made chemicals. For example, the tropics' warm, humid climate often promotes fungal growth in stored feeds, leading to mycotoxin outbreaks that require specialized monitoring. Similarly, the region's rich biodiversity includes unique venomous snakes and insects rarely seen elsewhere. By bringing together case studies and data relevant to these tropical hazards, this book aims to be an essential reference for any veterinarian practicing in hot, humid regions.

My hope is that *Tropical Veterinary Toxicology* will serve as a practical, scientifically grounded guide. Veterinarians, animal health officers, and students will find in it the tools they need to recognize tropical poisonings, perform appropriate diagnostics, and apply effective treatments. Equally, this work is intended to strengthen interdisciplinary collaboration: By linking toxicology insights with ecology, food safety, and One Health perspectives, we can improve animal production and public health across the tropics. It is my sincere wish that this book will support practitioners on the front lines of tropical veterinary medicine, enabling them to safeguard animal and human health in challenging environments.

Preface

I wrote *Tropical Veterinary Toxicology* because the realities of tropical practice rarely fit the contours of temperate-centric references. Working in hot, humid environments, I saw the same gaps recur: poisonous local plants that never appear in standard lists; monsoon-driven feed spoilage and mycotoxins; heat stress and dehydration that shift pharmacokinetics; residues and counterfeit products circulating through porous supply chains; and aquatic or wildlife exposures that blur the lines between domestic, feral, and free-ranging species. This book is my attempt to address those gaps with a resource built for the tropics.

My aim is practical and evidence-guided: shorten the time from suspicion to sound management; help clinicians choose the right matrices at the right time; and reduce preventable losses through better prevention and communication. Where literature is sparse, I pair the best available evidence with field-tested reasoning and clear limits to inference. Throughout, the book adopts a One Health lens – because in tropical systems, animal toxicology, food safety, and environmental health are inseparable.

How to Use This Book

Early chapters establish foundations you can apply at the bench or in the field: how toxic agents enter, distribute, transform, and exit the body; and how species, age, nutrition, genetics, and environment modulate response. Mid-book chapters translate those principles into practice – diagnostics, sampling, and interpretation – and then into hazard domains that dominate tropical casework (pesticides and agricultural chemicals, heavy metals, and natural toxicants). Later chapters consolidate learning through case-based applications and quick-reference material. The Appendix gathers units, conversions, and bedside tables to keep calculations and sampling choices error-free under time pressure.

Each topic balances mechanism with action: brief context for the why, followed by the what-to-do – first-hour priorities, matrix selection tips, monitoring suggestions, and prevention points that can be communicated to producers, wildlife teams, and regulators. Where withdrawal periods, residues, or environmental externalities matter, those flags are called out so that clinical decisions align with public health and trade realities.

Audience

The primary reader is the veterinarian or student working in (or with) the tropics. The material will also serve laboratory personnel, toxicologists, wildlife officers, producers, and public-health teams – anyone who must recognize patterns quickly, stabilize safely, collect defensible samples, and communicate risk clearly. Educators will find case summaries and figures designed for teaching in resource-variable settings.

Organization

The book begins with core principles (exposure, ADME [absorption, distribution, metabolism, and excretion], and modifiers of toxicity), proceeds to diagnostics and sampling in real-world conditions, and then treats major hazard domains: pesticides and agricultural chemicals; heavy metals; and natural toxicants across plants, fungi, bacteria, and animals. Drug-related toxicities are grouped by therapeutic class and toxidrome for rapid bedside use. A closing chapter integrates lessons through cases and practical tools.

Scope and Limits

This is a guide to decision-making, not a substitute for national regulations or specialist consultation. Trade names are minimized in favor of generic names; concentrations are given in SI units; and examples reflect regional realities while encouraging local adaptation. Where evidence is evolving, I note the uncertainty and emphasize conservative, safety-first practice.

If this book helps you recognize a toxidrome sooner, select the correct matrix, avoid a common pitfall, or prevent the next incident, then it has achieved its purpose. My hope is simple: safer animals, stronger livelihoods, and healthier ecosystems across the tropics.

Acknowledgments

I am deeply grateful to John Wiley & Sons – the editors, production staff, and permissions team – for shepherding this project with care and professionalism. I owe heartfelt thanks to my family for their unwavering encouragement: my wife, Zaharah, and our daughters, Nurain Qisitina and Nuryn Izzaty, who have endured long stretches of writing and fieldwork with patience and love. My parents, Mohd Noor Md Yusop and Zauya Jaafar, instilled a love of learning and a work ethic that sustained every chapter of this book.

Special gratitude goes to the late Professor Dato' Dr. Abdul Salam Abdullah, a pioneering and formative mentor whose scholarship and teaching helped establish veterinary toxicology in Malaysia; his example continues to set the standard for rigor and service. I also thank Professor Dr. Mohd Ali Rajion, distinguished professor of animal physiology at the Faculty of Veterinary Medicine, Universiti Putra Malaysia, for his generous counsel and for reminding me to anchor clinical decisions in physiology and evidence. Finally, I am indebted to the many colleagues, students, laboratory teams, producers and farmers, and field veterinarians who shared cases, questions, and data; their real-world insight is the backbone of this book. Any shortcomings that remain are mine alone.

1

Introduction to Veterinary Toxicology

The production and utilization of hazardous chemicals in both developed and developing countries have increased significantly over the past few decades. With the world population continuing to grow, the demand for food is rising; consequently, the use of pesticides and other potentially toxic chemicals is also expected to increase. Recent data exemplifies this trend: In Malaysia, the agrochemicals market was estimated at USD 679.59 million in 2024 and is projected to reach USD 849.33 million by 2029, growing at a compound annual growth rate (CAGR) of 4.56% during that period (Figure 1.1).

Industrial growth will also require a greater variety and amount of industrial chemicals and metallic compounds that are potentially toxic. The combined interactions of population growth, urbanization, and industrialization, coupled with poor sanitation, malnutrition, inadequate health care, and lack of regulatory control over the use of potentially dangerous chemicals, particularly in developing countries, will undoubtedly have significant impacts on the environment and subsequently on human health (Landrigan et al., 2018; Fuller et al., 2022; Kuddus et al., 2020; Briffa et al., 2020). Thus, urgent and decisive action is required to ameliorate the situation before it gets worse and unmanageable. The least one can do is to identify and understand the properties of any potentially toxic chemical or substance they are handling. Therefore, sufficient data on the toxicological properties of chemicals and their hazardous effects on the environment and human health should be made readily accessible to the general public.

Toxicology, as a scientific discipline, traces its roots back thousands of years – its earliest documentation being in ancient texts from China, Egypt, and India, where naturally derived poisons from plants and animals were used for both medicinal and malicious purposes. Over time, the study of toxic substances evolved from a primitive understanding of symptoms into a complex science that now encompasses molecular biology, chemistry, veterinary medicine, environmental science, and even social policy (Figure 1.2).

In today's context, veterinary toxicology has taken on a new urgency. The growing interconnection between animal and human health, accelerated by climate change, globalization, and transboundary trade, has placed toxicants at the forefront of One Health concerns. This is especially critical in tropical countries, where high humidity, intense rainfall, and pest proliferation encourage frequent use of agrochemicals – often with limited regulatory oversight. Unfortunately, the lack of comprehensive toxicovigilance systems in many developing nations makes animals – both domesticated and wild – early victims of unmonitored chemical exposure.

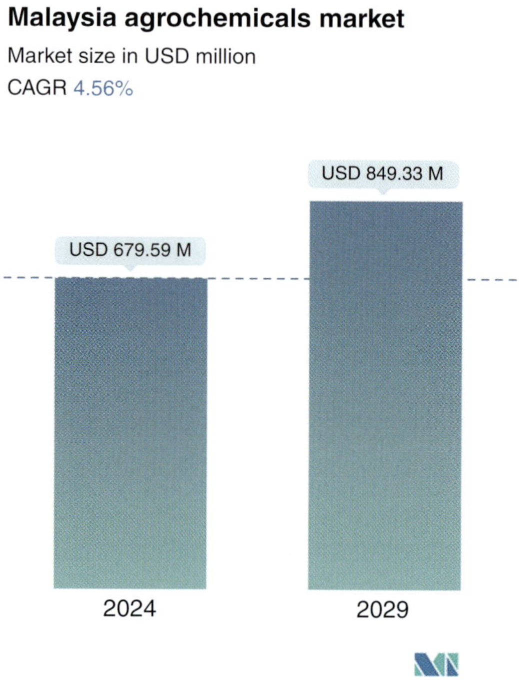

Figure 1.1 Agrochemical market size for Malaysia. *Source:* Malaysia Agrochemicals Market Size & Share Analysis - Growth Trends and Forecast (2025–2030)/ Mordor Intelligence.

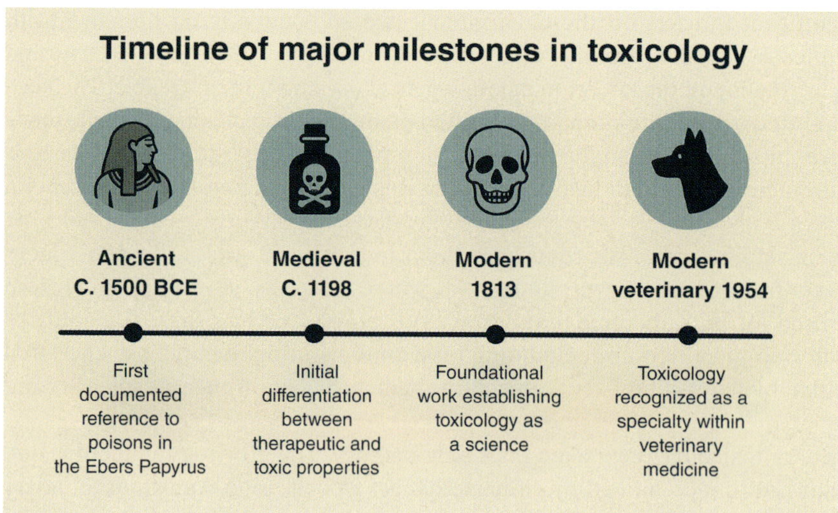

Figure 1.2 Timeline infographic of major milestones in toxicology (ancient → modern veterinary).

From a veterinary perspective, the presence of chemical contaminants in water sources, feed, pasturelands, or air has profound implications. In livestock, subclinical levels of mycotoxins can reduce reproductive efficiency and immune competence, leading to economic losses that remain hidden for years. In poultry and aquaculture, feed contamination can decimate entire production cycles. Meanwhile, wildlife face cumulative risks from bioaccumulated toxins such as organochlorines and heavy metals, particularly in ecologically sensitive regions like wetlands, mangrove belts, and marine sanctuaries.

The impact is not just biological – it is also economic and societal. In regions where animal husbandry contributes significantly to food security and rural livelihood, mass poisoning events can cripple income streams and food supply chains. The most alarming aspect is that many of these exposures are preventable through education, regulation, and better diagnostic infrastructure. This book seeks to fill that gap – not just by presenting the science of poisons, but also by contextualizing it within the tropical realities faced by veterinarians, researchers, and policymakers alike.

Moreover, the integration of modern toxicology into veterinary curricula and diagnostic services is still uneven across countries. There is a pressing need to strengthen regional toxicology laboratories, develop locally relevant reference values, and train more veterinary professionals in diagnostic toxicology – especially those working in field settings or in remote rural regions. Without these investments, many poisoning cases will go undiagnosed or misdiagnosed, and valuable lessons will be lost.

Veterinary toxicology must also evolve to respond to twenty-first-century challenges: climate-driven emergence of new toxic plants, the increasing use of synthetic supplements in animal feed, and the potential for pharmaceutical residues in the environment due to improper disposal of veterinary drugs. These complex challenges require a new generation of veterinarians who are not just diagnosticians but also advocates for safe chemical practices and sentinels of ecosystem health.

What Is a Poison?

A poison is defined as any chemical agent that can cause a deleterious response in a biological system or is capable of seriously affecting normal biological function or destroying life. It is a relative term because it requires definition of the biological system in which the deleterious effect is produced and the circumstances and conditions under which exposure to the poison occurs (Gupta, 2018; Hayes & Kruger, 2021). Feed-grade urea is a good example of this. Although urea is used as a feed ingredient as a substitute for natural protein in cattle, it is poisonous and highly lethal under certain nutritional conditions or improper utilization. For this reason, urea is normally included in cattle rations at the rate of approximately 1% of the total ration to avoid the occurrence of urea poisoning in cattle (Plumlee, 2013).

The term poison has a harsh meaning and historical significance. Toxicologists prefer to use the term toxicant because substances intended for use as feed additives, agricultural chemicals, or therapeutic drugs become poisons only when they are mishandled (Klaassen, 2021). Poisons can be of biological origin, such as the aflatoxins from the fungus *Aspergillus flavus*; nicotine from tobacco; muscarine from the poisonous mushroom *Amanita muscaria*; chemicals intended for human use, such as therapeutic drugs and agricultural chemicals; or naturally occurring chemical substances like lead and copper (Gupta, 2018). The term toxin is used to describe poisons released through biological processes, such as

Table 1.1 Conversion of percentage to parts per million (ppm) and parts per billion (ppb).

Percentage	Parts per million (ppm)
1	10,000
0.1	1,000
0.01	100
0.001	10
0.0001	1
0.00001	0.1 ppm = 100 ppb
0.000001	0.01 ppm = 10 ppb
0.0000001	0.001 ppm = 1 ppb
ppb – (parts per billion)	

the endotoxins and exotoxins released by bacteria, phytotoxins from plants, and zootoxins from animals. These toxins are generally referred to as biotoxins.

The introduction of any new chemical, whether intended for use in humans, agriculture, or industry, is subjected to rigorous and stringent safety evaluations to determine its potential hazards. These hazardous effects are usually evaluated using experimental animals such as rats and primates. A few terminologies are used in safety testing. One of them is the median lethal dose, abbreviated LD_{50}, which is the minimum dose required to kill 50% of the population (Hayes & Kruger, 2021).

Toxicologists must understand the nature and effects of the poison, the biological system and environment in which it occurs, and the level of contamination or concentration of the toxicant in the biological system, environment, or in food or water to relate with the clinical symptoms exhibited in any case of suspected poisoning. The level of contamination or concentration of the toxicant is usually expressed as parts per million (ppm) or parts per billion (ppb). In metric units, 1 ppm is equal to 1 mg/kg and 1 ppb is equal to 1 μg/kg. In simple terms, 1 ppm is one part of substance X in 999,999 parts of substance Y on a weight-per-weight basis. The concentration of a toxicant can also be expressed as a percentage on a weight-per-weight basis, especially when dealing with high concentrations. The relationship between percentage and ppm is given in Table 1.1. To convert percentage to ppm or vice versa, the decimal point is moved four places to the right or left, respectively (Gupta, 2018).

In veterinary toxicology, identifying what constitutes a poison becomes more complex due to the diversity of species involved. A compound that is harmless to one species may be fatal to another, which emphasizes the importance of species-specific risk assessments. For example, grapes and raisins, which are innocuous to humans, can cause acute renal failure in dogs, while theobromine in chocolate can cause multiple organ failure in dogs (Plumlee, 2013). *Lilium* spp. (true lilies) are highly nephrotoxic to cats, even in minute amounts. Avocado contains persin, which is toxic to birds and some ruminants but safe for humans. These examples reflect the critical need to evaluate toxicants in the context of the affected species' physiology (Figure 1.3).

Equally important is the route of exposure, which can significantly affect toxicity. A compound may be lethal when ingested but relatively harmless on dermal exposure. This is particularly relevant in field

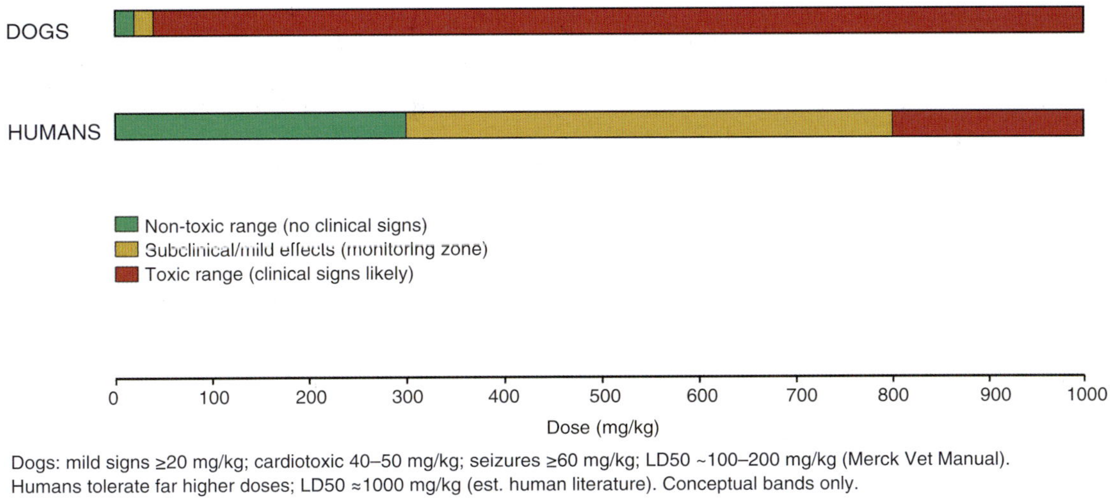

Figure 1.3 Example of a toxic vs. nontoxic doses of substances across species.

conditions where animals may encounter substances in contaminated soil, water, or vegetation. For instance, organophosphate insecticides can cause cholinergic overstimulation if absorbed through the skin in livestock, especially when improperly diluted or applied during hot weather that promotes dermal absorption (Gupta, 2018; Klaassen, 2021).

The form of the compound – its chemical state – also plays a pivotal role. Elemental mercury is far less toxic when ingested than methylmercury, which readily crosses the blood–brain barrier. Similarly, ferrous sulfate, an iron supplement, is safe at therapeutic doses but potentially fatal if accidentally ingested by piglets or puppies in large amounts (Plumlee, 2013).

Understanding poisons also demands consideration of the animal's health status. Nutritional deficiencies, dehydration, pregnancy, or preexisting disease may all predispose an animal to increased susceptibility. For example, ruminants suffering from molybdenum deficiency are far more prone to chronic copper poisoning due to impaired excretion (Gupta, 2018).

Finally, the term "poison" in public discourse often carries fear and finality, but toxicologists recognize that it is often a matter of context, dose, and preparedness. With proper awareness, even potentially lethal substances can be handled safely and put to productive use. The goal is not to eliminate all toxicants from animal environments – an impossible task – but to understand, anticipate, and manage the risks they present.

What Is Toxicology?

Toxicology, as a discipline, fundamentally revolves around the principle that "the dose makes the poison." This emphasizes that any substance, even water or oxygen, can exert harmful effects if exposure exceeds safe thresholds (Hayes & Kruger, 2021; Klaassen, 2021). Understanding the pathways of exposure – whether ingestion, inhalation, or dermal absorption – is essential in assessing risk and guiding a clinical response. The severity and manifestation of toxicosis often depend not only on dose and route but also on the species, age, health status, and environmental context of the affected animal (Gupta, 2018).

It is subdivided into:

Environmental toxicology deals with the toxic effects of chemicals contaminating the environment (atmosphere, food, and water) as either accidental or occupational hazards (Hayes & Kruger, 2021).

Economic toxicology deals with the hazards of chemicals purposely applied to living organisms to achieve a specific purpose. This includes the toxic effects of:

- therapeutic drugs for human and veterinary use
- chemicals used as food preservatives and cosmetics
- pesticides and herbicides used in agriculture (Gupta, 2018; Peterson and Talcott, 2013)

Forensic toxicology addresses the diagnosis, treatment, and legal consequences of poisoning – whether intentional or accidental.

In the veterinary context, toxicology is not merely an academic discipline – it is an essential clinical tool that informs diagnosis, treatment, prevention, and even policy formulation. Understanding how toxicants behave in biological systems is vital to addressing common scenarios encountered in practice, such as adverse drug reactions, environmental poisonings, or unexplained deaths in livestock herds (Plumlee, 2013).

One of the cornerstones of toxicological assessment is the ADME model: absorption, distribution, metabolism, and excretion. These four processes determine how a substance moves through and interacts with an animal's body. Each step varies significantly among species, age groups, and physiological states (Klaassen, 2021). For example, the gastrointestinal absorption of fat-soluble toxicants like organochlorines is enhanced in neonates due to increased gut permeability, while metabolic detoxification pathways may be underdeveloped in young animals, increasing their susceptibility (Figure 1.4).

Absorption refers to the route and efficiency by which a toxicant enters the bloodstream – through ingestion, inhalation, dermal contact, or injection. Distribution determines where the toxicant goes – whether it accumulates in fat, crosses the blood–brain barrier, or binds to plasma proteins. Metabolism often transforms lipophilic compounds into hydrophilic metabolites for easier excretion, though in some cases, these metabolites may be more toxic than the parent compound (e.g., acetaminophen in cats; Plumlee, 2013). Excretion occurs mainly through urine, bile, sweat, or milk – posing secondary risks to nursing offspring and humans consuming animal products (Figure 1.5).

Another critical concept is toxicodynamics – the interaction between the toxicant and cellular targets. Some agents inhibit enzymes, disrupt cell membranes, or trigger oxidative damage. Aflatoxins, for example, bind to DNA and cause mutations, making them both acutely hepatotoxic and chronically carcinogenic (Gupta, 2018). Ionophores like monensin disrupt ion gradients across membranes, affecting skeletal and cardiac muscle cells, particularly in horses (Peterson and Talcott, 2013).

Veterinary toxicology also interfaces with risk assessment and hazard characterization. A hazard is the inherent potential of a substance to cause harm, whereas risk is the likelihood of that harm occurring under specific exposure conditions. Thus, while copper is an essential trace element, it becomes

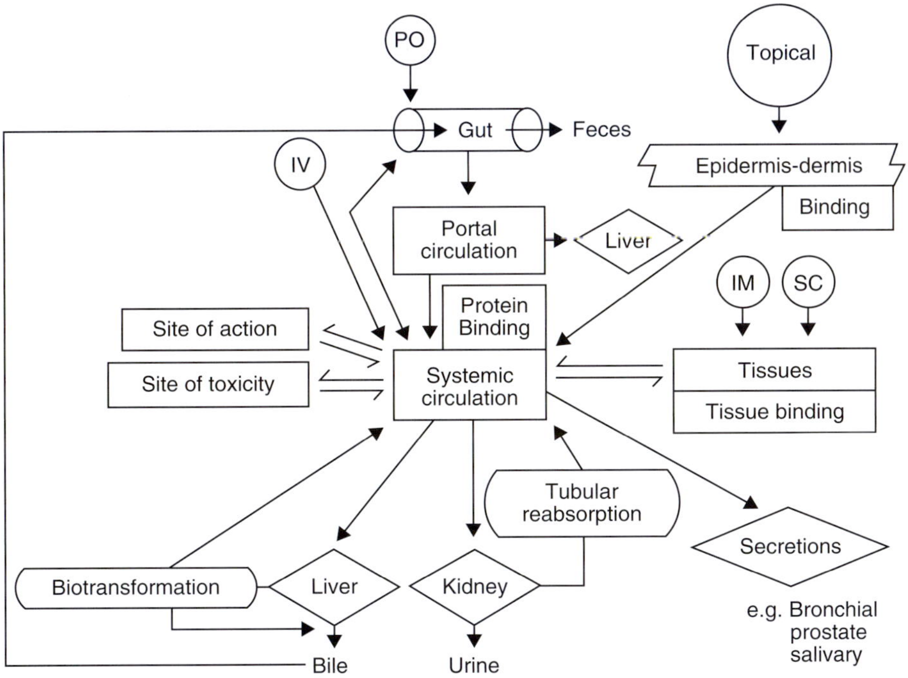

Figure 1.4 Basic schema by which drug is absorbed, distributed, metabolized, and excreted from the body. These processes are those that form the basis for developing pharmacokinetic models (Riviere and Papich, 2018).

Figure 1.5 Dose-response curve illustration (e.g., hormesis and NOAEL). *Source:* Author's original figure (conceptual basis consistent with standard toxicology texts).

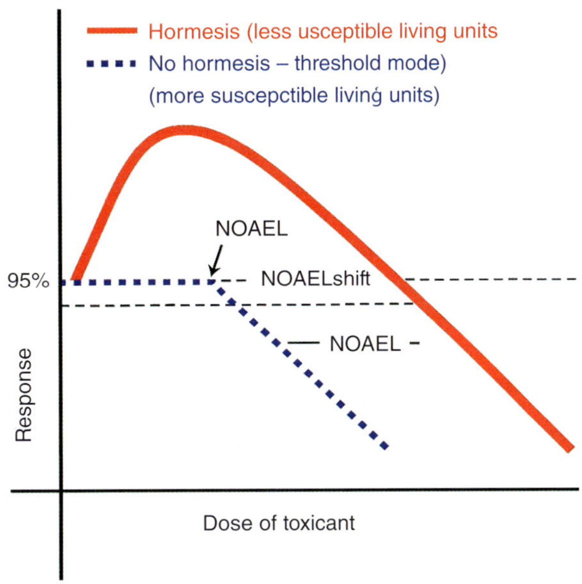

hazardous at certain thresholds – particularly in sheep, which are genetically less efficient at copper excretion (Hayes & Kruger, 2021).

Emerging branches of toxicology further enrich its relevance. Ecotoxicology evaluates how toxicants affect animal populations and ecosystems, such as pesticide runoff impacting aquatic fauna (Klaassen, 2021). Pharmacovigilance and residue toxicology ensure that therapeutic agents do not persist in meat, milk, or eggs beyond acceptable limits, protecting consumers (WHO, 2019). Nanotoxicology is also gaining traction, as nanoparticles used in animal feed or diagnostics may behave differently at the molecular level, warranting fresh scrutiny (Peterson and Talcott, 2013).

Importantly, toxicology serves not only animals but also the communities that depend on them. During environmental disasters – oil spills, chemical plant explosions, or flooding – veterinary toxicologists play a vital role in assessing exposure risks and mitigating fallout for both animals and food chains. They also contribute to One Health frameworks, linking animal and human toxicological surveillance to predict and prevent cross-species exposure to harmful substances (Rumbeiha, 2012).

Ultimately, veterinary toxicology is both a preventive and reactive discipline. It enables the development of withdrawal intervals, safe feeding guidelines, poisoning management protocols, and regulatory benchmarks. It also guides veterinarians to think critically when faced with atypical clinical presentations – recognizing that toxicoses may masquerade as infectious, metabolic, or nutritional diseases (Gupta, 2018; Plumlee, 2013).

Relevance to Wildlife, Livestock, and Companion Animals Globally

Veterinary toxicology plays a critical role in safeguarding animal health across all major species categories. In wildlife, exposure to environmental pollutants such as lead, mercury, or organochlorine pesticides can disrupt reproductive systems, impair neurologic function, and even threaten species conservation efforts (Klaassen, 2021). For example, marine mammals and raptors have been widely documented to suffer from bioaccumulation of persistent toxicants (Gupta, 2018).

In livestock, the improper use of agrochemicals, contaminated feed, or inadequate withdrawal periods can lead to poisoning events that compromise not only animal welfare but also food safety and public health (Peterson and Talcott, 2013). Meanwhile, companion animals face poisoning risks due to their close proximity to humans. Common household items such as chocolate, xylitol, antifreeze (ethylene glycol), and certain medications can be highly toxic to pets (Plumlee, 2013; Figure 1.6).

Thus, a global perspective on toxicological threats is essential, especially as human activity continues to shape the health of animal populations across different ecological zones.

Wildlife: Sentinels of Environmental Health

Wildlife species are often the first to exhibit the effects of environmental contamination, making them invaluable biological sentinels. In the tropics, waterbirds inhabiting mangrove and estuarine ecosystems accumulate mercury and other heavy metals from mining runoff and industrial waste (Hayes & Kruger, 2021). Raptors, such as hawks and eagles, suffer from secondary poisoning after consuming prey that have ingested rodenticides or insecticide-laced carrion – a phenomenon well-documented in both tropical and temperate countries (Ogada et al., 2012).

(a)

(b)

(c)

(d)

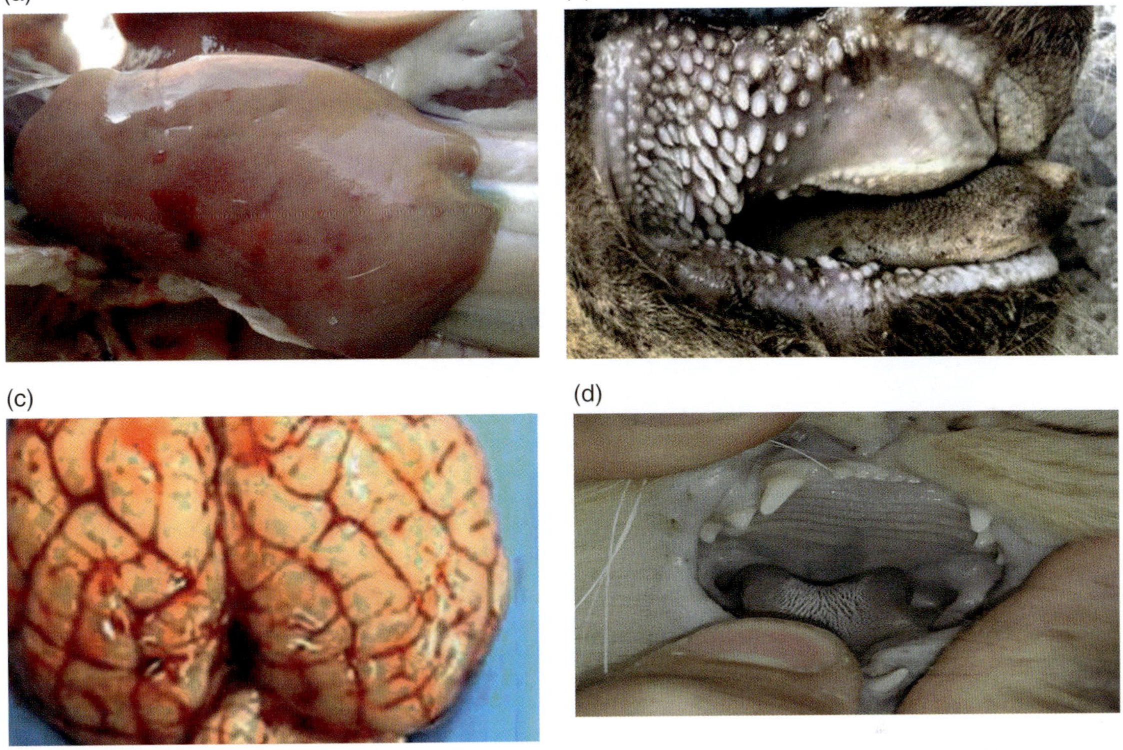

Figure 1.6 Comparative photos of toxicoses in different animals (details will be in subsequent chapters). (a) Aflatoxicosis (broiler) – pale, greasy liver with hemorrhages. (b) Nitrate poisoning (cattle) – muddy/cyanotic oral mucosa from methemoglobinemia. (c) Organophosphate poisoning (sheep) – congested meninges with hemorrhages. (d) Acetaminophen toxicity (cat) – cyanotic gums due to methemoglobinemia. *Source:* (a) Cide Intelligence Solutions / https://www.veterinariadigital.com/en/post_blog/aflatoxicosis-in-broilers/ / last accessed on Dec 17, 2025; (b) Flock & Herd / https://www.flockandherd.net.au/cattle/ireader/nitrate-toxicity-cattle.html / last accessed on Dec 17, 2025; (c) Rizzo et al. (2024) / The Scientific Electronic Library Online (SciELO) / CC BY 4.0; (d) Pet Health Club (2024) / Independent Vetcare Ltd.

One of the most striking examples is the decline of vulture populations in South Asia due to exposure to diclofenac, a nonsteroidal anti-inflammatory drug (NSAID) used in cattle. Although effective in livestock, diclofenac causes acute renal failure in vultures that scavenge on treated carcasses. The impact has been catastrophic, with population declines exceeding 95% in some regions (Green et al., 2004; Oaks et al., 2004; Shultz et al., 2004).

In aquatic wildlife, algal blooms driven by agricultural runoff can lead to the production of biotoxins such as microcystins. These toxins are fatal to fish, turtles, and marine mammals and can enter the food chain, posing risks to larger predators, including humans (Gupta, 2018).

In tropical rainforests, indigenous animals like fruit bats and primates are at risk of ingesting naturally toxic plants or fungal metabolites, especially during dry seasons when food is scarce. Bioaccumulation and the biomagnification of persistent pollutants are long-term ecological threats, particularly for top predators with slow reproductive rates (Hayes & Kruger, 2021) (Figures 1.7 and 1.8).

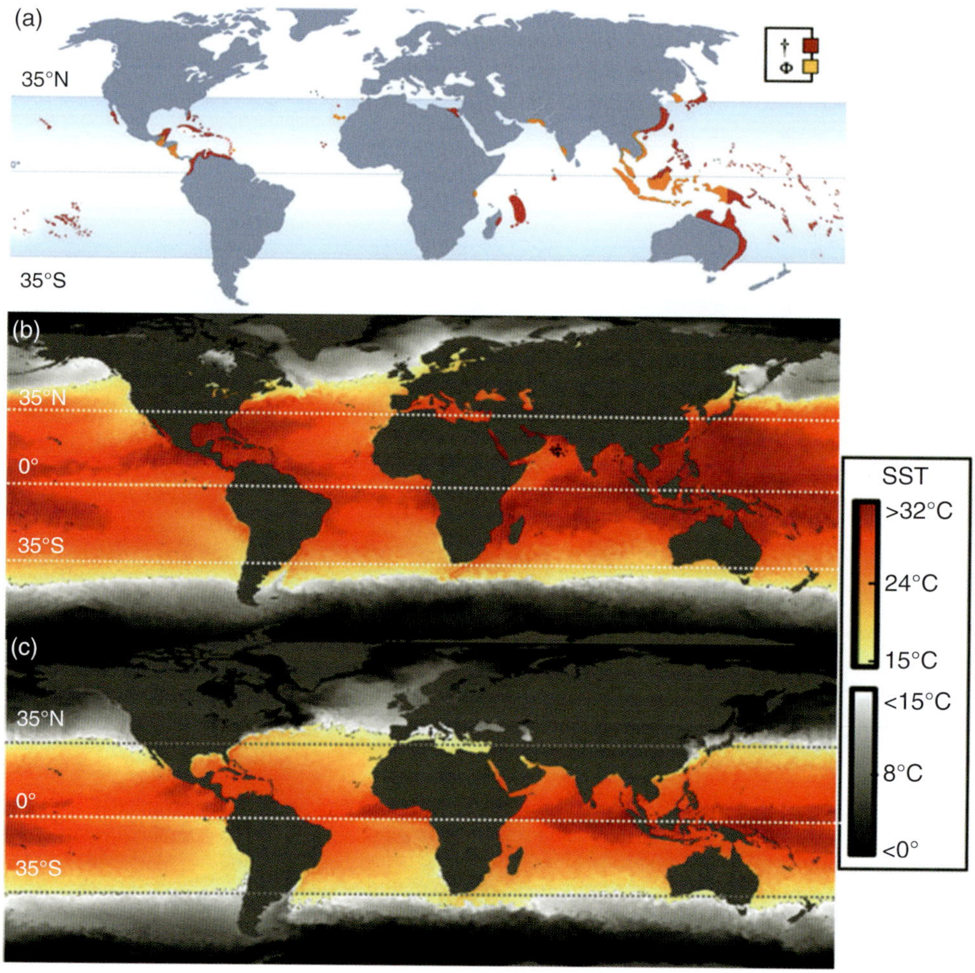

Figure 1.7 Global distribution of ciguatera fish poisoning and associated sea-surface temperatures (SSTs): (a) global map showing regions where ciguatera fish poisoning has been reported (mainly tropical and subtropical coastal/island areas); (b) global SST distribution under warmer conditions; and (c) global SST distribution under cooler conditions, illustrating the temperature envelope associated with the reported geographic distribution.

Livestock: Productivity and Food Chain Security

In livestock systems – especially in tropical developing countries – poor feed storage, weak regulation, and inadequate farmer training are major contributors to toxicoses. Mycotoxins such as aflatoxins, fumonisins, and zearalenone contaminate feed grains stored in humid conditions. Chronic exposure leads to immunosuppression, hepatotoxicity, reduced fertility, and stunted growth, often without overt clinical signs (Warnatzsch et al., 2020; Peterson and Talcott, 2013).

Ruminants are susceptible to nitrate and nitrite poisoning when consuming forage heavily fertilized with nitrogenous compounds, especially after drought or cloudy weather that impairs photosynthesis

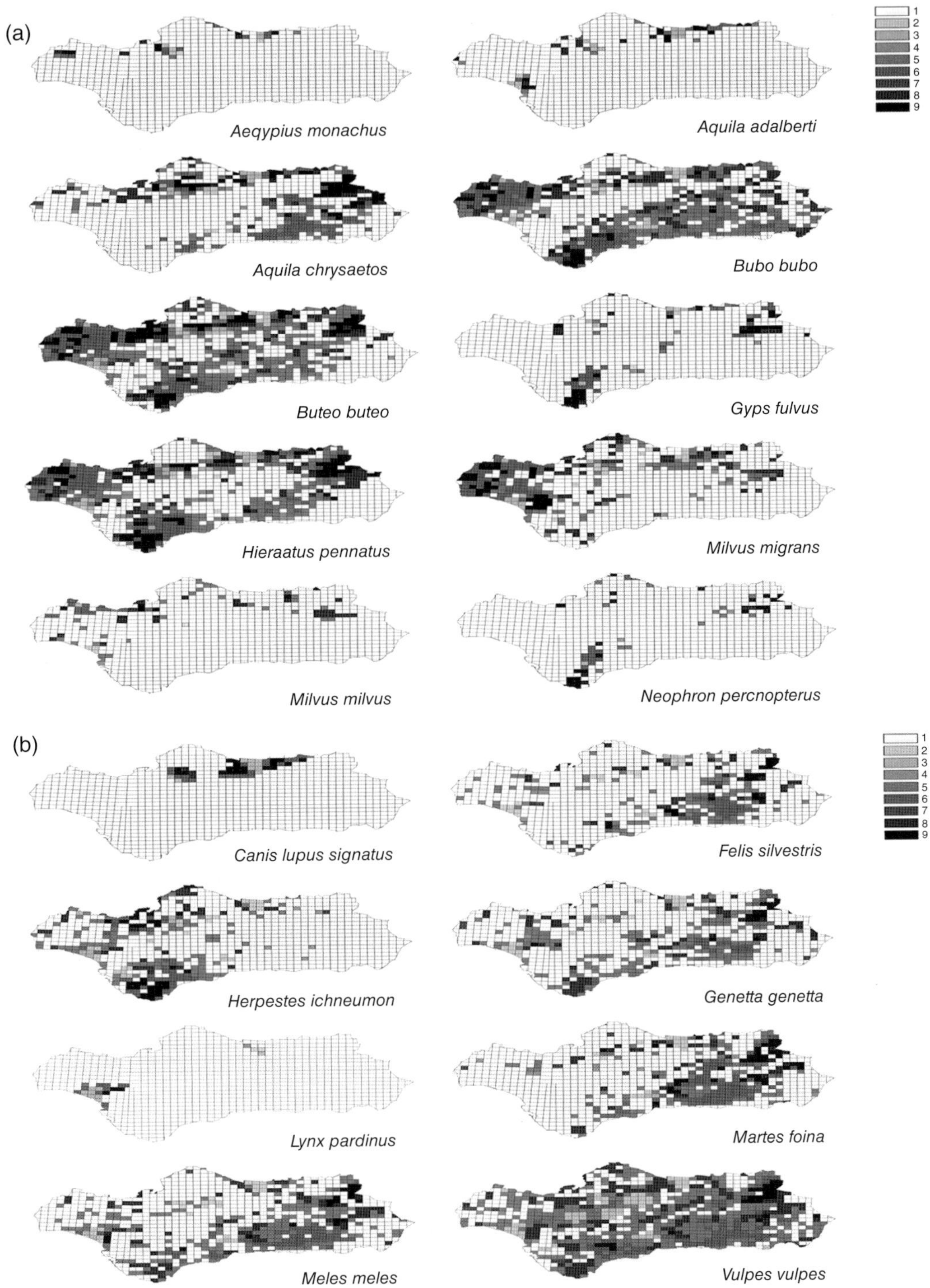

Figure 1.8 Conflict zones for wildlife poisoning incidents in specific regions. (a) Regional overview map highlighting conflict-affected areas associated with reported wildlife poisoning incidents; (b) zoomed-in/hotspot view showing clustering of incidents within the conflict zone(s) for clearer geographic interpretation.

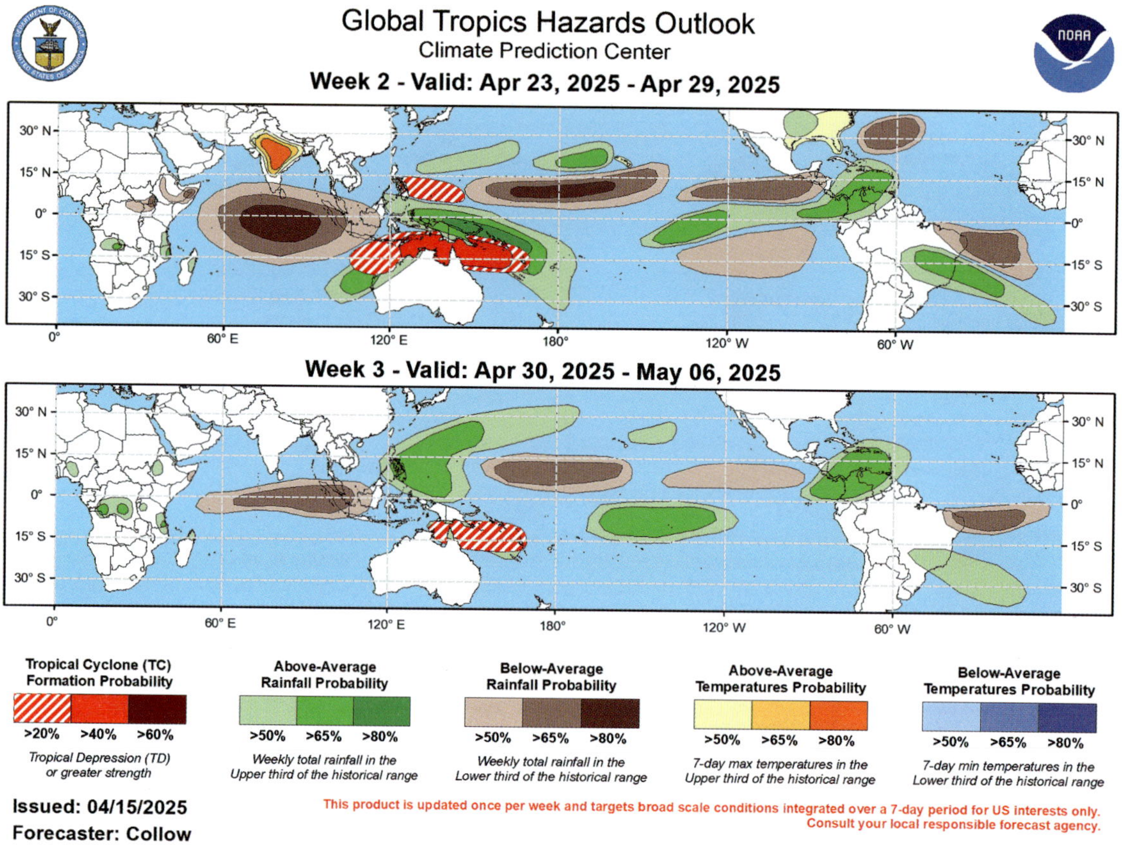

Figure 1.9 NOAA's forecast of climate-related hazards across the global tropics. *Source:* Weeks 2–3 Global Tropics Hazards Outlook/NOAA/Public Domain.

(Gupta, 2018). In tropical pastures, the presence of toxic plants such as *Lantana camara* or *Indigofera* species can result in hepatic and neurological toxicoses, respectively (Klaassen, 2021).

A unique challenge in tropical livestock farming is the accidental exposure to pesticides used for tick and pest control. Improper dilution, frequency, or use of banned organophosphates and carbamates can result in subacute toxicity that manifests as poor weight gain, photosensitization, or sudden death. These cases often go unreported or misdiagnosed due to the lack of diagnostic labs (FAO, 2021).

Moreover, failure to observe appropriate withdrawal periods for drugs like ivermectin, oxytetracycline, or albendazole results in detectable residues in meat and milk – posing public health concerns and leading to rejected export shipments in countries with strict residue surveillance systems (WHO, 2019) (Figure 1.9).

Companion Animals: Hidden Dangers in the Home

Pets, particularly dogs and cats, are frequently exposed to substances not intended for them. Common culprits include xylitol-containing gum, acetaminophen, grapes and raisins, essential oils, and nonprescription

NSAIDs (Plumlee, 2013). Many of these exposures are unintentional – owners may offer foods or medications that are safe for humans but deadly for animals.

Cats, due to their unique glucuronidation pathways, are highly susceptible to certain drugs and chemicals. A single tablet of acetaminophen can induce methemoglobinemia and hepatotoxicity in a cat. Similarly, ingestion of lilies – even licking pollen – can cause fatal acute kidney injury.

In dogs, chocolate toxicosis remains common. Theobromine levels in dark chocolate can cause tachycardia, tremors, and seizures. Antifreeze (ethylene glycol) toxicity is another notorious household hazard, with just a few milliliters being fatal due to oxalate crystal formation in the kidneys (Peterson and Talcott, 2013).

In multi-pet households, exposure to topical flea medications intended for dogs, such as permethrin-based products, can lead to life-threatening seizures in cats that groom each other. These scenarios emphasize the need for pet-specific toxicology education for both owners and clinicians.

Zoonotic and Public Health Implications

Veterinary toxicology is intricately tied to public health. Toxins that affect animals often have implications for humans through milk, meat, eggs, or water contamination. This is particularly crucial in rural settings where livestock and humans share the same water sources. Cyanobacteria blooms in stagnant ponds, for instance, pose risks not only to livestock but also to families using the water for washing or drinking (Hayes & Kruger, 2021).

In tropical zones, backyard poultry is often treated with antibiotics or pesticides without veterinary guidance. These birds, if slaughtered or consumed without observing withdrawal periods, become vectors for antimicrobial resistance (AMR) and chemical residues (WHO, 2019).

Moreover, the improper disposal of veterinary pharmaceuticals – especially in commercial farms – can lead to environmental contamination, bioaccumulation, and antibiotic leaching into soil and waterways. This contributes to the broader global issue of environmental toxicology and One Health disruption (Rumbeiha, 2012; OIE, 2021).

Terminologies in Toxicology

There are several terminologies one should be familiar with when dealing with poisons or incidents of poisoning. The effect of the toxicant on a biological system is described as toxic, but the disease state following exposure to a toxicant is termed toxicosis (Gupta, 2018; Klaassen, 2021). For example, excessive hemorrhage is a toxic effect of warfarin, but a dog poisoned with this rodenticide is described as suffering warfarin toxicosis. The term toxicity refers to the amount of toxicant required to trigger toxic effects under a specific set of conditions.

The toxicity of a compound is normally expressed in terms of the average or LD_{50}, which indicates the smallest dose required to produce a lethal effect in 50% of the population (Hayes & Kruger, 2021).

Key Terms Explained

Toxicant: A man-made or naturally occurring substance that causes harm when introduced into a living organism. Example: Carbofuran is a toxicant that causes acute cholinergic crisis in birds and mammals (Peterson and Talcott, 2013).

Table 1.2 Definitions and species-specific real-world examples for key toxicological terms.

Term	Definition	Real-world example (by species)
Toxin	A toxic substance produced by a living organism	Botulinum toxin causing paralysis in horses
Toxicant	A toxic substance produced by human activities	Rodenticide ingestion in dogs
Toxicity	The degree to which a substance is harmful	Higher toxicity of lilies in cats vs. dogs
Toxicosis	Disease caused by exposure to a toxin or toxicant	Organophosphate toxicosis in small ruminants
Hazard	The potential of a substance to cause harm	Storage of chocolate in homes with dogs
Risk	The likelihood of harm occurring under conditions of exposure	Risk of nitrate poisoning increases during drought in cattle
Dose	The amount of a substance required to cause harm	Acetaminophen overdose causing methemoglobinemia in cats
LD_{50}	The dose lethal to 50% of a test population	LD_{50} of sodium nitrite in pigs is ~175 mg/kg

Toxin: A specific subclass of toxicants that are produced by living organisms. Example: Botulinum toxin from *Clostridium botulinum* is one of the most potent biological toxins known (Klaassen, 2021).

Poison: A general term referring to any substance that can cause harm. In veterinary medicine, its use is typically reserved for substances that are clearly harmful in small quantities. Example: A rodenticide like zinc phosphide is termed a poison because of its lethality in minute doses (Gupta, 2018).

Toxicosis: The clinical condition resulting from exposure to a toxicant. Example: A horse suffering from monensin ingestion is said to have ionophore toxicosis (Plumlee, 2013).

Toxicity: A quantitative measurement of how poisonous a substance is – often expressed through metrics like LD_{50} or NOAEL (No Observed Adverse Effect Level; Hayes & Kruger, 2021).

Hazard: The inherent potential of a substance to cause harm. Example: Even water can be a hazard under conditions of overhydration, leading to electrolyte imbalances (Klaassen, 2021).

Risk: The probability that harm will occur from a particular exposure scenario. Example: The hazard of aflatoxin in cattle feed may be high, but the risk is low if feed storage is optimized (FAO, 2021) (Table 1.2).

Classification of Degrees of Toxicity

Toxic substances may be classified based on their degrees of toxicity. Six degrees of toxicity, in decreasing order, are described as follows: (i) extremely toxic, (ii) highly toxic, (iii) moderately toxic, (iv) slightly toxic, (v) practically nontoxic, and (vi) relatively harmless (Gupta, 2018; Hayes & Kruger, 2021). In order to differentiate these categories, the estimated lethal dose for man, dog, and cow in common units of measurement are tabulated in Table 1.3.

Toxicity classifications are crucial for understanding how much of a substance it takes to cause harm or death in various species. This allows veterinarians, farmers, and pet owners to anticipate risk and design appropriate safety measures in drug administration, feed formulation, pest control, and environmental exposure (Peterson and Talcott, 2013).

Table 1.3 Degree of toxicity and estimated single-dose oral lethality with household-volume equivalents in humans, a 20-kg dog, and a 450-kg cow.

			Lethal dose (volume)		
Toxicity rating	**Category dose**	**Single oral**	**Man**	**Dog (20 kg)**	**Cow (450 kg)**
1	Extremely toxic	1 mg or less/kg	A taste or 1 grain	0.004 teaspoon	0.09 teaspoon
2	Highly toxic	1–5 mg/kg or 4 mL	1 teaspoon	0.2 teaspoon	4.5 teaspoons
3	Moderately toxic	50–500 mg/kg	1 oz	2 teaspoons	1 cup
4	Slightly toxic	0.5–5 g/kg	1 pint	0.45 cup	2.5 quarts
5	Practically nontoxic	0.5–15 g/kg	1 quart	1.34 cups	2 gallons
6	Relatively harmless	>15 g/kg	1 quart	>1.34 cups	>2 gallons

Toxicity categories span from extremely toxic (≤1 mg/kg; "a taste" in humans) to relatively harmless (>15 g/kg), with approximate teaspoon–cup–gallon conversions provided for rapid clinical reference.
Sources: Gupta (2018); Hayes and Kruger (2021).

One of the most widely used benchmarks for classifying toxicity is the LD_{50}, which refers to the amount of a substance (typically in mg/kg body weight) that will kill 50% of a population upon a single exposure. The smaller the LD_{50}, the more toxic the substance (Klaassen, 2021).

Examples Across Species

- Permethrin (in cats): Extremely toxic – LD_{50} <100 mg/kg; even topical exposure can be fatal due to poor hepatic metabolism (Plumlee, 2013).
- Chocolate (in dogs): Moderately toxic – Theobromine LD_{50} ~300 mg/kg; a few squares of dark chocolate can induce seizures (Plumlee, 2013).
- Monensin (in horses): Highly toxic – LD_{50} ~1.4 mg/kg; a dose tolerated by ruminants can be fatal to equines (Plumlee, 2013).
- Copper (in sheep): Slightly toxic to moderately toxic depending on breed; predisposing dietary factors affect accumulation.
- Table salt (in dogs): Practically nontoxic in low quantities, but ingestion >4 g/kg can lead to hypernatremia and seizures (Gupta, 2018).

Why LD_{50} Isn't Everything

Although LD_{50} is a useful starting point, it's not always the best indicator of clinical toxicity:

- Sublethal toxicity: Chronic exposure to a toxicant may not cause death but may induce severe organ damage over time (e.g., aflatoxin B1 causing chronic liver failure in poultry; Hayes & Kruger, 2021).
- Species variability: The same compound may be highly toxic in one species and virtually harmless in another (e.g., xylitol is safe for humans but hepatotoxic in dogs; Plumlee, 2013).

- Formulation effects: Some drugs or poisons are more harmful depending on how they're formulated (e.g., injectable vs. oral ivermectin).

Veterinary Application of Toxicity Classes

Toxicity classifications guide veterinarians in choosing safe treatment options. For example:

- A drug with a narrow therapeutic index (difference between effective dose and toxic dose) must be dosed with caution – like digoxin or aminoglycosides.
- Feed additives like ionophores (monensin, salinomycin) are used safely in poultry and ruminants, but are fatal in equines (Peterson and Talcott, 2013).
- Knowing a substance's toxicity class helps in triage: An animal exposed to something in the "extremely toxic" class needs urgent decontamination, supportive care, and possibly antidotal therapy (Klaassen, 2021).

Classification of Toxic Reactions

Toxic reactions may be classified as acute, subacute, or chronic, based on the rate of onset of symptoms as well as the rate and duration of exposure to the poison or toxic agent (Gupta, 2018; Hayes & Kruger, 2021). In acute toxicity, symptoms that result in death typically develop rapidly following a single or sudden intake of a toxic dose. For example, ingestion of a large amount of phenobarbital, a central nervous system depressant, can lead to profound respiratory depression and death within hours. Similarly, death can occur within minutes of exposure to carbon monoxide or hydrogen cyanide, both of which impair cellular respiration (Klaassen, 2021). Carbon monoxide binds to hemoglobin with nearly 300 times the affinity of oxygen, while cyanide forms a stable complex with cytochrome oxidase enzymes, halting oxidative phosphorylation.

The difference between acute and subacute toxicity is based on the frequency and concentration of exposure. In subacute cases, the individual is subjected to repeated exposures over hours or days to doses insufficient to cause toxicity if administered once (Peterson and Talcott, 2013). For instance, a farmer spraying organophosphate pesticides over several days without proper protection may accumulate toxic levels via skin or respiratory absorption.

Chronic toxicity results from repeated or continuous exposure over weeks or months to substances with long biological half-lives (Gupta, 2018). These include heavy metals like lead, mercury, and copper, which accumulate in tissues and may not be efficiently excreted. A classic example is lead poisoning in children and livestock due to ingestion of contaminated materials like old paint chips.

Notably, chronic toxicity is not limited to slow-excreting compounds. Substances like benzene, although rapidly metabolized, can still lead to cumulative hematopoietic damage upon repeated exposure, impairing bone marrow function and increasing leukemia risk (Hayes & Kruger, 2021). Benzene toxicity exemplifies how both acute and chronic presentations can result from the same agent under different exposure conditions.

Toxic Reactions Are Not One-Size-Fits-All

The nature, intensity, and duration of exposure determine the clinical, pathological, and public health implications of a toxic reaction. A comprehensive classification is essential for diagnosis, management, and prevention.

Acute Toxicity: The Rapid Kill

Veterinary examples:

- Strychnine in dogs: Causes rapid-onset seizures and death (Plumlee, 2013).
- Ionophore toxicity in horses: Acute cardiac failure from contaminated poultry feed (Peterson and Talcott, 2013).
- Zinc phosphide ingestion: Produces phosphine gas in the stomach, causing fatal pulmonary and cardiac collapse (Gupta, 2018).

These cases require immediate decontamination and aggressive supportive care, such as administration of activated charcoal, oxygen, and specific antidotes where applicable.

Subacute Toxicity: The Stealth Threat

Veterinary examples:

- Organophosphate exposure in livestock or humans: Subclinical cholinergic syndrome from repeated dermal/inhalational absorption (Hayes & Kruger, 2021).
- Blue-green algae (cyanobacteria) ingestion in cattle: Causes progressive liver damage.
- Subacute aflatoxicosis in pigs and poultry: Leads to suppressed immunity and stunted growth.

These conditions often mimic infectious or nutritional deficiencies, making early recognition and differentiation vital.

Chronic Toxicity: The Slow Poison

Chronic toxicoses are insidious and may only be detected after irreversible damage is done. This is especially true in food-producing animals, where residues pose risks to consumers.

Veterinary examples:

- Copper accumulation in sheep: Often unnoticed until sudden hepatic failure (Gupta, 2018).
- Lead poisoning in cattle: Progressive ataxia and rumen stasis after ingestion of batteries (Hayes & Kruger, 2021).
- Mycotoxin ingestion: Reproductive and hepatic dysfunction in pigs and poultry.
- Pyrrolizidine alkaloid exposure in horses: Liver fibrosis and photosensitization from chronic plant ingestion (e.g., *Senecio* spp.) (Figure 1.10).

Other Types of Toxic Reactions Worth Mentioning

- Delayed toxicity: Effects manifest days or weeks post-exposure. *Example:* Organophosphate-induced axonopathy (Klaassen, 2021).
- Idiosyncratic reactions: Non-dose-dependent and unpredictable. *Example:* Sulfonamide-induced keratoconjunctivitis in genetically predisposed Dobermans.

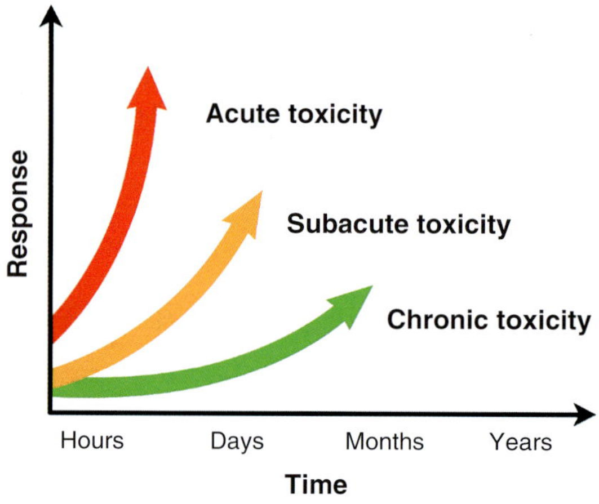

Figure 1.10 Timeline diagram of acute vs. subacute vs. chronic toxicity.

Table 1.4 Comparative table of common veterinary toxicants by reaction type (selected).

Reaction type	Toxicant	Species affected	Example/clinical sign
Hepatotoxic	Aflatoxin	Poultry, dogs	Liver enlargement, hepatic necrosis
Nephrotoxic	Ethylene glycol	Dogs, cats	Acute renal failure, crystalluria
Neurotoxic	Organophosphates	Cattle, sheep, dogs	Salivation, tremors, seizures
Hemotoxic	Zinc	Dogs, birds	Hemolytic anemia, vomiting
Respiratory	Paraquat	Cats, dogs	Pulmonary fibrosis, dyspnea
Cardiotoxic	Oleander	Ruminants, horses	Arrhythmias, sudden death
Gastrointestinal	NSAIDs (e.g., Ibuprofen)	Dogs	Gastric ulceration, vomiting, diarrhea

- Carcinogenicity and teratogenicity: Long-term exposure may lead to cancer or birth defects. *Example:* Aflatoxin B1 and dioxins as chronic mutagens and teratogens (Table 1.4).

The Role of Veterinary Toxicologists in Tropical Practice

Veterinary toxicologists occupy a unique space at the intersection of animal health, public health, and ecosystem management (Peterson and Talcott, 2013). In tropical regions, their role becomes even more significant due to frequent pesticide usage, climate-sensitive toxic exposures, and limited veterinary infrastructure. They conduct outbreak investigations, contribute to establishing maximum residue limits (MRLs), and help shape regulatory frameworks for drug safety (WHO, 2019; Rumbeiha, 2012). Their responsibilities span teaching, diagnostics, field investigation, and policy advocacy. For example, after monsoon flooding in parts of Southeast Asia, toxicologists played a key role in tracking aflatoxin contamination in feed and advising on emergency decontamination protocols (FAO, 2021). Furthermore, they collaborate with environmental agencies to assess lead or mercury contamination in livestock areas near mining zones. In academia, they publish vital data on indigenous plant toxicants and provide evidence for updating veterinary drug withdrawal times.

One of the primary responsibilities of veterinary toxicologists in the tropics is outbreak investigation and diagnosis. When livestock die suddenly or wildlife exhibits unexplained morbidity, toxicologists are often the first responders, tasked with identifying the causative agent and tracing its source. They utilize a blend of clinical acumen, analytical chemistry, pathology, and epidemiology to determine whether a toxicant is involved and to advise on treatment, decontamination, or culling protocols.

In addition to reactive roles, these professionals engage in preventive strategies. This includes setting MRLs for drugs and pesticides, advising on safe withdrawal periods, and training farmers and veterinarians in the safe handling of agrochemicals, feed additives, and pharmaceuticals. Their input is essential when formulating national guidelines for veterinary drug registration, feed-safety monitoring, and environmental toxin surveillance.

Moreover, veterinary toxicologists play key roles in disaster response. In flood-prone tropical countries, disasters often mobilize toxic contaminants, including pesticides, sewage, and industrial effluents. Toxicologists help assess risk to animals, secure water supplies, and prevent secondary outbreaks caused by toxin-induced immunosuppression.

They also contribute to the One Health movement, supporting joint surveillance systems with physicians, environmental scientists, and public health experts to tackle cross-species threats such as lead poisoning, zoonotic pesticide residues, or marine biotoxins.

In academia and research, they advance knowledge by conducting studies on indigenous toxic plants, emerging contaminants, and locally used herbal preparations, ensuring that veterinary medicine in tropical zones is supported by evidence-based toxicology (Figure 1.11).

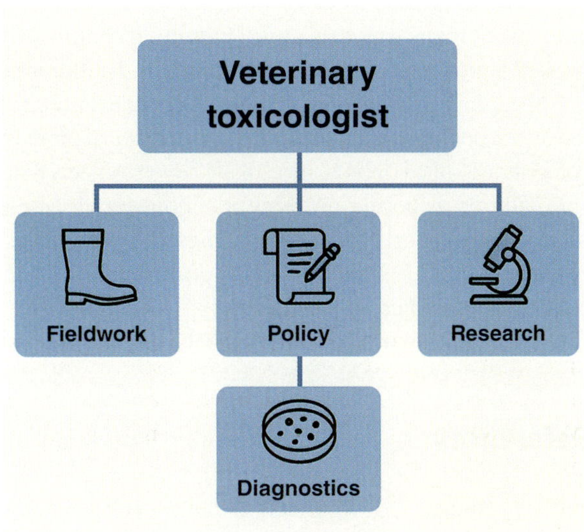

Figure 1.11 Veterinary toxicologists' role across fieldwork, policy, research, and diagnostics.

Emerging Toxic Threats in Tropical Countries

The toxicological landscape in tropical regions is changing rapidly. Once dominated by classical pesticide and plant toxicities, today's threats are increasingly diverse, often stemming from the very changes meant to drive development – urbanization, intensification of agriculture, and globalization of trade.

As agriculture intensifies in the tropics, toxic exposures are becoming more diverse and harder to regulate. Key threats include mycotoxins, nitrate accumulation during droughts, and cyanobacterial blooms (World Bank, 2022). For instance, recent studies in the Philippines, Malaysia, and Ghana have linked changing rainfall patterns to rising aflatoxin levels in stored corn and poultry feed (Warnatzsch et al., 2020). Additionally, misuse of growth promoters and antiparasitics – especially in smallholder farms – can lead to tissue residues and AMR (WHO, 2019). Tropical countries also face a growing influx of counterfeit veterinary drugs. These often contain banned substances or incorrect dosages, exacerbating toxicity risks in both animals and humans (OIE, 2021). Another overlooked issue is urban pet poisoning. With increased indoor pet keeping, there's been a documented rise in accidental exposures to detergents, rodenticides, and essential oils (Pet Poison Helpline, 2023). Veterinary toxicologists are vital in researching these evolving hazards and advising both local veterinarians and policymakers.

One of the most prominent threats is antimicrobial and anthelmintic resistance arising from sublethal chemical exposure. In many tropical countries, veterinary drugs are available over the counter without prescription, leading to unregulated use. Animals are often overdosed or treated with unapproved substances, resulting in cumulative toxicoses and long-term tissue damage. Additionally, improper disposal of expired drugs and syringes contaminates soil and water, affecting both animals and humans.

Climate change is also altering the dynamics of toxic exposures. Increased rainfall and humidity facilitate the growth of mycotoxin-producing fungi in feed and grain. Drought, meanwhile, may lead to nitrate accumulation in plants and sudden outbreaks of nitrate poisoning in ruminants. Warmer waters in coastal zones promote the spread of harmful algal blooms (HABs) that affect fish, turtles, and marine mammals through ingestion of cyanotoxins and saxitoxins.

The rise in urban animal keeping – especially backyard poultry and goats – creates new interfaces between animals, humans, and toxicants. Household chemicals, improperly stored rodenticides, and cleaning agents present a growing threat to both animals and children in low-income tropical settlements.

Also alarming is the increased use of nonconventional feed ingredients such as palm kernel cake, fermented food waste, or herbal mixtures whose toxicological profiles are not well studied. In these contexts, veterinary toxicologists are called upon to investigate adverse effects that range from organ damage to reproductive failure.

Finally, cross-border movement of counterfeit veterinary products has introduced a shadow market of unregistered, poorly formulated drugs and pesticides. These not only lack efficacy but may contain contaminants that are directly toxic to animals.

The solution lies in strengthening toxicovigilance systems, building local laboratory capacity, and investing in collaborative research between tropical nations to generate region-specific toxicological data.

References

Briffa, J., Sinagra, E., & Blundell, R. (2020). Heavy metal pollution in the environment and their toxicological effects on humans. *Heliyon*, *6*(9), e04691. https://doi.org/10.1016/j.heliyon.2020.e04691

FAO. (2021). *Emergency response to aflatoxin outbreaks in Asia-Pacific livestock systems*. Food and Agriculture Organization of the United Nations.

Fuller, R., Landrigan, P. J., Balakrishnan, K., Bathan, G., Bose-O'Reilly, S., Brauer, M., et al. (2022). Pollution and health: a progress update. *The Lancet Planetary Health*, *6*(6), e535–e547. https://doi.org/10.1016/S2542-5196(22)00090-0

Green, R. E., Newton, I., Shultz, S., Cunningham, A. A., Gilbert, M., Pain, D. J., & Prakash, V. (2004). Diclofenac poisoning as a cause of vulture population declines across the Indian subcontinent. *Journal of Applied Ecology*, *41*(5), 793–800. https://doi.org/10.1111/j.0021-8901.2004.00954.x

Gupta, R. C. (2018). *Veterinary toxicology: Basic and clinical principles* (3rd ed.). Academic Press.

Hayes, A. W., & Kruger, C. L. (Eds.). (2021). *Hayes' principles and methods of toxicology* (7th ed.). CRC Press.

Klaassen, C. D. (Ed.). (2021). *Casarett & Doull's toxicology: The basic science of poisons* (10th ed.). McGraw-Hill.

Kuddus, M. A., Tynan, E., & McBryde, E. (2020). Urbanization: a problem for the rich and the poor? *Public Health Reviews*, *41*, 1. https://doi.org/10.1186/s40985-019-0116-0

Landrigan, P. J., Fuller, R., Acosta, N. J. R., Adeyi, O., Arnold, R., Basu, N., et al. (2018). The Lancet Commission on pollution and health. *The Lancet*, *391*(10119), 462–512. https://doi.org/10.1016/S0140-6736(17)32345-0

Oaks, J. L., Gilbert, M., Virani, M. Z., Watson, R. T., Meteyer, C. U., Rideout, B. A., et al. (2004). Diclofenac residues as the cause of vulture population decline in Pakistan. *Nature*, *427*(6975), 630–633. https://doi.org/10.1038/nature02317

Ogada, D. L., Keesing, F., & Virani, M. Z. (2012). Dropping dead: Causes and consequences of vulture population declines worldwide. *Annals of the New York Academy of Sciences*, *1249*(1), 57–71. https://doi.org/10.1111/j.1749-6632.2011.06293.x

OIE (WOAH) (2021). Substandard and falsified veterinary products. World Organisation for Animal Health (WOAH), 17 Feb 2021. Available at: https://rr-europe.woah.org/app/uploads/2021/03/2_substandard-falsified-veterinary-products_en.pdf (accessed 15 January 2026).

Pet Poison Helpline (2023). 2023 Annual Report Card (Report Card 2). Pet Poison Helpline. Available at: https://www.petpoisonhelpline.com/report-card/2023-annual-report-card-2/ (accessed 15 January 2026).

Peterson, M. E., & Talcott, P. A. (2013). *Small Animal Toxicology* (3rd ed.). Elsevier Saunders.

Plumlee, K. H. (2013). *Clinical veterinary toxicology* (2nd ed.). Elsevier Health Sciences.

Riviere, J. E., & Papich, M. G. (Eds.). (2018). *Veterinary Pharmacology and Therapeutics* (10th ed.). John Wiley & Sons.

Rizzo, H., Silveira Filho, M. E. M., Jesus, T. K. S., Soares, L. L. S. & Silva Junior, V.A. (2024). Organophosphate poisoning in sheep: case report. *Arquivo Brasileiro de Medicina Veterinária e Zootecnia*, *76*(6), e13276. https://doi.org/10.1590/1678-4162-13276

Rumbeiha, W. K. (2012). Toxicology and "one health": Opportunities for multidisciplinary collaborations. *Journal of Medical Toxicology*, *8*(2), 91–93. https://doi.org/10.1007/s13181-012-0224-4

Shultz, S., Baral, H. S., Charman, S., Cunningham, A. A., Das, D., Ghalsasi, G. R., et al. (2004). Diclofenac poisoning is widespread in declining vulture populations across the Indian subcontinent. Proceedings of the Royal Society of London. *Series B: Biological Sciences*, *271*(suppl_6), S458–S460. https://doi.org/10.1098/rsbl.2004.0223

Warnatzsch, E. A., Reay, D. S., Camardo Leggieri, M., & Battilani, P. (2020). Climate Change Impact on Aflatoxin Contamination Risk in Malawi's Maize Crops. *Frontiers in Sustainable Food Systems*, *4*, 591792. https://doi.org/10.3389/fsufs.2020.591792

WHO. (2019). *Critically important antimicrobials for human medicine – 6th revision*. World Health Organization.

World Bank (2022). Pollution management for healthier communities: Egypt makes strides in managing hazardous chemicals. World Bank (Results), 13 Dec 2022. Available at: https://www.worldbank.org/en/results/2022/12/13/pollution-management-for-healthier-communities-egypt-makes-strides-in-managing-hazardous-chemicals (accessed 15 January 2026).

2

Factors Affecting Toxicity

Manifestation of toxicity is initiated when sufficiently high concentrations of poisons or their toxic metabolites are present in a biological system. The amount of a toxicant entering the system depends largely on the dose, route, and duration of exposure. Thus, changes in dose, route, or duration of exposure can directly influence the biological response to a toxic substance. These are considered extrinsic factors. However, the ultimate response to a toxicant by an individual also depends on intrinsic factors that influence the absorption, distribution, biotransformation, or excretion of the toxicant. This chapter reviews these and other factors that have been shown to influence the toxic response to an agent in biological systems.

Toxic responses can vary greatly among individuals and species due to the dynamic interplay between extrinsic and intrinsic factors. A classic toxicological principle – "the dose makes the poison," coined by Paracelsus – still holds true and underpins how exposure dose, frequency, and duration influence toxic manifestations (Hayes & Kruger, 2021). However, toxicity is not solely dose-dependent. A toxicant's chemical nature, stability, and interaction with the host's physiology also contribute to its overall toxicokinetics and toxicodynamics (Klaassen, 2021).

Some compounds exhibit cumulative toxicity, wherein repeated sublethal exposures can eventually result in severe toxicity even if individual doses are low. Lead, for instance, accumulates in bones and soft tissues and can cause progressive damage to the nervous and hematopoietic systems over time (Assi et al., 2016). The rate at which a toxicant accumulates, distributes, or is excreted often depends on both the chemical's properties and the physiological state of the host.

Furthermore, the route of entry plays a critical role. Inhalation can produce rapid systemic exposure for volatile compounds, whereas dermal absorption may result in a delayed but prolonged effect. Oral ingestion is a common route in both accidental and intentional poisoning of animals, and its effects are modulated by factors such as gut microflora, food content, and gastrointestinal (GI) motility (Gupta, 2018).

In summary, the toxicity of any given agent is influenced by (i) the properties of the agent itself, (ii) the conditions of exposure, and (iii) the characteristics of the exposed subject. Subject-related factors can be subdivided into inherent (internal) factors and external (environmental) factors. In the following sections, we examine how the nature of the toxic agent, the exposure conditions, and the subject's own biological traits each affect toxic outcomes.

Poison or Toxic Agent

The intrinsic properties of a chemical or toxic compound play a central role in determining its toxicological potential. The chemical structure of the agent influences its interactions with cellular receptors, enzymes, and transport systems. Structural analogs can differ drastically in potency due to minor molecular substitutions, as seen with certain organophosphate pesticides or synthetic pyrethroids (Klaassen, 2021). The presence of specific functional groups or anions, a compound's pK_a, and its acid–base dissociation properties can all influence solubility and absorption across biological membranes.

Physical characteristics, including particle size and formulation (solid, liquid, aerosol), also determine the rate and extent of uptake. Fine particles, for example, are more readily inhaled into alveoli and can rapidly enter systemic circulation. Liquids may be more rapidly absorbed orally, while solids may need to dissolve in GI fluids before significant systemic absorption occurs (Hayes & Kruger, 2021). Excipients or formulation additives (such as emulsifiers or solvents) can further modify a toxicant's bioavailability. Some excipients serve as enhancers of membrane permeability or stabilizers of the active compound, but they may also introduce independent toxicity if not properly evaluated.

The lipid solubility of a compound is among the most critical determinants of its distribution in the body. Lipophilic toxicants easily cross cell membranes and tend to accumulate in adipose tissue or the central nervous system, contributing to long-term persistence and delayed clearance. Organochlorine pesticides such as dichlorodiphenyltrichloroethane (*DDT*) are prime examples of persistent lipophilic toxicants with bioaccumulative properties.

Another crucial factor is the stability of the compound, especially under varying conditions of temperature, light, and pH. Unstable compounds may degrade into other toxic or even more toxic metabolites, or conversely, they may lose efficacy or toxicity upon degradation. For example, the organophosphate insecticide parathion is metabolically activated to paraoxon, a breakdown product that is significantly more toxic than the parent compound due to its stronger cholinesterase-inhibiting activity. On the other hand, some compounds become less harmful upon degradation or metabolism. In tropical environments, where high humidity and heat are common, chemical stability (or instability) becomes especially relevant to toxicity outcomes (FAO, 2021).

Exposure

The manner in which a toxicant enters and encounters the body profoundly affects its toxicokinetic profile. The dose, concentration, and exposure duration largely determine whether an exposure remains subclinical or escalates into acute toxicosis. The route of administration – whether oral, dermal, inhalational, or parenteral – influences both the rate and the site of absorption. For example, intravenous administration leads to immediate systemic availability, while dermal or oral exposures may be partially mitigated by protective barriers or first-pass metabolism (e.g., the skin or the liver) before the toxicant reaches systemic circulation (Gupta, 2018).

The frequency and rate of exposure also help determine the toxic outcome. A single large (bolus) dose may overwhelm detoxification pathways and cause acute toxicity, whereas slow or continuous exposure might allow time for partial elimination or physiological adaptation. The site of administration is important as well; for instance, an intraperitoneal injection can bypass some aspects of first-pass hepatic metabolism and thus may produce more exaggerated toxicity than an equivalent oral dose.

Additionally, the presence of other chemicals or drugs can modulate a toxicant's effects. Interactions between multiple substances may be synergistic or antagonistic. For example, one compound might induce metabolic enzymes that enhance the activation of another toxicant, or conversely, a concurrently administered chemical could inhibit detoxification enzymes and increase the toxicity of the first compound. Such chemical interactions are an important extrinsic factor in real-world exposures and can significantly change toxic outcomes, although their specifics are often complex and case-dependent.

Environmental Factors

Environmental conditions can significantly influence toxicity outcomes, and these factors are considered extrinsic to the organism. Climate and housing conditions – such as ambient temperature, humidity, ventilation, and even social stressors – can modulate how a toxicant affects an animal. High ambient temperatures may increase dermal absorption of chemicals (due to increased cutaneous blood flow and skin permeability) and can also alter biotransformation rates by affecting metabolic enzyme activity. Poor housing ventilation can concentrate airborne toxins (e.g., fumes or gases), thereby increasing respiratory exposure. Meanwhile, overcrowding or other stressors can alter an animal's neuroendocrine and immune function, potentially exacerbating susceptibility to toxic insults (Brunton et al., 2018). These environmental influences often act in concert with the properties of the toxicant and the physiology of the subject.

For a summary of key environmental factors that modulate toxic responses, see Table 2.1.

Subject Factors (Intrinsic)

Subject-related (intrinsic) characteristics of the animal account for much of the variability in response to poisons among individuals of the same species, as well as across different species. Species, breed, and genetic makeup are major determinants of how a toxicant is metabolized and tolerated. For instance, cats are known to be deficient in certain hepatic glucuronidation enzymes, making them highly susceptible to

Table 2.1 Comparative table: factors by category.

Category	Key factors	Example
Toxic agent	Chemistry, lipid solubility, excipients, stability	DDT (lipophilic), aflatoxin B1 (unstable in heat)
Exposure	Dose, route, volume, site, rate	Inhaled vs. oral pesticide exposure
Subject (inherent)	Species, genetics, age, nutrition, health	Cats (deficient UDP-glucuronosyltransferase [UGT] enzyme), Neonates (immature liver)
Subject (external)	Housing, temperature, humidity, social conditions	High temp → ↑ dermal absorption

acetaminophen (paracetamol) poisoning (Gupta, 2018). Similarly, some dog breeds (e.g., Collies) exhibit extreme sensitivity to the antiparasitic ivermectin due to mutations in the *MDR1* gene, which encodes the P-glycoprotein drug transporter. Such a mutation allows higher levels of certain drugs to penetrate the brain, leading to neurotoxicity in affected dogs. Differences in metabolic enzymes or membrane transporters across species (and even among individuals of the same species) can dramatically influence the toxicity of a given compound.

The individual's immune and physiological status also influences toxic outcomes. Immunocompromised animals, or neonates with immature immune systems, may be less able to cope with toxic insults, leading to more severe or unusual manifestations of toxicity. Nutritional status plays a dual role: An antioxidant-rich, vitamin-sufficient diet can bolster defenses against oxidative toxins, whereas protein or micronutrient deficiencies can impair hepatic detoxification pathways and exacerbate toxic effects. Health status is equally important – preexisting liver or kidney dysfunction will reduce the metabolism and excretion of toxicants, often resulting in exaggerated or prolonged effects. Additionally, unique physiological states like pregnancy can alter hepatic enzyme activity and blood flow patterns (for example, pregnancy often increases the metabolism of certain drugs and changes their volume of distribution), thereby affecting the susceptibility of an animal to some toxicants.

Because of these inherent biological factors, individual animals can occasionally respond to a poison in an atypical or idiosyncratic manner, differing from the expected response in the majority of a population. Below, we discuss several key intrinsic factors – age, sex, and nutrition – that have significant impacts on toxicity.

Age, Maturity, and Body Weight

Age and body size are among the most significant biologic factors influencing an animal's response to toxic agents. In neonates and juvenile animals, immature liver and kidney function, underdeveloped enzymatic systems, and a more permeable blood–brain barrier increase susceptibility to many toxicants (Figure 2.2). For instance, in young ruminants, exposure to even low levels of nitrates can result in life-threatening methemoglobinemia due to limited metabolic detoxification capacity – a classic example of age-specific toxicity (Klaassen, 2021). Conversely, geriatric animals may show altered sensitivity to poisons as well, due to age-related physiological changes such as decreased hepatic metabolism, reduced renal clearance, and cumulative lifetime exposure. In veterinary pharmacology, for example, aged dogs have been observed to clear certain NSAIDs more slowly, increasing the risk of dose-related complications like GI ulceration and nephrotoxicity.

Body weight is closely interlinked with dosing and toxicokinetics. Smaller animals (or those with very low body weight) are at higher risk of relative overdose because a given amount of toxicant represents a larger dose per unit body mass, and standard dose calculations may overshoot safe levels for them. On the other hand, obese animals have a greater proportion of adipose tissue, which can act as a reservoir for lipophilic toxicants. Such toxicants may bioaccumulate in fat, leading to prolonged retention of the substance and delayed systemic clearance. In practice, age and body weight factors necessitate careful adjustment of dosages and heightened monitoring for signs of toxicity in both very young animals and in older or extremely small/large patients. *(Figures 2.1 and 2.2 illustrate age-related differences in susceptibility to toxicants.)*

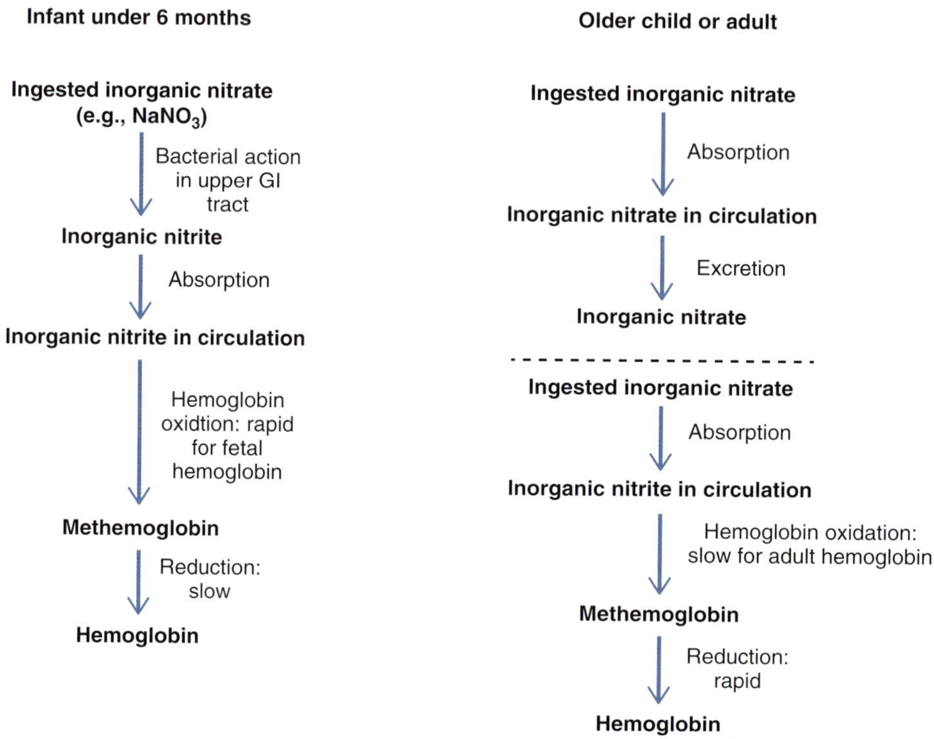

Figure 2.1 Effect of age on the potential toxicity of inorganic nitrates and nitrites.

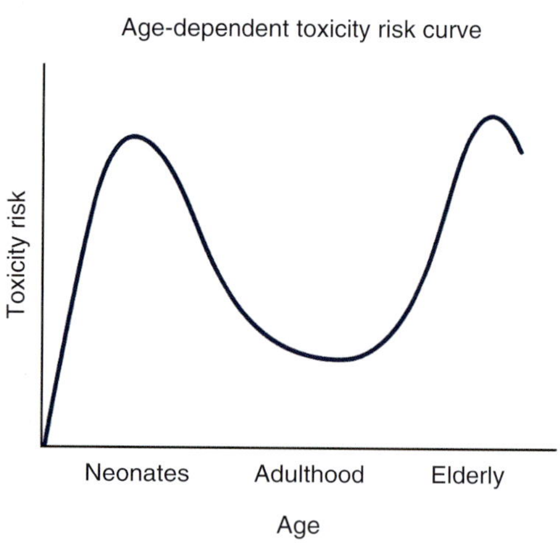

Figure 2.2 Age-dependent toxicity risk curve.

Sex and Hormonal Effects

Sex-based differences in toxicological responses are well documented, with hormonal and metabolic distinctions between males and females affecting xenobiotic metabolism, immune function, and tissue sensitivity. Female animals often exhibit slower biotransformation of certain chemicals, partly due to the influence of estrogens on the regulation of hepatic enzymes. Conversely, males may express higher levels of certain cytochrome P450 (CYP450) enzymes, which can accelerate the metabolism of specific compounds – sometimes leading to toxication (bioactivation to more toxic metabolites) rather than detoxification.

Studies have demonstrated clear examples of these differences. Male rats, for instance, show significantly higher liver biotransformation capacity for certain

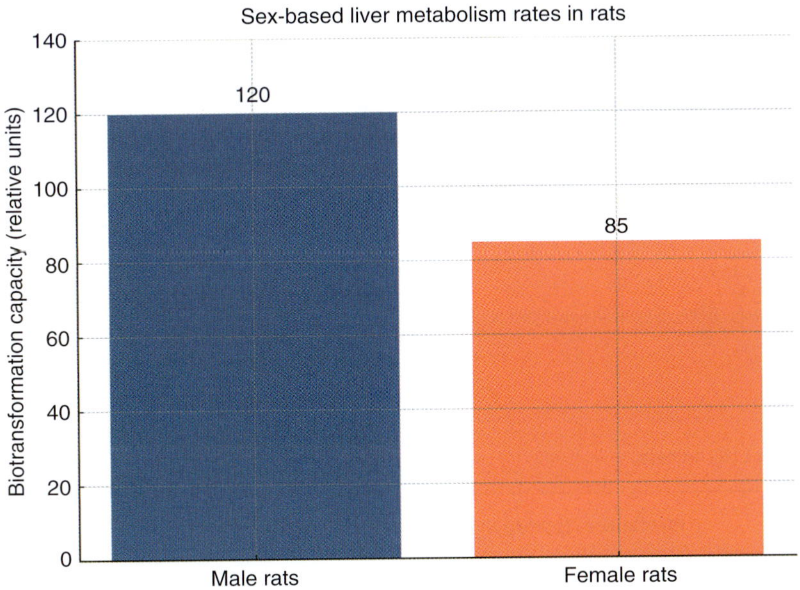

Figure 2.3 Sex-based liver metabolism rates in rats showing higher biotransformation capacity in male rats compared to females – based on hypothetical relative units representing cytochrome P450 activity.

substrates compared to females, due in part to elevated expression of specific hepatic enzymes such as cytochrome P450 2C11 (CYP2C11) and cytochrome P450 3A2 (CYP3A2) that are predominantly expressed in males (Kwekel et al., 2010; Ryan & Levin, 1994). Females, in contrast, have greater expression of CYP2C12. This sexual dimorphism in hepatic enzyme expression means that male and female rats – and by extension, males and females of other species – may metabolize certain drugs and toxicants at different rates. Such enzyme-profile differences underscore the importance of including both sexes in toxicity testing and risk assessment, as one sex may be more vulnerable to a given compound than the other (Figure 2.3).

This sex difference becomes evident in classic toxicity assessments: for example, median lethal doses (LD_{50} values) for various compounds often differ between male and female animals. Tables 2.2 and 2.3 illustrate this discrepancy, showing that male rats have a higher tolerance (i.e., higher LD_{50}) for certain toxicants like parathion compared to females, consistent with their faster metabolic clearance of the compound.

Furthermore, some toxicants exhibit sex-specific effects in susceptibility or severity. A notable example is aflatoxin B_1 – studies have found that male rodents are more susceptible to the carcinogenic effects of aflatoxin B_1 than females. This is possibly due to androgen-driven enhancement of the CYP450 enzymes that bioactivate aflatoxin B_1 into its reactive epoxide form. Such sex–toxin interactions continue to be an area of active research because of their implications for food safety and mycotoxin regulation (Abdel-Wahhab & Kholif, 2008; Alshannaq & Yu, 2017; Fink-Gremmels, 2008; Tables 2.2 and 2.3).

Table 2.2 Effect of sex on acute oral LD_{50} in rats.

	LD_{50} (mg/kg)	
Compound	**Female**	**Male**
Digitoxin	56	94
Trifluperidol	140	360
Dieldrin	119	213
Parathion	3.6	9

Source: Data from Gupta (2018).

Table 2.3 Effect of sex on acute oral LD_{50} in rats.

	Metabolism (ppm/g liver)	
Gender	**1 h**	**6 h**
Male	1,200	10,500
Female	270	3,200

Source: Data from Gupta (2018).

Nutritional Status and Dietary Factors

Nutrition acts as an important modulating factor in toxicity through multiple mechanisms. Adequate protein intake, for example, supports the hepatic detoxification enzyme systems – including glutathione-S-transferases, CYP450s, and sulfotransferases – that metabolize and eliminate toxicants. Conversely, protein-deficient animals may show impaired hepatic function and increased susceptibility to hepatotoxic effects from common feed-borne contaminants (Klaassen, 2021). Deficiencies in specific nutrients (such as selenium or vitamins that serve as enzyme cofactors) can likewise compromise detoxification pathways.

In addition, various dietary components may act as chemical modifiers. Some nutrients and phytochemicals function as natural detoxicants. For example, plant-derived flavonoids and polyphenols can neutralize free radicals or bind (chelate) heavy metal ions, thereby reducing the systemic toxicity of those agents. On the other hand, certain dietary factors can enhance toxicity. A high dietary fat content, for instance, can facilitate the absorption of lipophilic toxicants from the gut, leading to greater systemic distribution of those toxicants. Thus, animals on lipid-rich diets might absorb more of a fat-soluble poison than those on low-fat diets.

Overall diet quality can therefore sway toxic outcomes. One illustrative case is the protective effect of a high-protein diet: Laboratory studies have shown that rats fed a 20% casein (high-protein) diet were protected against arsenic-induced reproductive toxicity compared to rats on a standard protein diet

(Mondal et al., 2013). On the other hand, poor diet quality or malnutrition – whether due to imbalanced nutrition, feed contamination, or caloric restriction – tends to increase an animal's vulnerability to many toxic substances by weakening metabolic and reparative capacities. *(Figure 2.4 exemplifies how nutritional status can modulate toxicity.)*

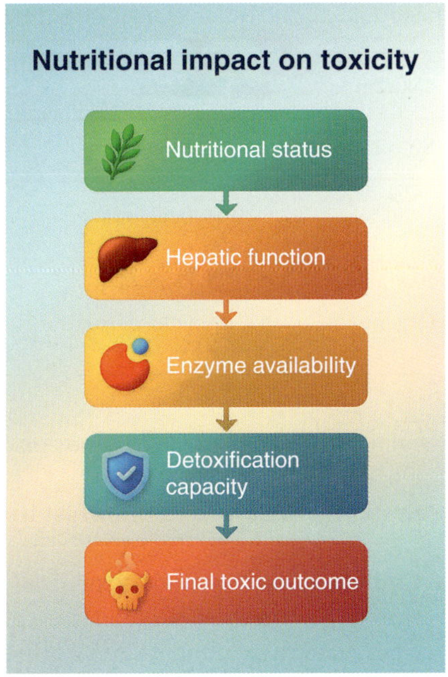

Figure 2.4 Nutritional impact on toxicity.

Sites of Toxic Reaction

In addition to the factors described above, the site of toxic action – whether a toxicant causes effects locally at the point of contact or systemically throughout the body – is an important aspect of toxicity. Certain chemical and exposure factors determine whether a poison causes damage primarily at the entry site or after being absorbed and distributed to distant organs.

The nature of the toxicant often dictates the local vs. systemic pattern of toxicity. Some chemicals cause local toxicity, meaning the toxic effect is limited to the site of initial contact with the body (such as the skin, respiratory tract, or GI tract). For example, strong caustic or corrosive substances are nonselective irritants that cause immediate injury to any cells they contact, with the severity of damage proportional to the concentration of the substance. Strong acids (e.g., hydrochloric acid, sulfuric acid, nitric acid) and strong alkalis (e.g., sodium hydroxide, potassium hydroxide, ammonium hydroxide) belong to this group of toxicants; they cause severe tissue necrosis at the site of contact. Similarly, irritating gases such as sulfur dioxide or nitrogen dioxide (present in polluted air) can produce toxic reactions in the upper respiratory tract and lungs by converting to strong acids upon contact with the moist mucosal surfaces.

- Dermal contact: Phenol and other phenolics, as well as strong acids and bases, can cause severe local skin corrosion and necrosis at the site of contact.
- Inhalation: Chlorine gas, ammonia, and nitrogen dioxide primarily cause local irritation and inflammation of the respiratory tract (from the nasal passages to the lungs).
- Oral/GI exposure: Ingestion of caustic substances like sodium hydroxide (lye) or bleach can lead to immediate burns of the mouth, esophagus, and stomach; even certain pesticides or household cleaners can cause localized GI injury upon ingestion.

For a comparative summary of local versus systemic toxic effects, see Table 2.4.

By contrast, most other toxic substances (except for those extremely reactive compounds mentioned above) produce systemic toxicity, meaning their harmful effects occur at sites distant from the point of initial contact. Systemic effects require that the toxicant be absorbed into the bloodstream and distributed throughout the body. These effects are often more insidious or delayed in onset, since they depend on reaching and accumulating in a target organ. Whether a toxicant causes predominantly

Table 2.4 Classification of toxic effects by site of action.

Toxicant	Route	Local effects	Systemic effects
Sulfur dioxide	Inhalation	Respiratory tract irritation	Pulmonary acidification
Lead	Oral/inhaled	GI irritation (rare)	Central nervous system, kidneys, hematopoietic toxicity
Phenol	Dermal	Skin corrosion	Hepatorenal toxicity (high dose)
Organophosphates	Oral/dermal	Minor local effect	Central nervous system (CNS) (acetylcholine crisis)

local or systemic damage depends on its ability to penetrate biological barriers and its stability inside the body.

Systemic toxicity can manifest in various ways, but there are some common patterns:

- Cumulative toxicity: The toxin gradually builds up in the body with repeated exposures, eventually reaching a threshold for toxicity (e.g., heavy metals like lead or cadmium, and persistent organochlorines, tend to accumulate and cause chronic effects).
- Organ-specific targeting: The toxin preferentially affects certain organs or tissues after distribution (for example, aflatoxin B_1 is primarily hepatotoxic, targeting the liver; organophosphate insecticides are neurotoxic, chiefly affecting the nervous system by inhibiting acetylcholinesterase).

As noted earlier, lead is a prime example of a heavy metal that produces systemic toxicity. It is stored primarily in bones, where it can reside for years, yet it exerts toxic effects on other systems such as the hematopoietic system, nervous system, and kidneys (Assi et al., 2016). Similarly, organophosphate compounds, once absorbed, act on multiple organs by inhibiting cholinesterase activity, which leads to neurologic dysfunction throughout the body. *(Figure 2.5 illustrates how a systemic toxicant can affect multiple organ systems.)*

Target organ susceptibility is influenced by several factors:

- Blood perfusion rate: Organs that receive a high proportion of the blood flow (e.g., liver, kidneys, brain) are delivered more of the toxicant per unit time, which can make them more vulnerable to systemic poisons.
- Biotransformation capacity: Organs with high metabolic enzyme activity (notably the liver, and to a lesser extent the kidneys and lungs) may convert toxins into reactive intermediates on site, sometimes increasing local damage in those organs.
- Bioaccumulation tendency: Some tissues have an affinity for certain chemicals – for example, fat stores sequester fat-soluble toxins, bone stores lead – causing the toxicant to concentrate in those locations over time.

These principles help explain why certain organ systems (central nervous system, liver, kidney, etc.) are more frequently affected in systemic toxicity, whereas others (such as bone or skeletal muscle) are less commonly harmed directly, except as sites of storage.

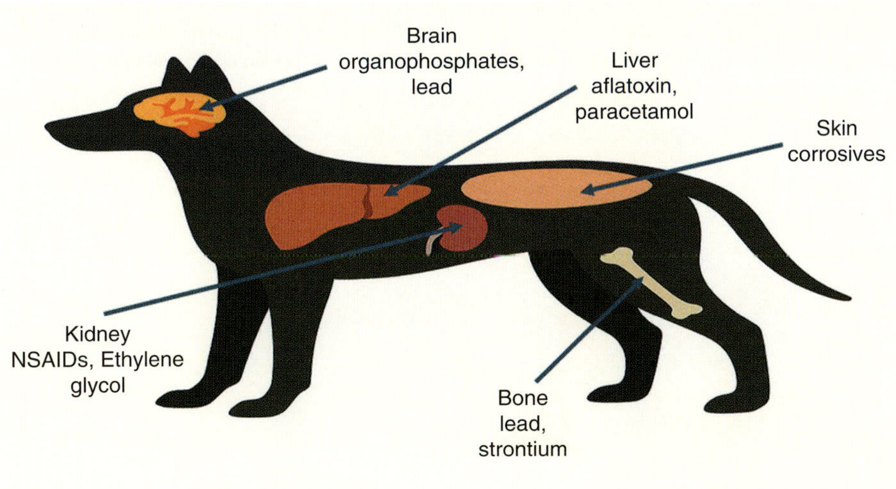

Figure 2.5 Systemic distribution and target organs of common toxicants.

Special Considerations in Tropical and Subtropical Contexts

In tropical and subtropical regions, environmental and management factors can influence the manifestation of toxicity in ways that differ from temperate settings. High ambient temperature and humidity, for example, can accelerate the deterioration of feed and promote fungal growth, leading to increased contamination by mycotoxins (especially aflatoxins). These conditions are common in poorly stored feedstuffs and are frequently encountered in smallholder farming systems in the tropics. Furthermore, heat stress in animals – accompanied by changes such as reduced feed intake, altered gut motility, and increased respiration – may affect the rates of absorption, distribution, metabolism, and excretion of toxicants. The widespread use of agrochemicals and traditional herbal remedies with minimal regulatory oversight in many tropical regions may also increase the risk of exposure to potentially toxic substances. It is therefore essential to consider these regional factors when evaluating the risk and impact of toxic substances in veterinary practice in hot, humid climates (Ráduly et al., 2020). *(Figure 2.6 provides an illustration of climate-related toxicological challenges in tropical systems.)*

One of the most pressing toxicological concerns in tropical environments is the high prevalence of mycotoxins, particularly aflatoxin B_1, fumonisins, and ochratoxins. These toxins are produced by fungi such as *Aspergillus flavus* and *Fusarium* spp., which thrive in hot, humid conditions common in regions like Southeast Asia, sub-Saharan Africa, and parts of South America. Mycotoxins are often present in staple feed ingredients (e.g., maize, groundnuts, rice bran) when preservation is poor, and chronic ingestion by livestock leads to syndromes such as liver damage, immunosuppression, and poor reproductive performance (FAO, 2021; Ráduly et al., 2020). Climate change may further exacerbate these risks by lengthening fungal growing seasons and making weather patterns more erratic. For instance, rising temperatures and periods of heavy rainfall followed by drought can increase the likelihood of mold growth and toxin production in stored feeds. Moreover, thermal stress in livestock (due to high heat loads)

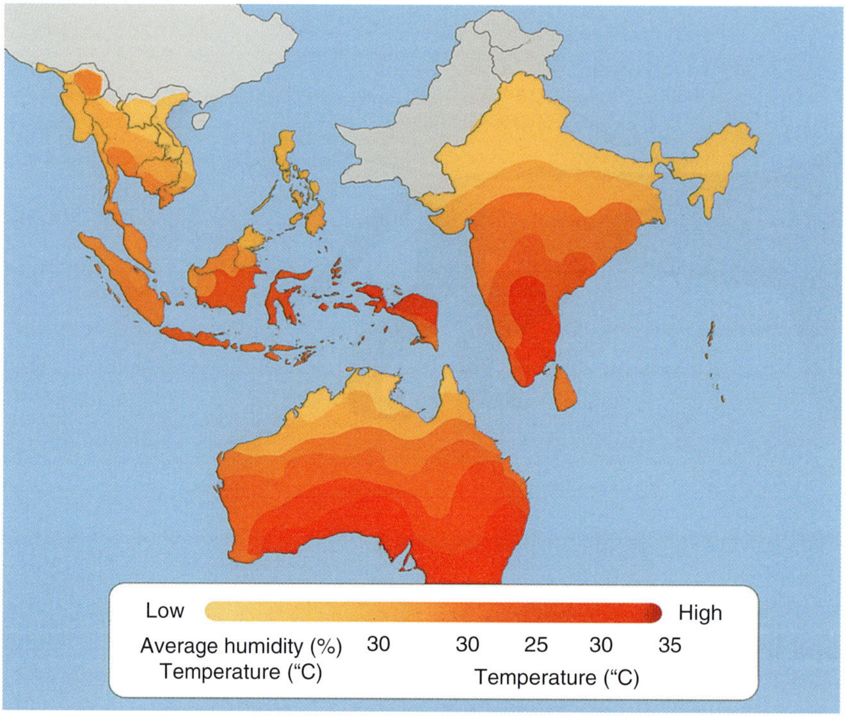

Figure 2.6 Climatic risk zones for mycotoxin proliferation.

reduces feed intake, alters gut integrity, and compromises mucosal immunity, all of which make animals more vulnerable to orally ingested toxins (Bernabucci et al., 2010).

In tropical veterinary settings, the use of traditional herbal remedies and ethnoveterinary preparations is widespread, especially in rural areas. While some of these preparations have genuine pharmacological effects, others may be contaminated with heavy metals or pesticide residues, or they may contain naturally occurring toxic constituents (Shaban et al., 2016). Poorly regulated herbal products have been associated with chronic problems like hepatotoxicity, reproductive failure, and photosensitization in ruminants and horses.

Another regional concern is toxicity from endemic poisonous flora. Toxic plants such as *Jatropha curcas*, *Leucaena leucocephala*, *Ipomoea carnea*, and *Eupatorium adenophorum* are more common in the tropics and are frequently implicated in accidental livestock poisoning, particularly during droughts or periods of feed scarcity when animals graze unfamiliar plants. In goats, for example, ingestion of *Ipomoea* (morning glory) species can lead to neurologic syndromes due to the neurotoxin swainsonine, while *Leucaena* (lead tree) can cause hair loss and infertility in cattle due to the mimosine content. *(Figure 2.7 shows examples of some toxic plants prevalent in tropical regions.)*

Tropical regions also bear a disproportionate burden of parasitic infestations (e.g., liver flukes, GI helminths, and blood parasites), which can indirectly increase toxicity risks. Heavy parasite loads may impair organ function or alter drug metabolism and nutrient absorption, thereby changing how animals handle toxicants. For example, chronic infection with the liver fluke *Fasciola hepatica* causes liver damage and reduced detoxification capacity, and it has been shown to exacerbate the toxic effects of aflatoxin B_1 in livestock (Osuna et al., 1977).

From a policy perspective, many tropical countries face challenges in enforcing food and feed safety regulations. Surveillance of feed mills, enforcement of proper pesticide uses and withdrawal times in food animals, and regulation of imported agrochemicals may be inconsistent due to infrastructure and governance limitations. These gaps in regulatory frameworks make it even more critical to have region-specific toxicovigilance systems and diagnostic protocols in place. Veterinary professionals in tropical and subtropical areas must remain vigilant for toxicity cases that may stem from these unique environmental, biological, and socioeconomic factors, and adapt prevention strategies accordingly.

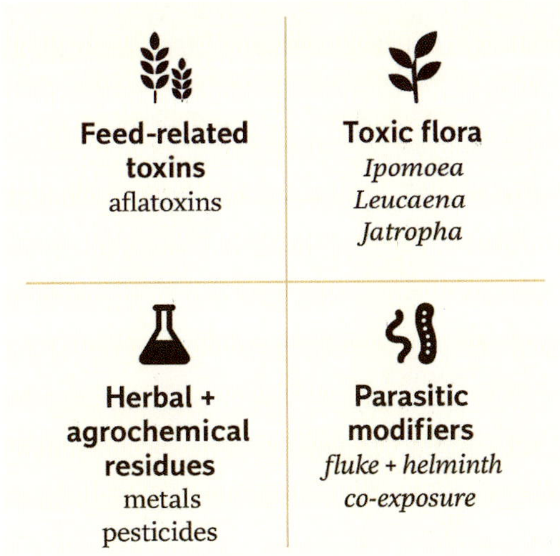

Figure 2.7 Toxicological challenges in the tropics.

References

Abdel-Wahhab, M. A., & Kholif, A. M. (2008). Mycotoxins in Animal Feeds and Prevention Strategies: A Review. *Asian Journal of Animal Sciences*, *2*(1), 7–25. https://doi.org/10.3923/ajas.2008.7.25

Alshannaq, A., & Yu, J. H. (2017). Occurrence, toxicity, and analysis of major mycotoxins in food. *International Journal of Environmental Research and Public Health*, *14*(6), 632. https://doi.org/10.3390/ijerph14060632

Assi, M. A., Hezmee, M. N. M., Haron, A. W., Sabri, M. Y., & Rajion, M. A. (2016). The detrimental effects of lead on human and animal health. *Veterinary World*, *9*(6), 660–671. https://doi.org/10.14202/vetworld.2016.660-671

Bernabucci, U., Lacetera, N., Baumgard, L. H., Rhoads, R. P., Ronchi, B., & Nardone, A. (2010). Metabolic and hormonal acclimation to heat stress in domesticated ruminants. *Animal*, *4*(7), 1167–1183. https://doi.org/10.1017/S175173111000090X

Brunton, L. L., Hilal-Dandan, R., & Knollmann, B. C. (Eds.). (2018). *Goodman and Gilman's: The pharmacological basis of therapeutics* (13th ed.). McGraw-Hill.

FAO. (2021). *Emergency response to aflatoxin outbreaks in Asia-Pacific livestock systems*. Food and Agriculture Organization of the United Nations.

Fink-Gremmels, J. (2008). The role of mycotoxins in the health and performance of dairy cows. *The Veterinary Journal*, *176*(1), 84–92. https://doi.org/10.1016/j.tvjl.2007.12.034

Gupta, R. C. (Ed.). (2018). *Veterinary toxicology: Basic and clinical principles* (3rd ed.). Academic Press.

Hayes, A. W., & Kruger, C. L. (Eds.). (2021). *Hayes' principles and methods of toxicology* (7th ed.). CRC Press.

Klaassen, C. D. (Ed.). (2021). *Casarett and Doull's toxicology: The basic science of poisons* (10th ed.). McGraw-Hill.

Kwekel, J. C., Desai, V. G., Moland, C. L., Branham, W. S., & Fuscoe, J. C. (2010). Age- and sex-dependent changes in liver gene expression during the life cycle of the rat. *BMC Genomics*, *11*, 675. https://doi.org/10.1186/1471-2164-11-675

Mondal, S., Mukherjee, S., Chaudhuri, K., Kabir, S. N., & Kumar Mukhopadhyay, P. (2013). Prevention of arsenic-mediated reproductive toxicity in adult female rats by high protein diet. *Pharmaceutical Biology*, *51*(11), 1363–1371. https://doi.org/10.3109/13880209.2013.792846

Osuna, O., Edds, G. T., & Blankespoor, H. D. (1977). Toxic effects of aflatoxin B_1 in male Holstein calves with prior infection by flukes (*Fasciola hepatica*). *American Journal of Veterinary Research*, *38*(3), 341–349.

Ráduly, Z., Szabó, L., Madar, A., Pócsi, I., & Tóth, B. (2020). Toxicological and medical aspects of *Aspergillus*-derived mycotoxins entering the feed and food chain. *Frontiers in Microbiology*, *10*, 2908. https://doi.org/10.3389/fmicb.2019.02908

Ryan, D. E., & Levin, W. (1994). Age- and gender-related expression of rat liver cytochrome P450. In R. Klinger (Ed.), *Handbook of experimental pharmacology* (Vol. 105, pp. 239–284). Springer.

Shaban, N. S., Abdou, K. A., & Hassan, N. E.-H. Y. (2016). Impact of toxic heavy metals and pesticide residues in herbal products. *Beni-Suef University Journal of Basic and Applied Sciences*, *5*(1), 102–106. https://doi.org/10.1016/j.bjbas.2015.10.001

3

Absorption and Distribution of Toxicants

Most toxic substances must enter the body before producing deleterious effects, and the extent of the damage will depend significantly on the concentration of these toxicants within the body tissues. The effective concentration of any given toxicant at its site of action depends not only on the quantity of a toxicant that an individual absorbs, inhales, or otherwise takes in, but also on the efficiency and rate of absorption, on distribution mechanisms within the body, on biotransformation processes, and on eventual excretion. Each of these factors can profoundly alter the magnitude and duration of the toxic response (Hodgson, 2010; Klaassen, 2013a).

Absorption refers to the entry of toxicants into systemic circulation from the site of exposure. This initial stage critically influences toxicity because a substance must typically enter systemic circulation to affect distant organs and tissues. The route through which a toxicant enters the body often dictates the absorption rate and extent, subsequently influencing toxicity levels and the manifestation of clinical signs (Klaassen, 2013b). For instance, absorption via inhalation can lead to rapid distribution into the bloodstream due to the extensive vascularization and large surface area of the pulmonary alveoli. In contrast, oral ingestion often involves absorption through the gastrointestinal tract, where several factors such as gastric pH, gastrointestinal motility, and presence of food can significantly alter absorption rates (Klaassen, 2013a).

Distribution is the subsequent movement of toxicants throughout the body via systemic circulation to various tissues and organs. Distribution patterns are greatly affected by the physicochemical properties of the toxicant such as lipid solubility, molecular size, and ionization, as well as physiological parameters including blood-flow rates to different tissues and the presence of specific binding proteins (Gibaldi & Perrier, 2007). For example, highly lipid-soluble compounds such as organochlorine insecticides predominantly accumulate in fatty tissues. They can remain stored there for extended periods, slowly releasing back into the bloodstream and prolonging toxic effects.

Biotransformation, also known as metabolism, involves biochemical modifications of toxicants primarily in the liver, although other organs like kidneys, lungs, and gastrointestinal mucosa also participate significantly. The primary purpose of biotransformation is to convert lipid-soluble toxicants into water-soluble metabolites that are more readily excreted. However, this metabolic process occasionally produces metabolites that are more toxic than the parent compound. For example, the insecticide parathion is metabolized to the more toxic paraoxon (Parkinson and Ogilvie, 2008).

Excretion is the final phase in toxicant kinetics, involving the removal of toxic substances and their metabolites from the body. This can occur through various routes, including renal excretion via urine, hepatic excretion via bile into feces, pulmonary excretion through exhaled air, and to a lesser extent, through sweat, tears, and breast milk. The efficiency of excretion can significantly impact the toxicity and duration of action of toxic substances, especially those with longer half-lives that undergo enterohepatic circulation or extensive reabsorption processes (Hodgson, 2010).

Various routes of toxicant exposure critically determine the initial absorption and subsequently affect distribution, metabolism, and excretion processes. The primary routes include inhalation, ingestion, dermal absorption, and injection.

Inhalation exposure involves toxicants entering the respiratory tract, often resulting in rapid systemic absorption. Industrial solvents, pesticides, and gaseous pollutants exemplify substances frequently encountered via inhalation. Ingestion typically relates to contaminated food and water, oral medications, or accidental intake of hazardous materials. Heavy metals, foodborne toxins, and certain drugs predominantly enter systemic circulation through this pathway.

Dermal absorption, or percutaneous exposure, is influenced by the condition of the skin barrier, the toxicant's lipophilicity, and environmental conditions such as temperature and humidity. Organophosphate pesticides and solvents are examples that efficiently penetrate intact skin, leading to systemic toxicity. Injection exposure, although less common environmentally, can be critically significant in medical or veterinary scenarios, involving direct introduction of substances into systemic circulation, bypassing absorptive barriers (Figure 3.1).

Understanding the intricacies of these processes is essential for effective toxicological risk assessment, management of poisoning cases, and the establishment of safety guidelines for environmental,

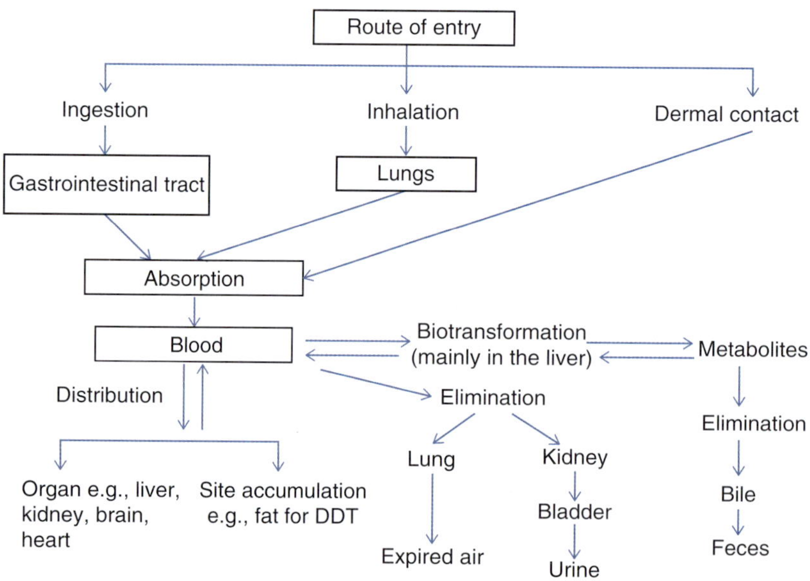

Figure 3.1 Schematic representation of absorption, distribution, and elimination of toxicants from the body.

occupational, and veterinary settings. Subsequent sections will further elaborate on species-specific pathways in wildlife and domestic animals, alongside comparative discussions across diverse regional contexts.

Cell Membrane Structure

Toxicants must pass through various biological barriers to achieve sufficient concentrations at their target sites. These barriers include membranes of skin cells, epithelial cells lining the gut, and the endothelium of blood vessels. All cell membranes share a basic trilaminar structure, consisting mainly of proteins and lipids arranged distinctly in three layers. The central lipid layer primarily comprises lecithin, cephalin, and cholesterol, surrounded by protein layers forming the outermost and innermost surfaces. This trilaminar structure is crucial because it restricts or facilitates the penetration of toxicants based on their chemical characteristics (Barrett et al., 2019; Rang et al., 2019) (Figure 3.2).

The lipid bilayer component of the cell membrane plays a particularly critical role in toxicant permeability. Lipid-soluble (lipophilic) toxicants, such as organochlorines and organophosphates, readily diffuse through this lipid bilayer due to their affinity for hydrophobic environments. Once these lipophilic toxicants penetrate the cell membrane, they can distribute widely within the body, especially accumulating in lipid-rich tissues like adipose tissue, the brain, and nervous tissue, leading to prolonged toxic effects (Figure 3.3).

Conversely, water-soluble (hydrophilic) toxicants face difficulty crossing the lipid bilayer directly due to the hydrophobic nature of the membrane's interior. However, certain small hydrophilic molecules can

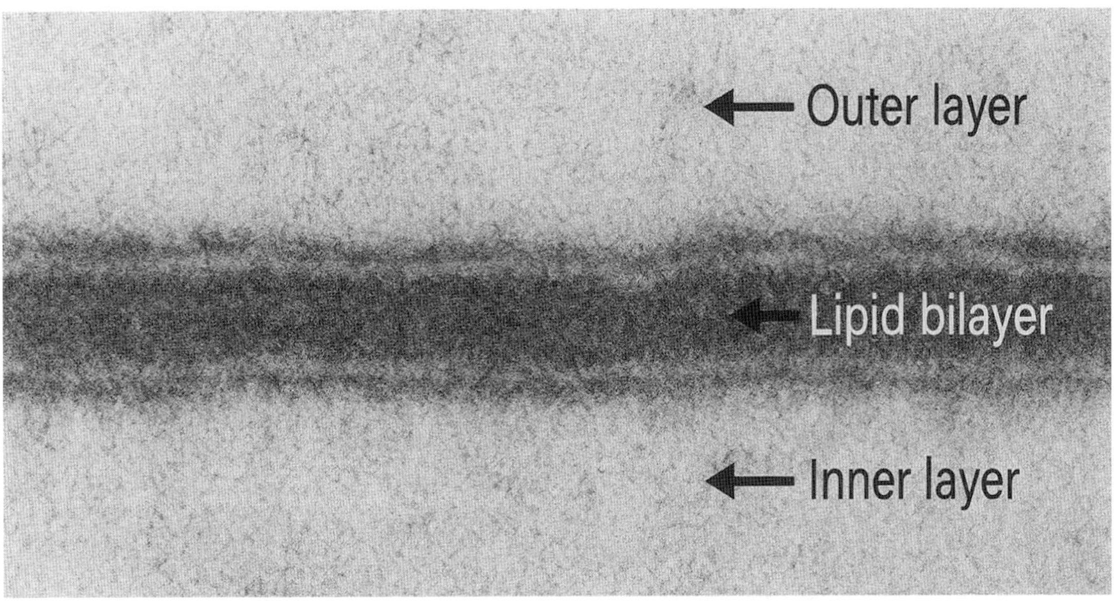

Figure 3.2 Electron micrograph clearly depicting the trilaminar structure of the plasma membrane.

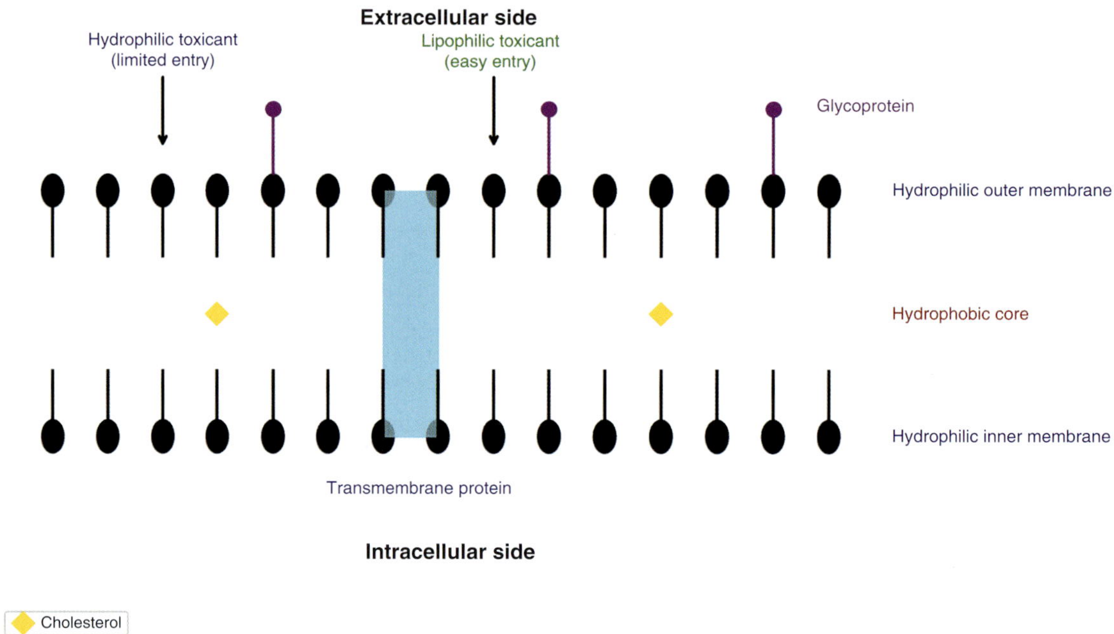

Figure 3.3 Interactions of lipophilic and hydrophilic toxicants with the lipid bilayer of the cell membrane. Lipophilic toxicants diffuse readily through the hydrophobic core, whereas hydrophilic toxicants require carrier proteins for entry. *Source:* Hodgson (2010); Klaassen (2013a).

pass through specific transport proteins embedded within the cell membrane via facilitated diffusion or active transport. For example, heavy metals such as lead and cadmium can exploit ion channels and transporters typically used for calcium or zinc, allowing them to bypass the lipid barrier.

Toxicants that are ionized at physiological pH generally have reduced membrane permeability because charged molecules are poorly soluble in lipids. The degree of ionization is dictated by the compound's inherent chemical properties (pK_a value) and the pH of the local environment. For instance, weak acids like aspirin are absorbed more efficiently in the acidic environment of the stomach because they remain non-ionized and thus lipid-soluble, allowing easier passage through the gastric mucosal membranes.

In addition to chemical interactions, the integrity of the cell membrane itself influences toxicant absorption. Damaged or compromised membranes – such as those affected by abrasions, burns, or disease conditions – significantly increase permeability and enhance toxicant entry into systemic circulation. This mechanism underscores the importance of intact biological barriers in mitigating exposure to harmful substances.

Biotransport

The movement of chemicals across biological barriers is known as biotransport. This can occur by passive diffusion or specialized transport mechanisms (Levine, 1973).

Passive Diffusion

Passive diffusion involves the transfer of a chemical across a biological barrier from higher to lower concentration without cellular energy expenditure. It is influenced by several key factors:

- Lipid/water partition coefficient: Highly lipid-soluble compounds (e.g., organophosphate pesticides like methyl parathion) diffuse readily through cell membranes.
- Degree of ionization: Weak acids and bases are more permeable when non ionized. Aspirin, a weak acid, is absorbed rapidly in the acidic gastric environment.
- Concentration gradient: A larger gradient increases the diffusion rate.
- Molecular size: Smaller molecules diffuse more efficiently.

Specialized Transport

Several specialized transport mechanisms enable the selective transfer of substances across cell membranes:

Facilitated diffusion: Utilizes carrier proteins to move substances like glucose and amino acids along the concentration gradient. Toxicants structurally similar to nutrients, such as dinitrophenol, can exploit this pathway (Figure 3.4).

Active transport: Requires energy (adenosine triphosphate [ATP]) to move substances against the concentration gradient. For example, cells actively pump essential ions such as calcium to maintain homeostasis. Some toxicants can hijack these pathways – for instance, heavy metals like lead can mimic calcium and enter neurons through calcium channels, disrupting neurological function (Figure 3.5).

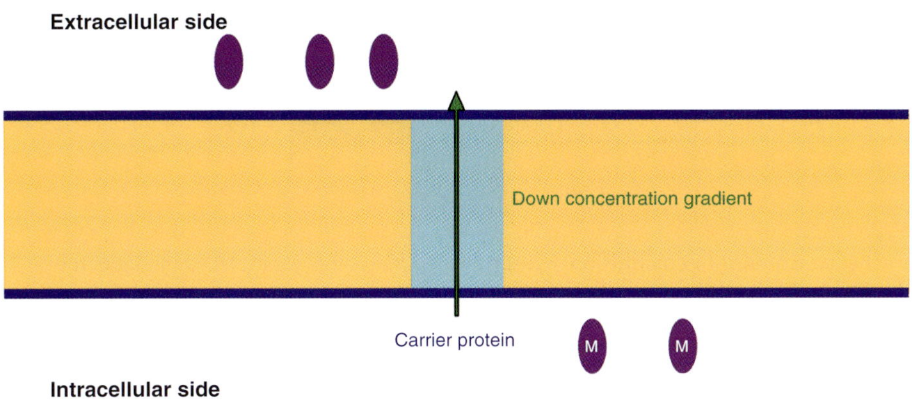

Figure 3.4 Schematic of facilitated diffusion across a lipid bilayer, showing the role of carrier proteins in moving toxicants down their concentration gradient without energy expenditure. *Source:* Barrett et al. (2019); Gibaldi and Perrier (2007).

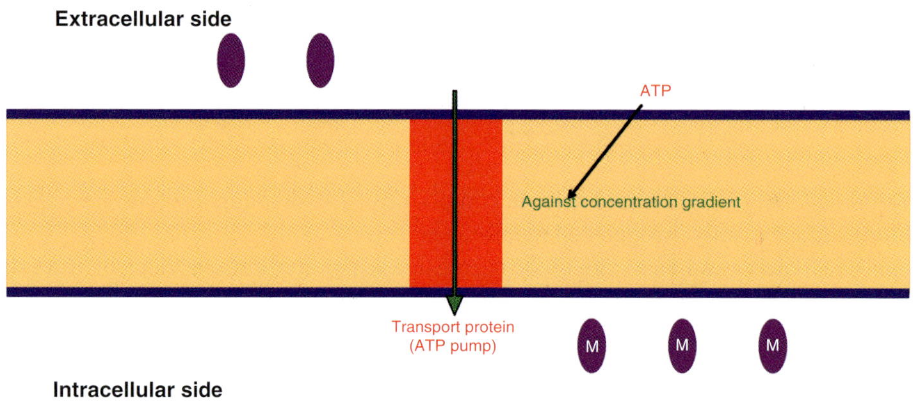

Figure 3.5 Schematic of active transport across the lipid bilayer. Toxicants are transported against their concentration gradient via ATP-dependent pumps. *Source:* Parkinson & Ogilvie (2008); Rang et al. (2019).

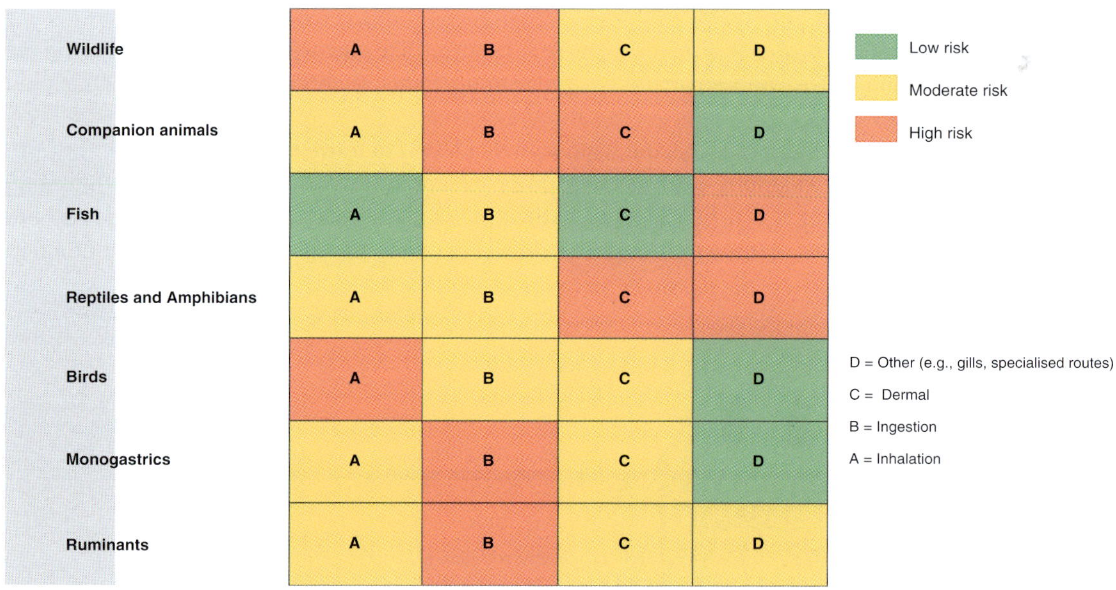

Figure 3.6 Combined schematic of facilitated diffusion, active transport, and pinocytosis. This highlights the multiple mechanisms by which xenobiotics enter cells, including carrier-mediated, energy-dependent, and vesicular uptake. *Source:* Klaassen (2013a); O'Brien & Cousins (2015).

Pinocytosis: Involves the engulfment of extracellular fluid by cell-membrane invaginations, enabling uptake of macromolecules and nanoparticle toxicants. For example, nanoparticles used in drug-delivery systems often utilize this pathway.

Figure 3.6 provides a combined illustration of these specialized transport mechanisms.

Pathways in Wildlife and Domestic Species

Ruminants: Ruminants like cattle, sheep, and goats possess a complex forestomach (rumen) that significantly influences toxicant absorption. The rumen microbial ecosystem can metabolically alter xenobiotics, reducing or occasionally enhancing their toxicity. For example, nitrate poisoning occurs frequently in cattle due to the microbial conversion of nitrates into toxic nitrites. Conversely, certain mycotoxins are detoxified by ruminal microbes, highlighting both protective and harmful microbial roles.

Monogastrics: Monogastric species including pigs, horses, and dogs exhibit more rapid absorption of orally administered toxicants due to a single acidic gastric chamber and rapid intestinal transit times. For instance, acute poisoning by deoxynivalenol, a prevalent mycotoxin, is commonly reported in pigs, causing severe gastrointestinal disturbances and weight loss due to rapid and extensive absorption.

Birds: Birds have a highly efficient respiratory system and relatively thin skin, increasing their susceptibility to inhaled and dermal toxicants. Birds rapidly accumulate lipophilic substances such as dichlorodiphenyltrichloroethane (DDT) and organophosphate insecticides in their adipose and brain tissues. Case studies involving avian species exposed to fumigants like phosphine have demonstrated rapid-onset neurological dysfunction and high mortality rates due to efficient respiratory absorption and central nervous system distribution.

Reptiles and amphibians: Reptiles and amphibians typically exhibit slow metabolism and elimination processes. Amphibians, with their permeable skin, are particularly susceptible to dermal absorption of pesticides and heavy metals from aquatic habitats. A notable example is the widespread amphibian decline linked to the dermal absorption of agricultural runoff containing atrazine, which disrupts endocrine function, leading to reproductive abnormalities.

Fish and aquatic wildlife: Fish directly absorb waterborne toxicants through their gills, a process accelerated by extensive gill surface area and constant exposure to contaminated water. Lipophilic compounds accumulate predominantly in adipose tissues and liver, whereas hydrophilic substances tend to concentrate in the kidneys. Mercury bioaccumulation in predatory fish like tuna exemplifies toxicant biomagnification, impacting both ecosystem health and human consumers.

Companion animals (dogs and cats): Companion animals frequently encounter toxicants through accidental ingestion or dermal exposure to household chemicals and veterinary pharmaceuticals. Cats are particularly sensitive to toxins such as permethrin-based flea treatments due to deficient hepatic glucuronidation pathways, resulting in severe neurotoxic effects even at low exposure levels. Dogs frequently present with clinical signs of poisoning from anticoagulant rodenticides, characterized by severe hemorrhaging due to disruption of vitamin K-dependent clotting factors.

Wildlife case studies: Elephants consuming water contaminated with heavy metals demonstrate prolonged bioaccumulation in their bones and tusks, leading to chronic renal failure and compromised health. Raptors ingesting anticoagulant rodenticides through prey exhibit secondary poisoning characterized by internal bleeding and increased mortality rates, highlighting the risks of bioaccumulative toxins in predator–prey food chains.

Bioaccumulation patterns vary widely among taxa: Elevated mercury levels are found in predatory fish (Ali et al., 2019). Lead and cadmium accumulate in waterbirds (Rahman et al., 2017). Secondary poisoning from anticoagulant rodenticides has been observed in raptors (Nakayama et al., 2019). Freshwater fish exhibit high pesticide residues (Islam et al., 2025). Amphibians show notable atrazine uptake (Hayes et al., 2002). These species-specific differences necessitate adjusted therapeutic doses, varied withdrawal periods for veterinary drugs, and careful extrapolation of toxicity data from laboratory to wildlife species (Figures 3.7 and 3.8).

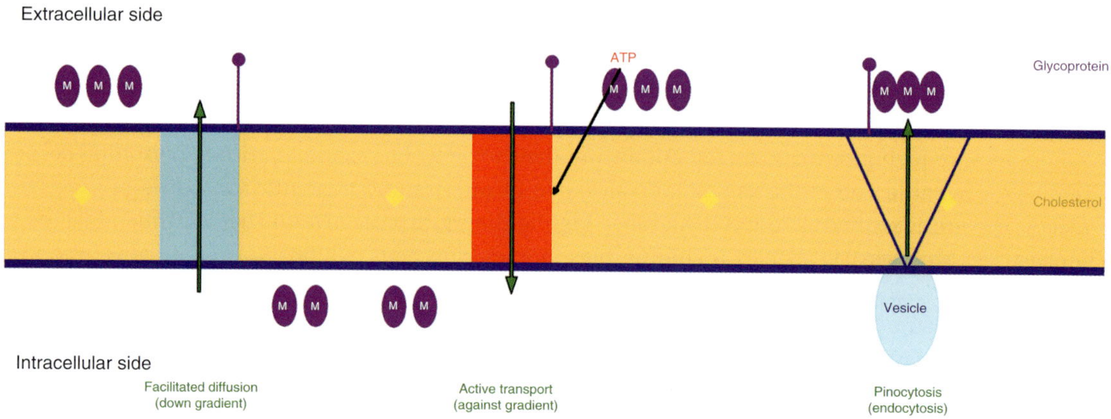

Figure 3.7 Comparative absorption pathways across species. Species differ in their dominant routes of exposure (e.g., ingestion, dermal, inhalation), reflecting physiological and ecological adaptations. *Source:* O'Brien & Cousins, (2015); Walker et al., (2012).

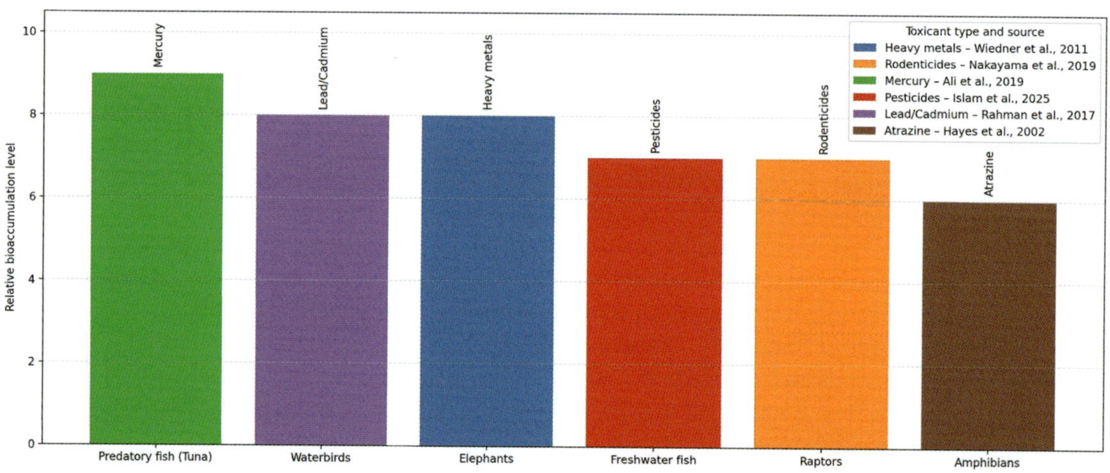

Figure 3.8 Bioaccumulation case studies across species. Examples include mercury in predatory fish, lead and cadmium in waterbirds, and atrazine in amphibians, highlighting species-specific vulnerabilities. *Source:* Ali et al. (2019); Hayes et al. (2002); Islam et al. (2025); Nakayama et al. (2019); Rahman et al. (2017); Wiedner et al. (2011).

Comparative Aspects Across Regions

Tropical regions: In tropical climates, high temperatures and humidity substantially enhance the dermal absorption of toxicants. Agricultural practices often involve extensive use of pesticides due to continuous pest pressure, resulting in significant bioaccumulation in local wildlife. Southeast Asia exemplifies this with high pesticide use in rice paddies, contributing to elevated levels of chlorpyrifos and carbofuran residues in freshwater fish and aquatic organisms. Furthermore, the rapid microbial degradation rates in tropical soils influence the environmental persistence of chemicals differently compared to temperate regions.

Temperate regions: Temperate regions, characterized by moderate climates and distinct seasonal variations, display different toxicant behavior patterns. Pesticides used in temperate agricultural systems, such as herbicides (glyphosate) and fungicides (azoxystrobin), tend to persist longer in soils during colder seasons due to reduced microbial activity. Consequently, spring runoff and snowmelt can transport accumulated toxicants into aquatic ecosystems, posing seasonal risks to aquatic wildlife and drinking-water sources in North America and Europe.

Arid regions: Arid and semiarid environments, prevalent in parts of Africa and the American Southwest, exhibit unique toxicant dynamics. Limited rainfall concentrates toxicants such as heavy metals and pesticides in diminishing water resources, increasing the risk of chronic intoxication for wildlife and livestock dependent on these sources. Case studies from sub-Saharan Africa highlight frequent occurrences of heavy-metal poisoning in wildlife around evaporating watering holes contaminated by mining runoff, causing renal and hepatic toxicities.

Aquatic regions: Aquatic ecosystems, encompassing freshwater and marine habitats, are particularly sensitive to toxicant pollution due to the constant and direct exposure of aquatic organisms. Coastal areas in Southeast Asia have significant problems with pesticide and industrial pollutant runoff, impacting fish and marine mammals. Persistent organic pollutants (POPs) such as polychlorinated biphenyls (PCBs) and heavy metals like mercury bioaccumulate in marine food webs, as seen in dolphins and predatory fish species, posing significant ecological and public health concerns.

Veterinary and ecological implications: Regional differences profoundly influence veterinary and ecological health outcomes. In Africa, wildlife veterinarians frequently encounter cases of lead poisoning in scavenging species, linked to contaminated hunting grounds. In temperate Europe, domestic animals frequently present veterinary challenges associated with antifreeze (ethylene glycol) poisoning during colder months. In North America, cases of chronic pesticide exposure in migratory birds correlate strongly with agricultural land-use patterns, highlighting the need for tailored wildlife-management strategies.

Regulatory frameworks and management practices: Regulatory frameworks and management practices vary significantly across regions, affecting toxicant exposure and bioaccumulation patterns. Developed regions such as Europe and North America generally enforce stringent regulations on pesticide usage, industrial discharge, and heavy-metal emissions, significantly reducing environmental contamination risks. Conversely, developing regions in Africa and Asia often struggle with enforcement due to limited resources and infrastructure, resulting in higher environmental and wildlife exposure to toxicants. Examples include differences in pesticide regulatory frameworks between the EU's stringent registration system versus less regulated markets in many Southeast Asian countries.

Management practices also differ substantially, with integrated pest management (IPM) approaches widely adopted in temperate regions but less prevalent in tropical and developing regions, where pesticide reliance remains high. Effective management and regulatory frameworks significantly reduce environmental and wildlife exposure risks, emphasizing the importance of region-specific strategies for mitigating toxicological impacts (Figures 3.9 and 3.10).

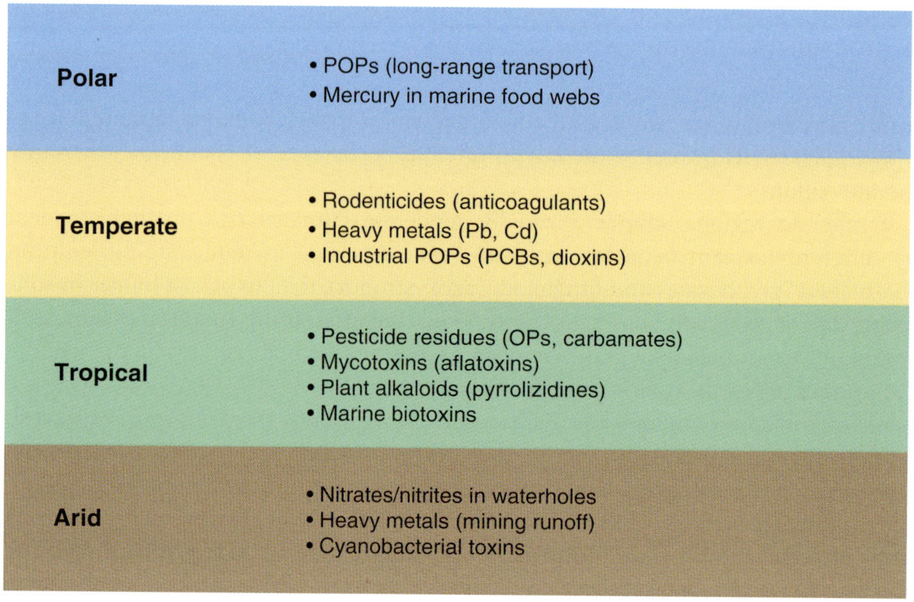

Figure 3.9 Simplified schematic showing the distribution of common toxicants across major climatic regions. Polar regions are characterized by persistent organic pollutants (POPs) transported over long distances and mercury bioaccumulation in marine food webs. Temperate regions often report rodenticide exposure, heavy metals such as lead (Pb) and cadmium (Cd), and industrial persistent organic pollutants (POPs) including polychlorinated biphenyls (PCBs) and dioxins. Tropical regions are associated with pesticide residues (e.g., organophosphates, carbamates), mycotoxins such as aflatoxins, plant-derived alkaloids (e.g., pyrrolizidines), and marine biotoxins. Arid regions frequently encounter nitrate/nitrite contamination in waterholes, heavy metals from mining activities, and cyanobacterial toxins.

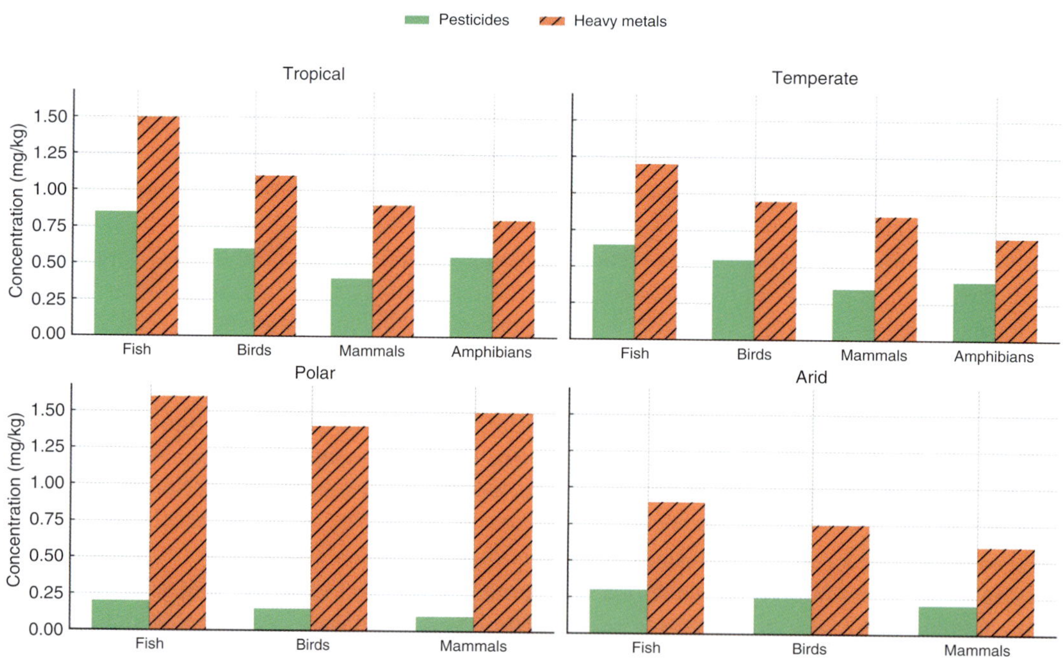

Figure 3.10 Species are shown only where they naturally occur in each climate zone. Polar regions include marine mammals (e.g., seals, polar bears) and seabirds, with no amphibians. Arid regions typically lack amphibians. Values are plausible estimates from literature trends, with higher pesticide residues in tropical and temperate agricultural systems, and higher heavy metal concentrations in polar marine food webs due to bioaccumulation.

References

Ali, H., Khan, E., & Ilahi, I. (2019). Environmental chemistry and ecotoxicology of hazardous heavy metals: Environmental persistence, toxicity, and bioaccumulation. *Journal of Chemistry*, *2019*, 6730305. https://doi.org/10.1155/2019/6730305

Barrett, K. E., Barman, S. M., Brooks, H. L., & Yuan, J. X. J. (2019). *Ganong's review of medical physiology* (26th ed.). McGraw-Hill Education.

Gibaldi, M., & Perrier, D. (2007). *Pharmacokinetics* (2nd ed.). Informa Healthcare.

Hayes, T. B., Collins, A., Lee, M., Mendoza, M., Noriega, N., Stuart, A. A., & Vonk, A. (2002). Hermaphroditic, demasculinized frogs after exposure to the herbicide atrazine at low ecologically relevant doses. *Proceedings of the National Academy of Sciences*, *99*(8), 5476–5480. https://doi.org/10.1073/pnas.082121499

Hodgson, E. (2010). *A textbook of modern toxicology* (4th ed.). Wiley-Blackwell.

Islam, M. A., Amin, S. M. N., Aziz, D., Ismail, M. F. S., Brown, C. L., Juraimi, A. S., Halim, M. A., Uddin, M. K., Mahmud, Y., Rahi, M. L., & Arshad, A. (2025). Multicompartmental monitoring and associated health risks estimation of some selected pesticides in the aquatic ecosystems of Sungai Besar, Sekinchan, Malaysia. *Environmental Science and Pollution Research*, *32*(35), 21198–21216. https://doi.org/10.1007/s11356-025-36913-3

Klaassen, C. D. (Ed.). (2013a). *Casarett & Doull's toxicology: The basic science of poisons* (8th ed.). McGraw-Hill Education.

Klaassen, C. D. (2013b). *Casarett and Doull's essentials of toxicology* (3rd ed.). McGraw-Hill Education.

Levine, R. R. (1973). *Pharmacology: Drug actions and reactions* (3rd ed.). Little, Brown and Company.

Nakayama, S. M. M., Morita, A., Ikenaka, Y., Mizukawa, H., & Ishizuka, M. (2019). A review: poisoning by anticoagulant rodenticides in non-target animals globally. *Journal of Veterinary Medical Science*, *81*(2), 298–313. https://doi.org/10.1292/jvms.17-0717

O'Brien, J., & Cousins, R. J. (2015). Comparative toxicokinetics: An overview. In E. Hodgson (Ed.), *A textbook of modern toxicology* (4th ed., pp. 127–144). Wiley-Blackwell.

Parkinson, A., & Ogilvie, B. W. (2008). Biotransformation of xenobiotics. In C. D. Klaassen (Ed.), *Casarett and Doull's toxicology: The basic science of poisons* (7th ed., pp. 161–304). McGraw-Hill.

Rahman, F., Ismail, A., Omar, H., & Hussin, M. Z. (2017). Exposure of the endangered Milky stork population to cadmium and lead via food and water intake in Kuala Gula Bird Sanctuary, Perak, Malaysia. *Toxicology Reports*, *4*, 502–506. https://doi.org/10.1016/j.toxrep.2017.09.003

Rang, H. P., Ritter, J. M., Flower, R. J., & Henderson, G. (2019). *Rang & Dale's pharmacology* (9th ed.). Elsevier.

Walker, C. H., Sibly, R. M., Hopkin, S. P., & Peakall, D. B. (2012). *Principles of ecotoxicology* (4th ed.). CRC Press.

Wiedner, E. B., Takeuchi, N. Y., Isaza, R., & Barber, D. (2011). Baseline levels of trace metals in blood of captive Asian elephants (Elephas maximus). *Journal of Zoo and Wildlife Medicine*, *42*(2), 360–362. https://doi.org/10.1638/2011-0010.1

4

Biotransformation and Fate of Toxicants

Biotransformation (metabolism) and the subsequent fate of toxicants in the body are central to understanding toxicology in veterinary species. Toxicokinetic processes dictate how a toxic substance is absorbed, distributed to tissues, metabolized into other compounds, and ultimately excreted (Schmid & Brutlag, 2024). Biotransformation generally serves to make lipophilic xenobiotics more water-soluble for elimination, often detoxifying them. However, in some cases metabolism can produce more reactive or toxic metabolites (a phenomenon historically termed "lethal synthesis") (Schmid & Brutlag, 2024). For example, ethylene glycol itself has little direct toxicity, but hepatic metabolism generates glycolic acid, glyoxylic acid, and oxalic acid – metabolites responsible for fatal metabolic acidosis and renal failure (Schmid & Brutlag, 2024). Understanding these pathways is critical for recognizing and treating poisonings. Equally important are the fate processes – how toxicants distribute in an animal's body (sometimes accumulating in specific tissues) and how they are excreted via kidneys, bile, or other routes (Schmid & Brutlag, 2024).

Veterinarians in tropical regions face unique toxicological challenges. Many plant and fungal toxins are more prevalent in warm, humid climates, and tropical livestock and wildlife often encounter endemic toxic plants, mycotoxins, and agrochemicals. Species common to tropical animal agriculture – ruminants (cattle, sheep, goats, buffalo), poultry (chickens, ducks), fish (both farmed and wild tropical fish), and companion animals (dogs, cats) – may exhibit distinct biotransformation capacities or vulnerabilities. This chapter focuses on the metabolic pathways of toxicants, highlighting common principles as well as species-specific and regional variations in tropical environments. We also emphasize how these processes inform the diagnosis of toxicoses (for instance, selecting the appropriate tissue for analysis based on distribution) and the treatment of poisoned animals (such as choosing therapies that alter metabolism or enhance elimination). By deepening our understanding of Phase I and Phase II metabolism, factors that affect these pathways, and how toxicants move through and out of the body, veterinarians can improve diagnostic accuracy and tailor interventions for toxic exposures. Throughout, special attention is given to tropical scenarios – from plant poisons degraded by rumen microbes to fish with temperature-dependent metabolism – ensuring relevance to practitioners and researchers in tropical veterinary medicine (Figure 4.1).

Metabolic Pathways: Commonalities and Regional Variations

Metabolism of toxicants is classically divided into two phases. Phase I (functionalization) reactions include oxidation, reduction, and hydrolysis processes that often introduce a polar functional group or reveal an active site on the molecules (Schmid & Brutlag, 2024). These reactions, chiefly catalyzed by hepatic enzymes (especially the cytochrome P450 [CYP450] monooxygenases), frequently produce a slightly more polar metabolite that can be conjugated in Phase II (Schmid & Brutlag, 2024). Phase I metabolism sometimes inactivates a compound but in other cases yields an activated toxic metabolite. Phase II (conjugation) reactions involve coupling the toxicant (or its Phase I metabolite) to an endogenous substrate such as glucuronic acid, sulfate, acetate, glycine, or glutathione (Schmid & Brutlag, 2024). Conjugation greatly increases water solubility and usually produces a less toxic, readily excretable product. In general, metabolism transforms lipophilic xenobiotics into hydrophilic forms that can be eliminated via urine or bile. However, these pathways seldom operate in isolation or completion – often a fraction of a xenobiotic is excreted unchanged while the rest undergoes multiple metabolic steps (Schmid & Brutlag, 2024). Notably, there are important species commonalities in these pathways – for instance, glucuronidation and sulfation are ubiquitous Phase II routes across mammals, birds, and other vertebrates (Kolanczyk et al., 2024). Yet there are also striking species differences and even regional (geographic or dietary) variations that affect metabolism, which are particularly relevant in tropical animal populations.

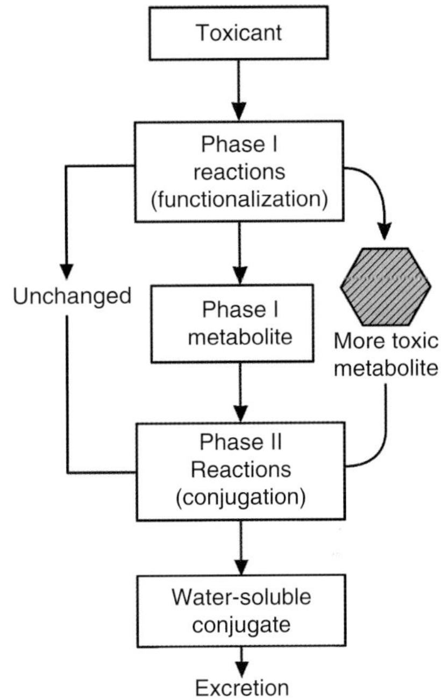

Figure 4.1 Overview of xenobiotic biotransformation. Schematic flowchart illustrating the two phases of biotransformation: Phase I reactions (functionalization) introduce or expose polar functional groups on the toxicant (often converting a lipophilic compound into a more reactive intermediate), and Phase II reactions (conjugation) attach endogenous polar molecules to Phase I metabolites, yielding water-soluble conjugates that can be readily excreted.

Phase I Biotransformation of Toxicants

Phase I reactions are predominantly oxidative and are catalyzed by enzyme systems such as CYP450 monooxygenases, flavin-containing monooxygenases (FMO), esterases, and reductases in the liver and other tissues. By adding or exposing functional groups (e.g., —OH, —NH_2, —COOH), Phase I often prepares a molecule for Phase II conjugation (Schmid & Brutlag, 2024). These reactions tend to be rapid and can significantly alter a toxicant's activity. In many cases, Phase I is detoxifying – for example, hydrolysis of an organophosphate insecticide by esterases can render it inactive. However, Phase I can also convert innocuous precursors into reactive toxins. This metabolic bioactivation underlies the toxicity of several important tropical poisons:

- Aflatoxin B_1: This mycotoxin, common in moldy tropical feeds like peanuts and corn, requires Phase I activation to exert its carcinogenic effects. In the liver, CYP enzymes (especially of the CYP3A family) metabolize aflatoxin B_1 to an exo-8,9-epoxide, a highly reactive intermediate that can bind to DNA and cause hepatocellular carcinoma (Diaz et al., 2010). Animals vary in susceptibility to aflatoxin due in part to differences in this bioactivation process. For instance, poultry and trout are extremely sensitive to aflatoxin-induced liver cancer, whereas some mammals have more efficient detoxification of the epoxide via conjugation. Ruminants have a partial defense: certain rumen microbes can biotransform aflatoxin B_1 into less toxic metabolites such as aflatoxicol and aflatoxin D_1 (Loh et al., 2020). These microbial Phase I reactions (likely reductions) in the rumen mean that cattle and goats can convert a portion of ingested aflatoxin to safer forms before absorption. Nonetheless, if exposure is high or rumen flora is unadapted, aflatoxin B_1 can overwhelm defenses, leading to liver damage, reduced productivity, and residues in milk. The hot, humid conditions of the tropics predispose feedstuffs to aflatoxin contamination, making this metabolic activation pathway especially pertinent to tropical veterinary practice.
- Organophosphate (OP) insecticides: Widely used in tropical agriculture and parasite control, many OP compounds (e.g., parathion) are relatively nontoxic as applied but are oxidatively desulfured by CYP450 in the liver to yield an "oxon" metabolite (e.g., paraoxon) that is a potent acetylcholinesterase inhibitor. This Phase I oxidation greatly increases toxicity. Species differences in the activity of hepatic paraoxonase/A-esterases (enzymes that can hydrolyze and inactivate oxon metabolites) partly explain differential OP susceptibility. For example, birds generally have low levels of paraoxonase and are quite sensitive to certain OPs, whereas some mammals can hydrolyze paraoxon faster. In tropical regions where OP use is common, understanding these metabolic steps is vital: A case of parathion poisoning in a cow might involve delayed onset of clinical signs as metabolism converts it to paraoxon; treatment may involve preventing bioactivation (e.g., using atropine early and supportive care while the liver processes the compound).
- Pyrrolizidine alkaloids (PAs): These hepatotoxic compounds, found in tropical and subtropical plants like *Crotalaria*, *Senecio*, and *Heliotropium*, are not directly toxic until metabolized. In the liver, CYP enzymes convert PAs into highly reactive pyrrolic metabolites (pyrrole derivatives) that alkylate proteins and DNA, leading to hepatocyte damage (megalocytosis) and hepatic fibrosis. Both monogastric and ruminant herbivores are affected by PA toxicosis (Loh et al., 2020). Notably, the common metabolic pathway (CYP-mediated dehydrogenation of the alkaloid to a pyrrole) exists across species – a shared vulnerability. However, ruminants often show more chronic poisoning, as their rumen microflora can partially detoxify PAs. Sheep and goats, for instance, are relatively resistant to acute PA toxicity, rarely showing sudden liver failure; instead, they develop chronic damage after prolonged intake (Loh et al., 2020). Rumen microbes in adapted animals can metabolize PAs to less toxic conjugates or breakdown products, especially after prior exposure allows microbial populations to adjust (Loh et al., 2020). Studies in Australia have isolated bacteria (e.g., *Peptostreptococcus heliotrinreducens*) that reduce PAs to nontoxic 1-methylene derivatives (Loh et al., 2020). These findings have even prompted research into probiotic inoculation – transferring PA-degrading microbes from resistant sheep to susceptible animals as a protective measure (Loh et al., 2020). Such regional

adaptations illustrate how Phase I metabolic capacity can vary based on local diets and microbial ecosystems. In tropical husbandry, where PA-containing weeds may contaminate forage, recognizing that cattle or horses new to an area lack the adapted rumen flora is important in preventing poisoning. The commonality is that Phase I liver CYPs activate PAs in all animals; the variation lies in the degree to which non-hepatic microbes can preempt or reverse this activation.

- Microbial Phase I metabolism in the gut: This can significantly influence toxicity. Ruminant livestock in the tropics often consume forages with natural toxins that monogastric animals cannot tolerate. For example, the tropical legume *Leucaena leucocephala* contains mimosine, a nonprotein amino acid toxin. In Australian cattle lacking prior exposure, mimosine is initially degraded by rumen microbes to 3,4-DHP (3,4-dihydroxypyridine), which is still toxic and causes ill-thrift, hair loss, and goiter. However, cattle in Hawaii and other regions where Leucaena has long been used have developed rumen bacterial consortia (including *Synergistes jonesii*) that perform further Phase I-like metabolism: they isomerize and hydroxylate 3,4-DHP to nontoxic 2,3-DHP and beyond, preventing poisoning (Loh et al., 2020). By inoculating Australian ruminants with rumen fluid from Hawaiian cattle (containing *S. jonesii*), researchers enabled them to safely eat *Leucaena* without developing mimosine toxicosis (Loh et al., 2020). This is a compelling case of regional variation in metabolic capability – the metabolic pathway (degradation of mimosine) is achievable by ruminants everywhere if the appropriate microbes are present, but it was only naturally found in certain locales. Tropical veterinarians should be aware that transferring "experienced" rumen fluid can confer metabolic tolerance to local plant toxicants, highlighting how Phase I biotransformations may extend beyond the host's own enzymes.

From these examples, we see that Phase I metabolism is broadly conserved (most animals have CYP-mediated oxidation systems) but also exhibits quantitative differences across species. Carnivores vs. herbivores: Many herbivores have evolved robust Phase I detoxication enzymes due to their plant toxin-rich diets, whereas felids (obligate carnivores) have a more limited complement of some detox enzymes. Birds and fish vs. mammals: Birds generally possess CYP enzymes similar to mammals, though with fewer isoforms in some cases; for instance, avian species rely heavily on CYP1A and CYP2-like enzymes for pesticide metabolism and can produce similar Phase I metabolites as mammals (Kolanczyk et al., 2024). Fish have functional Phase I systems, but their metabolic rate is influenced by water temperature (being poikilotherms) and oxygen availability. Many tropical fish species have comparable Phase I pathways to temperate fish, yet warm water can accelerate enzyme kinetics up to a point. Some fish are surprisingly slow at metabolizing certain chemicals; they may accumulate Phase I metabolites more slowly, contributing to higher sensitivity. For example, tropical tilapia exposed to an organophosphate pesticide had prolonged effects partly because their metabolic breakdown of the compound was slow, causing the toxicant to persist longer in tissues (Saha & Dutta, 2024). In one study, fish retained the pyrethroid insecticide bifenthrin much longer than mammals did due to comparatively lower biotransformation rates (Saha & Dutta, 2024). Thus, fish in aquaculture may suffer toxicity from doses of insecticides that a mammal of similar weight could clear more rapidly. Recognizing such differences is crucial in tropical aquaculture settings when using chemicals for parasite control – fish may require lower doses or longer withdrawal times because their Phase I metabolism and elimination are less efficient.

In summary, Phase I pathways are common across vertebrates in principle, but species-specific enzyme expression and activity can lead to major differences in toxicant susceptibility. Cats famously lack certain Phase I and II capacities (making them vulnerable to drugs like acetaminophen), whereas ruminants, thanks to both hepatic enzymes and symbiotic flora, often withstand plant toxins that would harm monogastrics (Loh et al., 2020; Thompson, 2024). Tropical conditions can further modulate Phase I metabolism: High ambient temperatures can increase metabolic enzyme activity to a degree (as seen in warm-water fish), whereas dietary factors (e.g., consumption of plant secondary compounds) can induce certain CYPs over time; conversely, nutrient deficiencies (common with low-protein diets) might reduce metabolic efficiency. Moreover, genetic polymorphisms in metabolic enzymes may cluster in certain regions or breeds – for example, some cattle breeds in the tropics might exhibit slower drug metabolism due to genetic variants, although this is an area of ongoing research.

Phase II Biotransformation of Toxicants

Phase II conjugation reactions act on functional groups (either those present on the parent toxicant or introduced by Phase I) to form water-soluble xenobiotic conjugates. Major Phase II pathways include glucuronidation (conjugation with glucuronic acid via uridine diphosphate [UDP]-glucuronosyltransferases [UGTs]), sulfation (addition of sulfate via sulfotransferases), acetylation (via N-acetyltransferases), amino acid conjugation (e.g., glycine conjugation of benzoates), glutathione conjugation (via glutathione-S-transferases, yielding mercapturic acids), and methylation (less common for xenobiotics, often for endogenous toxins). Phase II generally renders the molecule much more polar and usually biologically inactive. There are, however, exceptions where a conjugate can be toxic (for instance, acyl-glucuronides of NSAIDs can be reactive and trigger immune-mediated hepatotoxicity in some animals, and sulfate conjugates of certain aromatic amines can decompose to reactive intermediates in the bladder). By and large, however, conjugation is a detoxification step.

Commonalities: Glucuronidation and sulfation are among the most universal conjugation mechanisms in vertebrates. Most mammals, birds, and reptiles can form glucuronides of phenols, alcohols, and carboxylic acids, and sulfate esters of phenols and aliphatic alcohols. Glutathione conjugation of electrophilic intermediates (like epoxides or quinones) is another crucial protective mechanism shared broadly – for example, the reactive metabolite N-acetyl-p-benzoquinone imine (NAPQI) from acetaminophen is neutralized by glutathione in many species. The importance of Phase II is evident in the example of acetaminophen (paracetamol): normally, this drug (and toxicant at high doses) is mainly eliminated by glucuronide and sulfate conjugation to nontoxic metabolites (Center, 2024). Only a small fraction is metabolized via Phase I to NAPQI, which is then detoxified by glutathione conjugation.

Species differences in Phase II: A well-known veterinary example is the domestic cat (*Felis catus*). Cats have limited Phase II glucuronidation capacity because they lack certain UDP-UGT isoforms. As a result, cats form glucuronide conjugates poorly for substances like phenolic drugs. For instance, cats are deficient in glucuronidation of acetaminophen, morphine, and many nonsteroidal anti-inflammatory drugs (NSAIDs) (Loh et al., 2020). Instead, cats rely more on sulfation (which has a lower capacity) or produce alternate metabolites. Consequently, toxic para-aminophenol and NAPQI build up, causing methemoglobinemia and liver injury in cats given acetaminophen. This stark species variation explains why a dose of acetaminophen safe for a dog or human can be lethal to a cat. Another deficiency is in acetylation: dogs completely lack the cytosolic N-acetyltransferase 2 (NAT2) enzyme. Studies show dogs have no functional NAT enzymes (Center, 2024). Therefore, they cannot acetylate aromatic amines or hydrazines. A practical outcome is that dogs are unable to detoxify certain sulfonamide antibiotics via acetylation, making them prone to sulfonamide toxicosis (and causing sulfa drugs to persist longer, potentially leading to immune-mediated reactions) (Center, 2024). In fact, trimethoprim-sulfa has caused idiosyncratic hepatotoxicity in dogs partly because they cannot rapidly eliminate the hydroxylamine metabolites by acetylation (Center, 2024). Likewise, isoniazid (a hydrazide compound) is extremely dangerous in dogs – their inability to acetylate isoniazid means it must be cleared by alternate pathways that are easily overwhelmed (Oh, 2021). By contrast, most other mammals (and even cats, which have NAT1) can perform some acetylation.

Among herbivores, there are differences in conjugation preferences: for example, pigs have very high capacity for sulfation but relatively low capacity for glucuronidation of some xenobiotics, whereas ruminants often glucuronidate well but may form atypical conjugates (like glutamine conjugates for certain plant compounds) to handle dietary toxins. Avian species generally lack the enzyme UGT1A6, making them less efficient at glucuronidating planar phenols; instead, birds may rely more on sulfation. Chickens, for instance, more readily sulfate certain toxins (such as phenolic mycotoxins) rather than glucuronidate them. In one comparative study, bird species metabolized the model compound pyrene to similar Phase I hydroxypyrene as mammals, but then excreted mainly sulfate conjugates in urine (Saengtienchai et al., 2018). Fish possess functional glucuronosyltransferases and sulfotransferases as well (Kolanczyk et al., 2024). In fact, as in mammals, glucuronidation is a major Phase II route in fish (Kolanczyk et al., 2024). However, capacity varies by species and water temperature. Many fish have lower absolute conjugation rates at colder temperatures, but tropical fish living in warm waters may have higher baseline Phase II enzyme activity. A fascinating case of a Phase II difference conferring selective toxicity is the lampricide TFM (3-trifluoromethyl-4-nitrophenol) used in fisheries: It is significantly more toxic to sea lamprey than to other fish because lamprey have a reduced capacity to glucuronidate and eliminate TFM (Kolanczyk et al., 2024). Other fish can conjugate TFM into a glucuronide more efficiently, whereas lamprey accumulate the active compound, succumbing to its effects. This demonstrates how even within aquatic species, a deficit in a single Phase II pathway can be exploited for selective poisoning of a pest species (Kolanczyk et al., 2024).

In the tropics, Phase II pathways can be affected by diet and environmental factors. Many tropical forages are rich in plant secondary metabolites that may induce or compete for conjugation pathways. For instance, if a herbivore's diet contains high levels of tannins or phenolics, the liver might upregulate glucuronidation enzymes (or conversely, the conjugation capacity might become saturated). Nutritional status also plays a role: conjugation reactions require co-substrates (e.g., sulfate conjugation requires adequate sulfur/amino acids; glucuronide formation requires UDP-glucuronic acid, which depends on glucose metabolism). Malnutrition or mineral deficiencies common in some tropical regions (such as low dietary sulfur) could theoretically limit Phase II conjugation efficacy, making animals more susceptible to toxicosis. Young animals of all species have lower Phase II enzyme expression – for example, neonatal ruminants and foals cannot conjugate chloramphenicol effectively (leading to "gray baby syndrome"-like effects). Tropical husbandry often involves young stock exposed to various stressors and pathogens requiring medication, so understanding that neonates have immature conjugation systems is important (e.g., a young calf might be less able to glucuronidate certain pesticides compared to an adult).

Overall, Phase II metabolism is a critical detoxification stage with generally conserved mechanisms but species-specific strengths and weaknesses. Veterinary clinicians must be mindful of these differences: what is a harmless conjugate in one species could be impossible to form in another, leading to toxicity. A practical example: giving a feline patient a drug primarily cleared by glucuronidation (like aspirin or acetaminophen) is hazardous (Schmid & Brutlag, 2024), whereas the same dose in a goat

Table 4.1 Species differences in metabolic pathways among tropical species. Illustration comparing major Phase I and II detoxification capabilities: for example, cats have low UDP-UGT activity (poor glucuronidation) (Schmid & Brutlag, 2024), dogs lack N-acetyltransferase 2 and cannot acetylate certain xenobiotics (Center, 2024), ruminants benefit from rumen microbes that degrade toxins like mimosine and PAs (Loh et al., 2020), and fish metabolize some chemicals more slowly, leading to prolonged toxin persistence (Saha & Dutta, 2024). All species possess the core metabolic enzyme systems, but quantitative differences influence their susceptibility to toxicants.

Species/group	Notable metabolic traits
Cats	Limited glucuronidation capacity (lack certain UGT enzymes) – cannot effectively conjugate some drugs (e.g., acetaminophen).
Dogs	Lack N-acetyltransferase 2 – unable to acetylate specific drugs (e.g., sulfonamides, isoniazid).
Ruminants (cattle, sheep, goats)	Symbiotic rumen microbes degrade certain toxins (e.g., pyrrolizidine alkaloids, mimosine), aiding detoxification.
Birds (poultry)	Rely more on sulfation (missing some UGT isoforms); excrete uric acid (some drugs concentrate in kidneys, causing gout in extreme cases).
Fish (tropical species)	Slower metabolic rate at equivalent temperatures; high lipid stores lead to bioaccumulation of lipophilic toxins.

might be handled readily. Conversely, a drug producing a potentially toxic glucuronide (like certain NSAIDs) might cause more issues in a dog (which readily glucuronidates and accumulates the reactive conjugate in bile) than in a bird (which might sulfate it instead) (Table 4.1).

Factors Influencing Xenobiotic Metabolism

The efficiency and route of toxicant biotransformation can be influenced by a variety of intrinsic and extrinsic factors. Understanding these factors is essential as they help explain why even within a species some individuals succumb to a toxicant while others do not or why an animal might handle a toxin 1 day but not the next. Key factors include:

- Genetic and species/breed factors: As described above, genetics determine the presence or absence of certain enzymes (e.g., UGT isoforms in cats, NAT in dogs). Within a species, different breeds or populations might have polymorphisms affecting metabolism. For example, there are breed differences in certain drug-metabolizing enzymes in pigs and cattle (Helke et al., 2016), and wild species often have unique adaptations (e.g., insectivorous bats with high detox capacity for insect toxins). In tropical regions, indigenous breeds (such as *Bos indicus* cattle or village chickens) may have evolved metabolic traits to cope with local dietary toxins or climate stressors. Additionally, idiosyncratic genetic deficiencies occur: some individual animals may have unusually low levels of a detox enzyme (as seen in human pharmacogenetics and likely in animals too, though less documented).
- Age: Neonates and juveniles have immature metabolic enzyme systems. At birth, liver CYP450 content is low; Phase II conjugation pathways (glucuronidation especially) ramp up over the first weeks to months of life. This is why young animals are often more sensitive to certain toxicants – for instance, newborn ruminants are more susceptible to organophosphate insecticides or to chloramphenicol

toxicity due to limited metabolic clearance. Geriatric animals may also metabolize drugs and toxins more slowly due to decreased liver mass, blood flow, and enzyme activity (Boothe, 2016). An older animal might accumulate higher toxin levels or take longer to eliminate them, prolonging effects. In practical terms, a very young goat or an elderly cow in the tropics might be less tolerant of a given plant toxin exposure than a prime-age adult, necessitating extra care in dosing treatments or in preventing exposure.

- Sex: Gender can influence metabolism because of hormonal regulation of enzymes. In some species (notably rodents), males have higher expression of certain CYP enzymes than females due to androgen effects. In domestic species, sex differences are generally modest, but there are examples: for instance, male rats and possibly male livestock have greater capacity for metabolizing some compounds via CYP2E1 or CYP3A. In contrast, female hormones can upregulate or downregulate certain pathways. In veterinary contexts, sex is not usually a dramatic factor, but one might observe, say, intact male goats metabolize a toxin slightly faster than females or castrates due to hormonal influences. Additionally, pregnancy can alter metabolism: Late gestation may reduce biotransformation rate (due to decreased enzyme expression or organ displacement reducing hepatic blood flow), whereas lactation can increase Phase II conjugation of some xenobiotics as part of enhanced clearance (and some conjugates may be excreted in milk). Pregnancy also introduces the fetus as a sensitive subunit – some metabolites cross the placenta and can harm the fetus even if the dam is unaffected (e.g., certain PA metabolites causing fetal poisoning or birth defects) (Loh et al., 2020).
- Diet and nutritional status: Nutrition profoundly affects metabolism. High-protein diets can increase hepatic CYP content (since enzymes are proteins and ample amino acids are available), whereas protein-calorie malnutrition reduces metabolism. Animals on energy-poor diets may have lower UDP-glucuronic acid stores, impairing glucuronidation. Mineral and vitamin cofactors are crucial: for example, glutathione conjugation depends on selenium and sulfur-containing amino acids. If an animal is deficient in selenium or methionine, its glutathione stores might be low, compromising its ability to detoxify peroxides and electrophiles. In the tropics, periods of drought or poor pasture can lead to malnutrition that exacerbates toxicity of plants normally tolerated when nutrition is adequate. One example is copper poisoning in ruminants – normally copper is excreted via bile (which involves conjugation to glutathione), but on diets low in molybdenum or sulfur (common in some tropical forages), copper accumulates in the liver. The reduced molybdenum (a copper antagonist) means more free copper is absorbed, which eventually causes hepatic oxidative damage when released. Diet can also modulate the rumen environment – high-carbohydrate feed can lower rumen pH and potentially shift microbial populations, possibly reducing the biodegradation of toxins (for instance, a cow suddenly switched from roughage to grain might lose some ability to degrade nitrite or certain alkaloids). On the other hand, certain dietary supplements can induce metabolic enzymes: compounds with phenobarbital-like effects or natural inducers in feed (e.g., indoles in cruciferous vegetables) may ramp up CYP expression.
- Environmental factors: Ambient temperature, day length, and housing conditions can affect metabolism. Temperature is especially relevant for ectothermic species (like fish and reptiles). A tropical fish at 30°C will metabolize a toxin much faster than at 20°C, because enzyme kinetics increase with temperature. However, beyond thermal optima, stress can set in and metabolism may become less efficient. Circadian rhythms exist for certain liver enzymes – metabolism might be faster during the active phase of the animal's daily cycle. In farm animals, some evidence suggests higher metabolic

activity during daytime feeding versus nighttime. In tropical management systems, if animals experience heat stress (extremely high temperatures and humidity), blood is shunted away from the viscera (to the skin for cooling), potentially reducing hepatic clearance. Thus, severe heat stress could decrease toxin metabolism and excretion, worsening toxicosis.

- Disease states: The health of metabolic organs is critical. Liver disease (from any cause) can markedly impair both Phase I and II metabolism, making an animal much more sensitive to toxicants. For instance, a dog with subclinical liver fibrosis may not tolerate an insecticide exposure that a healthy dog handles, because it cannot metabolize and eliminate it efficiently. Renal disease can indirectly affect metabolism by causing retention of conjugated toxins (if the kidney doesn't excrete a conjugate, it might be hydrolyzed and the toxin re-enters circulation) and by causing uremia, which can inhibit enzymes. Endocrine disorders (like hypo- or hyperthyroidism) can alter metabolic rate and enzyme levels too. In tropical regions, parasitic diseases and chronic infections are common and can suppress metabolic enzyme expression (an effect known as "inflamed liver" downregulation of P450). For example, chronic trypanosomiasis or liver fluke infestation in cattle could reduce their drug-metabolizing ability, making them more prone to toxicity from routine dosages.
- Prior and concurrent chemical exposures (enzyme induction and inhibition): Xenobiotic metabolism is adaptive. Prior exposure to certain chemicals can induce metabolic enzymes, increasing the metabolism of subsequent exposures. This is often seen with drugs: e.g., phenobarbital induces CYP450 enzymes in the liver; a dog on phenobarbital for seizures may develop tolerance to certain toxicants because it clears them faster (or, conversely, may convert a protoxin to a toxin faster – induction can increase toxic metabolite formation of other compounds) (Center, 2024). In toxicology, induction can confer tolerance: animals preexposed to small doses of a toxic plant may survive a later larger dose as their metabolizing enzymes are upregulated. Notably, guinea pigs are relatively resistant to the rodenticide bromethalin not because of prior induction but because they inherently cannot metabolize bromethalin into its toxic N-desmethyl metabolite (Schmid & Brutlag, 2024). On the other hand, enzyme inhibition by a co-exposed chemical can dramatically increase toxicity. For instance, if an animal is given an antifungal like ketoconazole (a strong CYP inhibitor) and simultaneously exposed to a pesticide that needs metabolism for detoxification, the pesticide's toxicity will be enhanced. A real scenario: Dogs receiving ketoconazole and the sedative midazolam show prolonged sedation because ketoconazole blocks midazolam's metabolism. In a toxicology context, if a dog ingested a pyrethroid insecticide while on ketoconazole therapy, it might experience more severe neurologic signs due to reduced detoxification. Another example is chloramphenicol, an antibiotic that inhibits CYP2B enzymes – if a bird is exposed to an organophosphate at the same time, chloramphenicol might slow the bird's hydrolysis of the OP, worsening cholinergic toxicity. Thus, polypharmacy and environmental chemical mixtures (common in areas with high pesticide use) are important considerations. Induction and inhibition are mechanisms behind herb–drug and drug–drug interactions in animals. In tropical smallholder farms, one might encounter this when, for example, a farmer treats chickens with a synthetic pyrethroid for mites and also feeds them a herbal remedy; some herbal compounds (like piperine in black pepper) can inhibit metabolism and cause the insecticide to be more toxic than anticipated.

In sum, xenobiotic metabolism is not a static process – it is influenced by who the animal is (species, breed, genetics), what stage of life it's in (age, pregnancy), its lifestyle and environment (diet, climate, stress), its health status, and what other chemicals are on board. Tropical veterinarians must often contend with multiple factors at once: for instance, a malnourished, parasitized cow in the dry season (nutritional stress, liver stress) may drink from a pesticide-contaminated puddle. That cow's fate could be very different from that of a healthy, well-fed cow encountering the same pesticide. Knowledge of these factors guides more cautious management – e.g., avoiding certain drugs in the very young or very old, adjusting doses for animals in poor condition, ensuring adequate nutrition to support metabolism and staggering treatments to avoid harmful interactions.

Distribution and Tissue Retention of Toxicants

Once absorbed into the bloodstream, toxicants distribute throughout the body to varying degrees. Distribution refers to the reversible transfer of a substance from the circulation to tissues and organs. It is governed by factors such as blood flow to tissues, the chemical's affinity for tissue components, the permeability of tissue barriers, and the compound's physicochemical properties (lipid solubility, ionization, size). All animals share the same basic principles of distribution, but differences in physiology (ruminants vs. monogastrics, mammals vs. birds, etc.) can influence where a toxicant goes and how long it stays.

- Water-soluble vs. lipid-soluble distribution: Hydrophilic toxicants (e.g., ionized salts like nitrate) tend to stay in the aqueous compartments – blood plasma and interstitial fluid – and are often rapidly excreted by the kidneys (Schmid & Brutlag, 2024). They have a relatively small volume of distribution. Lipophilic toxicants (e.g., organochlorine pesticides, bromethalin rodenticide) readily penetrate cell membranes and accumulate in tissues like fat, nervous tissue, and liver (Schmid & Brutlag, 2024). Such compounds often have a large apparent volume of distribution (Vd) and can linger in the body for long periods (Schmid & Brutlag, 2024). For example, the pesticide dichlorodiphenyltrichloroethane (DDT) (now banned but historically important) is very lipophilic and was notorious for concentrating in adipose tissue of cattle and chickens. During periods of weight loss or lactation (fat mobilization), such stored toxicants can be released into the bloodstream, a phenomenon known as redistribution. Rapid weight loss in an animal can mobilize lipophilic toxins from fat, leading to renewed or increased toxicity as vital organs get dosed from the fat reserves (Jandacek et al., 2024; La Merrill et al., 2013). This means that an obese dog who ingested bromethalin might initially show only mild signs as the toxin is "stored" in fat, but if that dog then loses weight quickly, the toxin could redistribute and cause delayed CNS signs. Storage depots like adipose tissue can thus be a double-edged sword: initially sequestering a toxin and protecting target organs, but later releasing it and prolonging poisoning (Schmid & Brutlag, 2024).
- Plasma protein binding: Many toxicants reversibly bind to plasma proteins (albumin, globulins). Only the free (unbound) fraction can distribute into tissues or be filtered by the kidneys. If an animal has low plasma protein (common in malnutrition or liver disease in the tropics), more free toxicant is available, potentially increasing tissue uptake and toxicity. Conversely, competition for binding sites can occur: e.g., two drugs may displace each other from albumin, suddenly raising free concentrations.
- Special barriers: The blood–brain barrier (BBB) protects the central nervous system by limiting entry of many toxicants. It consists of tight capillary endothelial junctions and efflux transporters (like P-glycoprotein) that pump out foreign substances. Lipid-soluble, small molecules can still cross the BBB and cause neurotoxicity (e.g., many pesticides, toxic solvents). Notably, some breeds (like MDR1-mutant Collies) have defective P-glycoprotein, leading to increased brain distribution of ivermectin and other

drugs – an example of genetic variation in distribution. In general, distribution to the brain is more restricted than to other tissues, but once a toxin is in the CNS, damage can be severe. The placental barrier is another consideration: in livestock, many toxicants cross into the fetus, but some larger polar compounds do not. For instance, anticoagulant rodenticides cross the placenta and can cause fetal hemorrhage, whereas extremely large protein toxins might not. Tropical plant toxins such as methylazoxymethanol (from cycad seeds) have been shown to cross into cow fetuses, causing birth defects; similarly, nitrates cross and cause methemoglobinemia in fetuses (Thompson, 2024). Knowledge of placental transfer is important when treating pregnant animals (choosing antidotes that will also protect the fetus if needed).

- Tissue affinities: Certain toxicants have a predilection for specific tissues due to chemical affinity. Calcium-binding chemicals (like lead and fluoride) accumulate in bone and teeth. Lead deposits in bone (by substituting for calcium in hydroxyapatite); indeed, bone ends up containing the highest concentration of lead in a chronically exposed animal (Schmid & Brutlag, 2024). However, bone is not the site of lead's toxic action (which is mainly neural and hematopoietic), and bone lead is relatively inert (Schmid & Brutlag, 2024). This illustrates an important point: The tissue with the highest toxicant concentration is not necessarily the target organ of toxicity (Schmid & Brutlag, 2024). Lead can be sequestered in bone for years with minimal effect, but if mobilized (e.g., during osteoporosis or eggshell formation in birds), it can then cause acute poisoning. Another example: iodine accumulates in the thyroid gland (due to active uptake by iodide transporters), so radioactive iodine or iodine-based toxins concentrate there, causing thyroid dysfunction. Melanin affinity is observed with polycyclic aromatic hydrocarbons and some drugs – they bind to pigmented tissues like the eye and skin. In heavily pigmented tropical animals, melanin binding could act as a sink for certain toxins (some insecticides show higher toxicity in albino vs. pigmented mice because melanin binding reduces free toxin levels). Fat-soluble vitamins (e.g., Vitamin D_3 when in excess) can deposit in adipose and muscle. Organs like the liver and kidney often accumulate toxins because they are highly perfused and rich in binding proteins; these organs are common sites of toxin damage, especially for metals (copper, iron) and compounds with metallothionein affinity (e.g., cadmium accumulates in kidney cortex).
- Volume of distribution (Vd): This pharmacokinetic concept quantifies how extensively a toxicant disperses into tissues. If a toxicant has a small Vd (on the order of plasma volume), it is mostly confined to blood (e.g., a very polar large molecule or a highly protein-bound compound). If Vd is enormous (much larger than total body water), it suggests extensive tissue binding/sequestration. Digoxin, for example, has a huge Vd because it binds widely to muscle Na^+/K^+ ATPase – in digoxin poisoning, blood levels might be low while tissue levels are high. In toxicology, we exploit distribution characteristics in treatment: for a toxin with low Vd largely confined to blood, interventions like plasma exchange or hemodialysis may be effective. For toxins with a high Vd in fat or tissue, those methods won't work well; instead, we need antidotes that reach those tissues or strategies to carefully mobilize the toxin.

Species differences in distribution: most anatomical and physiological features affecting distribution are similar across mammals, but there are notable differences:

- Ruminants vs. monogastrics: Ruminants have a large forestomach where ingested toxicants can pool or be released slowly. Fat-soluble toxicants can dissolve in rumen contents or bind to feed particles, altering absorption kinetics and initial distribution. Also, a ruminant's compartmentalized stomach leads to some peculiarities in distribution (e.g., lead objects can sit in the reticulum causing chronic absorption; soluble oxalates might bind rumen calcium and precipitate, reducing systemic distribution compared to a horse where oxalate is swiftly absorbed). Additionally, ruminants generally have a higher volume of distribution for water-soluble compounds (per kg body weight) due to a larger gut fluid volume and a higher fraction of body weight as extracellular water.

- Birds: Birds have a higher cardiac output and different blood flow patterns (e.g., a renal portal system), which might influence distribution. They also have higher baseline body temperatures (~41°C in chickens), which can increase tissue perfusion. Birds' bones are hollow (pneumatized) and connected to air sacs – not directly relevant to distribution of most chemicals, but interestingly, inhaled toxins can get into bones via the air sacs. Birds excrete uric acid via kidneys that have some differences in blood flow (their dual renal portal system can cause certain substances to concentrate in the kidney). Certain toxins (like aminoglycoside antibiotics) in birds concentrate heavily in renal tissue due to this system (a distribution + excretion quirk).
- Fish: Fish have the added dimension of gill distribution. Waterborne toxicants can enter and leave the body through the gills. Gills are highly perfused; a toxin may distribute into gill tissue and be directly excreted back to the water. Additionally, fish often have a higher lipid content in the body (especially in the liver for some species or in muscle for oily fish), so lipophilic contaminants (PCBs, organochlorines, etc.) massively concentrate in these tissues. This is why bioaccumulation is a major issue in aquatic food chains – fish can have toxin levels orders of magnitude above the water concentration due to distribution into fat. Tropical fish in warm waters often reach distribution equilibrium faster but also face repeated exposure due to contaminated water; hence, they accumulate toxins like mercury or pesticides in muscle and organs, which is a food safety concern (Ray & Shaju, 2023).
- Invertebrates: Although beyond our main scope, distribution differences exist in invertebrates as well (e.g., in bees or other insects, toxins might remain in hemolymph or concentrate in the fat body differently than in vertebrates).

From a diagnostic perspective, understanding distribution is critical. It guides which tissue or fluid to sample when a toxicosis is suspected. For example, if nitrate/nitrite poisoning is suspected in a ruminant, one of the best postmortem samples is ocular fluid for nitrate analysis (Thompson, 2024), because nitrite distributes rapidly into the aqueous humor and remains relatively stable there after death. If lead poisoning is suspected, analyzing kidney cortex or liver is more informative than bone in acute cases, even though bone has the highest lead burden – bone lead reflects chronic exposure and is not bioavailable (Schmid & Brutlag, 2024). For anticoagulant rodenticide poisoning, liver is the tissue of choice to assay, as these compounds concentrate in the liver. In a neurotoxic syndrome, sampling brain or cerebrospinal fluid may be necessary for substances that primarily distribute to the CNS (e.g., the desmethylbromethalin metabolite of bromethalin). Knowing the depot sites also helps in treatment decisions. For instance, if a toxin is known to accumulate in fat and the animal is obese, aggressive measures like liposome-based binding agents or even surgical removal of fat (in extreme cases) could be contemplated; more realistically, one would avoid causing sudden weight loss in that animal and instead administer repeated doses of activated charcoal over time to catch toxin re-released into the gut via bile (a strategy used for lipophilic, recirculating toxicants). In heavy metal poisoning, chelation therapy works by redistributing metal from tissues to blood for excretion – chelators must reach the storage sites (e.g., calcium disodium ethylenediaminetetraacetate [Ca-EDTA] can mobilize lead from bone matrix, albeit slowly).

Toxicant distribution also has food safety implications in food-producing animals. Certain tissues must be tested or have extended withdrawal times after toxin exposure. For example, persistent organic

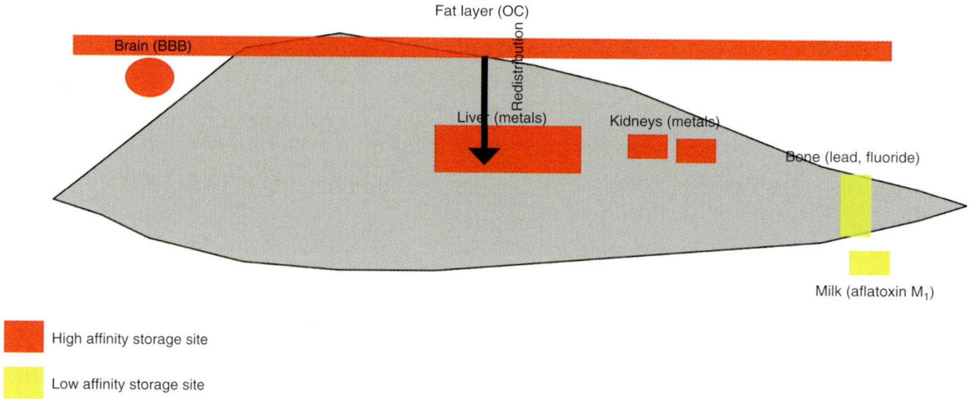

Figure 4.2 Deposition and tissue retention of toxicants in an animal. Illustration of how certain chemicals concentrate in specific tissues: e.g., lipophilic compounds accumulate in adipose tissue and can be released during fat mobilization; heavy metals such as lead deposit in bone; various toxins may concentrate in the liver and kidney. Such distribution patterns can prolong the presence of a toxicant in the body and inform treatment strategies (by targeting the organs that serve as toxin reservoirs).

pollutants often accumulate in adipose tissue – so even if an animal's blood is cleared, its fat (and milk) can contain residues. An animal might recover clinically from a toxin, but its liver or kidneys might retain residues that pose a risk if those organs enter the food chain. As the Merck Veterinary Manual notes, "violative residues of toxic agents can occur in food-producing animals; knowledge of this possibility is important when determining the outcome of an animal product intended to enter the food chain" (Schmid & Brutlag, 2024). This means veterinarians may have to recommend euthanasia or extended withdrawal periods for animals with certain distributions of toxicants (for instance, heavy metals sequestered in the kidneys, which could condemn a carcass).

In summary, distribution determines where a toxicant goes in the body and for how long. Common patterns exist (lipophilic compounds into fat, polar compounds in extracellular water, etc.), but the nuances of each species' anatomy and physiology, as well as chemical-specific affinities, create a mosaic of possible outcomes. Recognizing these patterns enables more accurate prognoses (e.g., if a toxin deposits in bone, the animal might survive the acute phase but could suffer chronic effects or relapses) and more targeted interventions (like focusing treatment on protecting or decontaminating a specific organ known to accumulate the toxin) (Figure 4.2).

Excretion and Elimination Pathways

Excretion is the removal of the toxicant (and its metabolites) from the body. The primary excretory routes are renal (urine) and hepatobiliary (feces via bile), with minor routes including exhalation (for volatile compounds), sweat, saliva, tears, and milk. In veterinary species – especially those in tropical production systems – excretion is critical not only for terminating the toxicant's action in the animal but also because excreted residues can affect human food safety (e.g., drug residues in milk) or cause environmental contamination (e.g., pesticide in manure affecting fish downstream).

Renal excretion: The kidneys are the main route for most water-soluble toxins and metabolites. Renal elimination involves three processes:

- Glomerular filtration: Passive filtration of small, unbound molecules from blood into the urine filtrate.
- Tubular reabsorption: Passive or active reuptake of substances from the filtrate back into blood (toxins that are lipophilic or that resemble nutrients might be reabsorbed).
- Tubular secretion: Active transport of certain molecules from blood into the urine (notably organic acids and bases via transporters in the proximal tubules).

Many veterinary toxicants (e.g., aminoglycoside antibiotics, many mycotoxin metabolites, ethylene glycol metabolites) are excreted largely unchanged or as metabolites in urine. Urine pH can influence excretion: Herbivores have more alkaline urine (favoring excretion of weak acids, which stay ionized and trapped in urine), while carnivores have acidic urine (favoring excretion of weak bases). This principle is exploited in treatment: For acidic toxicants like aspirin or phenobarbital, one can alkalinize the urine to enhance excretion; for basic toxins like amphetamines, carefully acidifying the urine can increase elimination. In tropical climates, where dehydration is common, reduced glomerular filtration can slow excretion and increase toxin retention. Ensuring adequate hydration and diuresis is a mainstay of treating many toxicoses (for example, giving IV fluids to a dehydrated animal that ate nephrotoxic plants in order to flush out toxins).

Renal excretion is also intimately linked to renal toxicity. The kidney, in concentrating and excreting toxins, often bears the brunt of their toxic effects. As the Merck Manual notes, "damage to the kidney from excretion of xenobiotics is specific to the anatomical location where excretion occurs … The proximal convoluted tubule is the most common site of toxic injury" (Schmid & Brutlag, 2024). For example, oxalate crystals from ethylene glycol metabolism precipitate in renal tubules, causing mechanical damage; aminoglycosides accumulate in proximal tubular cells via pinocytosis, causing necrosis; and melamine-cyanuric acid complexes crystallize in distal tubules. Each example corresponds to where those compounds concentrate during excretion. Veterinarians should monitor kidney function in any poisoning case, and certain therapies aim to protect the kidney (e.g., IV fluids to promote flushing, sodium thiosulfate to detoxify oxalate in situ, or bicarbonate to prevent hemoglobin precipitation in renal tubules during hemolysis). Extra-renal routes in some species: Birds excrete uric acid in a semisolid urate; their kidneys actively secrete urates and other compounds. They also have cloacal excretion where some reflux of urine into the colon can allow further water reabsorption (complicating things like drug elimination and residues in eggs).

Hepatobiliary excretion: The liver is unique in that it both metabolizes and excretes substances. Many conjugated toxicant metabolites (glucuronides, glutathione conjugates, etc.) are excreted in bile. Hepatocytes secrete these conjugates into bile canaliculi, which deliver them to the intestine via the gallbladder. Once in the gut, conjugates can be eliminated in feces. However, a critical phenomenon is enterohepatic circulation (EHC). Some conjugated toxins can be deconjugated by gut bacteria (e.g., bacterial β-glucuronidase can cleave glucuronide conjugates), releasing the original toxin or its Phase I metabolite, which can then be reabsorbed across the intestinal wall back into the bloodstream (Schmid & Brutlag, 2024). This creates a recycling loop. An "enterohepatic cycle" occurs when compounds are excreted from the liver via bile, reabsorbed from the intestine, and returned to the liver (Schmid & Brutlag, 2024). EHC effectively extends the half-life of a toxicant in the body and can lead to secondary peaks of toxicity after the initial exposure. Many plant and drug toxins undergo EHC: for example, phosphorus-based pesticides or indoxacarb (a flea-control agent) in dogs undergo EHC that can prolong neurotoxic effects; digitalis glycosides from oleander or yellow oleander undergo EHC, making their cardiotoxicity persist; and notably, cyanobacterial toxins like microcystin are excreted in bile but can be reabsorbed, causing prolonged liver damage. A classic example in large animals is organophosphate or carbamate insecticides in ruminants – they may be metabolized and excreted in bile but then reabsorbed, which is why multiple doses of activated charcoal are often needed to interrupt cycling.

Implications of biliary excretion and EHC for treatment:

- We often administer activated charcoal in repeated doses to bind toxins in the gut as they are excreted in bile, preventing reabsorption (multiple-dose activated charcoal therapy).
- Cholestyramine, an anion exchange resin, can bind certain compounds (like NSAIDs, blue-green algae hepatotoxins, or amatoxins from poisonous mushrooms) in the gut and halt enterohepatic recirculation. For instance, in dogs with severe ibuprofen or naproxen toxicosis (both undergo EHC), cholestyramine has been shown to hasten elimination by trapping the drug in the gut (Center, 2024). Similarly, in a reported ketoconazole overdose, cholestyramine was recommended to help remove the drug undergoing EHC (Center, 2024).
- Knowing a toxin undergoes EHC informs the monitoring period – animals may have a biphasic illness, seeming to improve then worsening as the toxin recycles. We maintain treatment (e.g., cholinesterase reactivators in OP poisoning, IV fluids, etc.) longer in such cases to cover those secondary peaks.

Minor routes:

- Pulmonary excretion: Gases and volatile substances are excreted via the lungs. This includes anesthetic gases (important in inhalant toxicosis) as well as toxic volatile metabolites like acetone (in isopropanol poisoning) or carbon dioxide (from metabolic acidosis). In ruminants, eructation can also expel volatile toxins (like fermentative ethanol or methane, though those are not typically considered "toxicants"). During heatstroke or heavy exercise, panting can eliminate more volatile compounds; for instance, if an animal ingests a large amount of formaldehyde or cyanide, some could be exhaled.
- Sweat and saliva: These are minor excretory pathways in most animals (who sweat less than humans). Horses do sweat appreciably; heavy metals like arsenic or iodine can be excreted to a degree in sweat (iodine toxicity can be detected by the odor of iodine on a horse's sweat). Salivary excretion of toxins can lead to oral lesions – for example, mercury can be excreted in saliva, causing stomatitis.
- Milk: Lactating animals can excrete many xenobiotics into milk – a route of concern for nursing offspring and for people consuming the milk. Milk is rich in fats and proteins; thus fat-soluble toxins (e.g., organochlorines, brominated flame retardants) readily partition into milk fat, and certain heavy metals or alkaloids may chelate with milk proteins. For example, aflatoxin B_1 ingested by cows is metabolized to aflatoxin M_1, which is excreted in milk – a significant public health issue in tropical countries where feed aflatoxin contamination is high (Loh et al., 2020). The presence of toxins in milk means that when treating a lactating animal for poisoning, one must consider discarding the milk for a suitable withdrawal period. It also means neonates can be secondarily intoxicated (e.g., a mare on toxic pasture could excrete plant alkaloids in milk that poison the foal).
- Eggs: In laying poultry, some toxins are deposited in eggs. For instance, certain organochlorine pesticides and heavy metals can appear in the yolk. This is relevant for food safety and also indicates how the hen's body may shunt some toxins into eggs as a route of elimination.

- Tears and hair: Traces of toxins (or their metal complexes) can be found in hair and feathers, which is sometimes exploited in forensic analysis for chronic exposures (e.g., arsenic in hair). Tears can carry irritant toxins; for example, animals with iodine toxicity may have excessive tearing with iodine detectable in the tear fluid.

The rate of elimination is often described by the half-life ($t½$) – the time required for half of the toxin to be eliminated from the body. Toxicants can exhibit first-order kinetics (a constant fraction eliminated per time) or saturable zero-order kinetics (a constant amount eliminated per time, typical when elimination pathways are saturated) (Schmid & Brutlag, 2024). If a toxin's metabolism or excretion pathway saturates (e.g., acetaminophen in cats – once glucuronidation/sulfation is maxed out, the remainder goes via the toxic pathway), elimination becomes zero-order and poisoning risk increases disproportionately with dose. In many cases, an initial rapid distribution phase is followed by a slower elimination phase (a two-compartment model) (Schmid & Brutlag, 2024). Clinically, this means blood toxin levels drop fast as the compound moves into tissues then persist longer as tissues gradually release the toxin back into blood for final elimination.

Species and individual differences in excretion: Most interspecies differences are quantitative rather than qualitative. Herbivores with alkaline urine may retain weakly basic toxins longer (since bases are more readily reabsorbed in alkaline urine), whereas carnivores with acidic urine retain weak acids longer. Birds excrete uric acid – if a toxin coprecipitates with uric acid, it might cause kidney gout (e.g., melamine in chicken feed led to visceral gout due to urate crystal formation). Some fish excrete ammonia through gills – interestingly, this can carry out small amine-containing toxins as well. For example, waterborne amines or ammonia-based toxins can be partially excreted by fish gills, a route mammals lack. Aquatic animals also have the advantage of constant water flow to help diffuse water-soluble toxins out through gills or skin. However, if the surrounding water is polluted with the toxin, that advantage is lost because there is no concentration gradient for elimination (a fish in contaminated water can't excrete a pollutant if the water is equally polluted). This underscores the importance of clean water in aquaculture – not only to prevent toxin uptake but to allow normal excretion of internal waste.

Finally, excretion can be exploited therapeutically: forced diuresis (IV fluids ± diuretics) enhances renal elimination (with care taken to avoid volume overload or pulmonary edema); peritoneal dialysis or hemodialysis can remove water-soluble, low-Vd toxins (commonly used for ethylene glycol or alcohol poisoning in small animals, and for certain plant toxicoses like lily poisoning in cats); urinary pH manipulation (ion trapping) as discussed above can speed excretion of ionizable toxins; and binding agents or cathartics can enhance fecal elimination (e.g., mineral oil can speed the passage of fat-soluble toxins through the gut to reduce absorption, and cholestyramine binds bile acids and certain toxins for removal in feces). In ruminants, one can perform a rumenotomy or rumen lavage to physically remove or dilute unabsorbed toxins from the forestomach – an "excretion" of sorts before the toxin is absorbed. In birds, crop lavage can similarly remove ingested toxins before they pass into the intestines (Figures 4.3 and 4.4).

Implications for Diagnosis and Treatment

Understanding the metabolic fate of toxicants is fundamental in veterinary toxicology because it underpins the entire process of diagnosing and managing toxicosis. While the specific diagnostic protocols and therapeutic interventions are discussed in detail in Chapter 6: "Toxicological Diagnosis" and

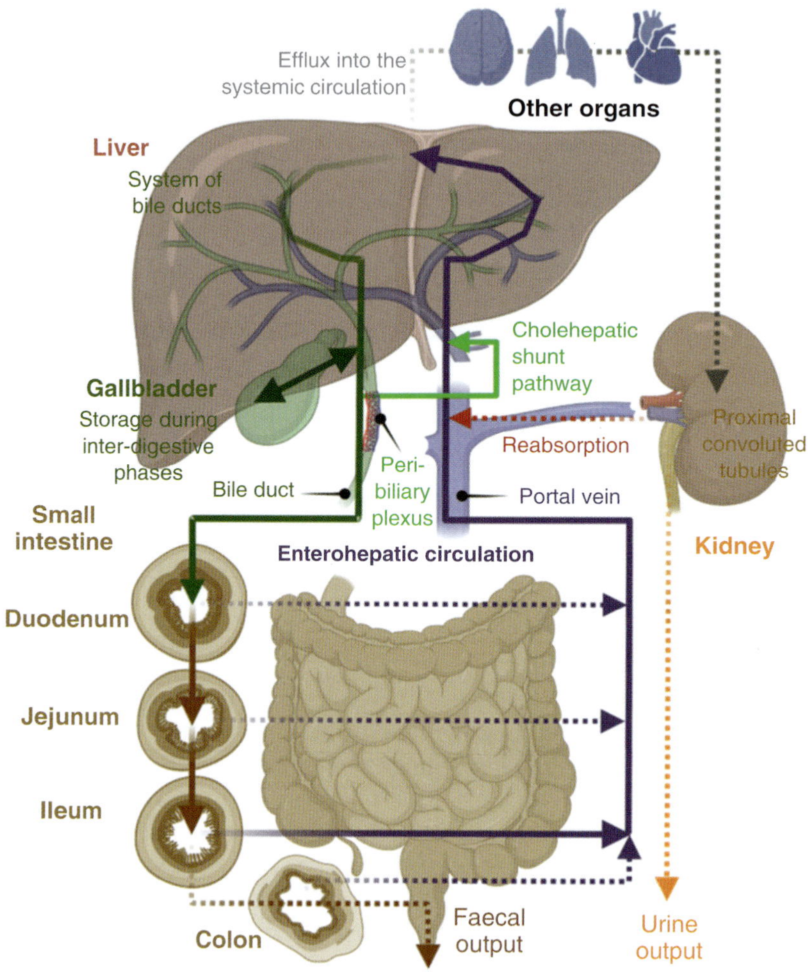

Figure 4.3 Diagram illustrating the enterohepatic circulation and related pathways, showing bile secretion from the liver and gallbladder into the small intestine, reabsorption into the portal vein, cholehepatic shunt, systemic distribution to other organs, and excretion via urine or feces (Durník et al., 2022).

Chapter 10: "Therapeutic Agents and Toxicity," the principles outlined here explain *why* such measures are chosen.

Knowledge of metabolic pathways – whether a toxicant undergoes rapid detoxification or is bioactivated into a more harmful metabolite – helps the clinician predict the course of intoxication, select the most relevant confirmatory tests, and anticipate potential complications. For example, recognizing that acetaminophen is poorly glucuronidated in cats alerts the veterinarian to the likelihood of a rapid onset of hepatic injury, guiding the choice of biochemical markers to monitor (see Chapter 6).

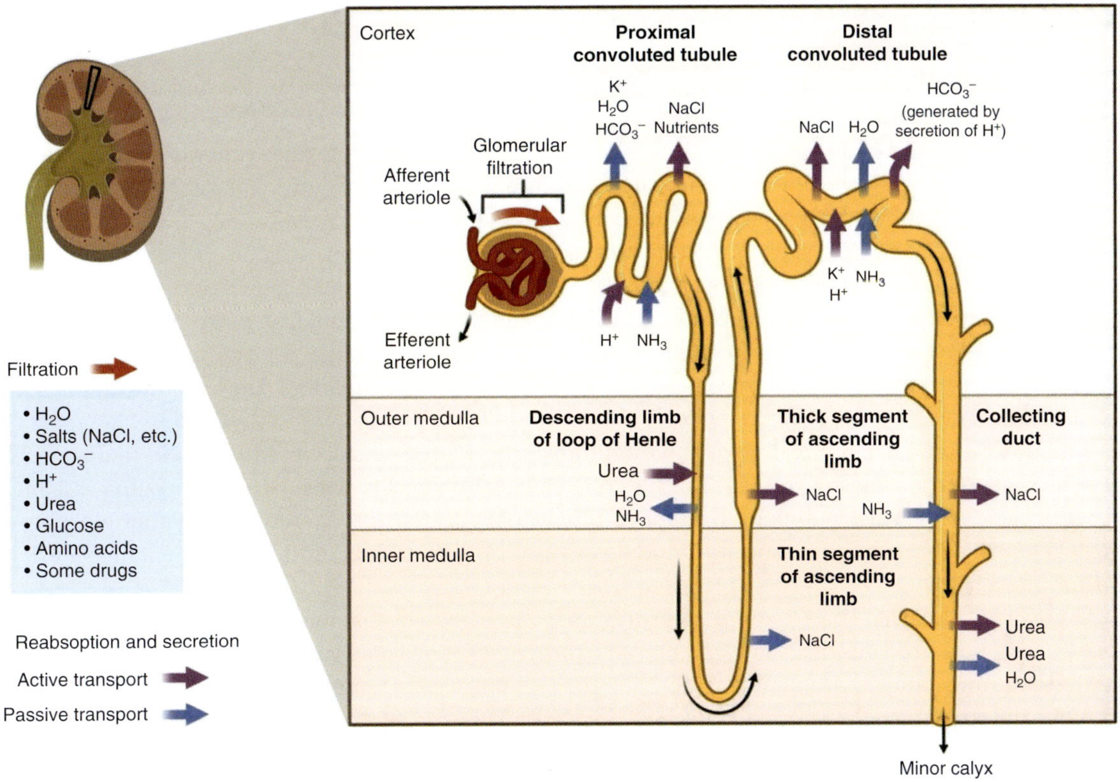

Figure 4.4 Schematic representation of renal handling of toxins through three main processes: **glomerular filtration** of water, unbound drugs, and metabolites into the nephron; **tubular secretion** of toxins from peritubular capillaries into the proximal tubule via active transport; and **tubular reabsorption** of lipid-soluble toxins back into the bloodstream, which can occur passively or actively. The proximal tubule is a common injury site for nephrotoxins, while the distal nephron is the final site for urinary excretion of toxins and their metabolites. The diagram also indicates that manipulation of urine pH can influence reabsorption through ion trapping, thereby enhancing toxin elimination.

Similarly, understanding that certain tropical fish species exhibit enhanced glutathione S-transferase activity compared to cold-water species can influence expectations of recovery time and the design of supportive care plans (see Chapter 10).

Biotransformation and excretion profiles also inform prognostic considerations: Species with slower detoxification rates or those prone to enterohepatic recirculation may require extended monitoring, even after the apparent cessation of clinical signs. This knowledge is particularly valuable in the tropics, where high environmental toxin exposure and limited laboratory resources demand prioritization of the most critical interventions.

In summary, while the "how-to" of diagnosis and treatment is detailed in later chapters, this chapter provides the metabolic and toxicokinetic foundation on which those practical steps rest.

Conclusion

Biotransformation and the fate of toxicants form the physiological foundation for understanding how poisons cause illness in animals and how recovery can be achieved. In tropical veterinary medicine – where animals face an extraordinary variety of natural toxins (plants, mycotoxins, venoms) and synthetic chemicals (pesticides, feed additives) under demanding environmental conditions – grasping the subtleties of metabolic pathways and species-specific differences is essential.

Metabolic commonalities, such as the universal phases of detoxification, provide reassurance that certain core interventions remain effective across species and regions. Yet the regional and species-specific variations shaped by evolution, environment, and husbandry practices demand a more tailored approach to each case. For example, a ruminant's rumen microflora can neutralize a pasture toxin, whereas a warm-water fish kill may result from pesticide runoff and bioaccumulation. These contextual factors shape clinical decision-making.

An informed understanding of toxicokinetics transforms both diagnosis and treatment. In diagnosis, it guides targeted testing and strategic sample collection, enabling clinicians to turn a puzzling case into a confirmed toxicosis. In treatment, it supports timely and effective interventions – whether blocking a toxic metabolic reaction with a specific antidote or sustaining an animal until natural clearance mechanisms prevail.

Ultimately, mastering Phase I and II pathways, appreciating the factors that influence metabolism, and recognizing how toxicants distribute and persist in different species help veterinarians better protect animal health. Integrating molecular insight with practical clinical skill enhances our ability to manage poisonings and strengthens preventive strategies, contributing to safer livestock production, healthier wildlife populations, and improved welfare for companion animals in both tropical and temperate regions.

References

Boothe, D. M (2016). *Factors affecting drug disposition*. Veterinary Key.

Center, S. A. (2024). *Hepatotoxins in small animals. MSD Veterinary Manual*. Merck & Co., Inc. Available at: https://www.msdvetmanual.com/digestive-system/hepatic-diseases-of-small-animals/hepatotoxins-in-small-animals (accessed 15 January 2026).

Diaz, G. J., Murcia, H. W., Cepeda, S. M., & Boermans, H. J. (2010). The role of selected cytochrome P450 enzymes on the bioactivation of aflatoxin B_1 by duck liver microsomes. *Avian Pathology*, *39*(4), 279–285. https://doi.org/10.1080/03079457.2010.495109

Durník, R., Šindlerová, L., Babica, P., & Jurček, O. (2022). Bile acids transporters of enterohepatic circulation for targeted drug delivery. *Molecules*, *27*(9), 2961. https://doi.org/10.3390/molecules27092961

Helke, K. L., Nelson, K. N., Sargeant, A. M., Jacob, B., McKeag, S., Haruna, J., Vemireddi, V., Greeley, M., Brocksmith, D., Navratil, N., Stricker-Krongrad, A., & Hollinger, C. (2016). Pigs in toxicology: Breed differences in metabolism and background findings. *Toxicologic Pathology*, *44*(4), 575–590. https://doi.org/10.1177/0192623316639389

Jandacek, R., Liu, M., & Tso, P. (2024). Interactions of body weight loss with lipophilic toxin storage: Commentary. *The Journal of Nutrition*, *154*(3), 801–803. https://doi.org/10.1016/j.tjnut.2024.01.018

Kolanczyk, R. C., Solem, L. E., Schmieder, P. K., & McKim, J. M., III. (2024). A comparative study of phase I and II biotransformation in salmonid fish. *Fishes*, *9*(7), 284. https:// doi. org/ 10. 3390/ fishes9070284

La Merrill, M., Emond, C., Kim, M. J., Antignac, J.-P., Le Bizec, B., Clément, K., Birnbaum, L. S., & Barouki, R. (2013). Toxicological function of adipose tissue: Focus on persistent organic pollutants. *Environmental Health Perspectives*, *121*(2), 162–169. https://doi.org/10.1289/ehp.1205485

La Merrill, M. (2012). Toxicological function of adipose tissue: Focus on its role in modulation of persistent organic pollutant (POP) toxicity. *Chemico-Biological Interactions*, *205*(1), 162–170. https://doi.org/10.1016/j.cbi.2013.07.002

Loh, Z. H., Ouwerkerk, D., Klieve, A. V., Hungerford, N. L., & Fletcher, M. T. (2020). Toxin degradation by rumen microorganisms: A review. *Toxins*, *12*(10), 664. https://doi.org/10.3390/toxins12100664

Oh, J. (2021). A case of isoniazid intoxication in a dog. *Journal of Veterinary Clinics*, *38*(4), 204–209. https://doi.org/10.17555/jvc.2021.38.4.204

Ray, S., & Shaju, S. T. (2023). Bioaccumulation of pesticides in fish resulting in toxicities in humans through the food chain and forensic aspects. *Environmental Analysis Health and Toxicology*, *38*(3), e2023017. https://doi.org/10.5620/eaht.2023017

Saengtienchai, A., Ikenaka, Y., Kawata, M., Kawai, Y., Takeda, K., Kondo, M., Bortey-Sam, N., Nakayama, S. M. M., Mizukawa, H., & Ishizuka, M. (2018). Comparison of xenobiotic metabolism in phase I oxidation and phase II conjugation between rats and bird species. *Comparative Biochemistry and Physiology Part C: Toxicology & Pharmacology*, *214*, 28–35. https://doi.org/10.1016/j.cbpc.2018.08.007

Saha, R., & Dutta, S. M. (2024). Pesticides' mode of action on aquatic life. *Toxicology Reports*, *13*, 101780. https://doi.org/10.1016/j.toxrep.2024.101780

Schmid, R. D. (2024). *Absorption, distribution, metabolism, and excretion of toxic agents in animals. MSD Veterinary Manual.* Merck & Co., Inc. Available at: https://www.msdvetmanual.com/toxicology/toxicology-introduction/absorption-distribution-metabolism-and-excretion-of-toxic-agents-in-animals (accessed 15 January 2026).

Thompson, L. J. (2024). *Nitrate and nitrite poisoning in animals. MSD Veterinary Manual.* Merck & Co., Inc. Available at: https://www.msdvetmanual.com/toxicology/nitrate-and-nitrite-poisoning/nitrate-and-nitrite-poisoning-in-animals (accessed 15 January 2026).

5

Toxicity Testing

Toxicity testing is conducted on new chemicals, drugs (human and veterinary), pesticides (herbicides, insecticides), feed additives, and industrial compounds before they are marketed. These tests, which often involve significant resources, determine whether a substance is safe under its intended conditions of use. They define a compound's potential to cause harm and help establish the highest dose that causes no adverse effect (the no-observed-adverse-effect level [NOAEL]). Toxicity testing assumes a suitable animal model is available and that a dose–response relationship can be demonstrated. Broadly, testing falls into general toxicity (acute, sub-chronic, chronic) and special tests (e.g., reproductive, skin/eye irritation, carcinogenic, teratogenic, genotoxicity). Compounds that may enter the environment (e.g., pesticides) must also be tested for effects on nontarget species such as fish and birds.

Modern toxicity testing uses both laboratory and field approaches. Controlled lab experiments (using animals or cell systems) are the cornerstone for identifying toxic effects under standardized conditions, while field studies and environmental monitoring evaluate effects in real-world settings. Regulatory agencies and international organizations have established guidelines (e.g., Organisation for Economic Co-operation and Development [OECD] test methods; World Health Organization [WHO]/Food and Agriculture Organization of the United Nations [FAO] frameworks) to harmonize these procedures. Such standards make data reliable and comparable worldwide and are increasingly adopted in tropical regions (e.g., Southeast Asia, sub-Saharan Africa, Latin America), where local conditions may modify toxicity. The following sections describe in vivo animal study design and specific test types and highlight global standards and tropical-context considerations.

Animal Studies (In Vivo Testing)

Animal studies remain a mainstay of toxicity testing despite the rise of in vitro methods. Live animal tests capture whole-organism responses and complex interactions among organs that simple cell systems cannot. They reveal clinical signs of toxicity (changes in behavior, neurological function, autonomic responses, etc.) that intact organisms exhibit. However, animals cannot report subjective symptoms as humans do. In contrast, in vitro (cell-based) assays have limitations:

Lack of systemic response: In vitro systems cannot show clinical symptoms or overt intoxication signs an intact animal would exhibit.

Poor prediction of complex effects: Interactions seen in vitro may not correlate with in vivo outcomes (e.g., cholinesterase inhibitor toxicity in cell culture may not fully predict animal effects).

No absorption, distribution, metabolism, and excretion (ADME) assessment: In vitro tests cannot measure whole-body absorption, distribution, metabolism, and excretion, which determine a toxicant's bioavailability.

Because of these gaps, animal testing is guided by principles that balance scientific need and ethics. Researchers follow animal welfare guidelines and apply the 3Rs (Replacement, Reduction, Refinement) to use alternatives when possible, use the minimum number of animals, and minimize their distress. Many regulatory bodies now accept or even prefer validated nonanimal methods for certain endpoints (such as skin or eye irritation) when available.

Field studies and epidemiological observations complement lab tests by revealing real-world effects. Field data (e.g., monitoring wildlife, livestock, or exposed human populations) can uncover outcomes that controlled lab tests might miss. For example, in sub-Saharan Africa, high pesticide exposures in farming communities have been correlated with health issues predicted by lab studies (Asefa et al., 2024; Isgren and Andersson, 2021; Sheahan et al., 2017). Recent surveillance among cotton farmers in Tanzania also highlights the burden of unintentional acute pesticide poisoning (Kapeleka et al., 2025).

Field observations also highlight how tropical factors, climate, nutrition, or co-exposures, modify toxicity. Heavy tropical rainfall can wash pesticides into waterways, requiring in situ assays (e.g., local aquatic species tests) to evaluate actual exposure effects (Lopes et al., 2007). Such examples underscore the importance of field-relevant toxicity testing in tropical regions.

Overall, comprehensive toxicity assessment often uses a tiered strategy: initial in vitro screens for obvious hazards, then in vivo animal studies for organism-level effects, and finally field or monitoring data for ecological and long-term human impacts.

Choice of Animal Model

Selecting the appropriate animal model is crucial. Factors include cost, availability, handling, species physiology, reproductive capability, housing requirements, and any known peculiarities of the species. No model perfectly replicates a human or target-animal species, but it should yield information that can be extrapolated with confidence. Ideally, the species should metabolize the compound similarly to humans or the target species, so the toxicokinetics are relevant.

Common laboratory models include rodents (rats, mice) and non-rodents (rabbits, guinea pigs, dogs, nonhuman primates). Rats are used extensively (low cost, well-characterized physiology); dogs (often beagles) are common in pharmaceutical studies because their metabolism complements rodent data. Other species are chosen for specific tests: rabbits for skin/eye studies (sensitive eyes/skin), guinea pigs for skin sensitization, and primates only when absolutely needed (due to cost/ethical constraints). In veterinary toxicology, the actual target livestock or companion animal may be tested (especially for safety of veterinary drugs), typically after initial screening in standard lab species.

Tropical regions add considerations: most lab strains are bred in temperate climates, so some tests may use local species to reflect ecosystem sensitivities. For instance, tropical native fish or invertebrates might be used in environmental toxicity tests. However, many tropical regulators still rely on OECD-recommended species for consistency (e.g., Malaysian guidelines reference OECD species). Ultimately, model choice balances scientific relevance, ethics, and regulatory acceptance.

Test Substances and Dosing

The test compound must be well-characterized and representative of the product that will be used. This ensures the results reflect the actual substance to which animals or humans will be exposed. Purity (or a detailed composition of impurities) is important because contaminants or metabolites may contribute to toxicity. The vehicle or solvent used to administer the compound should not react with it and should have minimal toxicity. A vehicle control group (receiving the vehicle without the active substance) is included in toxicity studies to distinguish effects of the test substance from any effects of the carrier.

Animals should be dosed via a route that mimics relevant exposure (e.g., oral for food contaminants, dermal for skin contact agents, inhalation for volatile substances). For pesticides expected to contact skin or be inhaled, dermal or inhalation routes are tested, respectively. In veterinary contexts, if a drug is given in feed or water, the oral route is used; if it's a pour-on or dip (ectoparasiticide), dermal dosing is used; and for inhalant anesthetics, inhalation studies are conducted.

Dosing schedules and levels are carefully planned to establish a dose–response relationship:

High dose: Chosen to produce clear toxicity or adverse effects (but not immediate lethality, except in some acute studies). It should reveal target organs and significant pathological changes. The high dose is often the maximum tolerated dose (MTD) that causes some toxicity without causing excessive early deaths.
Mid dose: Causes moderate effects, helping to define a gradient of response between high and low doses.
Low dose: The highest dose that causes no observable adverse effects (the NOAEL). Ideally, it yields no statistically or biologically significant toxicity, providing a safety margin below higher doses.

For practical and ethical reasons, the highest dose may be limited by multiples of expected human exposure or by the onset of severe toxicity. In an acute study the goal may be to find an approximate LD_{50} (dose lethal to 50% of animals); in sub-chronic and chronic studies, the goal is to identify a NOAEL and target organs for toxicity. Doses are adjusted for species size and metabolic rate (mg/kg for oral/dermal, mg/L for inhalation). In long studies, doses might be recalculated if animals gain weight or toxicity reduces feed intake, but any changes must maintain intended exposure levels.

Observations During Study

Animals are closely monitored during and after dosing. Standard practice is to observe animals at least once daily (and more often during critical periods) for clinical signs of toxicity. Observations typically include:

Behavioral changes: lethargy, hyperactivity, aggression
Neurological signs: tremors, convulsions, ataxia (gait abnormalities)
Autonomic signs: salivation, piloerection (raised hairs), pupil changes
Other visible signs: vomiting (in species that can), diarrhea, respiratory distress, changes in posture or activity

Body weight is recorded regularly (often weekly). Significant weight loss can indicate reduced food intake or systemic toxicity. Feed and water consumption are also tracked: A drop in intake may signal illness or unpalatability, whereas increased water intake can reflect metabolic disturbances (e.g., diabetes insipidus).

Periodically (e.g., monthly in sub-chronic/chronic studies), clinical pathology tests are performed. Blood is sampled for hematology and serum chemistry to detect organ-specific toxicity (e.g., elevated liver enzymes for hepatotoxicity, altered blood cell counts for bone marrow effects). Urinalysis may assess renal function, and specialized tests (ophthalmoscopic eye exams, audiometry, electrocardiograms, etc.) may be included for substances suspected of affecting specific systems.

Necropsy and Pathology

At the end of the study (and sometimes at planned interim points), animals are humanely euthanized for necropsy. A full gross pathological examination is conducted, and key organs (liver, kidneys, brain, heart, spleen, etc.) are weighed. Changes in organ weights (e.g., enlarged liver from hypertrophy) can sensitively indicate toxicity. Tissues are then examined histopathologically under the microscope to detect cellular-level damage (inflammation, degeneration, necrosis, hyperplasia, neoplasia, etc.). All collected data — including clinical observations, body weight and organ weight changes, and histology findings — are integrated to characterize adverse effects and establish dose–response relationships, helping define safe exposure levels for the test animals.

Interim Sacrifices

In longer studies (sub-chronic or chronic), one or more interim sacrifices may be included. This means a subset of animals in each group is euthanized before the planned end of the study (e.g., midpoint or other specified times). Interim data are valuable for observing the progression or reversibility of lesions or for obtaining early biochemical and pathological information. For example, in a 1-year study, one might sacrifice some animals at 6 months to check for early organ damage, while others continue to 12 months.

Interim sacrifices require adding extra animals at study start so that adequate group sizes remain at final sacrifice. Statistical planning must ensure that removing animals mid-study still leaves enough for valid end-point comparisons. Any interim findings (e.g., high-dose severe toxicity) could warrant adjusting the study (in rare cases leading to dose reduction or early termination on ethical grounds).

Interim euthanasia is also common in multi-generation reproductive studies (e.g., sampling a subset of weaned pups to assess development). Whenever interim sacrifices are planned, the protocol must justify their necessity and specify the timing and number of animals.

Preparation of Animal Subjects

Proper preparation of animals ensures consistency and welfare. Common preparatory steps include:

Selection and acclimation: Use healthy animals of specified age/weight. Acclimate them to the laboratory environment (typically 5–7 days) before dosing.

Weighing and identification: Weigh each animal before dosing. Assign a permanent ID (ear tag, microchip, etc.) and record initial body weight for dose calculations.

Fasting (if applicable): For oral studies (especially acute), animals may be fasted (usually ~12 hours) before dosing so the stomach is empty. This avoids food interfering with absorption. Water is usually provided ad libitum during fasting unless specified otherwise.

Skin preparation (for dermal tests): Clip or shave fur at the exposure site (e.g., ~10% of body surface or a defined area). Hair is trimmed short (millimeter length) to expose skin without injuring it. Some dermal tests include minor skin abrasion on part of the site to simulate damaged skin; abrasions should break the stratum corneum minimally (no bleeding) to test increased penetration.

Restraint during exposure: Ensure animals cannot remove the dose and are not harmed. For example, after applying a dermal patch, rabbits may be fitted with collars or bandages to prevent grooming or licking the site. Inhalation studies use specialized chambers or masks.

These preparations help deliver the dose consistently and protect animal welfare.

General Toxicity Tests (Acute, Sub-chronic, Chronic)

General toxicity tests evaluate the effects of a substance over different exposure durations, helping to establish its safety profile. The three main types are acute, sub-chronic, and chronic studies. Each yields distinct information:

Acute Toxicity

Acute toxicity studies involve short-term exposure (usually a single dose or two doses within 1 day) followed by observation for about 14 days. They are typically the first in vivo tests for a new compound and are designed to identify any immediate harmful effects. Acute studies also estimate the median lethal dose (LD_{50}), the dose expected to kill 50% of animals. Historically, finding the LD_{50} was a primary goal, but modern approaches de-emphasize exact LD_{50} determination in favor of identifying dose ranges and clinical signs while minimizing animal use.

Key points of acute testing:

Species and route: Usually at least one rodent species (rat or mouse) is tested, often plus a second species (e.g., dog) for pharmaceuticals. The administration route is chosen to match likely human/animal exposure. Oral dosing is common for systemic toxicity; dermal or inhalation routes are used if relevant (e.g., pesticides contacting skin or being inhaled).

Dosing and observation: Animals receive a single dose (or a split dose) and are observed for 14 days. Observations include daily checks for mortality and clinical signs. The 14-day period covers the time during which acute effects typically appear and either resolve or cause death/recovery.

A simplified flowchart (Figure 5.1) is often used to illustrate the acute test sequence: dose → immediate observation → periodic monitoring for 14 days → final necropsy of any animals that die (and gross examination of survivors).

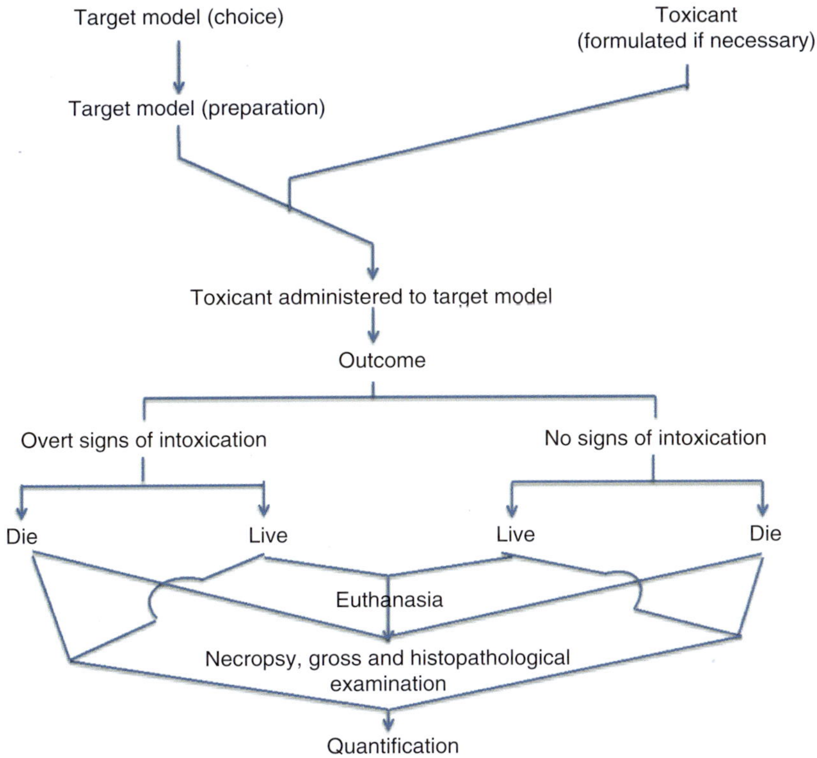

Figure 5.1 Acute toxicity testing – a flow diagram. *Source:* Adapted from Stephens et al. (2021).

Alternative methods: In place of the traditional multi-animal LD_{50} test, alternative procedures use fewer animals. For example, the OECD Up-and-Down Procedure (UDP) doses one animal at a time: if the first animal survives, the dose for the next is higher; if it dies, the dose is lowered (OECD, 2018). This process continues until enough data estimate toxicity with far fewer animals (Bruce, 1985). Other methods include the Fixed Dose Procedure and the Acute Toxic Class method (California Department of Pesticide Regulation, 2024). OECD guidelines (e.g., TG 423, 425) have replaced the older LD_{50} test in many regulatory systems, reflecting the 3Rs approach.

Acute testing outcomes: It reveals which organs are affected at high doses and establishes signs of toxicity. It also informs dosing for longer studies. For instance, if an acute study finds neurotoxic effects at 100 mg/kg, that dose may be chosen as the high dose in a subsequent 90-day study. Importantly, acute toxicity data are used for hazard classification. Systems like the UN Globally Harmonized System (GHS) and the WHO Recommended Classification of Pesticides use acute LD_{50} values (oral, dermal, inhalation) to categorize hazards. For example, a pesticide with rat oral LD_{50} <5 mg/kg is classified as WHO Class Ia (extremely hazardous). These classifications (often indicated by color-coded labels) facilitate risk communication, especially in areas where users may rely on simple hazard categories.

Sub-chronic Toxicity (28–90 Day Studies)

Subchronic toxicity studies involve repeated exposure for an intermediate duration, typically 28 or 90 days. They serve as a bridge between acute and chronic testing and are useful for identifying effects that take weeks to manifest. Key features:

Species and group size: Most often conducted in rodents (rats, and sometimes a non-rodent species like dogs for pharmaceuticals). In a 90-day rat study, group sizes are often ~10 animals per sex to ensure statistical power. Both sexes are included to detect any sex-specific effects.

Dosing regimen: Animals are dosed daily (7 days per week) for the study duration. Typically, three dose levels and a control group are used. The high dose is chosen to induce some signs of toxicity (but minimal mortality), the low dose is a presumed no-effect level, and a mid-dose is intermediate.

Observations: Animals are examined daily. Body weight and food/water consumption are recorded at least weekly. Clinical pathology (hematology and biochemistry) is performed at intervals (e.g., 4, 8, and 13 weeks) to detect trends (such as gradual anemia or liver enzyme elevations) that may not be overtly symptomatic.

Terminal procedures: At study end, animals are necropsied with full histopathology. Organ weights (e.g., liver, kidneys, heart) are compared to controls, as changes (enlargement or atrophy) can indicate target organ toxicity. Some protocols include a recovery group: animals are held for an additional 28 days after dosing stops to see if effects reverse.

Sub-chronic studies yield a 90-day NOAEL for the test substance, which is critical for risk assessment. The data help set dose levels for chronic studies and provide initial information on potential targets and safety margins.

Chronic Toxicity and Carcinogenicity (Long-Term Studies)

Chronic toxicity testing assesses long-term (often lifetime) exposure. In rodents, studies typically last 6 months to 2 years, with 2 years being standard for combined chronic toxicity and carcinogenicity bioassays in rats. The actual duration is chosen based on lifespan and expected human exposure. For example, a 1-year chronic toxicity study (without a carcinogenicity focus) is common, whereas a 2-year rat bioassay covers both chronic effects and tumor development. Chronic studies are considered the most relevant for assessing lifelong exposure risks, but they are the most costly, time-consuming, and ethically sensitive.

Design features: Chronic studies are similar to sub-chronic in that dosing is daily (7 days/week) and often the same species are used (rats, and often mice if tumors are evaluated; sometimes dogs for 1-year toxicity in drugs). Dose levels are typically based on sub-chronic results. For carcinogenicity studies, groups are large (e.g., 50 animals/sex/group in rodent bioassays) to provide statistical power to detect tumor incidence. Doses usually include a high dose that produces some toxicity (or benign tumors) but not excessive early deaths, and lower doses to define the NOAEL from sub-chronic studies.

During chronic studies, animals are observed daily and weighed regularly. Clinical pathology may be assessed at interim points (e.g., every 6–12 months) in chronic toxicity tests, but in a 2-year cancer bioassay, blood sampling may be limited after 1 year to avoid weakening the animals. The focus in long-term studies is on tumor detection and late-onset chronic effects (fibrosis, hypertrophy, degenerative changes).

At study end (and for any animals that died or were moribund), a full necropsy with histopathology of all major tissues is performed. Tumor incidence is recorded, and tissues are examined for both neoplastic (tumors) and nonneoplastic lesions.

A flow diagram can illustrate how acute versus chronic exposures differ. In acute exposure, high doses may cause immediate effects (possible death) or recovery (Figure 5.2). In chronic exposure, lower doses over time may accumulate and lead to chronic conditions (e.g., organ fibrosis or cancer) that would not appear in a short test.

Often, 2-year rodent studies will reveal tumors in high-dose groups. Determining human relevance of these tumors can be complex, as some rodent tumors are caused by rodent-specific mechanisms (e.g., male rat kidney tumors from α2u-globulin). Risk assessors evaluate such findings alongside mechanistic data. Chronic studies yield a chronic NOAEL and, if tumors are found, a carcinogenic potency estimate (such as TD50 or Benchmark Dose for a defined increase in tumor risk). These inform regulatory decisions: for example, if a pesticide is carcinogenic in rodents, authorities may apply extra safety factors or classify it as a possible human carcinogen. Many countries require at least two long-term studies (usually in rat and mouse) for pesticides and industrial chemicals (Takeda et al., 2023).

Because traditional 2-year bioassays are resource-intensive and raise ethical issues, alternatives have been sought (e.g., transgenic mouse models that develop tumors faster, in vitro cell transformation assays). These alternatives currently supplement but do not replace the animal tests. To date, chronic animal studies remain a cornerstone of long-term hazard assessment.

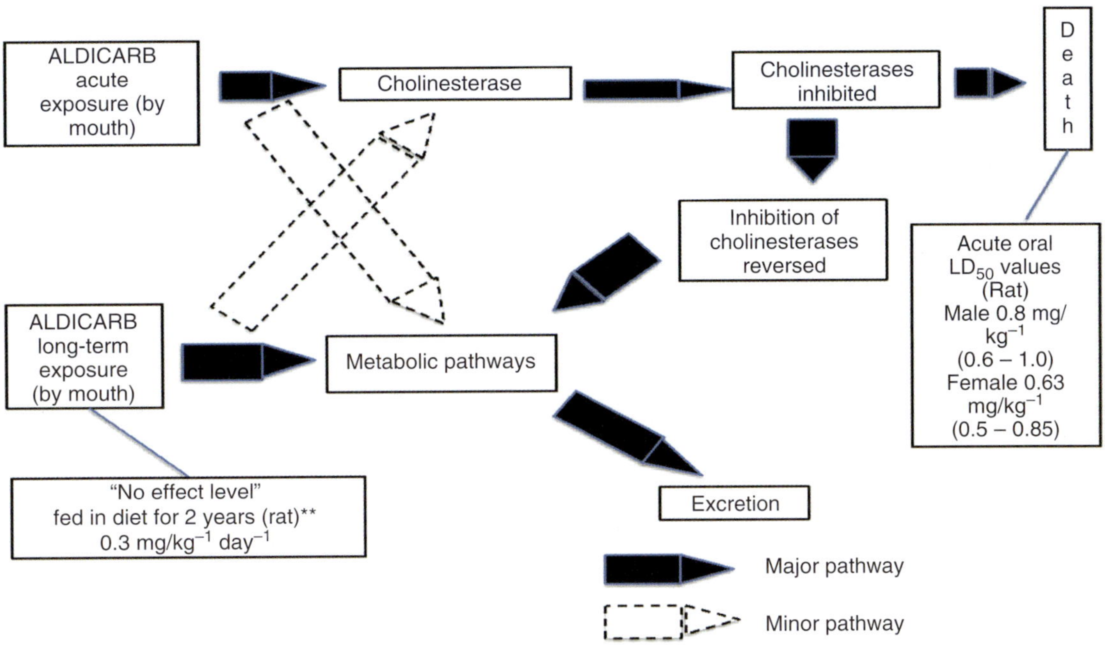

Figure 5.2 An example of difference between responses to acute and long-term exposure to a chemical (a simplified flow diagram). *Source:* Adapted from Stephens et al. (2021).

Carcinogenicity Testing: Carcinogenicity studies are essentially chronic studies with emphasis on tumors. They typically use both male and female rodents, aiming to last until late in life (often until survival in one group falls to ~20–25% or 2 years, whichever comes first). Dose selection targets the MTD as the high dose (the highest dose that does not significantly shorten lifespan from non-cancer toxicity). This ensures any carcinogenic potential is revealed, even if it means high-dose stress on cells. Lower doses help identify a dose–response or the highest noncarcinogenic dose. Results from carcinogenicity studies lead to categorizing chemicals under cancer hazard schemes (e.g., International Agency for Research on Cancer [IARC], the United States Environmental Protection Agency [US EPA]). Positive tumor results in two species typically indicate the substance is considered carcinogenic for humans, unless convincing evidence shows humans are not similarly affected.

Developmental and Reproductive Toxicity

Reproductive and developmental toxicity tests examine effects on fertility and offspring development. They typically involve multiphase or multi-generation studies:

Multi-generation studies (e.g., OECD TG 416): Rats (usually) are dosed for at least two successive generations. For example, in a two-generation study, parental animals (F0) of both sexes are dosed daily (often ~60 days) prior to mating to affect gametes. Dosing continues through mating, gestation, and lactation. The F0 produce the F1 generation; F1 animals (exposed in utero and via nursing) may be mated to produce F2, often on continued dosing. Endpoints include fertility indices, pregnancy outcomes, offspring growth, and survival. Some F1 pups may be sacrificed at weaning for developmental evaluation, while the rest are reared to breeding age. This design detects effects on reproduction and on the next generations.

Extended One-Generation Reproductive Toxicity Study (OECD TG 443): A newer protocol that can replace the traditional two-generation test. One generation of rats (F0 and F1) is dosed continuously, but if certain “triggers” (e.g., offspring fertility issues) are observed, an F2 generation is produced; otherwise, the study stops at F1. This reduces animal use while still detecting important reproductive effects (OECD, 2024).

Developmental (Teratology) tests (e.g., OECD TG 414): These focus on embryonic/fetal development. Pregnant females (usually rats or rabbits) are dosed during the critical organogenesis period. Fetuses are then examined for malformations or developmental variations. This identifies potential birth defects.

Each reproductive/developmental test has specific guidelines, but in general, they evaluate effects on mating, fertility, pregnancy, parturition, and offspring growth and morphology. Data from these studies inform risk assessment for reproductive hazards and help set guidelines (like no-observed-effect levels for developmental toxicity [NOAELs]).

Genotoxicity (Mutagenicity) Testing

Genotoxicity tests detect damage to genetic material (DNA) and serve as an early warning of carcinogenicity. A standard genotoxicity test battery includes (OECD, 2017; EFSA Scientific Committee et al., 2017; European Medicines Agency, 2012; Fowler et al., 2024):

Bacterial gene mutation test: The Ames test (OECD TG 471) uses strains of bacteria to detect point mutations caused by the chemical. Many human carcinogens show positive Ames results.

Mammalian cell assays: In vitro tests for chromosomal damage are used, such as the chromosomal aberration test (OECD TG 473) and the in vitro micronucleus test (OECD TG 487). These detect clastogens (that break chromosomes) and aneugens (that disturb chromosome number) in cultured cells (e.g., hamster ovary cells).

In vivo assays: Typically, a rodent bone marrow micronucleus test (OECD TG 474) is performed. The test chemical is administered to mice or rats, and their bone marrow or blood is examined for micronuclei (small chromosome fragments) in erythrocytes. This confirms whether DNA damage seen in vitro also occurs in a living animal. Other in vivo tests (e.g., comet assay, transgenic rodent mutation assays) may also be used.

Genotoxicity testing is usually done early in development of a compound. A positive result in any of these assays raises concern: If a chemical is clearly mutagenic in multiple tests, it may be treated as a carcinogenic risk (for drugs, it often halts development unless the benefit–risk is justified). Regulatory guidelines (OECD, ICH S2[R1]) harmonize these tests globally. WHO/FAO expert panels consider genotoxicity when evaluating pesticides and residues (if a pesticide is genotoxic, it may be assumed to have no safe threshold). From a tropical perspective, genotoxicity tests are also used as biomarkers (e.g., measuring micronuclei in cells of people exposed to pesticides) to monitor exposure. Overall, a battery of genotoxicity assays is used because no single test can detect all mechanisms. A combination of negative results across bacterial and mammalian assays provides confidence that a substance is not genotoxic.

Dermal (Skin) Irritation and Sensitization Tests

Dermal tests evaluate local effects on the skin. Advances in toxicology have developed many alternative methods to avoid animal use in these tests (Jirova et al., 2020), but the classic protocols remain instructive.

Primary skin irritation test: This test determines if a substance causes skin irritation or corrosion. Typically, albino rabbits are used (their skin is sensitive and they have been the standard model). The test substance (solid/moistened or liquid) is applied to a small area of shaved skin under a patch. Two sites are usually prepared on each animal: one intact and one slightly abraded (lightly scratched without bleeding). Patches remain in place for 4 hours (24 hours in some protocols), then are removed. The skin is observed at 1, 24, 48, and 72 hours post-exposure. Erythema (redness) and edema (swelling) are scored on a numerical scale from 0 (none) to 4 (severe). For example, erythema scoring might be: 0 = no redness, 1 = very slight, 2 = well-defined, 3 = moderate to severe, 4 = severe (beefy red) with necrosis. Edema is similarly scored (0 = none to 4 = severe swelling). These scoring systems (examples of which appear in Tables 5.1 and 5.2) are from regulatory guidelines (e.g., OECD TG 404 (OECD, 2023c)). An overall Primary Irritation Index (PII) is calculated as the average of erythema and edema scores at specified times. Based on the PII, the chemical is classified as non-irritant, mildly, moderately, or severely irritating, or as corrosive if tissue destruction occurs.

Limitations of animal skin tests (expense, time, and interspecies differences) have led to alternatives. Human volunteer patch tests (for low-risk substances) or in vitro reconstructed human skin models are now common. For example, OECD TG 439 describes an in vitro skin irritation test using human

Table 5.1 Scoring system for erythematous (and scar) lesions based on severity.

Erythematous (and scar) lesions:	Score
No erythema	0
Very slight erythema (barely perceptible)	1
Well-defined erythema	2
Erythema very marked	3
Severe erythema, crimson red with slight eschar formation (injuries in depth)	4

Table 5.2 Scoring system for edematous lesions based on severity.

Edematous lesions:	Score
No edema	0
Very slight edema (barely perceptible)	1
Slight edema (edges of area well-defined by definite raising)	2
Moderate edema (area raised approximately 1 mm)	3
Severe edema (raised more than 1 mm and extending beyond area of application)	4

epidermis tissues (OECD, 2021). In the EU and elsewhere, many skin irritation tests now use these non-animal methods (OECD TG 439).

Skin sensitization test: This assesses allergic contact dermatitis potential. Traditional methods included guinea pig assays (Maximization Test or Buehler Test), which have two phases: induction (exposing animal to substance, often with an adjuvant injection, to provoke an immune response) and challenge (applying the substance to see if an allergic reaction occurs). A more modern and popular method is the local lymph node assay (LLNA, OECD TG 429) in mice: The test substance is applied to both ears of a mouse for 3 consecutive days, and the proliferation of lymphocytes in the draining lymph nodes is measured; a significant increase indicates sensitization potential. The LLNA has largely replaced guinea pig tests because it is quantitative, quicker, uses fewer animals, and avoids adjuvants.

In chemico and in vitro methods have been developed as well (e.g., DPRA – direct peptide reactivity assay for protein binding reactivity; KeratinoSens assay for keratinocyte activation) (Hoffmann et al., 2018; Kleinstreuer et al., 2018). These are components of Integrated Approaches to Testing and Assessment (IATA) for skin sensitization. Recent OECD "defined approaches" combine such assays to predict sensitization without animals. Regulators increasingly allow waiving of animal tests if robust nonanimal data predict sensitization (European Chemicals Agency, 2013).

In summary, dermal tests check for local effects on skin: irritation, corrosion, and allergic sensitization. They are typically required for chemicals like pesticides, industrial chemicals, and some consumer products (unless justified otherwise). However, the field is moving toward alternatives: OECD now has guidelines for in vitro skin irritation (TG 439) and corrosion (TG 431) using human skin models, which are encouraged especially in regions like the EU and increasingly worldwide.

Eye Irritation (Ocular Test)

The standard eye irritation test (Draize test) evaluates damage to the eye (cornea, iris, conjunctiva). Traditionally, albino rabbits are used due to their sensitive, accessible eyes. A fixed dose (e.g., 0.1 mL of a liquid or 100 mg of a solid) is applied into the conjunctival sac of one eye; the other eye serves as a control. Rabbits are then observed at specific intervals (1, 24, 48, 72 hours, and often up to 21 days) for signs of irritation: redness, swelling, discharge, corneal opacity, and iris damage, which are scored on standard scales. The Draize eye test is ethically controversial, and alternatives (e.g., isolated eye tests, in vitro corneal models) have been developed, but it remains a reference method in many guidelines (OECD, 2023d).

In eye testing, three factors influence the extent of damage:

Contact duration: Longer contact in the eye causes more damage. Immediate flushing/rinsing greatly reduces injury, which is why first-aid advice is to wash eyes with water. In tests, chemicals may be rinsed after fixed times to assess injury potential.

Physical properties: A chemical's formulation affects penetration. Highly lipophilic liquids may penetrate the cornea more readily than aqueous solutions, and solids/particles may cause mechanical irritation.

Chemical reactivity: Corrosive chemicals (e.g., strong acids or bases, which release hydroxide or hydronium ions) chemically damage eye tissues, leading to keratitis, cataracts, or blindness.

Although rabbits are the standard model (because of sensitive eyes and ease of scoring), some severe cases in research have used nonhuman primates for confirmation due to closer human eye anatomy; however, primate use is extremely rare due to ethical constraints. Currently, validated in vitro and ex vivo alternatives (e.g., reconstructed corneal models, Bovine Corneal Opacity Test) are replacing animal tests in many testing programs.

WHO/FAO Standards and Guidelines

International bodies provide standards for classifying hazards and guiding risk assessment. The WHO Recommended Classification of Pesticides by Hazard categorizes pesticides into classes (Ia "extremely hazardous," Ib "highly hazardous," II, III, U) based primarily on acute rat LD_{50} values. For instance, a pesticide with rat oral LD_{50} <5 mg/kg (solid) or <20 mg/kg (liquid) is Class Ia. These classes are often indicated on product labels using color codes (red for Class Ia/Ib, yellow for II, blue for III). The WHO system (latest 2019 edition) is aligned with the UN GHS categories for acute toxicity. Many tropical countries adopt WHO hazard classes for regulation, banning, or restricting the most dangerous categories to protect farmers and users (World Health Organization, 2020) (Table 5.3).

WHO/FAO also identify highly hazardous pesticides (HHPs) by broader criteria, including chronic effects (e.g., carcinogenicity, endocrine disruption). The International Programme on Chemical Safety (IPCS) and the United Nations Environment Programme (UNEP) guidance on HHPs helps countries phase out pesticides that pose severe health or environmental risks beyond acute toxicity (United Nations Environment Programme, n.d.).

The Joint FAO/WHO Meeting on Pesticide Residues (JMPR) provides risk assessment for human exposure (FAO/WHO, 2021; Food and Agriculture Organization of the United Nations, n.d.). JMPR reviews all toxicity data on a pesticide and sets an acceptable daily intake (ADI) for chronic exposure and

Table 5.3 WHO hazard classification of pesticides based on oral LD_{50} values, with examples from tropical regions.

WHO hazard class	Description	Oral LD_{50} (mg/kg body weight)	Example pesticides (tropics)
Ia	Extremely hazardous	<5	Parathion, Aldicarb
Ib	Highly hazardous	5–50	Methamidophos, Monocrotophos
II	Moderately hazardous	50–500	Malathion, Carbaryl
III	Slightly hazardous	500–2,000	Pyrethrins, Propoxur
U	Unlikely to present acute hazard	>2,000	Bacillus thuringiensis (Bt) formulations

Source: Data from World Health Organization (2020).

an acute reference dose (ARfD) for short-term exposure. These are typically derived by dividing a NOAEL from animal studies by safety factors (Herrman & Younes, 1999). For example, JMPR might report: "ADI = 0.01 mg/kg/day based on a NOAEL of 1.0 mg/kg/day and a 100-fold uncertainty factor." Such ADIs then inform Codex Alimentarius Maximum Residue Limits (MRLs) for food, aiding international trade and consumer safety. Tropical countries often adopt Codex MRLs, saving resources by not retesting chemicals already evaluated internationally. Similarly, JECFA (FAO/WHO Committee on Food Additives) performs this role for veterinary drug residues and food additives.

For veterinary drugs, the World Organisation for Animal Health (OIE) and the Veterinary International Conference on Harmonization (VICH) coordinate toxicity and safety requirements. VICH guidelines (analogous to human ICH) specify target animal safety tests, including reproduction and residue evaluations, to ensure veterinary drugs are safe for animals and for humans consuming animal products.

FAO also supports risk assessment capacity. The FAO Pesticide Registration Toolkit includes modules on using toxicity data in exposure models (e.g., for operators, bystanders, dietary intake). FAO publishes guidance documents for tropical conditions (such as metabolic differences in warm-water fish) to help regulators interpret data under local environmental scenarios.

Tropical Context and Implementation

Many tropical countries implement these international standards. For example, Malaysia's pesticide registration guidelines explicitly reference OECD and FAO/WHO protocols (Department of Agriculture Malaysia, 2020a, 2020b). As an OECD Mutual Acceptance of Data (MAD) adherent, Malaysia accepts GLP-compliant studies from OECD countries, streamlining registration (OECD, 2020). However, regulators still require a complete toxicity data package. Real-world events have influenced policy: After severe monocrotophos (Class Ib) poisonings in 1990s Asian cotton fields, several Association of Southeast Asian Nations (ASEAN) countries re-evaluated organophosphate pesticides using WHO hazard categories and banned the most hazardous ones (Figure 5.3).

Unique tropical issues include traditional medicines and natural toxins. Some governments now require toxicity testing of herbal remedies or plant toxins used in folk medicine.

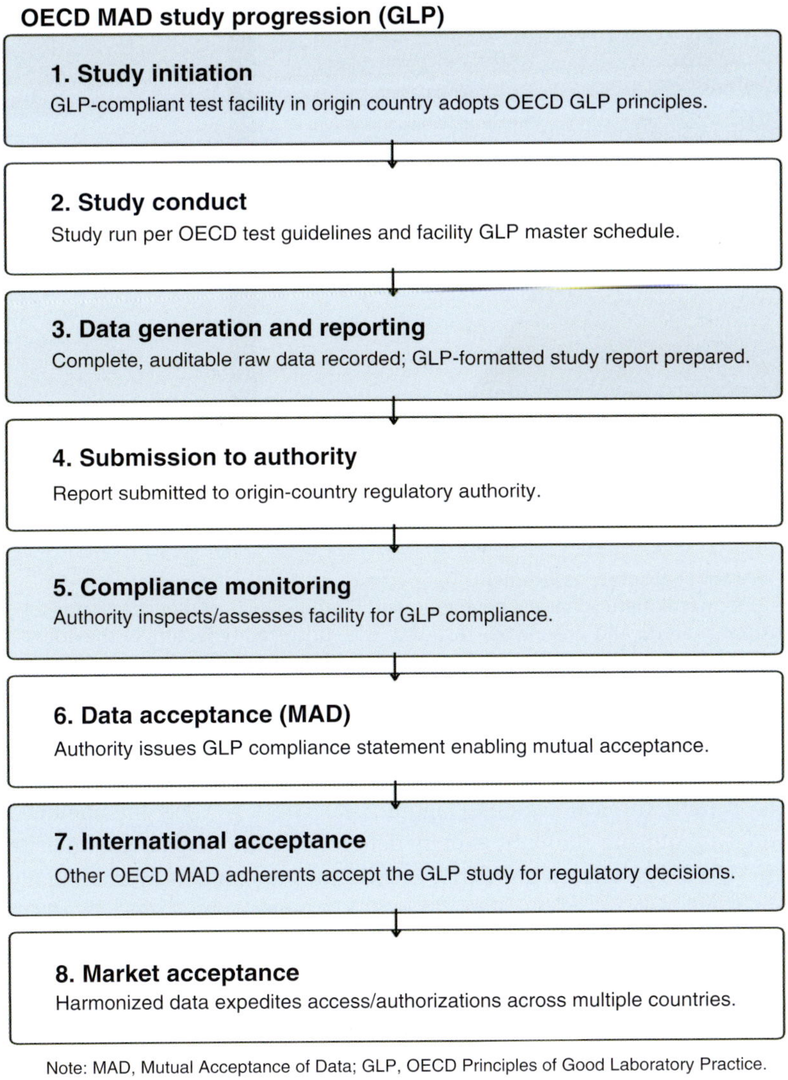

Figure 5.3 OECD mutual acceptance of data (MAD) study progression under good laboratory practice (GLP) principles. The diagram illustrates the sequential steps from study initiation in a GLP-compliant facility through data generation, regulatory submission, compliance monitoring, and national data acceptance, culminating in international recognition and market authorization. *Source:* Adapted from OECD GLP and MAD framework.

Regional cooperation has also arisen. In West Africa, countries (often via regional bodies) are collaborating on pesticide evaluation and may require local ecotoxicity tests on native species (e.g., local fish or invertebrates) to account for ecosystem differences. In Latin America, regulators adapt European risk models to local contexts (Niemeyer et al., 2017); many countries label pesticides with WHO hazard classes and incorporate them into farmer education, enhancing safe handling.

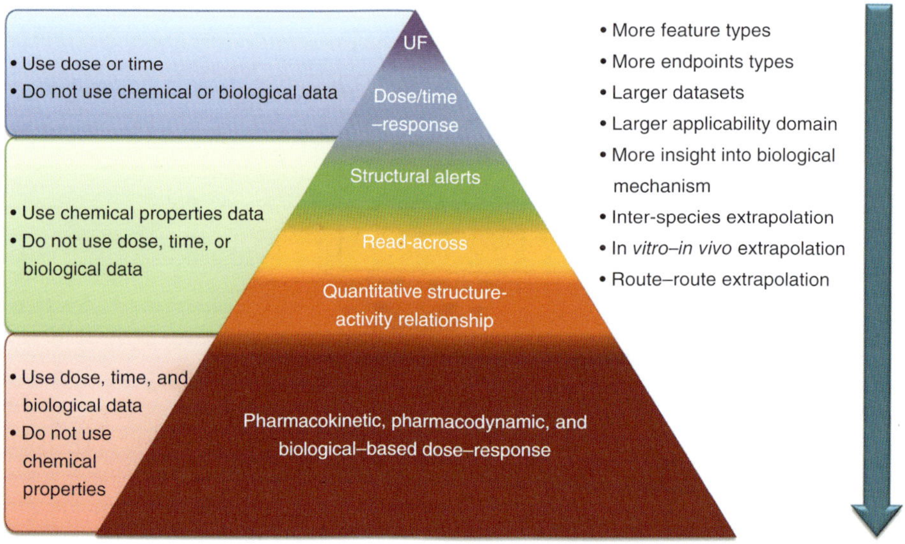

Figure 5.4 Tiered testing strategy for chemical safety assessment. The pyramid progresses from data-rich, mechanistic approaches at the base (pharmacokinetic, pharmacodynamic, and biologically based dose–response) through QSAR and read-across to structural alerts and dose/time–response with uncertainty factors at the apex. Side panels summarize what types of data are (or are not) used at each tier and highlight the increased feature types, endpoints, applicability domain, mechanistic insight, and extrapolation capability achieved as one moves down the pyramid. *Source:* Adapted from Raies and Bajic (2016).

Globally, harmonization trends benefit tropical regions (Figure 5.4). The UN GHS for chemical classification is being adopted widely, requiring standard toxicity data for labeling (e.g., acute toxicity categories align with OECD tests) (United Nations, 2019). OECD continues to expand internationally accepted methods, including nonanimal tests (skin/eye alternatives, IATA approaches) (OECD, 1981–2025; OECD, 2023b; ALTEX, 2021). This helps countries with limited animal testing resources adopt modern methods. For instance, a small lab in Asia may find a reconstructed skin assay more feasible than maintaining rabbits for a Draize test. We anticipate increased uptake of validated alternatives in Asia, Africa, and Latin America as technology and training advance.

International organizations have helped build capacity: For example, India and South Africa are now ISO/GLP-certified testing centers serving global clients, making them contributors to worldwide toxicology data. Regional harmonization initiatives (ASEAN, African Union) aim to align testing requirements and share data, reducing duplication (Asia-Pacific Economic Cooperation, 2024).

Conclusion

Toxicity testing is a dynamic discipline balancing scientific investigation, regulatory demands, and ethical responsibility. This chapter has outlined fundamental test types – acute, sub-chronic, chronic, and specialized assays for skin/eye irritation, sensitization, reproductive effects, and genotoxicity – and described how they are conducted and interpreted. From controlled animal studies establishing dose–response to cutting-edge in vitro and computational models reducing animal use, to field studies confirming real-world effects, the toolbox for toxicity assessment continues to grow (Gupta, 2018). International guidelines from OECD and others ensure scientists and regulators "speak a common language" of quality and protocol, while WHO and FAO translate toxicology data into public health actions (e.g., safe exposure limits, hazard labeling) to protect people, animals, and the environment.

Tropical regions face particular challenges and opportunities: They often deal with highly hazardous exposures (in agriculture, mining, etc.), require consideration of local species and conditions, and have the chance to adopt newer methods earlier. A veterinary toxicologist in the tropics must be skilled at interpreting data from lab studies (often conducted elsewhere) and at investigating local poisonings (e.g., mysterious livestock outbreaks or traditional toxicoses). Mastery of toxicity testing methodology and awareness of global standards empower professionals to make informed decisions and improve safety in their communities.

Looking ahead, emphasis on the 3Rs, adoption of harmonized methods, and learning from incidents (local and global) will drive the evolution of testing. Emerging tools like high-throughput screening, genomics, and artificial intelligence may soon complement or replace some conventional tests, making assessments faster and more predictive of human and environmental outcomes (Raies & Bajic, 2016). However, the core remains systematic hazard evaluation so that risks can be managed. This chapter provides a foundation; readers should consult the references for deeper exploration of specific topics introduced here.

References

ALTEX (2021). *OECD publishes defined approaches for skin sensitization integrating non-animal methods (NAMs).* ALTEX – Alternatives to Animal Experimentation.

Asefa, E. M., Damtew, Y. T., & Ober, J. (2024). Pesticide water pollution, human health risks, and regulatory evaluation: A nationwide analysis in Ethiopia. *Journal of Hazardous Materials*, *478*, 135326. https://doi.org/10.1016/j.jhazmat.2024.135326

Asia-Pacific Economic Cooperation. (2024). *Data for chemicals.*

Bruce, R. D. (1985). An up-and-down procedure for acute toxicity testing. *Fundamental and Applied Toxicology*, *5*(1), 151–157. https://doi.org/10.1016/0272-0590(85)90059-4

California Department of Pesticide Regulation. (2024). *The up-and-down procedure for acute toxicity testing.*

Department of Agriculture Malaysia. (2020a). *Guidelines on toxicological data requirements for pesticide registration (GP 2/2020).* Pesticides Board, Kuala Lumpur. (Demonstrates national adoption of OECD/WHO guidelines).

Department of Agriculture Malaysia. (2020b). *Garis panduan data toksikologi untuk pendaftaran racun makhluk perosak (GP2/2020) [Guidelines on toxicological data for pesticide registration (GP2/2020)].*

EFSA Scientific Committee, Hardy, A., Benford, D., Halldorsson, T., Jeger, M., Knutsen, H. K., More, S., Naegeli, H., Noteborn, H., Ockleford, C., Ricci, A., Rychen, G., Silano, V., Solecki, R., Turck, D., Younes, M., Aquilina, G., Crebelli, R., Gürtler, R., ... Schlatter, J. (2017). Clarification of some aspects related to genotoxicity assessment. *EFSA Journal*, *15*(12), e05113. https://doi.org/10.2903/j.efsa.2017.5113

European Chemicals Agency. (2013). *Advice on skin and eye irritation testing helps reduce animal tests.*

European Medicines Agency. (2012). *ICH guideline S2(R1) on genotoxicity testing and data interpretation for pharmaceuticals intended for human use: Step 5*. EMA.

FAO/WHO. (2021). *Joint FAO/WHO meeting on pesticide residues (JMPR) – summary report*. FAO Plant Production and Protection Division & WHO.

Food and Agriculture Organization of the United Nations. (n.d.). *Joint FAO/WHO meeting on pesticide residues (JMPR)*.

Fowler, P., Bearzatto, A., Beevers, C., Booth, E. D., Donner, E. M., Gan, L., Hartmann, K., Meurer, K., Schutte, M. E., & Settivari, R. S. (2024). Assessment of the three-test genetic toxicology battery for groundwater metabolites. *Mutagenesis*, *39*(2), 146–155. https://doi.org/10.1093/mutage/gead037

Gupta, R. C. (2018). *Veterinary toxicology: Basic and clinical principles* (3rd ed.). Academic Press.

Herrman, J. L., & Younes, M. (1999). Background to the ADI/TDI/PTWI. *Regulatory Toxicology and Pharmacology*, *30*(2, Pt. 2), S109–S113. https://doi.org/10.1006/rtph.1999.1335

Hoffmann, S., Kleinstreuer, N., Alépée, N., Allen, D., Api, A. M., Ashikaga, T., ... Schepky, A. (2018). Non-animal methods to predict skin sensitization (I): the Cosmetics Europe database. *Critical Reviews in Toxicology*, *48*(5), 344–358. https://doi.org/10.1080/10408444.2018.1429385

Isgren, E., & Andersson, E. (2021). An environmental justice perspective on smallholder pesticide use in Sub-Saharan Africa. *Journal of Environment & Development*, *30*(1), 68–97. https://doi.org/10.1177/1070496520974407

Jirova, D., Basketter, D. A., Liebsch, M., et al. (2020). Alternative methods for dermal toxicity testing: Current status and future prospects. *Regulatory Toxicology and Pharmacology*, *119*, 104829. https://doi.org/10.1016/j.yrtph.2020.104829

Kapeleka, J. A., Ngowi, A. V., Mng'anya, S., Willis, S. E., Salmon, J. P., Tyrell, K. F., Williamson, S., Eddleston, M., & Stuart, A. M. (2025). Assessment of unintentional acute pesticide poisoning (UAPP) amongst cotton farmers in Tanzania. *Toxics*, *13*(4), 300. https://doi.org/10.3390/toxics13040300

Kleinstreuer, N., Hoffmann, S., Alépée, N., Allen, D., Ashikaga, T., Casey, W., ... Schepky, A. (2018). *Non-animal methods to predict skin sensitization (II): an assessment of defined approaches. Critical Reviews in Toxicology*, *48*(5), 359–374. https://doi.org/10.1080/10408444.2018.1429386

Lopes, I., Moreira-Santos, M., da Silva, E. M., Sousa, J. P., Guilhermino, L., Soares, A. M., & Ribeiro, R. (2007). In situ assays with tropical cladocerans to evaluate edge-of-field pesticide runoff toxicity. *Chemosphere*, *67*(11), 2250–2256. https://doi.org/10.1016/j.chemosphere.2006.12.009

Niemeyer, J. C., Chelinho, S., & Sousa, J. P. (2017). Soil ecotoxicology in Latin America: Current research and perspectives. *Environmental Toxicology and Chemistry*, *36*(7), 1795–1810. https://doi.org/10.1002/etc.3792

Organisation for Economic Co-operation and Development. (1981–2025). *OECD guidelines for the testing of chemicals, sections 1–5 (periodic updates through 2025)*. OECD Publishing.

Organisation for Economic Co-operation and Development. (2017). *Overview of the set of OECD genetic toxicology test guidelines and updates performed in 2014–2015* (2nd ed.). OECD Publishing.

Organisation for Economic Co-operation and Development. (2018). *Guidelines for the testing of chemicals: Acute oral toxicity – up-and-down procedure*. OECD Publishing.

Organisation for Economic Co-operation and Development. (2020). *Data mutual acceptance: OECD mutual acceptance of data (MAD) in the assessment of chemicals*. OECD Environment, Health and Safety News, No, 32.

Organisation for Economic Co-operation and Development. (2021). *Test No. 439: In vitro skin irritation: Reconstructed human epidermis test method*. OECD Publishing.

Organisation for Economic Co-operation and Development. (2023b). *OECD guidelines for the testing of chemicals*. OECD. (Includes test guidelines accessible via OECD iLibrary)

Organisation for Economic Co-operation and Development. (2023c). *Test no. 404: Acute dermal irritation/corrosion*. OECD Publishing.

Organisation for Economic Co-operation and Development. (2023d). *Test No. 405: Acute eye irritation/corrosion*. OECD Publishing.

Organisation for Economic Co-operation and Development. (2024). *First commenting round on the draft updated test guideline on the extended one-generation reproductive toxicity study*. OECD.

Raies, A. B., & Bajic, V. B. (2016). *In silico toxicology: Computational methods for the prediction of chemical toxicity*. *WIREs Computational Molecular Science*, *6*(2), 147–172. https://doi.org/10.1002/wcms.1240

Sheahan, M., Barrett, C. B., & Goldvale, C. (2017). *Pesticide use and human health in Africa south of the Sahara (IFPRI Discussion Paper 01629)*. International Food Policy Research Institute (IFPRI).

Stephens, M. L., Mak, N., & Beauchamp, T. L. (2021). *Alternatives to animal testing: Past, present, and future* (1st ed.). Academic Press.

Takeda, T., Suzuki, M., Kano, H., Matsumoto, M., & Umeda, Y. (2023). Clear evidence of the carcinogenic potential of anthracene: A 2-year feeding study in rats and mice. *Environmental Toxicology*, *38*(4), 709–726. https://doi.org/10.1002/tox.23722

United Nations. (2019). *Globally Harmonized System of Classification and Labelling of Chemicals (GHS)* ((8th revised ed.). United Nations.

United Nations Environment Programme. (n.d.). *Highly hazardous pesticides (HHPs).*

World Health Organization. (2020). *The WHO recommended classification of pesticides by hazard and guidelines to classification* (2019th ed.). WHO.

6

Toxicological Diagnosis

The most important step in managing animal toxicosis is to achieve an accurate diagnosis. An accurate toxicological diagnosis determines specific treatment and prevention measures to cure affected animals and prevent further deterioration of their condition. Until a definitive diagnosis is made, only supportive and symptomatic treatments can be provided. Accurate diagnosis requires comprehensive case knowledge, reliable laboratory analysis of suspected toxicants from submitted specimens, and proper interpretation of lab results (Gupta, 2018). In tropical veterinary practice – especially for livestock and wildlife – this process involves systematic steps from field investigations through laboratory confirmation.

This chapter elaborates on each of these steps, with emphasis on practical approaches for tropical veterinary contexts. Special consideration is given to common tropical livestock poisons (mycotoxins, nitrates/nitrites, organophosphates, cyanide, and toxic plants). Brief notes on toxicological threats to wildlife (e.g., snakebite envenomation, mycotoxins in feed, and heavy metal contamination) are included. Proper sample collection and submission protocols are described, along with strategies to interpret laboratory results (Figure 6.1).

History

A thorough case history is the cornerstone of toxicological diagnosis. The circumstances of the case and the sequence of events, as narrated by the animal's owner or caretaker, provide critical clues. In tropical farm settings, the veterinarian should ask detailed questions about farm management and environment, including:

- Feeding practices: Type of feed (pasture, stored hay, concentrates), recent changes in feed or water sources, and storage methods. For example, feeding moldy or spoiled feed in warm, humid climates raises suspicion of mycotoxins (e.g., aflatoxin in maize or peanuts).
- Water sources: Access to potentially contaminated water, such as stagnant ponds with algal blooms or runoff from fertilized fields.

- Pesticide and agrochemical use: Recent use of insecticides (organophosphates, carbamates) or herbicides on the premises, including how and where they were applied. In smallholder farms, organophosphate pesticides are common, and accidental overexposure or improper storage can lead to livestock poisoning.
- Presence of toxic plants or materials: Check grazing areas for poisonous plants (cyanogenic plants like sorghum or cassava, nephrotoxic oxalate-accumulators, hepatotoxic plants like *Lantana camara*, etc.). Ask if animals have been seen eating unusual weeds. Also look for discarded chemicals: old motor batteries (lead), oil or fuel spills, paint chips, or garbage that animals could access.
- Animal management and housing: Whether animals are confined or free-roaming is important (e.g., a free-roaming dog might ingest household chemicals or rodenticides). Confinement limits exposure to the immediate area, whereas roaming animals have broader access to toxins.
- Timeline of events: When was the animal last normal, progression of symptoms (hours or days), and whether multiple animals are affected. A rapid onset of symptoms in several herd-mates suggests a common-source poisoning (such as toxic feed or water), whereas a single animal could indicate idiosyncratic ingestion or a small-scale exposure.
- Previous occurrences and treatments: Any past similar illness in the herd or treatments already given in this case. Prior treatments can mask or alter clinical signs. For instance, knowing an animal received atropine before the vet's arrival is crucial if organophosphate poisoning is suspected, as atropine could partially reverse muscarinic signs.

Owners may provide lengthy narratives, sometimes with irrelevant details. The veterinarian must listen carefully for key clues and verify the accuracy of the history, recognizing it may be incomplete. Important information can often be gleaned even from a convoluted story. It is helpful to cross-check the owner's observations with a direct examination of the site (pasture, feed bins, storage sheds) whenever possible.

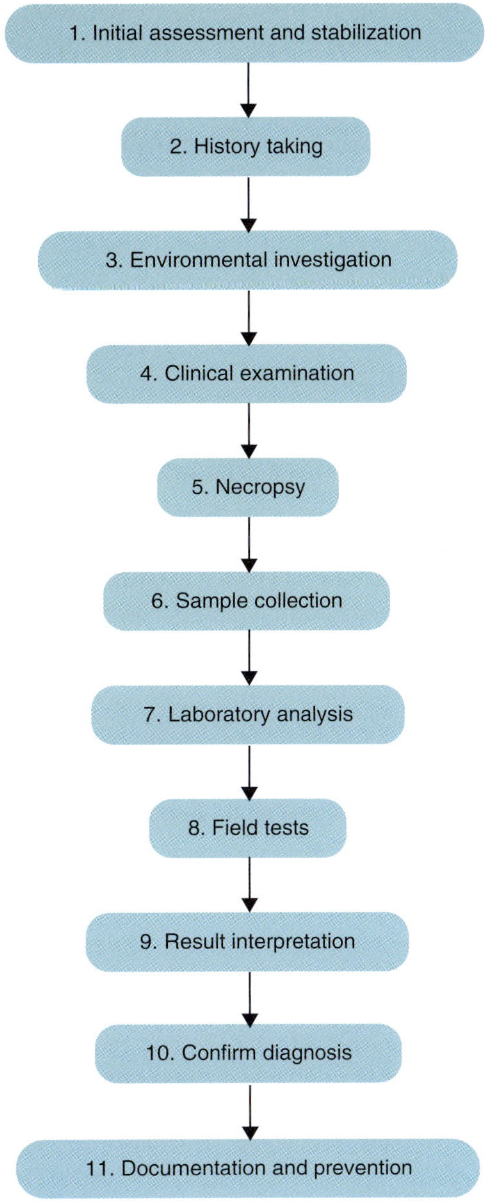

Figure 6.1 Stepwise diagnostic workflow for toxicological cases. A sequential approach from initial patient stabilization and history taking to final diagnosis, documentation, and preventive measures. Each step integrates clinical, environmental, and laboratory findings to ensure accurate identification of the toxic agent and implementation of corrective actions.

In wildlife or free-ranging animal cases, history may be limited or nonexistent. In such situations, environmental investigation becomes the primary "history." For example, if wild birds are found dead near a lake, inquire about recent algal blooms (cyanotoxins) or industrial runoff (heavy metals) in the area.

Information for laboratory submissions: When sending specimens to a lab, provide a concise case summary to guide the toxicologist. The submission form should include veterinarian and owner contact information, species/breed/age, number of animals at risk, detailed history of feed and management, observed clinical signs, and any treatments given. This context allows lab personnel to target likely toxicants, especially if initial tests are negative. A recommended list of information to include with submissions is given later under *Submission of Specimens*.

Clinical Signs

Careful observation and documentation of clinical signs are vital for both the field veterinarian and the toxicologist. The clinical presentation can provide strong clues about the toxin involved, although it must not be the sole basis for diagnosis. In tropical practice, where advanced diagnostics may be delayed, recognizing hallmark signs can facilitate timely intervention.

Describe clinical signs specifically. General terms like "GI disturbance" or "CNS signs" are not sufficient. Record exactly what is observed in each system, for example: profuse frothy salivation, muscle tremors, seizures, diarrhea, etc. Precise descriptions point to particular toxin categories:

- Neurological abnormalities: Note the type of tremors or convulsions, coordination issues, or behavior changes. For instance, opisthotonus (arching of the head and neck) and continuous convulsions in a dog strongly suggest metaldehyde (slug bait) poisoning (Blakley, 2021), whereas sudden tremors and seizures in cattle could indicate organochlorine pesticide exposure or tremorgenic mycotoxins from moldy feed.
- Gastrointestinal (GI) signs: Vomiting, bloat, diarrhea (note if hemorrhagic), tenesmus, etc. Irritant poisons (certain plants, arsenic) often cause severe diarrhea; organophosphate insecticides classically cause hypermotile diarrhea with abdominal pain due to cholinergic overstimulation (Gupta & Doss, 2024).
- Respiratory signs: Labored breathing (dyspnea), abnormal lung sounds, nasal discharge. Nitrate/nitrite poisoning causes rapid, open-mouthed breathing and brown/cyanotic mucous membranes (chocolate-brown blood) due to methemoglobinemia (Thompson, 2021; Hall, 2018). In contrast, cyanide poisoning may cause rapid breathing but bright red mucous membranes and sudden collapse (reflecting oxygenated venous blood). (Cyanide prevents cellular oxygen use.)
- Cardiovascular signs: Irregular heartbeat, weakness, collapse. Some plant cardiac glycosides (e.g., yellow oleander or *Taxus* yew) cause severe bradycardia or arrhythmias leading to acute collapse. Carbon monoxide (rare outdoors) or nitrite may cause chocolate-brown blood and weak pulses.
- Dermatologic signs: Primary or secondary photosensitization (sunburn-like lesions on unpigmented skin) suggests a hepatotoxic plant ingestion (e.g., *L. camara* or certain pyrrolizidine-alkaloid plants) causing liver failure and secondary photosensitivity.
- Urinary signs: Blood in urine or other renal findings may indicate specific toxins. For example, bracken fern poisoning causes hemorrhagic cystitis and bloody urine. Similarly, heavy metal exposure (arsenic) can lead to hemoglobinuria in severe cases (Garland, 2024).

- Other notable signs: Some poisonings have pathognomonic clues. The smell of vinegar or alcohol (acetaldehyde odor) in rumen contents is characteristic of metaldehyde toxicosis in livestock. A garlic-like odor on the breath may indicate organophosphate exposure (due to certain impurities) or phosphine gas from zinc/alkaline phosphide ingestion. Bright green vomitus can suggest colored rodenticide bait.

Remember that signs can evolve over time. A critical neurological sign might have resolved by the time of examination (e.g., transient seizures). Thus, obtaining the owner's report of initial signs – even seemingly minor ones – is important.

A syndromic approach can help: Match observed signs to toxin categories. Table 6.1 summarizes major toxins and their typical signs in livestock.

Table 6.1 Common toxic syndromes in tropical livestock: clinical signs, diagnostic remarks, and key references for major toxin categories.

Toxins	Clinical signs	Remarks	Citation(s)
Organophosphates and carbamates (insecticides)	Muscarinic signs – hypersalivation, lacrimation, urination, diarrhea (SLUD); nicotinic signs – muscle tremors, twitching, progressing to weakness, and paralysis; central signs – anxiety, seizures, coma; miosis, excessive bronchial secretion, colic in horses; death often due to respiratory failure.	Result from cholinesterase inhibition causing acetylcholine accumulation. Field test/ diagnosis: Markedly depressed blood cholinesterase activity supports diagnosis.	Gupta and Doss (2024)
Nitrate/nitrite (forage poisoning or fertilizer runoff)	Rapid onset hypoxia – tachypnea, tachycardia, exercise intolerance, muscle weakness, brownish/cyanotic mucous membranes; chocolate-brown blood in ruminants that fails to turn red on exposure to air; abortions may occur a few days after sublethal exposures.	Field test: Diphenylamine test on plant stems (dark blue = dangerous nitrate); test strips for nitrates in water or ocular fluid.	Thompson (2021); Hall (2018)
Plant toxins – *Lantana camara*	Hepatotoxicity → photosensitization (swelling/peeling of light-colored skin), depression, constipation → dark diarrhea, jaundice; ↑ liver enzymes	Diagnosis via history of exposure + elevated liver enzymes; plant material may be found in GI tract	Machado et al. (2023)
Plant toxins – *Brachiaria* (*Panicum*) grasses	Hepatogenous photosensitivity due to steroidal saponins	Common in tropical pastures; lesions in bile ducts	Low (2015)
Plant toxins – oxalate-accumulating plants (e.g., Napier grass on high N soils, setaria grass)	Acute hypocalcemia and nephrosis → tremors, weakness, recumbency, sudden death; Ca-oxalate crystals damage kidneys	Diagnose via kidney histology and oxalate crystal detection	Sidhu et al. (2014) Seawright et al. (1970).

(Continued)

Table 6.1 (Continued)

Toxins	Clinical signs	Remarks	Citation(s)
Plant toxins – cardiotoxic plants (yellow oleander, *Acokanthera*)	Cardiac arrhythmias, bradycardia, GI upset, sudden death	Confirm via oleandrin detection in GI content	Shridhar (2022) Van Wyk et al. (2002).
Plant toxins – Neurological plants (*Leucaena leucocephala)*	Causes alopecia, goiter, reduced fertility, growth retardation, and reproductive losses; effects are metabolic and reproductive rather than neurological.	Contains mimosine, metabolized to toxic pyridinediol compounds in susceptible ruminants lacking *Synergistes jonesii*. Diagnosis via plant identification + histopathology	Hammond (1995)
Plant toxins – Bracken fern	Prolonged ingestion → bone marrow suppression (anemia, leukopenia, hemorrhage) + polioencephalomalacia in monogastrics	Thiaminase activity in plants causes neuro signs in nonruminants	Tokarnia et al. (2002).
Cyanide (Prussic acid from plants like sorghums or industrial sources)	Peracute respiratory distress, excitement, muscle tremors, rapid collapse, convulsions; bright red venous blood; smell of bitter almonds (not always perceptible); death in minutes to hours.	Field test: Picrate paper test detects cyanogenic glycosides in plants/rumen (brick red color indicates cyanide release).	Cope (2021); Craigmill (1981)
Mycotoxins (Aflatoxins and others)	Aflatoxin: Chronic liver damage – ill thrift, reduced feed intake, icterus, anemia, hemorrhages; subacute – weakness, immunosuppression; acute high dose – sudden death with hemorrhages. Other mycotoxins: Ergot alkaloids – vasoconstriction, lameness, gangrene; Fumonisins – equine leukoencephalomalacia, pulmonary edema in pigs; Tremorgenic mycotoxins – tremors, ataxia, seizures.	Diagnosis: Demonstration of toxin in feed (lab analysis) with compatible lesions or clinical signs confirms mycotoxicosis.	Mostrom (2021)
Heavy metals	Lead – neurological signs (blindness, staggering, head pressing), GI stasis, anemia; copper – acute hemolytic crisis (icterus, hemoglobinuria); arsenic – violent gastroenteritis, dehydration, shock.	Diagnosis confirmed by elevated metal concentrations in blood/tissues (e.g., lead >0.35 ppm blood or >10 ppm liver in cattle; >8 ppm in liver can be fatal).	Assi et al. (2016) Blakley (2024) Garland (2024)

- Organophosphates and carbamates (insecticides): Muscarinic signs – excessive salivation, lacrimation, urination, diarrhea ("SLUD"); nicotinic signs – muscle tremors and fasciculations progressing to weakness and paralysis; central signs – anxiety, seizures, coma. Animals often have pinpoint pupils, bronchial secretions, and colic (in horses). Death is usually from respiratory failure. (Mechanism: cholinesterase inhibition leads to acetylcholine buildup.) Field test: markedly depressed blood cholinesterase activity supports diagnosis (Gupta & Doss, 2024).
- Nitrate/nitrite (forage or fertilizer poisoning): Sudden onset of hypoxia – rapid, labored breathing; muscle weakness; chocolate-brown mucous membranes. A classic sign is dark brown blood that does not redden when exposed to air (due to methemoglobin). Abortions can occur days later due to fetal hypoxia. Field test: diphenylamine paper on suspect plants – a rapid blue color indicates high nitrate. Commercial test strips can detect nitrates in water or bodily fluids (Thompson, 2021; Hall, 2018).
- Cyanide (prussic acid from plants like sorghum or industrial sources): Peracute respiratory distress and bright red venous blood (highly oxygenated but unusable). Animals may show excitement or tremors followed by rapid collapse and convulsions. A bitter-almond smell on rumen contents or breath (if present) supports cyanide exposure. Death can occur within minutes to hours. Field test: picrate paper on plant material or rumen contents – a brick-red color indicates cyanogenic glycosides (Cope, 2021; Craigmill, 1981).
- Mycotoxins (e.g., aflatoxin from moldy grains): Signs vary with toxin. Aflatoxin causes chronic liver damage: ill-thrift, anorexia, weight loss, jaundice, anemia, and bleeding due to hepatic failure (Mostrom, 2021). Immunosuppression leads to secondary infections. Acute high-dose exposure may cause sudden death with hemorrhages. Other mycotoxins: Ergot alkaloids (on grasses) cause vasoconstriction → lameness and gangrene; fumonisins (moldy corn) cause equine leukoencephalomalacia (neurological signs) and pig pulmonary edema; tremorgenic mycotoxins (e.g., from *Penicillium* fungi) cause fine muscle tremors, ataxia, and seizures. Diagnosis is confirmed by detecting the toxin in feed plus compatible lesions (Mostrom, 2021).
- Plant toxins (selected examples): Tropical regions host many poisonous plants. Examples include:
  - *L. camara*: Hepatotoxic – causes liver failure leading to secondary photosensitivity (swollen, peeling white areas on skin), jaundice, constipation followed by dark diarrhea, and weakness. Liver enzymes are markedly elevated (Machado et al., 2023).
  - *Brachiaria* (signal grass) and other *Panicum* grasses: Contain steroidal saponins; chronic ingestion causes hepatogenous photosensitivity (Low, 2015).
  - Oxalate-accumulating plants (e.g., *Napier grass* under high nitrogen, or *Setaria*): Cause acute hypocalcemia (tetany) and acute renal failure. Signs include severe muscle tremors, weakness, recumbency (similar to milk fever). Calcium oxalate crystals in kidneys may cause hemorrhagic nephritis, often with sudden death (Seawright et al., 1970; Sidhu et al., 2014).
  - Cardiotoxic plants (yellow oleander, *Thevetia*; *Acokanthera* spp.): Contain cardiac glycosides. Ingestion causes GI upset (vomiting, colic), bradycardia, arrhythmias, and acute collapse; often there are few lesions except for gastroenteritis. Diagnosis relies on history of access and detection of plant material in the stomach (Shridhar, 2022; Van Wyk et al., 2002).
  - *Leucaena leucocephala*: Contains mimosine, metabolized to toxic pyridinediols in ruminants. In animals lacking the bacterium *Synergistes jonesii*, metabolites cause alopecia, goiter, infertility, growth retardation, and high mortality, but no convulsions (Hammond, 1995).

- *Bracken fern*: Chronic ingestion causes bone marrow suppression in ruminants (anemia, leukopenia, hemorrhages) and polioencephalomalacia (neurological signs) in nonruminants (thiaminase action) (Tokarnia et al., 2002).

Diagnosis of plant poisonings relies on evidence of ingestion (finding plant material in the stomach or pasture) combined with compatible clinical and laboratory findings. Chemical analysis can detect some plant toxins (e.g., oleandrin from *Nerium oleander* in GI contents).

- Heavy metals (e.g., lead, copper, arsenic): Although not a "classic" tropical livestock toxin, heavy metal exposure is an emerging concern in tropical regions (informal mining, battery recycling). Clinical syndromes vary:
  - Lead: Often from ingested batteries or paint, causes neurological signs in cattle (blindness, staggering, head-pressing), GI stasis, and anemia. Subacute cases can show brain laminar cortical necrosis (polioencephalomalacia) detectable via UV fluorescence (Assi et al., 2016).
  - Copper: In sheep on high-copper diets, the liver accumulates copper that can suddenly release, causing acute hemolysis, hemoglobinuria, and jaundice (Blakley, 2024). Chronic copper poisoning may show hepatitis.
  - Arsenic: From old pesticides or contaminated water; causes severe gastroenteritis (vomiting, diarrhea), dehydration, and shock. Diagnosis is by elevated arsenic in blood or tissues (Garland, 2024).

Many of the syndromes above overlap, and animals may present with mixed signs if multiple organ systems are affected. Differential diagnoses (e.g., rabies, ketosis, colic) should be considered if they can mimic poisoning syndromes. Clinical signs guide the diagnostic process, but must be correlated with history and laboratory data.

Necropsy Findings

When an animal dies or is euthanized, necropsy is invaluable. Gross and microscopic findings can suggest a toxic cause or rule out other diseases. However, *not all poisons cause visible lesions*, and lesions, when present, may be nonspecific. Interpret necropsy findings cautiously:

- Extensive lesions (characteristic): Some toxins produce distinctive damage. For example, chronic copper toxicity leads to a yellow, friable liver and a gunmetal-gray kidney (from hemoglobin casts). Aflatoxin poisoning may cause a pale, fibrotic liver. *Lantana* ingestion can cause an enlarged cirrhotic liver. Anticoagulant rodenticides (more common in small animals) cause widespread hemorrhages.
- Minimal or no lesions: Many poisons leave little to see. Cyanide poisoning usually has no specific lesions (maybe pink tissues or bitter-almond odor). Urea (nonprotein nitrogen [NPN]) poisoning causes rapid bloat but no lesions. Strychnine causes violent convulsions but no lesions except trauma from injuries. Organophosphates typically do not leave gross lesions (maybe pulmonary congestion, GI motility evidence).

- Specific lesions: Some toxins have hallmark lesions. Calcium oxalate crystals may be visible in kidney tubules (oxalate poisoning). Lead can cause classic brain cortical necrosis. Zinc phosphide ingestion leaves a garlic-like odor and severe gastric mucosal hemorrhage.
- Histopathology: Microscopic examination often reveals clues. For instance, centrilobular hepatic necrosis is consistent with acute toxin-induced liver injury (seen in aflatoxicosis or phosphorus poisoning). Demyelination in the spinal cord may occur with chronic cyanide exposure or neurotoxic plant poisoning. Histopathology also rules out infection (e.g., granulomas for TB).

A full necropsy should be performed in suspected poisonings, especially if legal or commercial consequences are likely. Document all lesions carefully. Even if lesions are absent, the necropsy can provide alternative diagnoses or tissues for toxicology. In tropical climates, carcasses decompose rapidly, so prompt necropsy is critical. If delay is unavoidable, refrigerate (not freeze) the carcass or organs of interest, since freezing can create artifacts.

During necropsy, collect representative samples for toxicology (see *Sample Collection* below). For example, collect liver, kidney, brain, fat, stomach contents, etc., in appropriate containers. If a specific poison is suspected, sample target organs (e.g., whole brain for pesticides or heavy metals). Since some toxins distribute unevenly, multiple samples increase detection chances. In summary, necropsy findings can range from dramatic to subtle or absent; use them in concert with history, clinical signs, and lab analysis to reach a conclusion.

Chemical Analyses

Analytical chemistry is pivotal in confirming a toxicological diagnosis by detecting trace toxins in biological, feed, or environmental samples (Lee et al., 2021). However, lab results are not definitive proof on their own – they must fit the clinical picture. The most robust diagnoses come from findings consistent with history, signs, and necropsy. Key principles for chemical analysis include:

- Directed testing: Given the vast number of potential toxicants, testing should be targeted to likely suspects based on history and signs. Broad toxicology screens are time-consuming and costly. Use the case information to narrow possibilities. For example, if cattle die after grazing fertilized fields, test for nitrates/nitrites and cyanide before testing unrelated compounds.
- Avoiding false results: Proper sample selection and handling minimize false negatives/positives. False negatives can occur if the wrong tissue is tested (e.g., strychnine may be absent in liver but present in stomach contents). False positives may arise from laboratory contamination or misidentification. Laboratories should operate under quality systems (e.g., ISO/IEC 17025:2017) to ensure reliable results (ISO, 2017; UNODC, 1995).
- Sensitive and specific methods: Use analytical techniques suited to the toxin class. Gas chromatography–mass spectrometry (GC–MS) provides high sensitivity and specificity (detecting parts-per-billion) for volatile and semi-volatile organic compounds (Mbughuni et al., 2016). Liquid chromatography–tandem mass spectrometry (LC–MS/MS) allows analysis of polar, nonvolatile toxins (Kaufmann et al., 2011). Inductively coupled plasma mass spectrometry (ICP-MS) is ideal for trace metals (Beauchemin, 2002). Immunoassays (e.g., enzyme-linked immunosorbent assay [ELISA] and

radioimmunoassay [RIA]) are useful for certain toxins or rapid screening; for example, snake venom detection kits (immunoassays) exist in some regions (notably Australia) but are generally limited (Isbister et al., 2012).

- Turnaround time: Rapid results are often needed. Some tests (e.g., cholinesterase levels, dipstick color tests) can yield results in 2–4 days (Labcorp, 2024). In urgent cases, preliminary field tests can guide immediate action. However, comprehensive screens (e.g., full GC–MS panels) take longer – often several days in private labs or up to a month in public labs (DEA, 2021). Veterinarians should communicate urgency to the lab and take interim control measures (e.g., withholding suspect feed).
- Interpreting "none detected": A "no toxin detected" result does *not* prove absence of poisoning. The toxin might have been absent in that sample, metabolized/excreted, or below the assay's detection limit (Moeller et al., 2017). For example, cyanide is volatile and may disappear from blood after death. If clinical suspicion remains, consult the lab for more sensitive tests or alternate samples (e.g., test forage for cyanogenic potential).
- Interpreting "detected": Finding a toxin in a sample does not automatically mean it caused the illness. Low-level background residues of certain compounds (e.g., DDT in fat) can appear without causing acute disease (Lee et al., 2014; Pietrzak-Fiećko, 2018). Always ask: Is the detected concentration high enough to cause the observed signs? Labs often provide toxic reference ranges. For example, cattle liver lead >15 ppm is toxic (background <1 ppm), and milk aflatoxin >0.5 ppb is illegal in many countries (Mostrom, 2021). Compare results to known toxic thresholds.
- Multiple toxins: Sometimes more than one toxin is found. This could indicate multiple exposures or a single source with mixed contaminants (e.g., industrial waste). Evaluate levels and toxicities. Prioritize the compound present at a toxic concentration first.
- Differential diagnosis via lab: Toxicology labs can also help rule out other causes. For example, to distinguish nitrate poisoning from cyanide: Ocular fluid is best for nitrate analysis (Ensley & Carlson, n.d.; Kahn & Line, 2020). Nitrate causes methemoglobinemia (chocolate-brown blood), whereas cyanide yields cherry-red venous blood that resists oxygenation (Ensley & Carlson, n.d.; Kahn & Line, 2020). Combined with clinical signs and field tests, lab results can refine the diagnosis.

In summary, chemical analysis is a powerful diagnostic tool, but only when the right tests and samples are chosen, and results are interpreted in context. Veterinarians should work closely with the diagnostic lab, providing full case information to achieve meaningful results.

- Laboratory animal tests: Historically, biological assays using lab animals were used to confirm toxins (e.g., mouse bioassay for botulinum toxin; feeding suspect liver to test animals to elicit coagulopathy). A positive bioassay (e.g., chickens developing tremors after eating suspect feed) can confirm a toxin's presence. However, negative results do not guarantee safety (toxicity may be species-specific, dose-dependent, or the toxin may have degraded). Ethical and practical issues now limit such testing, and chemical analysis is preferred. Legal restrictions often prohibit intentional animal dosing for diagnostics.

  Laboratory animal tests may still be used in complex cases when a toxin is not identifiable chemically. For example, mysterious "tremorgenic syndromes" were historically confirmed by extracting feed and feeding it to mice to reproduce neurological signs (Pellett, 2019). In modern practice, such tests are rare and typically done by specialized labs under strict protocols.

Interpretation of Chemical Analysis Results

Interpreting toxicology lab data requires correlating lab findings with clinical observations. Lab results should never stand alone as proof of poisoning. Consider the following guidelines:

- Positive results: A detected toxin means the substance was found, but the **level** matters. Questions to ask: Is the concentration high enough to cause the illness? (e.g., liver lead at 15 ppm is clearly toxic in cattle). Are there regulatory or published thresholds? (e.g., milk aflatoxin M1 >0.5 ppb is illegal – presence above that confirms hazardous exposure, even if cows seem well). Could the finding be incidental? (e.g., trace levels of polychlorinated biphenyls (PCBs) in fat may reflect environmental exposure, not acute poisoning, unless clinical signs match.) Only if clinical signs and lesions align with the toxin should it be deemed causative.
- Negative results: "No toxin detected" is not the end. Check if the correct samples were tested – some toxins degrade rapidly in certain tissues. For example, cyanide dissipates quickly; a normal blood result may be due to delayed sampling or improper storage (Cornell University Animal Health Diagnostic Center, 2023). If suspicion remains, test other samples (water, rumen, ocular fluid) or use more sensitive methods. Remember assay detection limits; a toxin might be present below that threshold. Consulting the lab toxicologist is prudent when results conflict with clinical suspicion.
- Re-evaluation: If all tests for suspected toxins are negative, reconsider other causes (infectious or metabolic diseases). Labs can perform broad-spectrum unknown screens if poisoning is still suspected, but these are costly and time-consuming.
- Consult resources: Use reference texts or lab guidelines for toxic concentration ranges. The Merck Veterinary Manual (Kahn & Line, 2020) and Small Animal Toxicology (Peterson & Talcott, 2013) often list critical values (e.g., rumen ammonia-N >80 mg% suggests urea poisoning; blood acetylcholinesterase <25% of normal indicates organophosphate poisoning). Many diagnostic labs also provide interpretive comments on reports; use them and call the lab's toxicologist for clarification if needed.

Remember: Accurate diagnosis relies on the totality of evidence. The history (access to toxin), clinical signs (e.g., tremors in a dog plus finding of strychnine in stomach), necropsy findings, and lab data must all align. If contradictions arise (e.g., a toxin found that doesn't match the signs), re-examine the case. It is possible to encounter a coincidental disease outbreak with an unrelated low-level toxin exposure, so clinical judgment is key to synthesizing a final diagnosis.

Sample Collection and Submission Protocols

A successful toxicological investigation depends on proper sample collection and submission. In tropical regions, samples can degrade quickly, so special care (cold chain, clean containers) is needed. The goal is to provide the right specimen, in the right condition, to the lab. Guidelines for clinicians and researchers include:

General Guidelines for Sample Collection

- Personal protective equipment (PPE): Always wear gloves (and other protective gear) when handling potentially toxic samples. Many poisons can be absorbed or ingested by humans. Change gloves between handling different animals or samples to avoid cross-contamination.
- Choose appropriate specimens: Select samples based on the suspected toxicant, time since exposure, and whether the animal is alive or dead. Common samples include:
  - Live animals: Whole blood (5–10 mL in heparin **or** ethylenediaminetetraacetic acid (EDTA) tubes; more for broad screens), serum (for biochemistry or specific toxins; collect in trace-element-free tubes for metals), urine (5–10 mL), vomitus or gastric lavage fluid, feces, and any suspected materials the animal ingested (chewed plants, feed, bait).
  - Deceased animals: A full set of fresh tissues is ideal. Collect brain, liver, kidneys, heart blood (or clotted blood), bladder urine, stomach/rumen contents, intestinal contents, fat, and any lesions of interest. Also collect vitreous (aqueous) humor from the eye (2–3 mL if possible) – it is useful postmortem for nitrates, urea, etc. Preserve samples for histopathology (e.g., fixed liver and kidney) separately. Hair or skin can be submitted for chronic heavy metal or pesticide exposure (e.g., arsenic in hair).
- Sample size: Collect ample material. Toxicology tests often require more than routine samples. When in doubt, collect extra. For example, >100 g of suspect feed or rumen content; fist-sized (≥50 g) pieces of liver or kidney; 100+ mL of suspect water. If shipping a whole small animal, chill or freeze the intact carcass.
- Containers: Use clean, leak-proof, nonreactive containers. Glass jars with airtight lids are preferred for volatile toxins (cyanide, some organophosphates) to prevent losses. Plastic screw-top bottles or Whirl-Pak bags work for most samples. Do not reuse food containers. Label each container with animal ID, specimen type, and date.
- Avoid cross-contamination: Collect samples in order from cleanest to most contaminated. Draw blood first with clean syringes and vacutainers. Then collect urine. During necropsy, change gloves and use clean instruments for each sample. For example, remove the brain before opening the gut, because gut contents can contaminate tools. If collecting multiple environmental samples (soil, plants, water), use separate tools or sterilize between samples.
- Environmental samples: If poisoning is suspected, sample the environment. Collect feed (0.5–1 kg if mixed, or representative samples from different bales/bags). If moldy feed is involved, submit both moldy and normal portions (label them). Sample suspect pasture plants (a full plant sample including roots if possible). Water samples (500 mL^{-1} L) from drinking sources. Also consider paint chips, soil, engine oil, fertilizers, pesticides – any substances animals might contact. Document each sample's origin (e.g., "pond water at back of barn").

Preservation and Storage

Cold is your friend for toxicology samples (Michigan State University Veterinary Diagnostic Laboratory, 2023). Whenever possible, freeze fresh tissues and fluids (–20°C) soon after collection. Freezing halts microbial growth and enzyme activity that can degrade toxins (for example, cyanide and many plant toxins diminish in warm samples). Exceptions: Do not freeze whole blood or serum tubes before separating (they will hemolyze). Instead, keep blood refrigerated (4°C) if analysis is within a few days, or centrifuge and freeze serum/plasma for longer storage. Note: Some tests require fresh blood (e.g., cholinesterase activity assays should use fresh refrigerated blood within a few days).

For volatile toxins (cyanide, organophosphates), use airtight containers and freeze promptly. Some labs add preservatives (e.g., mercuric chloride drops) when freezing isn't possible (such as for ammonia in rumen fluid). Formalin is generally an enemy of chemical analysis – never place samples for toxin assays in fixatives. (Only collect formalin-fixed tissue for histopathology.) The only exception is if a laboratory's protocol specifically requests formalin (e.g., some labs ask for half the liver fresh and half in formalin or preserve kidney in formalin to allow microscopic examination for oxalate crystals).

Packaging and Shipping

Package specimens securely for transport: Primary containers (vials/bags) should be leak-proof, cushioned with absorbent material, inside a sturdy secondary container or cooler, and then placed in a rigid outer container with proper hazard labeling. Clearly mark packages "Diagnostic samples – not for human consumption." Use triple-layer packaging if shipping by air (according to IATA guidelines). Keep samples separated by type (wrap each organ individually to avoid contamination, e.g., gut contents seeping onto liver). Use ice packs or dry ice for frozen samples (follow shipping regulations and labeling). Ship samples to the lab as quickly as possible (overnight preferred).

Ice packs: Include enough to keep samples cold but ensure containers don't freeze solid unless appropriate. Clearly identify frozen vs. refrigerated shipments. Figure 6.2 illustrates recommended triple-layer packaging:

Submission Forms and Case Information

Accurate lab results depend on complete submission forms. Include all pertinent details, echoing the History checklist above: veterinarian and owner contacts; species/breed/age; number of animals exposed or affected; duration of illness; clinical signs; treatments given; and suspected toxicants or sources. If legal action or forensic requirements apply (e.g., malicious poisoning of livestock or wildlife), contact the lab beforehand to initiate a proper chain-of-custody procedure (sealed samples, documentation) (Table 6.2).

Table 6.3 provides quick-reference recommendations for preferred specimens, amounts, and handling for selected toxins (e.g., freeze whole blood, rumen content, and urine immediately for urea poisoning; collect ocular fluid and frozen samples for nitrates; use trace-element-free tubes for lead/methylmercury analysis).

Special Considerations: Tropical Wildlife

While this chapter focuses on livestock, tropical wildlife toxicology is an emerging concern and sometimes overlaps with livestock cases (e.g., birds, rodents sharing crops or pastures). Wildlife cases have unique challenges: often no history, the animal cannot be observed closely, and carcasses may

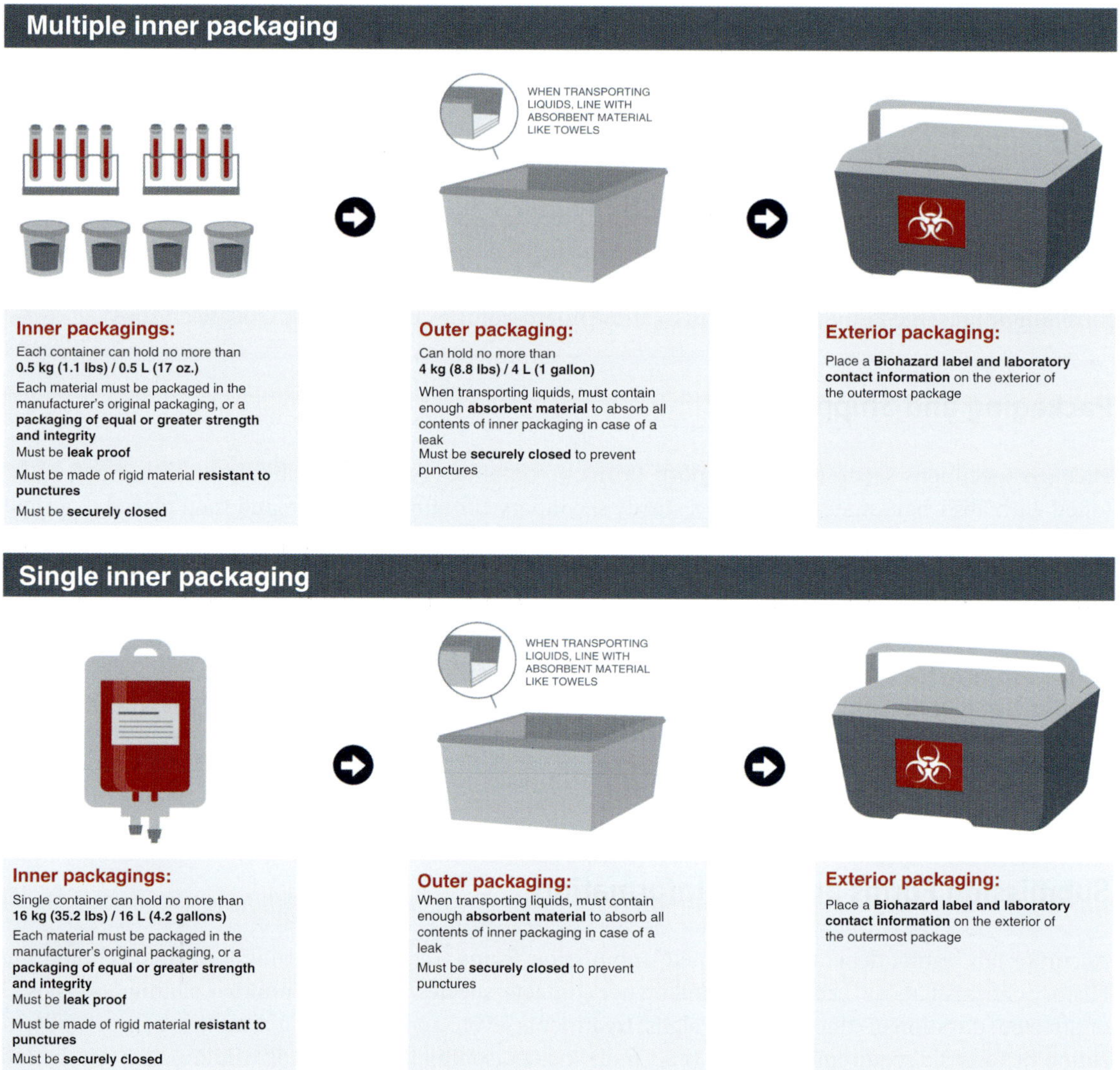

Figure 6.2 Triple-layer specimen packaging for veterinary diagnostics: a leak-proof primary container, absorbent secondary layer, and a labeled rigid outer box – ensuring safe transport and sample integrity (University of California, Davis, Environmental Health & Safety, 2025).

decompose rapidly in the field. Nonetheless, the same principles apply (environmental "history," clinical signs, necropsy, and testing).

Common wildlife threats in tropical regions include:

- Snakebite envenomation: Venomous snakes abound in the tropics, affecting domestic animals (dogs, horses) and wildlife (elephants, primates, antelope). Diagnosis is primarily clinical: history of snake

Table 6.2 Author-created quick guide to commonly submitted specimen types, typical diagnostic applications, and general handling/shipping practices for toxicology and related investigations. Guidance is compiled from publicly available veterinary diagnostic laboratory recommendations; specific requirements vary by laboratory and by test requested (Cornell University Animal Health Diagnostic Center, 2023; Michigan State University Veterinary Diagnostic Laboratory, 2023; University of Kentucky Veterinary Diagnostic Laboratory, n.d.).

Specimen (typical container)	Typical uses in suspected toxicosis	General handling and storage (diagnostic-lab guidance)	Shipping/submission notes
Whole blood (EDTA/heparin as requested)	Hematology; selected tox related tests	Keep **chilled/refrigerated**; protect from heat; follow receiving lab tube requirements	**Ship promptly (overnight preferred)**; include full history and suspected toxins
Serum/plasma (preferably separated)	Biochemistry; selected toxin/drug panels	Keep **refrigerated**; **freeze** where appropriate if shipping is delayed or long storage is needed	Ship promptly with cold packs; confirm fraction needed with lab
Citrated plasma	Coagulation (case-dependent)	Refrigerate and ship promptly; follow lab-specific processing instructions	Avoid temperature extremes
Urine (leak-proof)	Selected toxicology screening; adjunct urinalysis	Refrigerate; freeze if permitted and shipping is delayed	Prevent leakage; provide context
Gastric/rumen contents, vomitus, bait/unknown	Toxin screening/identification of ingesta	**Freeze when possible**; otherwise refrigerate and ship immediately	Double-bag; label clearly
Fresh tissues for toxicology (liver, kidney, brain, fat; case-dependent)	Confirmatory toxicology (organic compounds/metals)	**Freeze tissues when possible**; otherwise refrigerate and ship immediately	Separate containers; confirm preferred tissues/amounts with lab
Formalin-fixed tissues	Histopathology support	Fix in 10% neutral buffered formalin (standard histopath)	Keep separate from fresh/frozen specimens
Swabs (culture/PCR if requested)	Microbiology/molecular tests when indicated	Use appropriate transport medium; keep cool unless instructed otherwise	Follow lab kits/rules
Prepared slides	Cytology	Keep dry; protect from breakage	Stable if packed properly

encounter or fang marks, followed by syndromic signs. Neurotoxic bites (cobras, kraits) cause drooling, paralysis, respiratory failure; hemotoxic bites (vipers) cause painful swelling, edema, and coagulopathy (bleeding). Sea snakes cause muscle breakdown (myotoxicity), and some rattlesnakes combine effects. If a free-ranging animal is found neurological or bleeding, consider snakebite. Lab clues: incoagulable blood for viper bites; transient blood chemistry changes. Confirmatory tests (venom detection kits) exist in a few regions (e.g., Australia) but are generally limited (Seifert et al., 2022; Knudsen et al., 2021). Treatment (antivenom) should be given on suspicion. On necropsy, finding fang wounds with localized

Table 6.3 Recommended specimens, amounts, and submission requirements for selected poisons in veterinary toxicology.

Poisons or analysis	Specimens	Amount required	Submission requirements
Ammonia (urea/NPN poisoning)	Whole blood: refrigerate/chill (do not freeze) Rumen content/urine: freeze when possible; ship promptly	5 mL 100 g 5 mL	Freeze immediately. For rumen content, if immediate freezing not possible, add 1–2 drops saturated $HgCl_2$ per 100 g.
Urea/nonprotein nitrogen	Feed Rumen content	100 g each	Keep all specimens frozen.
Nitrates/nitrites	Forage/feed Water Eye fluid (aqueous humor) Serum/plasma	100 g 50–100 mL 2–5 mL 5 mL	Freeze plant and water samples. Refrigerate eye fluid and blood (do not freeze blood). Use field test strips as quick screen; confirm via lab.
Metals (Lead, mercury, arsenic, copper, zinc, etc.)	Whole blood (EDTA) Liver Kidney Urine (if As or Hg suspected) Suspect source (paint, soil, feed, water)	5–10 mL 50 g 50 g 50 mL 100 g/100 mL	Use royal-blue top trace element tubes. Freeze or refrigerate tissues; refrigerate blood. Avoid contamination – use stainless steel/plastic tools and new gloves.
Pesticides (Organochlorines, organophosphates, carbamates)	Brain Fat Liver Kidney Stomach/rumen content Blood/serum	½ brain (5–10 g) 50–100 g 50 g 50 g 100 g 10 mL	Freeze all except whole blood for cholinesterase test (keep refrigerated). For OP/carbamate, run blood cholinesterase test fresh.
Herbicides (paraquat, diquat)	Stomach/rumen content Urine Sprayed plant/hay	200 g 50 mL 100 g	Use plastic containers (paraquat adsorbs to glass). Freeze content and plant samples; refrigerate urine.
Cyanide	Whole blood Liver Suspect plants/feed Rumen content	10 mL 50 g 200 g leaves/100 g feed 100 g	Freeze immediately in airtight containers; keep frozen during transit.
Oxalate (plant-based nephrotoxins)	Whole plants (fresh forage) Kidney	5–6 plants Whole organ	Do not chop plants; freeze immediately. Keep one kidney in formalin for histopathology, freeze the other for chemical analysis.
Mycotoxins	Feed Stomach/rumen content	1–2 kg feed 100 g	Freeze feed and contents. For fungal culture, keep a portion of feed dry in paper bag.
Poisonous plants	Fresh plant samples (flowers, leaves, roots, seeds if present)	Sufficient for botanical ID	Send in sealed plastic bag with ice packs (not in direct sun). Do not add water. Double bag large branches/plants.

hemorrhage and tissue necrosis supports snake envenomation. Ongoing research aims for field venom tests, but diagnosis is currently mainly clinical (Seifert et al., 2022).

- Aflatoxicosis in wildlife: Wild animals can also ingest moldy feeds or garbage containing aflatoxins. Mortality in wild birds (ducks, pigeons) or captive primates has been traced to eating aflatoxin-contaminated grain or peanuts. Waterfowl die after consuming moldy corn in fields. Diagnosis mirrors livestock: Look for hepatic lesions (fatty change, hemorrhage) and test feed or GI content for aflatoxin. Wildlife may be more vulnerable if malnourished. In die-offs, submitting multiple carcasses or pooled samples increases detection likelihood.
- Heavy metals: Wildlife in tropical areas face environmental metal exposure. Lead poisoning is well known: Vultures and raptors suffer lead toxicosis from ingesting fragments of lead ammunition in carrion, and waterfowl ingest lead shot or mine runoff (Pain & Green, 2019). Clinical signs in birds include neurological impairment (ataxia, wing droop) and green diarrhea (from bile). Live birds with >0.2 ppm blood lead are considered poisoned; >0.5 ppm often lethal (Cornell Wildlife Health Lab, n.d.). Radiographs of bird gizzards can reveal ingested lead. Other metals: Mercury accumulates in fish and aquatic food chains; fur, feather, or egg testing can indicate exposure. Cadmium and arsenic poisonings occur in birds near mines or industrial waste (Cornell Wildlife Health Lab, n.d.).
- Pesticide poisonings: Illegal pesticide use can kill wildlife. Carbamate and organophosphate insecticides are sometimes deployed against predators (e.g., poison baits for wild cats), unintentionally killing scavengers (vultures, eagles). A cluster of dead raptors near poisoned carcasses is a red flag. Diagnosis is by chemical analysis of stomach contents/tissues for the pesticide and measuring cholinesterase activity in the brain of dead birds (low activity confirms OP/carbamate poisoning). Affected animals show convulsions, salivation, and paralysis.
- Plant and marine toxins: Wildlife encounter natural toxins too. For example, African bush elephants (*Loxodonta africana*) sometimes eat *Dichapetalum cymosum* ("gifblaar"), which causes fatal cardiac arrest from glycosides (Brain & Fox, 1994). Marine wildlife ingest algal biotoxins: fish-eating birds and mammals accumulate saxitoxin and domoic acid from algal blooms, leading to mass seabird and marine mammal die-offs (Rocke, 1999; Van Hemert et al., 2020). These cases require specialized tests (e.g., mouse bioassays, LC–MS for specific biotoxins). In wildlife investigations, a One Health perspective is useful: Diagnosing toxicoses in wildlife can prevent harm to livestock and humans. For instance, identifying pesticide poisoning in vultures prompted interventions to protect livestock and water sources.

Investigating wildlife poisonings often requires collaboration among veterinarians, biologists, and toxicologists. Maintain chain of custody if criminal activity is suspected (e.g., poisoning of protected species). Sample collection follows the same protocols, though obtaining fresh tissues or blood from wild animals may be challenging (e.g., capture vs. found carcass).

Conclusion

Toxicological diagnosis in tropical veterinary medicine requires a detective-like approach: combining thorough history-taking, detailed clinical observation, systematic sample collection, and sophisticated lab analysis. Clinicians must act pragmatically – stabilizing animals and preventing further exposure – while pursuing confirmatory tests. The structured approach outlined here (history, clinical signs, necropsy, sample submission, chemical analysis, and interpretation) will improve success in identifying poisoning causes in livestock and wildlife.

Preventive toxicology is equally important. Lessons from each diagnosis should inform future prevention: Educate farmers about safe feed storage to avoid mycotoxins, advocate alternatives to lead ammunition, promote judicious pesticide use, etc. Tropical regions pose unique challenges (high environmental toxin burdens, rapid carcass decomposition, limited laboratory access), but careful planning and communication with diagnostic laboratories can overcome these hurdles.

In all cases, maintain a critical thinking approach: consider differentials, confirm suspicions with evidence, and don't jump to conclusions. Toxicology is detective work – by gathering all clues and using the right tools, the veterinary investigator can crack the case, saving animal lives and protecting public health.

References

Assi, M. A., Hezmee, M. N. M., Haron, A. W., Sabri, M. Y., & Rajion, M. A. (2016). The detrimental effects of lead on human and animal health. *Veterinary World*, *9*(6), 660–671. https://doi.org/10.14202/vetworld.2016.660-671

Beauchemin, D. (2002). Inductively coupled plasma mass spectrometry. *Analytical Chemistry*, *74*(12), 2873–2894. https://doi.org/10.1021/ac020254y

Blakley, B. R. (2021). *Metaldehyde poisoning in animals*. MSD Veterinary Manual. Reviewed/Revised May 2021; Modified Mar 2025. Available at: https://www.msdvetmanual.com/toxicology/metaldehyde-poisoning/metaldehyde-poisoning-in-animals

Brain, C., & Fox, V. E. B. (1994). Suspected cardiac glycoside poisoning in elephants (*Loxodonta africana*). *Journal of the South African Veterinary Association*, *65*(4), 173–174. https://journals.co.za/doi/10.10520/AJA00382809_1512

Cope, R.B., 2021. Cyanide poisoning in animals. Merck Veterinary Manual. Available at: https://www.merckvetmanual.com/toxicology/cyanide-poisoning/cyanide-poisoning-in-animals (accessed 15 January 2026).

Cornell University Animal Health Diagnostic Center. (2023). Sampling for toxicology screens. Available at: https://www.vet.cornell.edu/animal-health-diagnostic-center/testing/testing-protocols-interpretations/sampling-toxicology-screens (accessed 15 January 2026).

Cornell Wildlife Health Lab. (n.d.). *Lead toxicosis*. Cornell University College of Veterinary Medicine. https://cwhl.vet.cornell.edu/disease/lead-toxicosis

Craigmill, A. L. (1981). Rapid field tests for detection of cyanide and nitrate in plants. *California Veterinary Toxicology Newsletter*, *1*(3), 1–4.

Drug Enforcement Administration (DEA). (2021). *2021 Toxicology Laboratory Survey Report (NFLIS-Tox)*. U.S. Department of Justice, Drug Enforcement Administration, Diversion Control Division. Available at: https://www.nflis.deadiversion.usdoj.gov/nflisdata/docs/NFLIS_2021ToxicologyLabSurvey.pdf. (accessed 15 January 2026)

Ensley, S., & Carlson, M. (n.d.). *Nitrate (NO_3) toxicosis*. University of Nebraska–Lincoln Veterinary Toxicology. https://vbms.unl.edu/nitrate-toxicosis

Garland, T. (2024). Inorganic arsenical toxicosis in animals. Merck Veterinary Manual. https://www.merckvetmanual.com/toxicology/arsenic-poisoning/inorganic-arsenical-toxicosis-in-animals

Gupta, R. C. (2018). *Veterinary toxicology: Basic and clinical principles* (3rd ed.). Academic Press.

Gupta, R. C., & Doss, R. B. (2024). *Organophosphate toxicosis in animals*. Merck Veterinary Manual. https://www.merckvetmanual.com/toxicology/insecticide-and-acaricide-organic-toxicity/organophosphate-toxicosis-in-animals

Hall, J. O. (2018). Nitrate- and nitrite-accumulating plants. In R. C. Gupta (Ed.), *Veterinary toxicology* (3rd ed., pp. 941–946). Academic Press.

Hammond, A. C. (1995). Leucaena toxicosis and its control in ruminants. *Journal of Animal Science*, *73*(5), 1487–1492. https://doi.org/10.2527/1995.7351487x

International Organization for Standardization. (2017). *ISO/IEC 17025:2017 – general requirements for the competence of testing and calibration laboratories*. ISO.

Isbister, G. K., Brown, S. G. A., Page, C. B., McCoubrie, D. L., Greene, S. L., Buckley, N. A., & The ASP Investigators. (2012). Snakebite in Australia: A practical approach to diagnosis and treatment. *Medical Journal of Australia*, *197*(2), 98–102. https://doi.org/10.5694/mja12.11172

Kahn, C. M., & Line, S. (2020). *The Merck veterinary manual* (11th ed.). Merck & Co., Inc.

Kaufmann, A., Butcher, P., Maden, K., Walker, S., & Widmer, M. (2011). Development of an improved high resolution mass spectrometry based multi-residue method for veterinary drugs in various food matrices. *Analytica Chimica Acta*, *700*(1–2), 86–94. https://doi.org/10.1016/j.aca.2010.11.034

Knudsen, C., Jürgensen, J. A., Føns, S., Haack, A. M., Friis, R. U. W., Dam, S. H., ... Laustsen, A. H. (2021). Snakebite envenoming: Diagnosis and diagnostics. *Frontiers in Immunology*, *12*, 661457. https://doi.org/10.3389/fimmu.2021.661457

LabCorp. (2024). *Cholinesterase, plasma test (Test 160200)*. https://www.labcorp.com/tests/160200/cholinesterase-plasma

Lee, D.-H., Porta, M., Jacobs, D. R., & Vandenberg, L. N. (2014). Chlorinated persistent organic pollutants, obesity, and type 2 diabetes. *Endocrine Reviews*, *35*(4), 557–601. https://doi.org/10.1210/er.2013-1084

Lee, J. S., Cha, Y. S., Yeon, S., Kim, T. Y., Lee, Y., Choi, J.-G., Cha, K.-C., Lee, K. H., & Kim, H. (2021). Changes in diagnosis of poisoning in patients in the emergency room using systematic toxicological analysis with the National Forensic Service. *Journal of Korean Medical Science*, *36*(18). https://doi.org/10.3346/jkms.2021.36.e118

Low, S. G. (2015). Signal grass (Brachiaria decumbens) toxicity in grazing ruminants. *Agriculture*, *5*(4), 971–990. https://doi.org/10.3390/agriculture5040971

Machado, M., Oliveira, L. G. S., Schild, C. O., Boabaid, F., Lucas, M., Buroni, F., Castro, M. B., & Riet-Correa, F. (2023). Lantana camara poisoning in cattle that took refuge during a storm in a forest invaded by this plant. *Toxicon*, *229*, 107124. https://doi.org/10.1016/j.toxicon.2023.10.124

Mbughuni, M.M., Jannetto, P.J., and Langman, L.J., 2016. Mass spectrometry applications for toxicology. *EJIFCC*, *27*(4), 272–287. Available at: https://pmc.ncbi.nlm.nih.gov/articles/PMC5282913/

Michigan State University Veterinary Diagnostic Laboratory. (2023). Toxicology sample collection and handling. Available at: https://cvm.msu.edu/vdl/laboratory-sections/toxicology/toxicology-sample-collection-and-handling (accessed 15 January 2026).

Moeller, K. E., Lee, K. C., & Kissack, J. C. (2008). Urine drug screening: Practical guide for clinicians. *Mayo Clinic Proceedings*, *83*(1), 66–76. https://doi.org/10.4065/83.1.66

Mostrom, M.S., 2021. Overview of mycotoxicoses in animals. Merck Veterinary Manual. Available at: https://www.merckvetmanual.com/toxicology/mycotoxicoses/overview-of-mycotoxicoses-in-animals (accessed 15 January 2026).

Pain, D. J., & Green, R. E. (2019). Effects of lead from ammunition on birds and other wildlife: A review. *Ambio*, *48*(9), 935–946. https://doi.org/10.1007/s13280-019-01159-0

Pellett, S. (2019). Critical analysis of neuronal cell and the mouse bioassay for detection of botulinum neurotoxin. *Toxins*, *11*(12), 713. https://doi.org/10.3390/toxins11120713

Peterson, M. E., & Talcott, P. (Eds.). (2013). *Small animal toxicology* (3rd ed.). Elsevier.

Pietrzak-Fiećko, R. (2018). Relationship between the content of chlorinated hydrocarbons and fatty acid composition of milk fat. *Journal of Veterinary Research*, *62*(1), 71–78. https://doi.org/10.2478/jvetres-2018-0010

Rocke, T. E. (1999). Biotoxins. In M. Friend & J. C. Franson (Eds.), technical editors*Field manual of wildlife diseases: General field procedures and diseases of birds* (pp. 173–178). U.S. Geological Survey, Information and Technology Report 1999-0001.

Seawright, A. A., Groenendyk, S., & Silva, K. I. (1970). An outbreak of oxalate poisoning in cattle grazing Setaria sphacelata. *Australian Veterinary Journal*, *46*(7), 293–296. https://doi.org/10.1111/j.1751-0813.1970.tb07900.x

Seifert, S. A., Armitage, J. O., & Sanchez, E. E. (2022). Snake envenomation. *New England Journal of Medicine*, *386*(1), 68–78. https://doi.org/10.1056/NEJMra2105228

Shridhar, N. B. (2022). Nerium oleander toxicity: A review. *International Journal of Advanced Academic Studies*, *4*(3), 23–32. https://doi.org/10.33545/27068919.2022.v4.i3a.813

Sidhu, P. K., Lamba, J. S., Kumbhar, G., Sekhon, G. S., Verma, S., & Gupta, M. P. (2014). Role of epidemiological factors in accumulation of oxalates in forage crops. *American International Journal of Research in Formal, Applied & Natural Sciences*, *7*(1), 48–52.

Thompson, L. J. (2021). *Nitrate and nitrite poisoning in animals*. Merck Veterinary Manual. Retrieved September 2024, from https://www.merckvetmanual.com/toxicology/nitrate-and-nitrite-poisoning/nitrate-and-nitrite-poisoning-in-animals

Tokarnia, C. H., Döbereiner, J., & Peixoto, P. V. (2002). Poisonous plants affecting livestock in Brazil. *Toxicon*, *40*(12), 1635–1660. https://doi.org/10.1016/s0041-0101(02)00239-8

United Nations Office on Drugs and Crime (UNODC). (2020). *Guidelines for quality assurance and good laboratory practices in forensic toxicology*. https://www.unodc.org/documents/scientific/Forensic_Toxicology_Guidelines.pdf

University of California, Davis, Environmental Health & Safety. (2025). *Triple packaging of diagnostic specimens*. https://safety.ucdavis.edu

University of Kentucky Veterinary Diagnostic Laboratory. (n.d.). Sample collection guidelines for toxicology analysis. Available at: https://vdl.uky.edu/sample-collection-guidelines-toxicology-analysis (accessed 15 January 2026).

Van Hemert, C., Schoen, S. K., Litaker, R. W., Smith, M. M., Arimitsu, M. L., Piatt, J. F., Holland, W. C., Ransom Hardison, D., & Pearce, J. M. (2020). Algal toxins in Alaskan seabirds: Evaluating the role of saxitoxin and domoic acid in a large-scale die-off of Common Murres. *Harmful Algae*, *92*, 101730. https://doi.org/10.1016/j.hal.2019.101730

Van Wyk, B.-E., Van Heerden, F. R., & Van Oudtshoorn, B. (2002). *Poisonous plants of South Africa*. Briza Publications.

7

Pesticides and Agricultural Chemicals

Pests are undesirable organisms that damage crops or injure or irritate animals or humans. Pests compete with people and food-producing animals for their food and can also transmit disease-causing organisms. As the world population increases and food security is threatened, farmers and public-health authorities often employ a range of tools, including chemical pesticides, to ensure that food supplies and livelihoods are protected and to help prevent diseases such as malaria and dengue.

The FAO/WHO International Code of Conduct on Pesticide Management defines pesticides as "any substance or mixture of substances intended for preventing, destroying or controlling any pest, including vectors of human or animal disease. The term includes substances intended for use as a plant regulator, defoliant, desiccant or agent for thinning fruit or preventing the premature fall of fruit and substances applied to crops either before or after harvest to protect the commodity from deterioration during storage, transport or marketing of food, agricultural commodities, wood and wood products or animal feedstuffs, or substances which may be administered to animals for the control of insects, arachnids or other pests in or on their bodies" (FAO and WHO, 2014; FAO and WHO, 2019).

In this chapter, we cover not only classical pesticides but also farm-related chemicals and feed-associated toxicants that are integral to tropical veterinary practice – notably nonprotein nitrogen (NPN) (urea), nitrate/nitrite accumulation, and sodium (salt) toxicosis – because these exposures often co-occur with pesticide use on farms and share overlapping risk pathways, diagnostics, and field management.

Pesticides can provide tremendous benefits when properly applied. Alongside other advances in agriculture, they have increased farmers' capability and productivity and contributed to lower food costs for consumers. However, when pesticides are carelessly used or abused, they may cause considerable harm to animals, humans, and the environment. Consequently, any pest-control program – chemical or bio-environmental – should be evaluated on economics, public health, and environmental protection. Programs deficient in any of these areas should be reconsidered, redesigned, or replaced (Table 7.1).

History of Pesticides

Although pyrethrins and nicotine were used as insecticides much earlier, various organic substances such as petroleum, creosote, kerosene, and turpentine were used to control mosquito larvae in the nineteenth century. Rotenone, a plant alkaloid, was used as an insecticide in the mid-twentieth century. Hydrogen cyanide (HCN) was first used in the late nineteenth century to kill scale insects; resistance

Table 7.1 Pesticides market in Asia in 2019 (Food and Agriculture Data by FAO [Food and Agriculture Organization of the United Nations]).

Country	Metric tonne
China	1,763,000
India	52,570
Korea Republic	20,043
Indonesia	1,597
Malaysia	67,288
Thailand	35,287

emerged decades later. In the late 1800s, salts of heavy metals such as copper, zinc, lead, thallium, and chromium were used against plant parasites; methyl bromide fumigation also gained importance. Plant extracts such as strychnine (used to kill rodents), hellebore, oleander, and pyrethrum were in common use around 1900; "high carbon acids" and anilines were used as herbicides, and mercurials and formaldehyde as fungicides. Other botanicals, such as sabadilla and derris, were used primarily as household and garden insecticides. Many of these compounds were no longer used due to poor efficacy or due to high mammalian toxicity, environmental persistence, or both.

The widely used insecticide dichlorodiphenyltrichloroethane (DDT) was first synthesized in 1874; its insecticidal properties were discovered in 1939 and it was patented for insecticidal use in 1942 (Klaassen, 2018). Organophosphorus insecticides were developed during World War II; tetraethyl pyrophosphate (TEPP) was among the earliest, followed by the more widely known parathion and methyl parathion a few years later. Carbamates were introduced for public use in 1957, despite experimental work beginning earlier. The use of organochlorine insecticides decreased dramatically after the 1960s due to their environmental persistence and potential toxicity to nontarget organisms. Fungicides include air-blown and dusting sulfur, Bordeaux mix, formaldehyde, and copper sulfate. Sulfur was used to prevent powdery mildews and rusts; Bordeaux mix (copper sulfate and slaked lime) was used for grapevine and potato blights; and formaldehyde (formalin) for cereal root rots and decay of sugar beets and potatoes. Some of these compounds are still in use, while several others have been replaced with more modern, less persistent chemicals. Since the 1950s, many new pesticides have been developed that are more effective against specific pests at lower doses and are less persistent than the older, more toxic organochlorines (Carson, 1962; European Commission, 2009; Klaassen, 2018).

Classes of Pesticides

Pesticides are chemical substances capable of selectively injuring or killing undesirable plant or animal pests. Unfortunately, most widely used pesticides are not highly selective and can be toxic to many non-target species, including humans and beneficial organisms.

The major classes of pesticides include insecticides, herbicides, fungicides, and rodenticides; pesticides may also include avicides, piscicides, molluscicides, nematicides, and acaricides (Table 7.2).

Table 7.2 Common pesticides available in the market.

Class	Group	Chemical name	Common name/trade name
Insecticides	Organochlorine (chlorinated hydrocarbon)	Dichlorodiphenylethanes	DDT
			DDD (Rothane)
			DMC (Dimite)
			Dicofol (kelthane)
			Methoxychlor
			Chlorbenzylate
		Hexachloro-cyclohexane	Lindane
			Benzane hexachloride
		Cyclodienes	Endrin
			Telodrin
			Isodrin
			Endosulfan
			Heptachlor
			Aldrin
			Dieldrin
			Chlordane
			Toxaphene
			Chlordecone
			Mirex
	Organophosphorus	Organosphosphates	Abate
			Bithion
			Temephos
		Azinphosmethyl	Guthion
			Gusathion
		Carbophenothion	Trithion
		Chlorfenvinphos	Supona
			Birlane
		Chlorpyrifos	Dursban
			Dowco
		Coumaphos	Co-Ral
			Asunthal
			Muscatox
		Crufomate	Ruelene
		Crotoxyphos	Ciodrin
		Demeton	Systox
		Diazinon	Diazinon

(Continued)

Table 7.2 (Continued)

Class	Group	Chemical name	Common name/trade name
		Dichlofenthion	V-C 13
		Dichlorvos	Vapona DDVP
		Dicrotophos	Bidrin
		Dimethoate	Cygon
		Diaxathion	Delnav
		Disulfoton	Di-syston
		Famphus	Warbex Famphos
		Fansulfothion	Dasanit
		Fenthion	Baytex Tiguvon
		Fonofos	Dyfonate
		Malathion	Cythion
Herbicides	Bipyridul compound	1, 1–dimenthyl–4, 4-bypyridylium dichloride	Paraquat and Diquat
	Chlorophenoxy compound	Dichlorophenoxyaceticacid, trichlorophenoxyaceticacid Dichloropropionic acid	2-4-D 2,4,5-T Downpon^{R}
	Dinitrophenols		
	Amide	2-chloro-N,N-diallyl acetamide and Trichlorobenzyl chloride	Randox-^{T}
	Substituted	3-(p-chlorophenyl) -1,1-dimethyl urea	Monuron (Telvar^{B})
		3-(3,4-Dichlorophenyl)-1 methoxymethyl urea	Linuron (Lorox^{R})
		3-phenyl-1, dimethyl urea	Fenuron (Dybar^{R})
		3-(3-4-Dichlorophenyl) 1,1-Dimethyl urea	Diuron (Karmex^{R})
Rodenticides		Strychnine	
		Warfarin	King Kong®
		Zinc phosphate	Tikusan®
Molluscicides		Metaldehyde	
		Methiocarb	
Fungicides			

Pesticides are also classified according to intended use or target species. For example, insecticides are applied to kill insect pests; fungicides control fungi; herbicides control weeds; and rodenticides target rodents. Fumigants are used mainly for the control of soil nematodes. The suffix "-icide" on these words indicates "killing" (Gupta, 2011).

Benefits and Risks

A benefit–risk evaluation of pesticides is challenging and remains a matter for public debate. It is essential to balance the expected benefits against possible hazards to human health and deleterious effects on environmental quality. Agricultural productivity and product quality can improve significantly with judicious pesticide use, reducing production costs and increasing farmers' income. In many production systems – both developed and developing – achieving reliable yields without any pesticides is currently not feasible.

The market share of pesticide types has shifted over time: herbicides have come to dominate many markets, and organochlorine insecticides have been largely replaced by organophosphates, carbamates, and newer chemistries. Public-health uses have also evolved, with tighter regulation of persistent compounds and increased emphasis on integrated approaches (FAO, 2024). Misuse can devastate wildlife and livestock. In 2013, 14 Bornean pygmy elephants in Sabah were found dead, with suspected poisoning linked to plantation practices (Motlagh, 2013). In another case, around 70 cattle in Malaysia died after grazing on recently treated pasture, consistent with paraquat exposure (New Straits Times, 1994, cited in International Labour Organization, 2011). These events emphasize the necessity of stewardship, appropriate selection of pesticide type, dose, and application method, and the use of nonchemical controls where feasible.

The following sections outline major pesticide groups – including insecticides, herbicides, rodenticides, and molluscicides – and add key farm chemical/feed-related toxicants (urea/NPN, nitrate–nitrite, and sodium/salt), covering sources, clinical signs, mechanisms of action, pathophysiology, diagnosis, and treatment.

Organochlorine Insecticides

Organochlorine insecticides (chlorinated hydrocarbons) are a diverse group subdivided into dichlorodiphenyltrichloroethanes (e.g., DDT), cyclodienes (e.g., aldrin, dieldrin), and cyclohexanes (e.g., lindane) (Table 7.3). Although largely phased out or restricted, legacy exposures persist in some regions.

Clinical Signs

Clinical signs typically develop within minutes to 24 hours after exposure. Acute or subacute toxicity may include paresthesia of the muzzle and tongue, apprehension, hypersusceptibility to stimuli, hyperirritability, dizziness, ataxia, tremors, running in circles, and tonic–clonic convulsions. Monogastric animals often vomit after ingestion, with profuse salivation and frothy oral secretions.

Table 7.3 Derivatives, structures, and examples of organochlorine insecticides.

Derivatives	Chemical structure	Examples
Dichlorodiphenyltrichloroethane	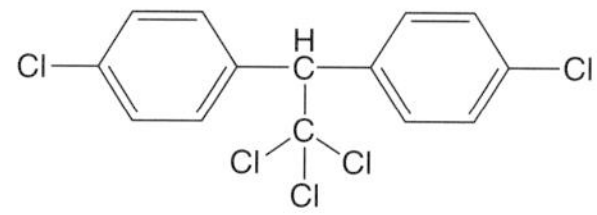	DDT, DDD, dicolol, perthano, methoxychlor, methiochlor
Cyclodienes	SDBS-NO = 7026 ALDRIN 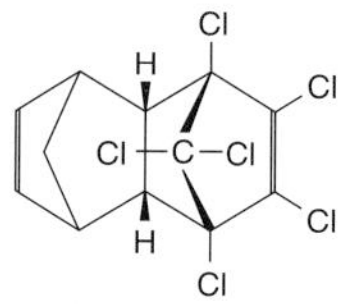	Aldrin, Dieldrin, Heptachlor, Chlordane, Endosulfan
Chlorinated Benzenes Cyclohexanes	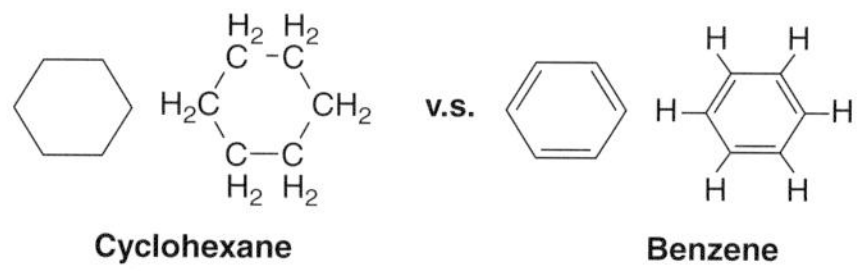	HCB, HCH, Lindane (% BHC)

Central nervous system (CNS) stimulation may be followed by depression; affected animals may be comatose for 1–2 days. Death can occur within 72 hours due to respiratory failure (Gupta, 2011).

Mechanism of Action

Primary sites of action include sensory and motor nerve fibers and the motor cortex. Studies on isolated neurons and nerve fibers show that DDT prolongs the negative afterpotential of nerve fibers (Figure 7.1). Four likely mechanisms, acting simultaneously, include:

- Prevention of potassium efflux across the membrane
- Inhibition of neuronal ATPases that transport sodium and potassium
- Alteration of sodium channels and interference with active sodium extrusion needed for repolarization and
- Inhibition of calmodulin's ability to carry Ca^{2+} necessary for neurotransmitter release

All of these effects prolong repolarization and lower the threshold for stimulation, increasing nerve firing rates. Cyclodiene and cyclohexane derivatives act somewhat differently (Timbrell, 2023). Their effects are localized primarily in the CNS. They antagonize the neurotransmitter γ-aminobutyric acid (GABA_A) at GABA_A receptors, which normally mediate chloride-ion influx (Figure 7.2). Inhibition of chloride ion uptake leads to partial depolarization and uncontrolled excitation. Cyclodienes also inhibit Ca^{2+}/Mg^{2+}-ATPase, an enzyme critical for calcium transport across nerve membranes; inhibition promotes acetylcholine release at cholinergic synapses, compounding the excitatory state (Timbrell, 2023).

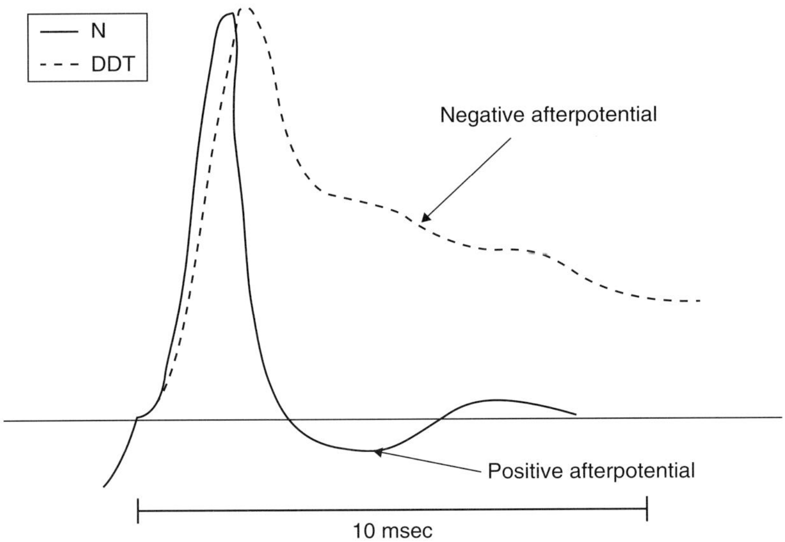

Figure 7.1 A schematic diagram of an oscilloscope recording to show the prolongation of the negative afterpotential induced by DDT(--) compared to the potential changes seen normally, N (-).

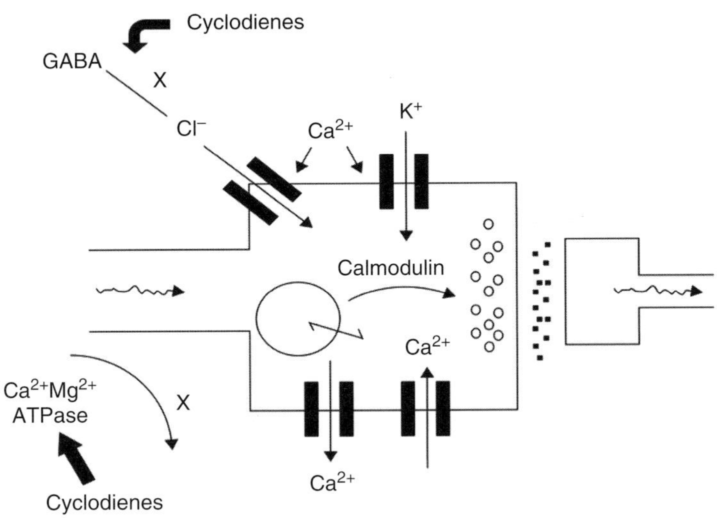

Figure 7.2 Cellular mechanism of action of the cyclodienes on chloride and calcium transport. Adapted from Matsumura (1975) and Ecobichon (1991).

Pathophysiology

Pathologic changes in acute/subacute organochlorine poisoning are minimal and nonspecific: petechial hemorrhages throughout the body (especially heart), congested/edematous lungs, and congested/edematous brain and spinal cord. Chronic exposure may lead to increased fat deposition, hepatocellular hypertrophy, and adrenal cortical atrophy (reported in dogs) (Gupta, 2011).

Diagnosis

A tentative diagnosis is based on exposure history with compatible neurologic signs (e.g., seizures). The absence of specific lesions on necropsy supports toxicosis. Confirmatory diagnosis relies on chemical analysis showing high organochlorine levels in liver and kidney, and possibly stomach contents or hair. Because organochlorines are cumulative, mere presence in tissues does not prove acute lethality; differential diagnoses (e.g., polioencephalomalacia, lead poisoning in cattle; water-deprivation sodium ion toxicosis) should be considered (Gupta, 2011).

Treatment

No specific antidote exists. Treat CNS stimulation with sedatives/anticonvulsants (e.g., chloral hydrate, long-acting barbiturates; diazepam as needed). If animals are dull and unresponsive, CNS stimulants are not indicated. IV calcium gluconate may help stabilize hyperirritable neurons. Prevent further absorption using saline cathartics or activated charcoal for oral exposure and thorough washing with soap/water for dermal exposure (Gupta, 2011).

Organophosphorus and Carbamate Insecticides

Organophosphorus (OP) and carbamate insecticides are widely used in tropical countries. OPs include aliphatic, carbocyclic, and heterocyclic phosphorus derivatives; carbamates are cyclic or aliphatic derivatives of carbamic acid. These compounds have systemic action and can be absorbed through intact skin (Gupta, 2011), gastrointestinal (GI) tract, and mucous membranes, distributing throughout the body in sufficient quantities to kill ticks, mites, and worms feeding on tissues or body fluids.

Clinical Signs

OPs/carbamates overstimulate the parasympathetic nervous system. Three groups of effects are recognized:

Muscarinic effects: Profuse salivation; GI hypermotility with colic, vomiting, and diarrhea; lacrimation; sweating; dyspnea/bronchoconstriction; miosis; pallor; cyanosis; and urinary incontinence.

Nicotinic effects: Twitching and fasciculations of small muscles (face, eyelids, tongue), progressing to larger limb and trunk muscles, producing tetany, ataxia, and staggering. Initial hyperactivity is followed by weakness and skeletal-muscle paralysis due to acetylcholine accumulation at neuromuscular junctions.

CNS effects: Species variability is marked. Food-producing animals may show hyperactivity but rarely seizures and usually become depressed. In dogs and cats, CNS stimulation may progress to convulsions. Death in all species is due to hypoxia from bronchoconstriction, excessive respiratory secretions, arrhythmias, and bradycardia (Gupta, 2011; Lotti & Moretto, 2005).

Mechanism of Action

OPs and carbamates competitively inhibit acetylcholinesterase (AChE) and butyrylcholinesterase (BChE) (pseudocholinesterase), which hydrolyze acetylcholine. AChE is present at cholinergic nerve endings, neuromuscular junctions, and in red blood cells; pseudocholinesterase is found in brain and plasma. OPs/carbamates inhibit by phosphorylating or carbamoylating the enzyme's active site (Figure 7.3). OP inhibition tends to be functionally irreversible over clinically relevant time frames; carbamate inhibition is reversible. OP-AChE complexes may age, becoming irreversibly resistant to oxime reactivation (Lotti & Moretto, 2005) (Figure 7.4).

Pathophysiology

Gross changes are often minimal and nonspecific. Excess salivation fills the mouth; excessive bronchial secretions and pulmonary edema cause dyspnea. Petechial/ecchymotic hemorrhages may be present in GI serosa/mucosa with luminal fluid (Figure 7.5). Acute pancreatitis has been reported in dogs (Frick et al., 1987) and humans (Harputluoglu et al., 2003; Peter et al., 2014) with OP poisoning. Diffuse endocardial hemorrhages may also occur.

Diagnosis

OP/carbamate toxicosis in cattle may be confused with urea toxicosis, nitrate/nitrite toxicosis, or cyanide poisoning. More broadly, any disease producing parasympathomimetic signs (dyspnea, muscle stiffness/paralysis, hypersalivation) is in the differential. A history of exposure within the past 48 hours, plus characteristic signs, supports diagnosis.

Because OPs/carbamates are cholinesterase inhibitors, confirm by testing for reduced cholinesterase activity in blood/tissues. Note that clinical signs reflect junctional AChE depletion; blood AChE is a surrogate. Tissue/chemical analyses for OPs/carbamates are often negative due to rapid biotransformation (Assis et al., 2018; Al-Jobory and Mohammad, 2005; Karami-Mohajeri and Abdollahi, 2013).

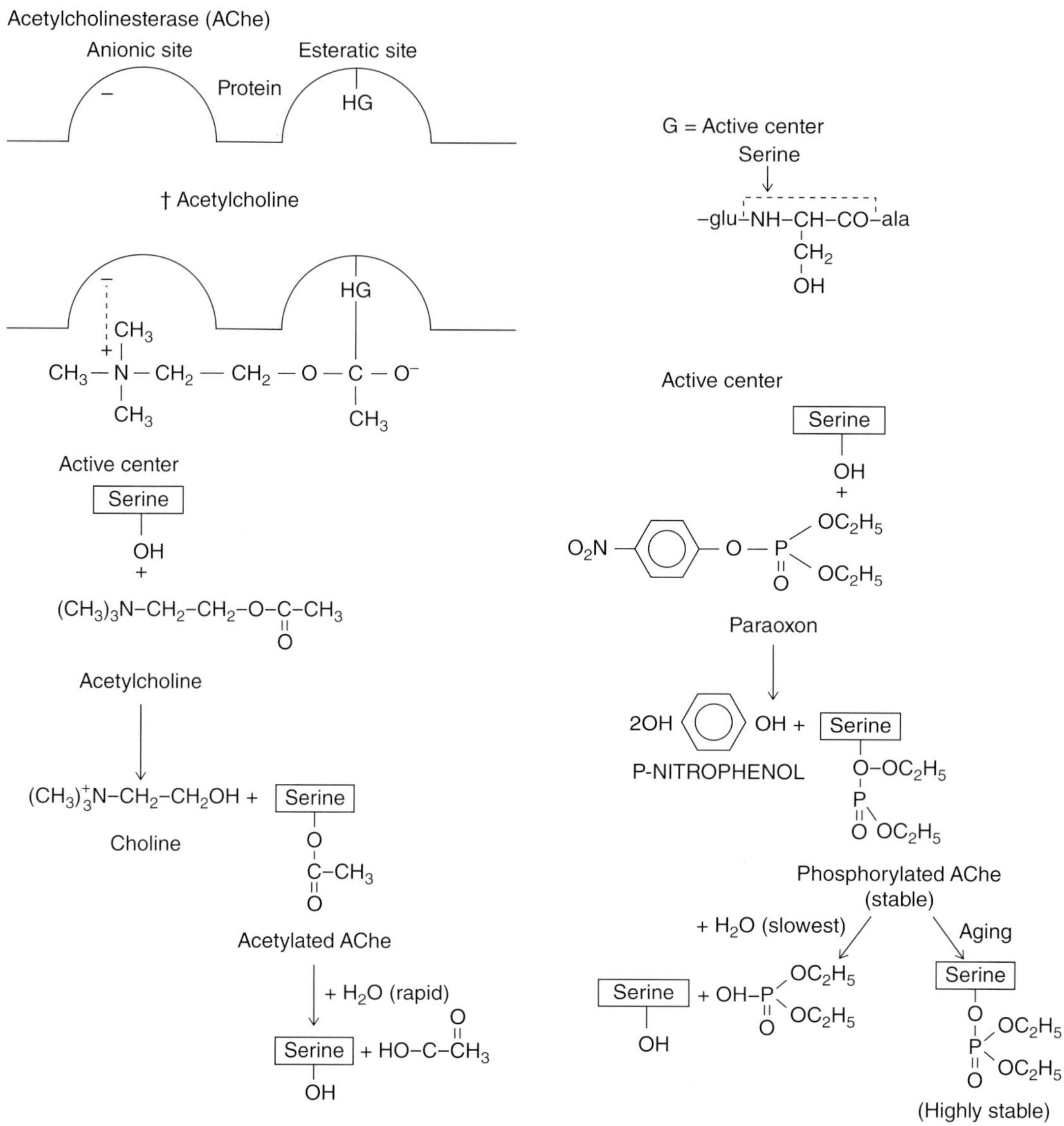

Figure 7.3 Hydrolysis of acetylcholine and paraoxon by acetylcholinesterase.

Determination of Cholinesterase Activity in Domestic Animals

Because AChE and BChE activities are routinely used as biomarkers of organophosphate/carbamate exposure, baseline and longitudinal interpretation is important (Strelitz et al., 2014). Several procedures measure blood cholinesterase, often via pH change after substrate hydrolysis (Assis et al., 2018;

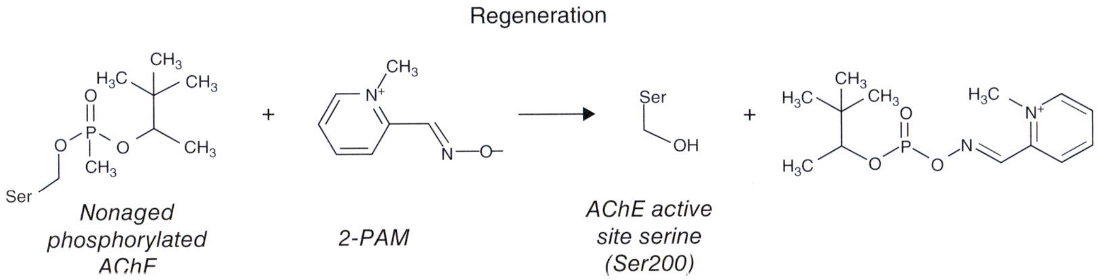

Figure 7.4 Reactivation of phosphorylated acetylcholinesterase by pralidoxime (2-PAM).

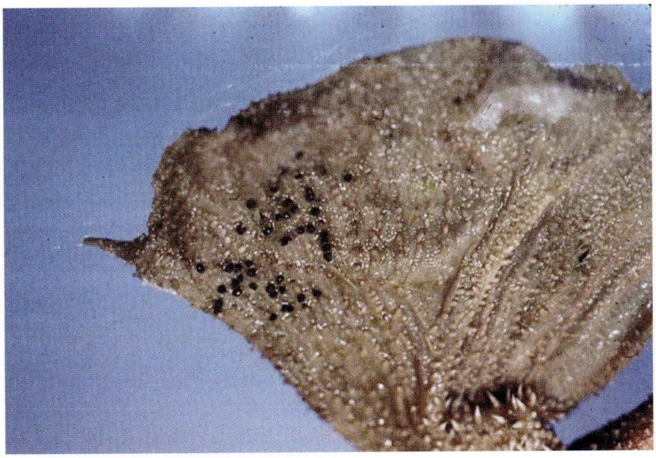

Figure 7.5 Gastrointestinal mucosa, bovine, suspected organophosphate poisoning – diffuse congestion with multifocal petechial hemorrhages ("peppery" appearance) consistent with acute hemorrhagic gastroenteritis. These gross changes are supportive but nonspecific; confirmation requires AChE inhibition and pesticide residue analysis. *Source:* Cornell Veterinary Medicine/ https://secure.vet.cornell.edu/nst/nst.asp/ / last accessed Oct. 30, 2025.

Karami-Mohajeri and Abdollahi, 2013). Large pH change indicates activity; a near-zero change indicates inhibition. Normal values (modified Michel method) are shown in Table 7.4.

Treatment

Atropine sulfate is highly effective for OP/carbamate poisoning: It antagonizes muscarinic effects of excess acetylcholine but does not reverse the biochemical lesion. Because parasympathomimetic effects are prolonged, higher-than-routine doses may be needed (e.g., approximately 0.5 mg/kg for ruminants; ~65 mg total for an average horse; ~2 mg total for an average dog). Administer ~25% IV and the remainder SC/IM; repeat every 3–4 hours for 1–2 days based on response.

Table 7.4 Percentage of total cholinesterase (Che) in erythrocytes and cholinesterase activity in whole blood of domestic animals.

Species	Percentage of total Che (%)	Activity (pH)
Cattle	90	0.30–0.75
Sheep	90	0.10–0.30
Goat	89	0.04–0.24
Horse	90	0.20–0.65
Dog	61	0.43
Pig	67–88	

Source: Karami-Mohajeri and Abdollahi, (2013)/with permission of John Wiley & Sons.

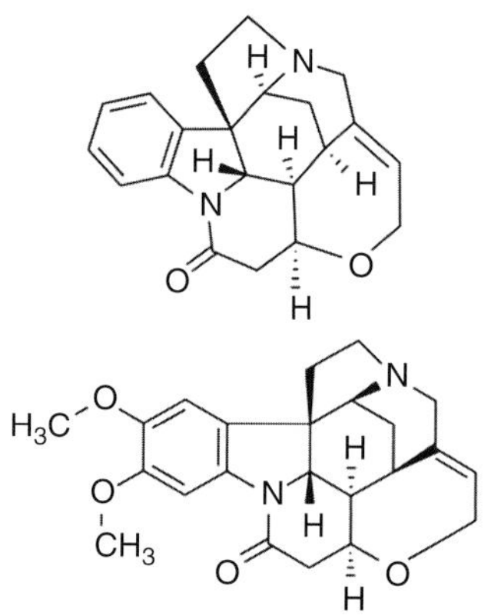

Figure 7.6 Chemical structure (strychnine and brucine).

Organophosphorus poisoning may also be treated with enzyme reactivators such as pralidoxime (2-PAM). 2-PAM cleaves phosphorylated AChE, freeing the enzyme; the bound OP is then hydrolyzed and excreted. Another oxime (diacetylmonoxime, DAM) has been recommended based on pharmacokinetics in buffaloes, 30 mg/kg IV initially, then 26 mg/kg at 14-hour intervals. Important: Oxime reactivators are contraindicated in pure carbamate poisoning (Jokanović & Prostran, 2009). In all cases, supportive care is essential (oxygen, ventilation, fluids, anticonvulsants, decontamination) (Gupta, 2011; Papich, 2019 Rodenticides – Strychnine

Strychnine is an indole alkaloid historically used as a rodenticide, commonly formulated as colored pellets. It is derived from the seeds of *Strychnos nux-vomica and Strychnos ignatii*. Brucine is structurally related with similar physiologic effects but is less potent. Structural formulas are shown in Figure 7.6.

Clinical Signs

Clinical signs appear within minutes after ingestion. Early signs in dogs include apprehension, excitement, nervousness, tenseness, and stiffness. Examination reveals rigid abdominal and cervical muscles and extensor rigidity. Violent tetanic convulsions may appear spontaneously or be triggered by noise, touch, or sudden bright light. Convulsions last seconds to a minute; intervals shorten as poisoning progresses. Pupils dilate and mucous membranes become cyanotic from anoxia. Apnea may occur during seizures; respiration resumes with clonic-tonic relaxation. Mortality is due to interference with exhalation during tonic spasm, causing asphyxiation. Tachycardia is common; temperature rises with repeated convulsions. Terminal hypothermia may occur rather than hyperthermia. In milder intoxication, signs may be limited to hyperirritability, slight stiffness, and extreme sensitivity to stimuli. A comatose stage may precede recovery, with complete return to normal afterward (Gupta, 2011).

Mechanism of Action

Strychnine selectively antagonizes glycine-mediated postsynaptic inhibition in the spinal cord and medulla, eliminating regulatory control and causing repetitive tetanic seizures and generalized rigidity. It reduces postsynaptic membrane permeability to glycine, abolishing inhibitory postsynaptic potentials. Strychnine does not cause structural neuronal damage.

Pathophysiology

Together, Figures 7.7 and 7.8 illustrate the exposure-to-lesion continuum. Figure 7.7 captures the recovered bait/ingesta – red-dyed cereal grains typical of commercial strychnine formulations – providing a rapid presumptive cue while toxicology is pending. Figure 7.8 then shows the gross gastric lesions with the same dyed grains embedded in the mucosa, linking field recognition of bait to the characteristic pattern of acute hemorrhagic–necrotizing gastritis and petechiae at necropsy. Using the pair side by side guides sample triage (stomach contents, any recovered bait, liver) and clarifies how gross pathology supports case confirmation rather than standing alone.

Diagnosis

Tentative diagnosis is based on history and characteristic signs. Similar signs may be seen with chlorinated hydrocarbons or lead poisoning, hypocalcemia, and acute massive hepatic necrosis; however, strychnine seizures are notably stimulus-evoked (touch, sound, light).

Confirm by detecting strychnine in vomitus, stomach contents, and liver via chemical analysis. A classic (historical) bioassay involves injecting a neutralized extract into a frog or mouse, producing typical convulsions within 2–5 minutes.

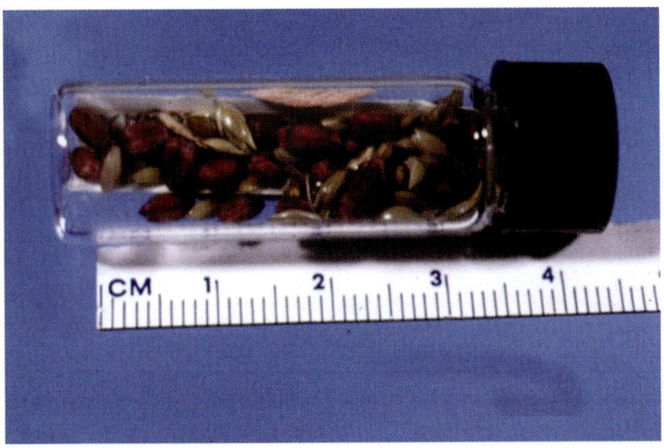

Figure 7.7 Stomach contents, dog – numerous red-dyed cereal grains (sorghum/milo) consistent with strychnine-treated bait recovered at necropsy. Presence of dyed grain strongly supports strychnine ingestion; confirmation requires toxicologic analysis. *Source:* Cornell Veterinary Medicine / https://secure.vet.cornell.edu/nst/nst.asp/ / last accessed Oct. 30, 2025.

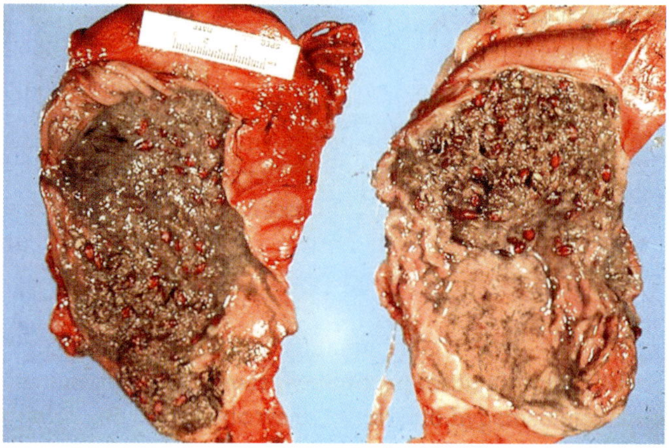

Figure 7.8 Stomach, dog – acute hemorrhagic and necrotizing gastritis with adherent red-dyed cereal grains. The mucosa is dark gray-black, thickened, and covered by necrotic exudate with multifocal petechiae/ecchymoses; numerous dyed grains consistent with commercial strychnine bait are embedded on the surface. *Source:* Cornell Veterinary Medicine / https://secure.vet.cornell.edu/nst/nst.asp/ / last accessed Oct. 30, 2025.

Treatment

No specific antidote exists. Priorities are sustained muscle relaxation and prevention of asphyxia. Deep sedation/anesthesia (benzodiazepines, barbiturates, inhalation anesthesia) and methocarbamol (150 mg/kg) may be used. Diazepam or glyceryl guaiacolate ether (2.5–20 mg IV or PO) can control convulsions. Decontaminate (induce emesis in early cases; gastric lavage) and administer activated charcoal and a cathartic (e.g., sodium sulfate). Forced diuresis (5% mannitol at 6.6 mL/kg/h) and urinary acidification may enhance elimination (Papich, 2019).

Anticoagulant Rodenticides

Discovery of anticoagulant activity (dicoumarol) in moldy sweet clover causing hemorrhagic disease in cattle in the early 1920s led to synthesis of warfarin and related agents (Gupta, 2018a). Vitamin K antagonism and newer anticoagulants differ in targets and reversal approaches (Levi et al., 2011). These "oral anticoagulants" are widely used as rodenticides and in human medicine.

Sources

Common anticoagulant rodenticides used by pest-control operators and the public are listed in Table 7.5. Most share a coumarin or indandione nucleus but differ in side chains, solubility, and toxicity. Because repeated warfarin exposures are often required before toxicity develops, resistance emerged in some rat strains, prompting the development of potent "superwarfarins" (e.g., brodifacoum, bromadiolone) (Stoytcheva and Zlatev, 2018).

Table 7.5 Chemical names and structural formula of common anticoagulant rodenticides.

Rodenticide	Chemical name	Chemical structure
Warfarin	3 (alpha-phenyl-beta-acetylethyl)-4-hydroxycoumarin	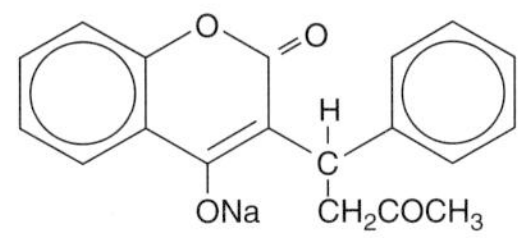
Pindone	2-pivalyl-1,3-indandione	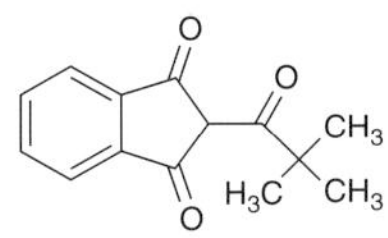
Diphacinone	2-diphenylacetyl-1,3-indandione	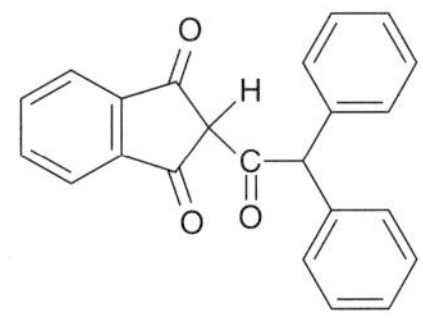
Brodifacoum	3-[3 (4′–bromo[1,1–biphenyl]-4-yl)–1,2,3,4–tetrahydro–1–napthalenyl]–4–hydroxyl–2H–1–bezopyran–2–one	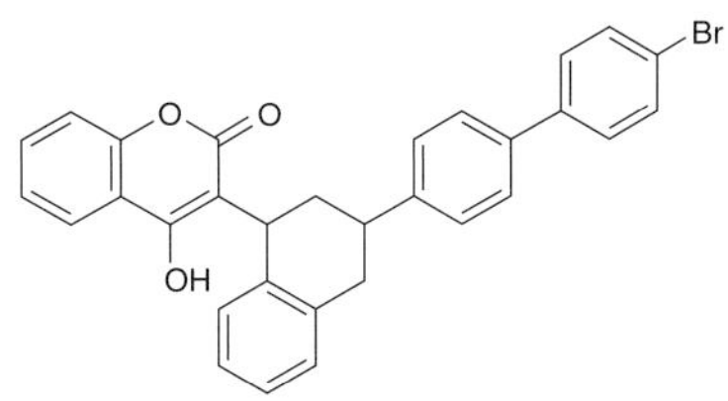

Toxicity

All mammals and birds are susceptible, with dogs, cats, and swine often affected. Toxic levels vary by species and compound (Table 7.6).

Contributing factors include decreased vitamin K synthesis after prolonged antibiotic therapy; hepatic disease (reduced prothrombin production); plasma-protein binding altering fate; increased receptor affinity; and stress or corticosteroid therapy increasing poisoning intensity.

Table 7.6 Toxic levels of warfarin in various species of domestic and laboratory animals.

Species	Single dose (mg/kg)	Repeated dose (mg/kg)
Rats	50–100	1 (for 5 d)
Dogs	50	5 (for 5–5 d)
Cats	5–50	1 (for 5–15 d)
Swine	—	0.05 (for 7 d)
Ruminants	—	50% of body weight of feed containing mg/kg

Source: Data from Gupta, (2018a).

Mechanism of Action

Anticoagulants inhibit vitamin K-dependent carboxylation of glutamate residues in prothrombin and factors VII, IX, and X. Resulting under-carboxylated proteins are inactive in coagulation. Anticoagulants also block reductive metabolism of vitamin K epoxide back to the active hydroquinone (Figure 7.9). Mutations in vitamin K epoxide reductase (VKOR) confer resistance in some rats and humans.

Clinical Signs

Findings include generalized hemorrhages and sudden death, sometimes without prior illness. Acute cases show cerebral, pericardial, and pleural hemorrhages. Subacute cases show severe anemia, weakness, pale mucous membranes, dyspnea, hematemesis, epistaxis, melena, and blood-tinged oral

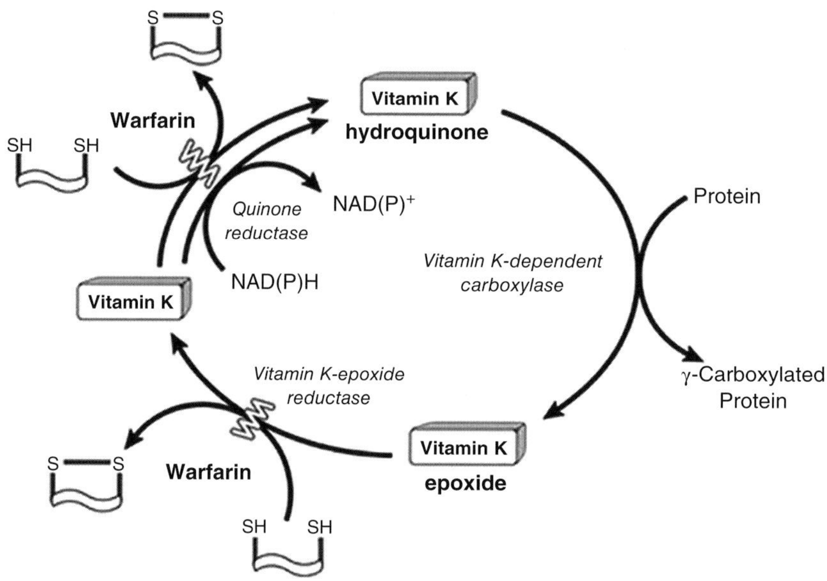

The reduced form of vitamin K (hydroquinone) donates a pair of electrons to the vitamin K-dependent carboxylase (known as γ-glutamyl carboxylase), which carboxylates glutamic acid residues in specific vitamin K-dependent proteins. The resultant oxidized form of vitamin K (epoxide) is converted back to hydroquinone in a two-step reaction. The first step, which converts vitamin K epoxide to vitamin K, is catalyzed by vitamin K-epoxide reductase; the second step is catalyzed by either vitamin K-epoxide reductase or most likely by another yet-to-defined reductase. This pathway is inhibited by the vitamin K antagonist and anticoagulant drug, warfarin. The reduction of vitamin K to hydroquinone is also possibly catalyzed by a NAD(P)H-dependent reductase that is resistant to warfarin.

Figure 7.9 Reduced vitamin K (vitamin K hydroquinone, KH_2) donates electrons to γ-glutamyl carboxylase (GGCX) to γ-carboxylate vitamin-K–dependent proteins, becoming vitamin K epoxide (KO). KO is recycled to vitamin K (quinone) and then back to KH_2, primarily by vitamin K epoxide reductase (VKORC1); **warfarin** inhibits VKOR, depleting KH_2 and blocking carboxylation. A warfarin-resistant NAD(P)H-dependent quinone reductase can also reduce vitamin K to KH_2. *Source:* Adapted from Tie and Stafford (2016); see Wallin and Martin (1987) and Whitlon et al. (1978).

froth. Conjunctival/intraocular hemorrhage may occur. Ataxia reflects anemia/weakness. Warfarin readily crosses the placenta and can induce fetal hemorrhages. Transplacental exposure to vitamin K antagonists has been associated with fetal hemorrhage in dogs (Munday et al., 2003).

Pathophysiology

Postmortem findings include generalized hemorrhages in the thoracic cavity, mediastinum, joints, subcutis, CNS, and GI tract. The heart may show severe hemopericardium with mediastinal hemorrhage and multifocal epicardial petechiae (Figure 7.10). The liver may show centrilobular necrosis from anemia/hypoxia; icterus can occur in prolonged cases.

Diagnosis

History of bait use with compatible signs is helpful. Laboratory abnormalities include prolonged bleeding/clotting times, prolonged one-stage prothrombin time (OSPT/PT) and activated partial thromboplastin time (APTT), with normal platelet and leukocyte counts but low packed cell volume (PCV). Differentials include other hemorrhagic disorders (aflatoxicosis, thrombocytopenia, infectious canine hepatitis) and dietary vitamin K deficiency (notably in swine/poultry). Confirm by measuring plasma warfarin/brodifacoum (live) or hepatic residues (postmortem).

Treatment

Keep animals warm and handle gently to minimize trauma. Sedation may reduce aggravation. Provide oxygen for respiratory distress or severe anemia. Fresh citrated whole blood (20 mL/kg) supplies clotting factors; administer half rapidly, then the remainder at ~20 drops/min. Administer vitamin K1

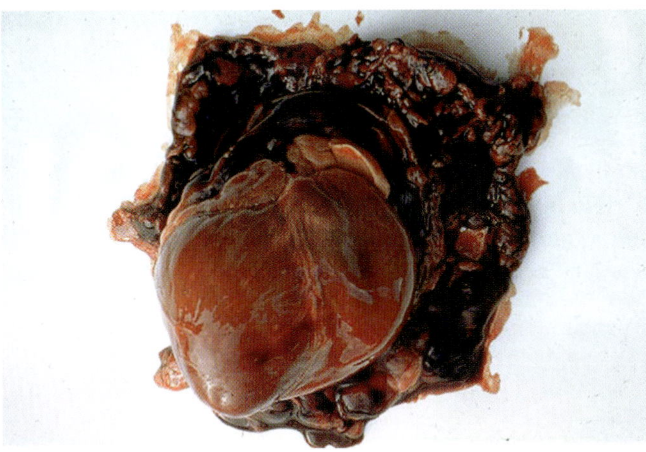

Figure 7.10 Heart, dog – severe hemopericardium (anticoagulant rodenticide). The pericardial sac and adjacent mediastinal tissues are suffused with dark red-to-black clotted and unclotted blood, compressing the heart (cardiac tamponade). The epicardium is smooth and glistening with scattered petechial-to-ecchymotic hemorrhages. *Source:* Cornell Veterinary Medicine / https://secure.vet.cornell.edu/nst/nst.asp/ / last accessed Oct. 30, 2025.

(phytonadione) IV (15–75 mg) and continue oral vitamin K1 (dogs/cats, 2–5 mg/kg/day in divided doses for ~2 weeks). Menadione (vitamin K3) is less effective (Papich, 2019).

Herbicide – Paraquat

Paraquat is a broad-spectrum, nonselective herbicide in the quaternary bipyridyl class (1,1-dimethyl-4,4′-bipyridinium dichloride). It was first synthesized in the nineteenth century; its herbicidal properties were recognized in the 1950s, and it has been marketed since 1962 (Dinis-Oliveira et al., 2008). Numerous human fatalities have occurred from accidental or suicidal ingestion; companion-animal cases are reported worldwide (Dinis-Oliveira et al., 2008; Williams et al., 2016).

Clinical Signs

Early signs include vomiting, anorexia, and lethargy, followed by acute respiratory distress. Breathing is often loud and noisy, with marked abdominal effort. The clinical hallmark is cyanosis due to inadequate arterial oxygenation (Gawarammana & Buckley, 2011). Affected dogs often assume sternal recumbency; rectal temperature is often normal but pulse may be elevated (150–160/min). Other signs include conjunctival congestion and mild to moderate dehydration. Respiratory distress may progress rapidly, leading to respiratory failure and death without prompt and aggressive treatment.

Mechanism of Action

Paraquat undergoes redox cycling, generating superoxide radicals that dismutate to hydrogen peroxide and, via metal-catalyzed reactions, produce highly reactive species (including singlet oxygen), causing lipid peroxidation in pulmonary tissues (Dinis-Oliveira et al., 2008). Membrane lipid hydroperoxides decompose into free radicals, initiating chain reactions (Figure 7.11).

Pathophysiology

Two stages characterize pulmonary lesions: a destructive stage (swelling and fragmentation of alveolar epithelium, alveolar edema, and acute inflammatory exudate) followed by a proliferative stage (intra-alveolar accumulation of fibroblasts maturing into fibrotic tissue), producing diffuse intra-alveolar pulmonary fibrosis (Figures 7.12 and 7.13). Extrapulmonary lesions include renal tubular necrosis, focal myocardial necrosis, and adrenal corticomedullary hemorrhages (Dinis-Oliveira et al., 2008; Subbiah and Tiwari, 2021; Williams et al., 2016).

Diagnosis

Diagnosis is difficult; history of access/ingestion with distinctive, rapidly progressive dyspnea is suggestive (Dinis-Oliveira et al., 2008). A sodium dithionite urine test can detect paraquat within ~48 hours of ingestion (Wang et al., 2021). Necropsy reveals characteristic lung changes.

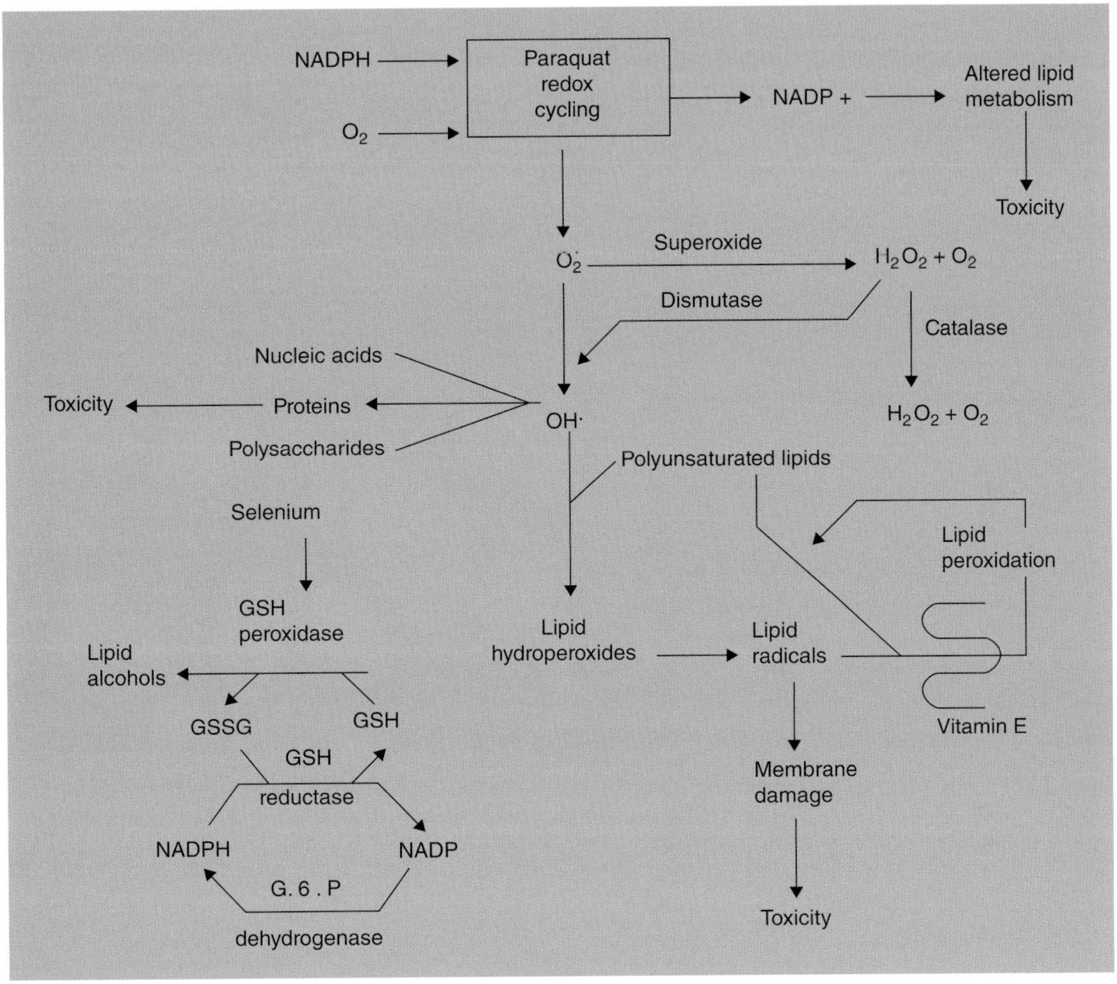

Figure 7.11 Paraquat redox cycling, oxidative injury, and antioxidant defenses. Paraquat (PQ^{2+}) undergoes one-electron reduction by NADPH-dependent reductases (e.g., NADPH–cytochrome P450 reductase) to $PQ^{\cdot+}$, which transfers an electron to O_2 forming superoxide ($O_2^{\cdot}$–). Superoxide is dismutated to H_2O_2, which yields ·OH in the presence of transition metals. These ROS initiate lipid peroxidation of polyunsaturated membrane lipids → lipid radicals/hydroperoxides → membrane damage → toxicity. Endogenous defenses include SOD, catalase, and selenium-dependent glutathione peroxidase (GPx); GPx uses GSH, which is regenerated by glutathione reductase using nicotinamide adenine dinucleotide phosphate (NADPH) supplied by G-6-P dehydrogenase. Vitamin E terminates lipid peroxyl radicals, limiting propagation. *Source:* Adapted from Bus et al. (1976); Dinis-Oliveira et al. (2008).

Treatment

Treatment must begin as soon as possible (ideally within 10 hours). Prevent absorption and hasten excretion: induce repeated emesis (if appropriate), administer adsorbents such as Fullers earth (30% w/v slurry or 7.5% bentonite) or activated charcoal (Gawarammana and Buckley, 2011). If clay is used, follow with a cathartic (e.g., magnesium sulfate) to maintain gut clearance. Forced diuresis may increase excretion,

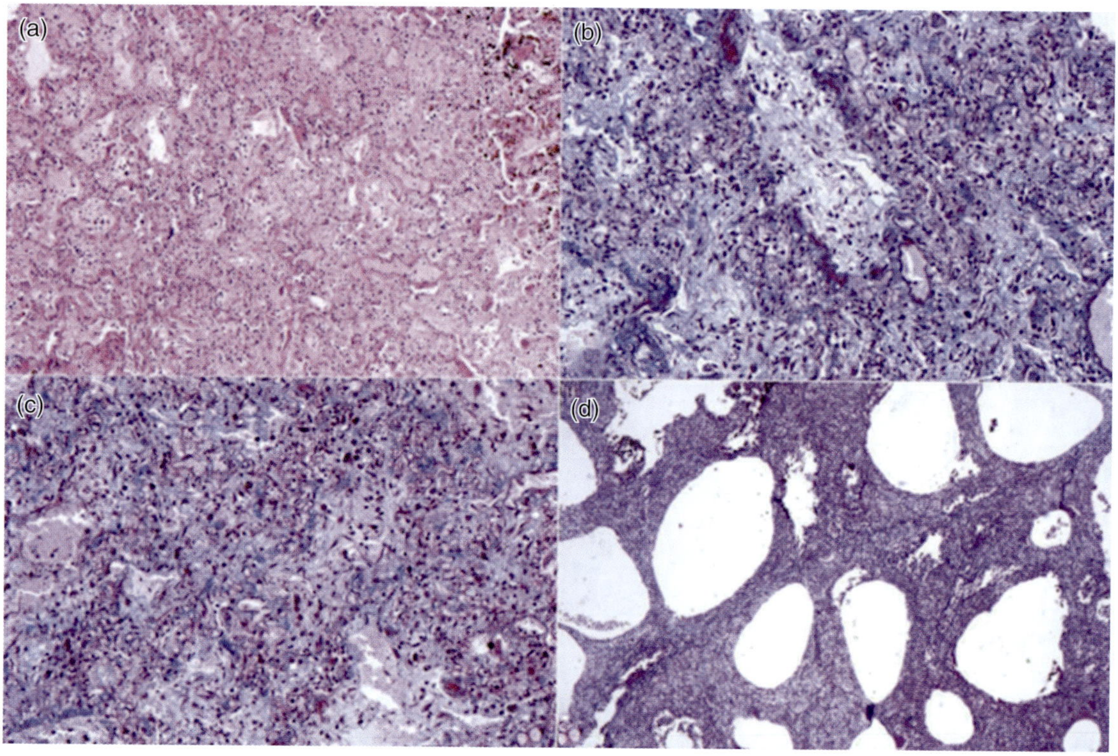

Figure 7.12 Lung, fatal paraquat poisoning – progression to fibrosis. (a) (H&E, 10×): Fibroblast infiltration with collagen deposition and obliteration of alveolar architecture. (b, c) (Masson's trichrome, 20×): Prominent intra-alveolar fibroblasts with collagen (blue) deposition. (d) (Masson's trichrome, 20×): Advanced "honeycomb" remodeling consistent with end-stage interstitial fibrosis. *Source:* Kumar et al., (2021)/Autops Case Rep/CC BY 4.0.

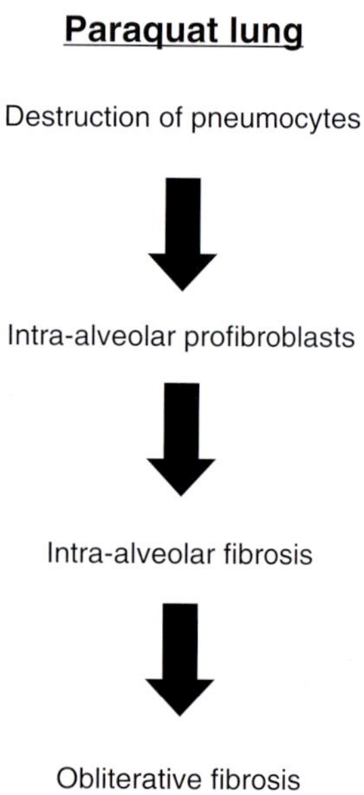

Figure 7.13 Paraquat lung – schematic of lesion progression. Following destruction of type I/II pneumocytes, proliferating intra-alveolar fibroblasts (fibroblastic plugs) organize the exudate, evolving into intra-alveolar/interstitial fibrosis and ultimately **obliterative** fibrosis ("honeycomb" remodeling (Dinis-Oliveira et al., 2008). *Source:* Adapted from Smith and Heath (1974), Fukuda et al.,1985).

provided renal function is adequate. Supportive care (oxygen, fluids) and, where feasible, antioxidants and anti-inflammatories may offer benefit; prognosis is grave once lung signs develop.

Molluscicides – Metaldehyde

Source

Metaldehyde, a cyclic polymer of acetaldehyde (Figure 7.14), is the active compound in many molluscicides. It is widely used worldwide to control snails and slugs in vegetable gardens, nurseries, and other settings where mollusks pose threats (Bates et al., 2012; Castle et al., 2017; National Pesticide Information Center, 2018).

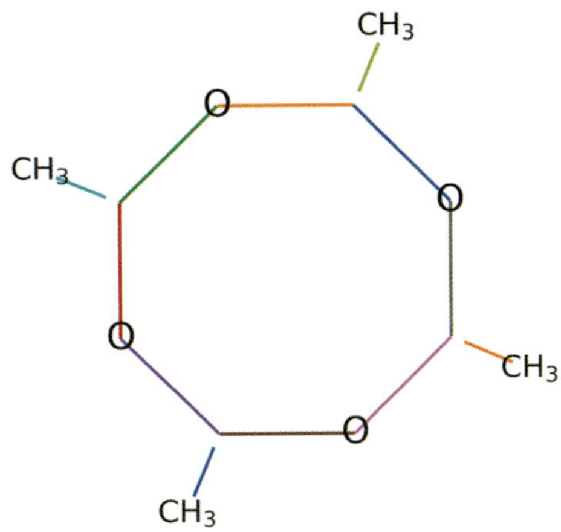

Figure 7.14 Metaldehyde ($C_8H_{16}O_4$) – cyclic tetramer of acetaldehyde and common molluscicide. Shown is the 1,3,5,7-tetraoxacyclooctane ring with four methyl-substituted carbons.

Commercial products are sold as liquids or pellets, typically containing ~1.5%–5% metaldehyde (Merck Veterinary Manual, 2025). Pelleted baits are attractive to dogs, cats, other domestic animals, and children and may be consumed in large quantities, resulting in toxicity and death. Poisoning has been reported in dogs (Bates et al., 2012), sheep (Tinson et al., 2017), horses (Sutherland, 1983), cattle (Stubbings, 1976; Valentine et al., 2007), geese and ducks (Andreasen Jr, 1993).

Toxicity

A few ounces of pelleted bait (≈75 mg metaldehyde) can cause acute, fatal poisoning in sheep (Tinson et al., 2017). A similar amount may be sufficient to poison a 15–25 kg dog (Gupta, 2018b).

Clinical Signs

Dogs: depression, hyperthermia, nausea, vomiting, hyperpnea, tachycardia, ataxia, hyperesthesia, tremors progressing to opisthotonus, and continuous convulsions; cyanosis, loss of consciousness, and death. Cats: nystagmus is described (Gupta, 2018b). Sheep: rectal temperature may rise to 43°C; dyspnea and head-pressing may occur.

Pathophysiology

Lesions include hepatic and renal hyperemia, hepatocellular and neuronal degeneration, and pulmonary interstitial hemorrhage/hyperemia (Figure 7.15). In sheep, the liver may be pale and friable; abundant froth can fill the respiratory tract (Tinson et al., 2017). Petechiae can be present in GI mucosa; stomach contents may smell of acetaldehyde.

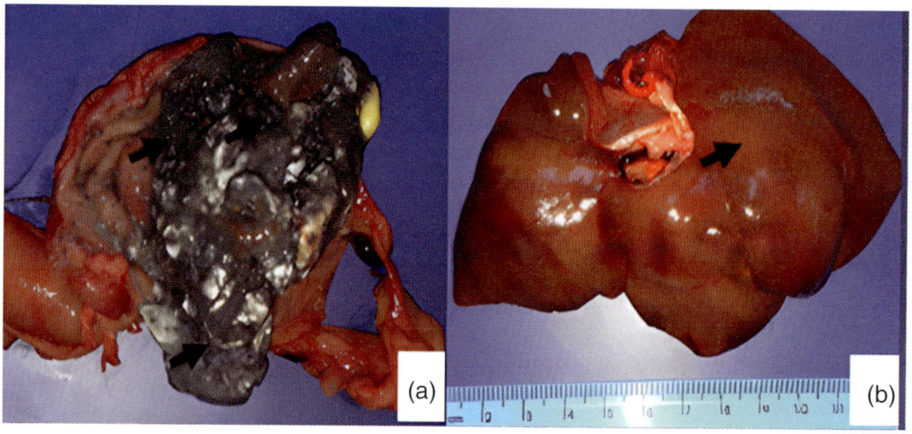

Figure 7.15 Necropsy lesions following ingestion of metaldehyde (dog). (a) Stomach: the mucosa is covered by a diffuse black–gray necrotic slough with adherent granular ingesta/bait (arrows), consistent with severe erosive–necrotizing **and** hemorrhagic gastritis after caustic/toxicant exposure. (b) **Liver**: enlarged, congested, and friable **with a** subcapsular hemorrhagic/necrotic focus (**arrow**), reflecting acute toxic hepatopathy secondary to systemic poisoning. *Source:* Botelho et al., (2020)/Springer Nature/CC BY 4.0.

Diagnosis

Tentative diagnosis is based on signs and history of bait use. Confirmation relies on detection of acetaldehyde (a metabolite) or metaldehyde in stomach contents via laboratory analysis.

Treatment

No specific antidote is available. Immediate removal of unabsorbed toxin is crucial (induce emesis or lavage), followed by seizure control and supportive care. Respiratory stimulants (e.g., nikethamide) are rarely used today; priority is aggressive anticonvulsant therapy (e.g., diazepam) and supportive fluids. Calcium borogluconate and dextrose-saline may support hepatic function. Tranquilizers such as acepromazine or diazepam may control convulsions and facilitate nursing (Merck Veterinary Manual, 2025; Plumlee, 2004). In a prospective cohort of 26 dogs with metaldehyde poisoning, common signs included ataxia, seizures, hypersalivation, and tremors; management was supportive (e.g., decontamination and anticonvulsants) with an overall survival of 81% (Dutil et al., 2023).

Molluscicides – Methiocarb

Source

Methiocarb, a carbamate cholinesterase inhibitor closely related to the insecticide carbaryl (1-naphthyl N-methylcarbamate), was introduced as a molluscicide following observations of molluscicidal properties in the late 1950s (Martinez & Evans, 2021). Common commercial preparations include Draza

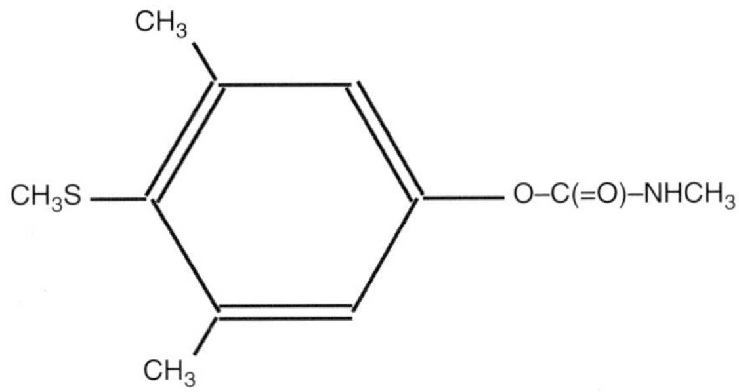

Figure 7.16 Methiocarb – 3,5-dimethyl-4-(methylthio)phenyl N-methylcarbamate.Skeletal formula showing the **carbamate group** (—O—C(=O)—$NHCH_3$) para to a methylthio substituent (—S—CH_3) and flanked by **3,5-dimethyl** ring positions. In veterinary toxicology, methiocarb (formerly used as slug/snail bait and seed treatment; trade name Mesurol) **is a** carbamate acetylcholinesterase inhibitor.

Forte (Bayer) and Slug Gard (Pan Britannica Industries), typically 4% methiocarb in cereal pellets dyed blue (Figure 7.16).

Toxicity

LD50 values: ~100 mg/kg (rat), ~40 mg/kg (guinea pig) (EFSA, 2018) and ~25 mg/kg (dog). Onset of clinical signs is typically 20–60 minutes after ingestion. While less commonly reported than metaldehyde, methiocarb poisoning occurs in dogs and sheep (Tinson et al., 2017; Corfield et al., 2008).

Mechanism of Action

Methiocarb competitively inhibits AChE and pseudocholinesterase, leading to acetylcholine accumulation and excessive muscarinic and nicotinic effects (Tinson et al., 2017; Corfield et al., 2008).

Clinical Signs

Dogs: profuse salivation, vomiting, severe diarrhea (often gelatinous/milky with blue streaks), tremors progressing to opisthotonus; miosis; mucous-membrane congestion; bradycardia; irregular pulse; and slow respiration (Tinson et al., 2017; Corfield et al., 2008). Sheep: depression, hypersalivation, diarrhea, dyspnea, blue dye stain on lips, hind-limb ataxia, and aimless walking (Gupta, 2018b).

Pathophysiology

Necropsy may reveal widespread petechiation (including the serosal surface of the small intestine, kidneys, and respiratory mucosa), congested/hemorrhagic lungs with frothy sanguineous fluid in the tracheobronchial tree – lesions consistent with respiratory distress.

Diagnosis

Diagnosis is based on history (presence of slug bait), clinical signs, and physical evidence (pellets/packaging).

Treatment

Treat as for carbamate/OP poisoning, except do not administer oximes (2-PAM). High-dose atropine (e.g., 2–4 mg for a dog) IV, repeated as necessary, plus benzodiazepines or other anticonvulsants for seizures. Provide oxygen or artificial ventilation for respiratory compromise (Tinson et al., 2017). Discharge after sustained stabilization with no relapse over 4–5 hours of observation.

Feed-Related and Agricultural Chemical Toxicoses

Nonprotein Nitrogen (Urea)

Sources

As shown in Figure 7.17, urea is commonly incorporated into ruminant rations, premixes, and molasses blocks as an NPN source to drive microbial protein synthesis. The same easily available prills can precipitate outbreaks when misformulated, introduced abruptly, accessed as fertilizer, or overconsumed in lick blocks – scenarios linked to urea (ammonia) toxicosis (Radostits et al., 2007; Gupta, 2018b).

Mechanism of Toxicity

Ruminal urease rapidly hydrolyzes urea to NH_3 and CO_2. As shown in Figure 58, when fermentable carbohydrate is adequate, NH_3 is captured into microbial protein and any surplus is detoxified via the hepatic urea cycle (green pathway). By contrast, with inadequate CHO or rapid intake, microbial

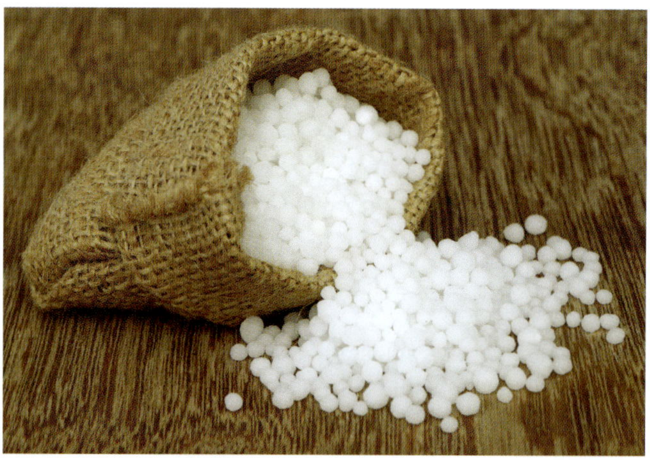

Figure 7.17 Urea prills used as a non-protein nitrogen (NPN) source. Typical feed/fertilizer urea granules ("prills") as handled from a bag. In ruminant nutrition they are blended into rations, premixes, or molasses blocks to support microbial protein synthesis; however, the same product poses a toxicosis risk if animals access fertilizer bags, if mixing is inaccurate, or if naïve, hungry stock over-consume urea blocks. *Source:* Swapan/Adobe Stock Photos.

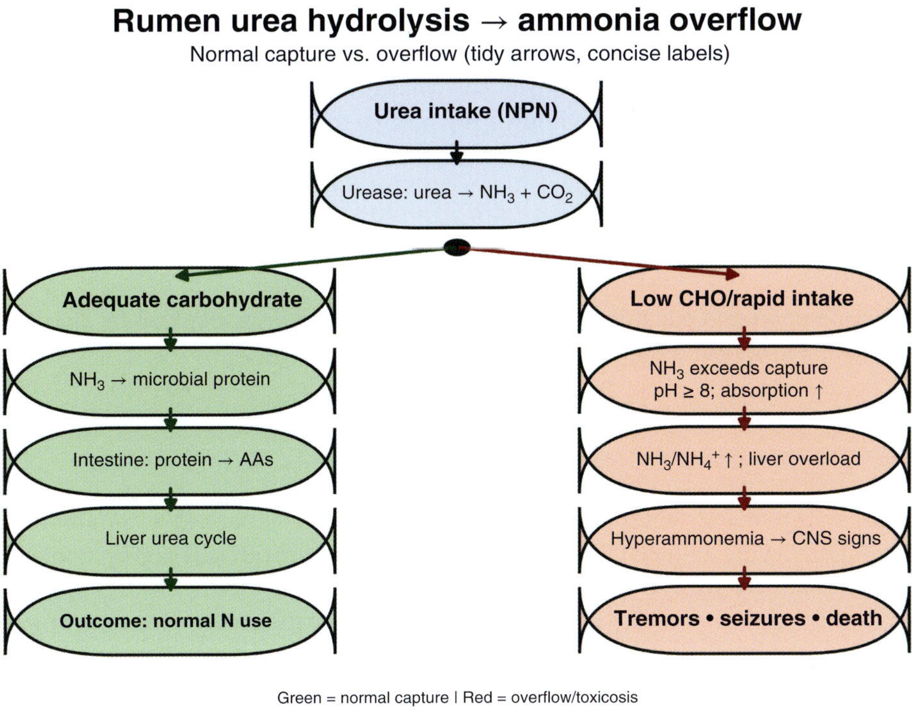

Figure 7.18 Rumen urea hydrolysis → ammonia overflow. Schematic of two fates for urea-derived ammonia after ruminal urease activity. The **green lane** (left) shows the normal capture pathway: adequate fermentable carbohydrate allows NH_3 to be incorporated into microbial protein, digested in the small intestine, and any surplus is handled by the hepatic urea cycle. The red lane (right) shows the overflow/toxicosis pathway: low CHO or rapid intake causes NH_3 to exceed microbial capture, rumen pH rises ($\geq$8) and absorption increases, the liver is overwhelmed, **hyperammonemia** develops, and neurological signs (tremors, seizures) may follow. Green, normal capture; Red, overflow/toxicosis.

utilization is exceeded; NH_3 accumulates, is absorbed across the rumen wall as pH rises, overwhelms hepatic detoxification, and leads to hyperammonemia with CNS dysfunction (red pathway) (Figure 7.18). With inadequate fermentable carbohydrate or excessive intake, microbial utilization is exceeded; NH_3 accumulates, is absorbed across the rumen wall, and overwhelms hepatic detoxification, resulting in hyperammonemia, metabolic alkalosis, CNS dysfunction, and respiratory failure.

Toxic/Lethal Doses and Risks

Minimum lethal doses in cattle are commonly cited around ~0.5–1.0 g/kg body weight (BW) urea, lower if ingestion is rapid or in unadapted animals; risk increases with fasting, dehydration, urease-rich feeds, and hot conditions that accelerate rumen kinetics (Gupta, 2018b).

Clinical Signs

Onset is rapid (20–60 minutes): restlessness, hypersalivation, colic, polyuria, tremors, ataxia, bellowing, bruxism, clonic convulsions, cyanosis, and death. Rumen pH is often alkaline (>8), bloat is common (Figure 7.19).

Diagnosis

History of access plus rapid onset and alkaline rumen pH support the diagnosis. Confirm by elevated ammonia in rumen fluid, blood, or ocular fluid (sample promptly).

Treatment

Immediate priorities are to dilute and acidify the rumen so that ammonia is trapped as ammonium ($NH_3 \rightarrow NH_4^+$), while stabilizing the animal. Give cold water with 5% acetic acid (vinegar) by stomach tube; in adult cattle, a pragmatic range is ~2–6 L of vinegar with copious cold water, delivered carefully to avoid aspiration. Provide supportive care – IV fluids to correct dehydration/alkalosis, control seizures and bloat – and, if a solid bolus was ingested or the response is poor, perform rumenotomy. Longer-term control is preventive: Introduce NPN gradually, pair urea with readily fermentable carbohydrate, and limit inclusion to ≤1% of the total ration DM with accurate mixing and constant water

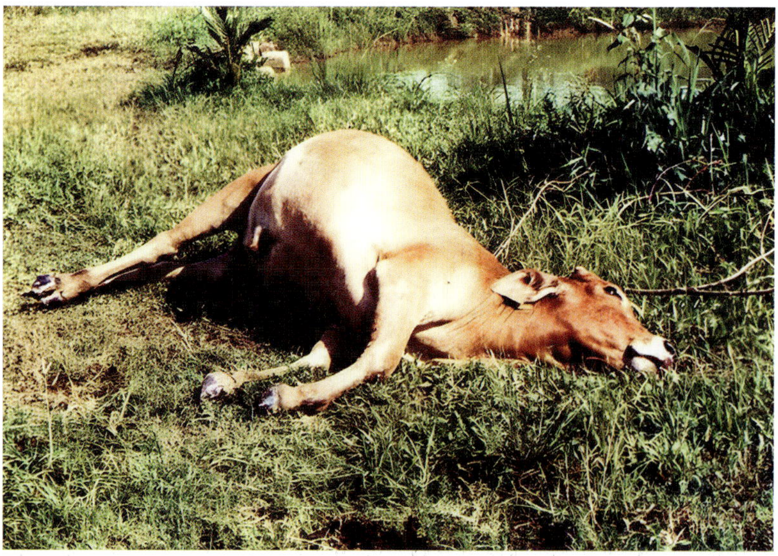

Figure 7.19 Peracute urea/ammonia toxicosis in a cow – field presentation. Adult bovine found in lateral recumbency with marked abdominal distension (bloat/ruminal tympany) and cyanotic muzzle, consistent with peracute death following ammonia overload. Bloat is a common terminal feature of urea poisoning.

Table 7.7 Limits reflect veterinary and regulatory guidance: ≤1% of complete feed dry matter (DM) for adapted ruminants European Food Safety Authority (EFSA), ≤2–3% of the concentrate and gradual acclimation over days–weeks (Merck Vet Manual). Daily safe intake around 0.3 g/kg BW/day corresponds to EFSA's adapted-animal benchmark; do not feed unadapted or hungry stock.

Guideline	Cattle (≈450–600 kg)	Sheep/goats (≈40–60 kg)	Notes
Maximum urea in total diet (DM basis)	**≤1.0%**	**≤1.0%**	Count **all** urea sources (premix, blocks, liquids).
Maximum urea in concentrate mix (DM)	**≤3%**	**≤3%**	Only when fed **with grain/ molasses** (readily fermentable CHO).
Daily maximum by body weight	**≤30 g/100 kg BW/day** (e.g., ≤150 g for 500 kg)	**≤30 g/100 kg BW/day** (e.g., ≤15 g for 50 kg)	Do **not** offer to hungry, unadapted stock.
Single-meal limit	**≤10 g/100 kg BW/meal**	**≤10 g/100 kg BW/meal**	Split across meals; never top-dress.
Adaptation (typical 2–4 wk)	Week 1: **0.25% DM** → Week 2: **0.5%** → Week 3: **0.75%** → Week 4 (if needed): **≤1.0%**	Same schedule, scaled to intake	Move up only if animals are eating well and manure is normal.
Essential pairing	Provide **readily fermentable CHO** (grain/molasses)	Provide **readily fermentable CHO**	Target rumen S:N ≈ **1:10–1:12**; maintain constant **fresh water** access.
Mixing and access	Dissolve in molasses/water before mixing; avoid "hot spots"	As at left	**Never** free-access for naïve/ starved animals; fence fertilizer urea.

* Limits and adaptation steps compiled from European Food Safety Authority (EFSA) Panel on Additives and Products or Substances used in Animal Feed (FEEDAP), 2012; Merck Veterinary Manual, 2024a; NASEM, 2016. European Food Safety Authority (EFSA) Panel on Additives and Products or Substances used in Animal Feed (FEEDAP), 2012; Merck Veterinary Manual, 2024a; National Academies of Sciences, Engineering, and Medicine, 2016; Food and Agriculture Organization of the United Nations, 2007.

access. Practical feeding limits and step-up schedules are summarized in Table 7.7 (European Food Safety Authority (EFSA) Panel on Additives and Products or Substances used in Animal Feed (FEEDAP), 2012; Food and Agriculture Organization of the United Nations, 2007; Merck Veterinary Manual, 2024a; National Academies of Sciences, Engineering, and Medicine, 2016), while field first-aid dosages and administration details are compiled in Table 7.8 (Merck Veterinary Manual, 2024a; Wilmar Sugar Australia, 2019).

Nitrate and Nitrite Poisoning

Sources

Annuals (sorghums, oats, millet, maize) and weeds (amaranth/pigweed, lambsquarters) accumulate nitrate under drought, heavy nitrogen fertilization, cloudy weather, or herbicide injury; contaminated well/pond water is another route. Poorly ensiled high-nitrate forage remains risky (Gupta, 2018b).

Table 7.8 Emergency treatment uses 5% acetic acid plus cold water delivered via stomach tube; volumes should be scaled to species/BW and clinical status (Merck Vet Manual). Some field guides specify ~45 L water followed by 2–6 L vinegar for adult cattle (Wilmar Sugar user guide); use veterinary judgment.

Species/BW	5% acetic acid (household vinegar)	Cold water (dilution/cooling)	Administration and notes
Adult cattle (450–600 kg)	2–6 L via stomach tube	20–40 L	Keep head/neck down to reduce aspiration; check rumen pH; may repeat once after 15–20 minutes if still alkaline. Decompress bloat if needed.
Growing cattle (100–250 kg)	0.5–2 L	5–20 L	Scale to size and severity.
Sheep/goats (40–60 kg)	0.5–1.0 L	2–5 L	Oral drench or small-bore tube; go slow.
If severe/bolus present	—	—	Rumenotomy can be lifesaving. Start IV fluids; control seizures; monitor acid–base status.

* *First-aid volumes collated from Merck Veterinary Manual,* 2024a; *Wilmar Sugar Australia,* 2019.
** ***Quick cautions:*** *These are pragmatic field ranges; adjust volumes for concentration if using acids* ***not*** *at 5% acetic strength; avoid over-acidification and aspiration; treatment does* ***not*** *replace urgent veterinary care (Merck Veterinary Manual,* 2024a*).*

Mechanism and Pathogenesis

As illustrated in Figure 7.20, rumen microbes normally reduce $NO_3^- \rightarrow NO_2^- \rightarrow NH_3$, but excess nitrite oxidizes hemoglobin to methemoglobin, impairing oxygen transport and producing chocolate-brown blood with clinical signs of hypoxia.

Clinical Signs and Diagnosis

Rapid/labored breathing, weakness, ataxia, brown mucosa, collapse, and death. Diagnosis is by methemoglobin measurement and nitrate/nitrite assays on suspect feed/water.

Treatment and Prevention

Thresholds for **forage and water nitrate** and the corresponding management actions are summarized in Table 7.9; values are adapted from NDSU Extension's interpretation guidelines (North Dakota State University Extension, 2020), with unit conversions per Nebraska Extension (University of Nebraska–Lincoln Extension, n.d.). When clinical signs indicate methemoglobinemia, administer methylene blue 1–2 mg/kg IV (titrated) (Agency for Toxic Substances and Disease Registry, n.d.; Merck Veterinary Manual, 2024b) and remove high-nitrate sources; longer-term control relies on testing/dilution and gradual adaptation (see Table 7.9 for thresholds that trigger action). Remove high-nitrate sources and offer good-quality forage; test suspect forages and adapt animals slowly; avoid heavy N fertilization before drought/cloudy periods (Gupta, 2018b).

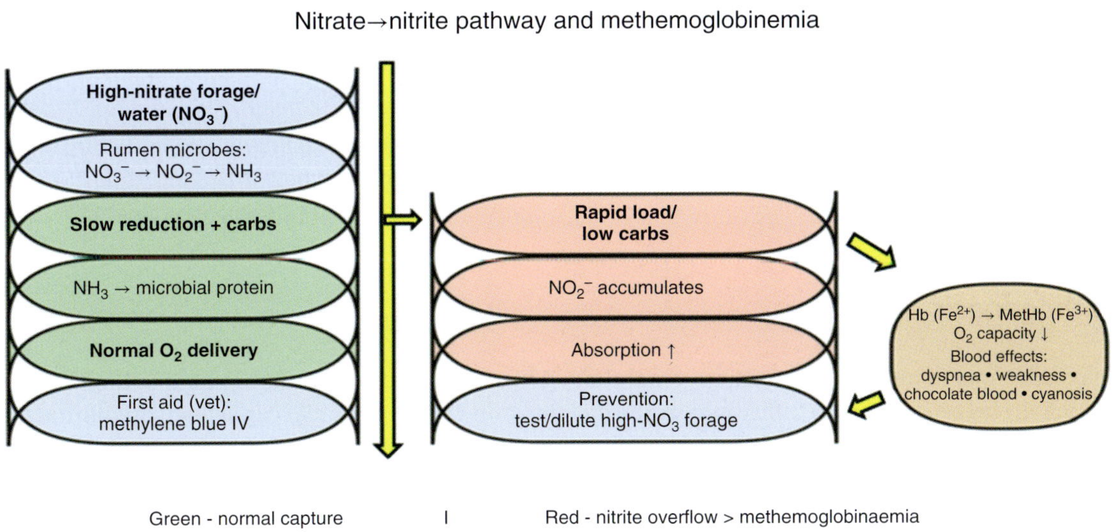

Figure 7.20 Nitrate → nitrite pathway and methemoglobinemia (ruminants). Schematic labels show rumen microbial reduction of nitrate (NO_3−) to nitrite (NO_2−) and then to ammonia. When NO_2− production outpaces its further reduction, nitrite accumulates, enters blood, and oxidizes hemoglobin $Fe^{2+} \rightarrow Fe^{3+}$, forming methemoglobin (MetHb) that cannot carry oxygen – resulting in hypoxia and the classic chocolate-brown blood appearance.

Table 7.9 Forage and water **nitrate thresholds** with suggested management actions (ruminants).

ForageNO_3 (ppm)	Water NO_3 (%)	Risk category	Management action
0–4,430	0–0.44	Generally safe	Feed normally.
4,430–6,645	0.44–0.66	Caution (pregnant stock)	Safe for nonpregnant animals; **limit to ≤50%** of ration DM for pregnant animals.
6,645–8,860	0.66–0.88	Caution (all stock)	**Limit to ≤50%** of ration DM for all animals.
8,860–15,505	0.88–1.55	High	**Limit to ~30–35%** of ration DM; **do not** feed to pregnant animals.
15,505–17,720	1.55–1.77	Very high	**Limit to ≤25%** of ration DM; **do not** feed to pregnant animals.
>17,720	>1.77	Dangerous	**Do not feed**.
NO_3-N (mg/L)	NO_3 (mg/L)	Risk category	Management action
0–100	0–443	Generally safe	Use normally, but consider additive nitrate from feed.
100–300	443–1,329	Caution	Monitor animals; **dilute** with low-nitrate water; reduce dietary nitrate.
>300	>1,329	Dangerous	**Do not use** for livestock; provide alternative source immediately.

Forage (dry-matter basis; reported as **nitrate ion, NO_3**, ppm)
Water (as received; livestock thresholds). Both units shown (1 mg/L ≈ 1 ppm; NO_3-N × 4.43 = NO_3) (North Dakota State University Extension, 2020).
Source: Data from NDSU, (2020).

Sodium (Salt) Toxicosis

Risk Scenarios

Occurs with high salt intake and limited water (or abrupt rewatering): brackish/seawater ingestion, inadequate trough supply, salt-polluted wells, high-salt feeds/mineral mixes, whey or isotonic fluids as sole water source. Species susceptibility: swine > poultry > ruminants; cats > dogs among pets (Gupta, 2018a).

Pathogenesis

Hypernatremia increases brain/cerebrospinal fluid (CSF) osmolality ("sodium trapping"). Rapid rehydration drives osmotic water influx into hyperosmotic brain cells → cerebral edema, increased intracranial pressure (ICP), seizures.

Clinical Signs and Lesions

Early: anorexia, abdominal pain, diarrhea, polydipsia/polyuria, blindness, seizures; swine show head-pressing, circling, intermittent seizures, sudden death. Lesions: meningeal congestion/edema; severe cases show cortical softening/necrosis (polioencephalomalacia).

Treatment

As shown in Figure 7.21, treatment prioritizes gradual rehydration with careful sodium correction over 24–48 hours, adding anticonvulsants if needed (Merck Veterinary Manual, 2024c). The flowchart highlights why rapid free-water intake must be avoided after salt/water deprivation, as it can precipitate cerebral edema and worsen the outcome. Table 7.10 complements this by outlining the main sodium salt sources, the species most at risk, and staged rehydration strategies applicable both in the field and clinical settings (Gupta, 2018b; Plumlee, 2004).

Usage, Risks, and Management Strategies in Diverse Climates

Pesticides and agricultural chemicals are indispensable tools for modern agriculture and public health, yet their usage patterns, risks, and management strategies differ across climates. In tropical regions like Malaysia, year-round pest pressure, warm temperatures, and heavy rainfall drive continuous pesticide use and create unique exposure and contamination pathways. In temperate regions, pest life cycles are seasonal, allowing more structured application and regulation, while arid regions face intermittent but intense outbreaks linked to irrigation and rainfall pulses (Daam & Van den Brink, 2010; Daam et al., 2019; FAO, 2024; Tudi et al., 2021).

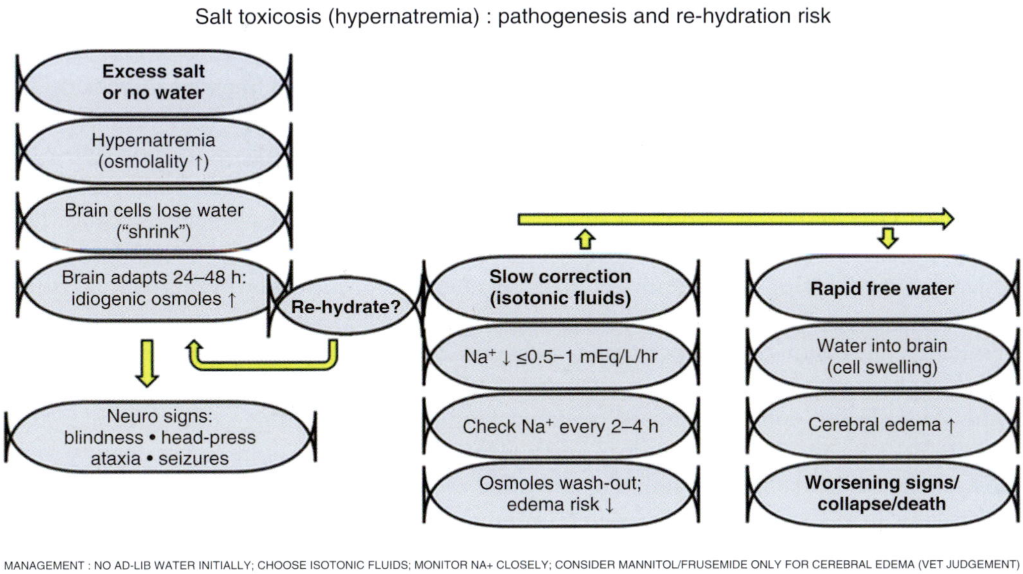

Figure 7.21 Salt toxicosis (hypernatremia) – management and rehydration flowchart. The diagram contrasts a slow, controlled rehydration lane – small, frequent water allowances and isotonic fluids with a planned sodium fall (≈ 0.5–1 mEq/L/h over 24–48 hours) – against the rapid free-water lane that risks cerebral edema and clinical deterioration. Adjunctive care includes anticonvulsants for seizures; prognosis is guarded once advanced neurologic signs are present.

Table 7.10 Sources of sodium salt exposure, species susceptibility, and staged rehydration protocols in salt toxicoses. The table highlights common exposure routes, clinical features, and evidence-based fluid correction strategies for different species.

Sources of sodium/ salt exposure	Species most susceptible	Clinical features	Staged rehydration protocol (field and clinical)	References
High-salt drinking water (brackish wells, boreholes)	Swine (most sensitive)	CNS signs: aimless wandering, blindness, seizures; cerebral edema histologically	• Remove salt source. • Give small, frequent water allowances (0.5–1% BW q1–2 h). • Avoid unrestricted water access.	Gupta (2018b), Plumlee (2004)
Salt-contaminated feed (fishmeal, whey, saline food waste)	Poultry, cattle	Neurological signs, depression, opisthotonus, watery diarrhea; cortical laminar necrosis	• Gradual correction of serum sodium (≤0.5–1 mEq/L/h over 24–48 h). • Use isotonic fluids cautiously; avoid rapid IV hypotonic fluids.	Plumlee (2004)
Water deprivation followed by unrestricted access	Swine, dogs, ruminants	Acute collapse, seizures, high mortality	• Controlled access to fresh water in divided doses. • Administer anticonvulsants if seizures occur.	Papich, 2019

Usage Patterns Across Climates

In tropical climates, insect, weed, and fungal pests thrive year-round, driving frequent insecticide and fungicide applications in crops such as oil palm, rice, and fruit orchards (Tudi et al., 2021). Public-health authorities also rely heavily on chemical interventions; organophosphates like malathion and pyrethroids such as cyphenothrin are routinely fogged in urban neighborhoods to control dengue vectors (Ministry of Health Malaysia, 2024; World Mosquito Program, 2024). Alongside pesticide exposure, livestock in these regions are vulnerable to agrichemical misuses, including urea misformulation, nitrate surges in drought–rainfall cycles, and sodium salt toxicoses after water deprivation events (Gupta, 2018b; Plumlee, 2004).

By contrast, temperate regions experience cyclical pest pressures tied to spring and summer, with fungicides and herbicides dominating veterinary exposure risks; anticoagulant rodenticides and molluscicides like metaldehyde are common causes of companion-animal poisoning (Caloni et al., 2016; McFarland et al., 2017; Ravindran et al., 2022). In arid and semiarid zones, pests are constrained by water scarcity, but episodic outbreaks follow rainfall or irrigation events, and salt toxicoses in livestock are a recurrent hazard due to brackish water or sudden rehydration.

These comparative patterns – spanning pesticides and agrichemicals – are summarized in Table 7.11, which contrasts tropical, temperate, and arid/semiarid climates in terms of pest drivers, agrochemical use, and veterinary toxicology risk profiles.

In the tropics, high temperatures and continuous forage growth amplify risks for urea misformulation and rapid rumen kinetics, while drought–rainfall cycles drive nitrate accumulation in annual forages; in arid zones, chronic water scarcity predisposes to salt toxicosis and dangerous rewatering events; in temperate regions, post-drought regrowth and heavy fertilization are classic nitrate risk windows. Field triage benefits from simple spot tests for nitrate in forages/water and conservative rehydration protocols after water deprivation (Gupta, 2018b). These patterns are summarized in Table 7.12, which links climatic triggers to urea, nitrate/nitrite, and salt toxicoses, and outlines simple first-response field measures to guide practitioners in tropical and temperate contexts (Gupta, 2018b; Plumlee, 2004).

Risks in Different Climates

Because pesticide risk pathways differ by climate, Figure 7.22 maps where exposures come from. In the tropics, intense rain mobilizes residues into rivers and wetlands (e.g., diuron/atrazine in Malaysian paddy irrigation water; Daam et al., 2019), while heat can revolatilize legacy organochlorines such as DDT (Unsworth et al., 1999). Wildlife impacts include the 2013 deaths of Bornean pygmy elephants after pesticide-laced palm fruit (Motlagh, 2013) and secondary anticoagulant exposures in barn owls and civets on oil-palm estates (Ravindran et al., 2022). In temperate regions, cold winters slow degradation but can preserve residues; in arid regions, irrigation networks can spread pesticides widely with limited dilution.

Table 7.11 Comparative pesticide- and agrichemical-use patterns across tropical, temperate, and arid/semiarid climates. Includes veterinary toxicology risks from pesticides (OPs, rodenticides, metaldehyde) and agrichemicals (urea, nitrate/nitrite, sodium salt). Qualitative synthesis of agronomic guidance, regulatory documents, and veterinary-toxicology references. Patterns reflect typical crops, targets, formulations, and exposure risks; they are **not** market-share data.

Dimension	Tropical	Temperate	Arid/semiarid
Agro climate drivers	Year-round warmth, high humidity and rainfall → continuous pest and disease pressure; drought–rainfall cycles promote nitrate accumulation.	Distinct seasons; winter off-season reduces some pest cycles but favors storage/seed treatments.	Heat, low rainfall, episodic pest outbreaks after rains; brackish water and sudden rehydration drive salt toxicoses.
Cropping calendars	Multi-cropping; perennial plantations (oil palm, rubber, cocoa, banana), rice double-crop.	Spring–summer annuals (cereals, potatoes, beet), orchards, and vineyards.	Rain-fed short seasons (millets, sorghum), irrigated vegetables; rangelands.
Dominant targets	Insects (lepidopterans, hemipterans), vector-borne diseases, fungal (leaf spots, blights), weeds; urea/nitrate-related forage risks.	Fungal diseases (rusts, mildews, scab, downy mildew), weeds in cereals/row crops, slugs/snails.	Locusts/grasshoppers, storage pests, weeds; livestock water–salt risks.
Common classes/agents	Pyrethroids, OPs/carbamates (declining but present), neonicotinoids, triazole and strobilurin fungicides, glyphosate/glufosinate; agrichemicals: urea fertilizers, nitrate-rich forages.	Fungicides (triazoles, SDHIs, copper, sulfur), selective herbicides, anticoagulant rodenticides, molluscicides (metaldehyde/ferric phosphate).	Pyrethroids and OPs for locust campaigns, phosphine for grain storage, phenoxy herbicides; salt exposure from brackish water and feeds.
Formulations favored	EC/Suspension concentrate (SC)/Water-dispersible granule (WG); rain-fastness & UV stability valued; ULV for vector control.	WG/SC/flowables; seed treatments; bait formulations.	ULV/Emulsifiable concentrate (EC) for aerial locust control; dusts and fumigants for storage.
Application pattern	Frequent/prophylactic in plantations; vector campaigns; forage fertilization risks.	Programmed sprays; herbicide rotations; seasonal rodenticide/metaldehyde use.	Pulsed apps tied to outbreaks; emergency locust campaigns; livestock rewatering.
Veterinary toxicology—frequent exposures	OP/carbamate insecticides (cholinergic crisis), pyrethroids in dogs/cats, rodenticides in plantation dogs; urea misformulation (ammonia toxicosis), nitrate surges (methemoglobinemia), salt toxicoses.	Anticoagulant rodenticides (hemorrhage), metaldehyde (tremors/seizures), fungicide solvents; occasional OPs.	Aluminum/magnesium phosphide (phosphine gas), OP/pyrethroid sprays, amitraz in dogs; recurrent salt toxicoses from water scarcity.
Regulatory tone (examples)	Malaysia: Pesticide Act 1974; stewardship programs (myGAP, MSPO); new uptake of biopesticides.	EU: hazard-based approvals; IPM mandated; strong wildlife & water protection.	Sub-Saharan Africa: heterogeneous; FAO-guided locust programs; limited control on agrichemicals.

LAAR, long-acting anticoagulant rodenticide; OP, organophosphate; QoI, quinone-outside inhibitor; SDHI, succinate dehydrogenase inhibitor; ULV, ultra-low volume.

Source: Department of Agriculture Malaysia. (2020), European Commission. (2009), Food and Agriculture Organization of the United Nations (2021), Food and Agriculture Organization of the United Nations & World Health Organization (2019), Fungicide Resistance Action Committee (FRAC) (2024), Insecticide Resistance Action Committee (IRAC) (2024), Kahn and Line (2010), National Pesticide Information Center (2018), Rattner et al. (2014), Schlipalius et al., 2008.

Table 7.12 Climate-linked triggers, common field scenarios, and first-response checklists for urea (NPN), nitrate/nitrite, and sodium salt toxicoses in food-producing animals. The table highlights how tropical heat and rainfall patterns, temperate post-drought regrowth, and arid water scarcity influence risk and guides practical field triage, screening, and initial stabilization measures. Adapted and compile by the references below:

Toxicant	Climate-linked trigger(s)	Common field scenarios	Key clinical risk window	First-response field checklist (triage)	Practical field test(s) / samples
Urea / non-protein nitrogen (NPN)	**Tropics:** heat accelerates rumen fermentation/ureolysis; year-round forage availability encourages frequent supplementation and mixing errors (Gupta, 2018b).	Misformulated ration or premix; sudden introduction of urea blocks; hungry/unadapted cattle access fertilizer bags; inadequate fermentable carbohydrate in the ration (Gupta, 2018b).	Often **20–60 min** after rapid intake; fastest and most severe in unadapted, hungry animals (Gupta, 2018b).	• **Remove** urea source immediately (feed, block, fertilizer access). • **Call for help early** (rapid progression). • If safe to do so, **rumen acidification/dilution** using **vinegar (acetic acid) + cold water** via stomach tube (field practice) to trap ammonia as NH_4^+ (Gupta, 2018b). • Control bloat, seizures, and provide supportive care while transporting (Gupta, 2018b).	• **Rumen pH** (often alkaline) and **rumen fluid ammonia** (where available). • Collect **rumen fluid** and **heparinized blood** promptly for ammonia (Gupta, 2018b). • In fatalities, collect **ocular (aqueous/vitreous) fluid** early if available (Gupta, 2018b).
Nitrate / nitrite	**Tropics:** drought–rainfall cycles and rapid regrowth increase nitrate in annual forages; heavy N fertilization + cloudy spells also increase accumulation (Gupta, 2018b). **Temperate:** classic post-drought regrowth and heavy fertilization risk windows (Gupta, 2018b).	Grazing high-risk crops/weeds (e.g., sorghum, millet, maize, amaranth/pigweed); feeding stressed forages or poorly made silage; contaminated well/pond water (Gupta, 2018b).	Acute hypoxia/methemoglobinemia can develop **within hours** of ingestion; sudden deaths may occur with very high nitrite load (Gupta, 2018b).	• **Stop exposure**: remove animals from suspect pasture/feed/water. • **Minimize exertion** (worsens hypoxia). • If available, treat under veterinary direction with **methylene blue** for methemoglobinemia (Gupta, 2018b). • Provide oxygen/supportive care and transport.	• **Spot test/dipstick** on forage and water (field screening) (Gupta, 2018b). • Collect **blood** (chocolate-brown suggests methemoglobin), plus **forage and water samples** for lab nitrate/nitrite (Gupta, 2018b). • In deaths, collect **ocular fluid** and representative **forage/water** samples (Gupta, 2018b).
Sodium salt (NaCl) / water deprivation–salt toxicosis	**Arid/semi-arid:** chronic water scarcity; brackish sources; dangerous **deprivation → sudden re-watering** events (Plumlee, 2004). **Also in tropics:** water interruptions in intensive units during heat stress (Gupta, 2018b).	Swine/poultry with restricted water; livestock drinking brackish water; high-salt rations, whey, saline food waste; sudden unlimited access after deprivation (Gupta, 2018b; Plumlee, 2004).	Neurologic signs often appear **after re-watering**, when cerebral edema develops; outbreaks can escalate quickly (Gupta, 2018b; Plumlee, 2004).	• **Do not allow unrestricted drinking** after deprivation. • **Controlled rehydration**: small, frequent water allowances. • Avoid rapid correction with hypotonic fluids; manage seizures as needed and transport (Gupta, 2018b; Plumlee, 2004).	• Check **serum sodium** if feasible; monitor neurologic status (Plumlee, 2004). • In fatalities, collect **brain (cerebrum/pons)** for histology and **serum/ocular fluid** where available (Gupta, 2018b; Plumlee, 2004).

1. Gupta, R. C. (Ed.). (2018b). *Veterinary toxicology: Basic and clinical principles* (3rd ed.). Academic Press.
2. Plumlee, K. H. (2004). *Clinical veterinary toxicology*. Mosby.

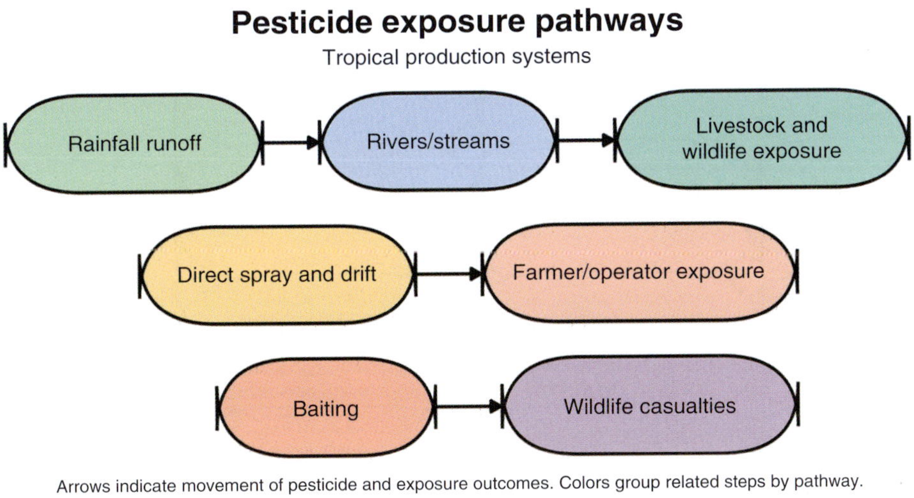

Figure 7.22 Pesticide exposure pathways in tropical production systems. Monsoonal rainfall and runoff carry pesticides into **streams/rivers**, exposing livestock and wildlife; direct spray and drift cause operator (farmer) dermal/inhalational exposure; and toxic baits lead to wildlife casualties (including secondary poisoning). Arrows depict major routes relevant to tropical settings – intense rain events → surface runoff/erosion → aquatic contamination and downstream watering points; spray applications without adequate PPE → acute human/animal exposures; and deliberate baiting in fields or around stores → primary and secondary wildlife poisonings. Add-on pathways (not shown) include mix–load spills, improper container disposal, irrigation channels, and fodder/crop residue ingestion.

Management Strategies in Diverse Climates

Integrated Pest and Agricultural Chemical Management (IPM/ACM)

Management strategies in diverse climates must encompass not only pesticide stewardship but also the risks posed by non-pesticide agricultural chemicals such as urea, nitrates, and sodium salts. Climate-driven triggers for these toxicoses underscore the importance of careful feed formulation, forage surveillance, and water access management alongside pest control. Integrated pest management (IPM) blends biological, cultural, and minimal chemical methods, remaining particularly vital in tropical settings. For example, in Malaysia, fruit growers demonstrate moderate knowledge but relatively low adoption of IPM despite awareness of environmental consequences (Chang et al., 2021). Practical adaptations include barn owl releases in oil-palm plantations to control rodents. In temperate zones, IPM adoption is generally higher, supported by well-developed extension services and precision agriculture tools (Staudacher et al., 2020).

As illustrated in Figure 7.23, integrated management frameworks across tropical, temperate, and arid regions now explicitly incorporate both pesticide and agricultural chemical toxicoses. This highlights how climate-linked triggers – such as monsoon-driven nitrate surges in the tropics, post-drought nitrate accumulation in temperate regions, and water deprivation salt crises in arid zones – demand equally climate-tailored first-response and stewardship strategies.

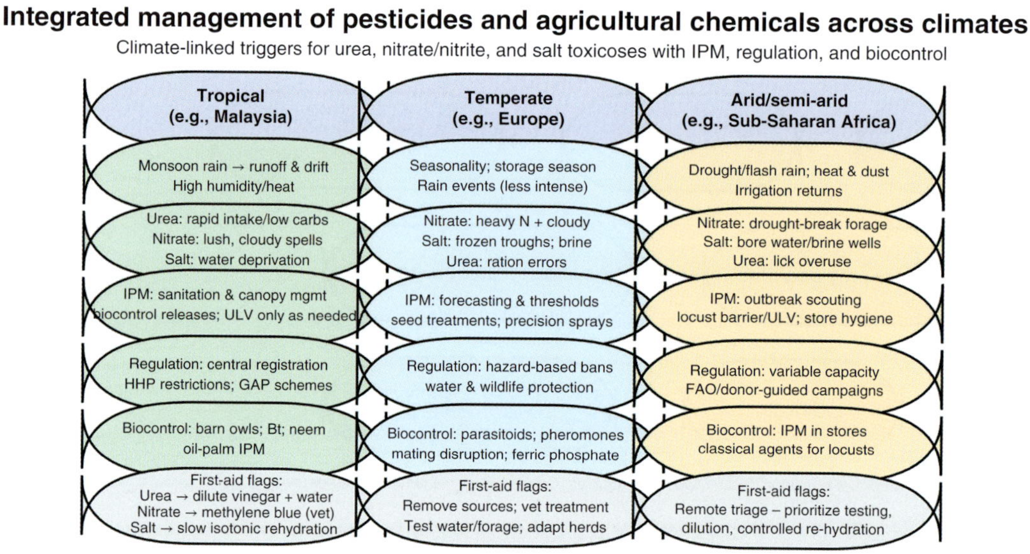

Figure 7.23 Integrated management of pesticides and agricultural chemicals across climates. The flowchart compares tropical (e.g., Malaysia), temperate (e.g., Europe), and arid/semiarid (e.g., sub-Saharan Africa) systems, linking climate-driven triggers for pesticide use and non-pesticide agricultural chemical toxicoses (urea, nitrate/nitrite, sodium salts) with corresponding IPM, regulatory frameworks, biocontrol approaches, and first-response field protocols (Daam & Van den Brink, 2010; European Commission, 2009; FAO & WHO, 2014/2019; FRAC, 2024; Gupta, 2018b; IRAC, 2024; Plumlee, 2004).

Regulatory Frameworks

Malaysia's Pesticide Act 1974 regulates imports and sales, supported by certification schemes such as myGAP, MSPO, and myOrganic (Sivapragasam & Goh, 2025). In contrast, the EU bans hazard-classified chemicals outright, while the United States employs risk-based re-evaluation (European Commission, 2009). Importantly, Malaysian regulations also guide safe handling of fertilizers and feed additives, recognizing their overlap with toxicological risks.

Biopesticides and Alternatives

Malaysia's registration pathway for low-risk products (GP7/2016) has spurred biopesticide uptake, including *Bacillus thuringiensis* and neem extracts (Sivapragasam & Goh, 2025). Adoption is growing but cost and familiarity remain barriers compared with temperate regions where biocontrol agents are widely mainstreamed.

Public Health Approaches

Vector management in the tropics is shifting toward integrated vector management (IVM). Malaysia has piloted *Wolbachia*-infected mosquitoes to combat dengue, reducing reliance on fogging with malathion and pyrethroids (Ministry of Health Malaysia, 2024; World Mosquito Program, 2024). Rotation of insecticide classes and environmental management (e.g., removing standing water) are vital for resistance control (WHO, n.d.; Hoffmann et al., 2024; Nurul-Nastasea et al., 2023; World Mosquito Program, 2024).

Case Studies

- Pygmy elephants (Sabah, Malaysia): 14 elephants fatally poisoned after consuming pesticide laced palm fruit bait (Motlagh, 2013).
- Paraquat in cattle (Malaysia): 70 cattle deaths after grazing on herbicide-treated pastures (New Straits Times, 1994, cited in International Labour Organization, 2011).
- Barn owls in oil-palm estates: Secondary anticoagulant rodenticide exposure documented in predators (Ravindran et al., 2022).
- Dengue vector resistance (Selangor, Malaysia): *Aedes aegypti* populations resistant to pyrethroids and malathion due to over-fogging (WHO, n.d.; Hoffmann et al., 2024; Nurul-Nastasea et al., 2023; World Mosquito Program, 2024).
- Urea misformulation in feedlot cattle (Tropics): Accidental over-supplementation led to acute ammonia toxicosis and sudden deaths (Gupta, 2018b).
- Nitrate surge after drought–rainfall cycles (Malaysia): Accumulated nitrates in forage caused acute methemoglobinemia and livestock mortality (Daam & Van den Brink, 2010).
- Salt toxicosis in swine (Arid/semiarid tropics): Water deprivation followed by unrestricted access triggered cerebral edema and high mortality (Plumlee, 2004) (Table 7.13).

Conclusion

Pesticides and agricultural chemicals remain indispensable in modern food and fiber production, yet their use in tropical regions presents unique toxicological challenges. In Malaysia and across comparable climates, year-round pest pressure, high humidity, and continuous cropping foster frequent chemical interventions that increase the likelihood of exposure incidents in livestock, wildlife, and companion animals. Misuse or misformulation of fertilizers and feed additives, such as urea and nitrate-rich forages, further amplifies risks, while recurrent water-deprivation and rehydration events predispose animals to sodium salt toxicoses.

The consequences are not confined to agriculture: Vector-control campaigns, plantation practices, and the encroachment of chemicals into aquatic and forest ecosystems extend these hazards to public health and biodiversity. Case studies from Malaysia – ranging from paraquat poisoning in cattle to rodenticide exposure in barn owls and resistance in *Aedes aegypti* – underscore the tangible intersection between agricultural practice and toxicological outcomes.

Yet, management strategies tailored to climate can mitigate many of these risks. IPM, judicious chemical stewardship, staged rehydration protocols, and biopesticide adoption illustrate pathways toward safer practice, provided they are supported by strong regulatory frameworks and farmer education. Regional contrasts also remind us that no single strategy suffices: While temperate systems lean on hazard-based bans and programmed sprays, tropical and arid regions demand continuous vigilance against both pesticides and agrichemicals under shifting environmental triggers.

Table 7.13 Case studies of pesticide- and agrichemical-related toxicoses in tropical regions, highlighting the impact on livestock, wildlife, and public health.

Case	Location	Toxicant/Chemical	Species affected	Outcome	Reference
Pygmy elephants poisoned by palm fruit bait	Sabah, Malaysia	Pesticide-laced palm fruit (suspected carbamate/organophosphate)	Asian elephant (*Elephas maximus borneensis*)	14 elephants fatally poisoned	Motlagh (2013)
Paraquat exposure in cattle	Malaysia	Paraquat herbicide	Cattle	70 cattle deaths after grazing treated pastures	New Straits Times, 1994, cited in International Labour Organization, 2011
Barn owls in oil-palm estates	Malaysia	Secondary anticoagulant rodenticides	Barn owl (*Tyto alba*)	Evidence of toxicant residues; ecological risk highlighted	Ravindran et al. (2022)
Dengue vector resistance	Selangor, Malaysia	Pyrethroids and malathion	*Aedes aegypti* mosquitoes	Documented insecticide resistance; reduced fogging efficacy	WHO, n.d.; Hoffmann et al., 2024; Nurul-Nastasea et al., 2023; World Mosquito Program, 2024
Urea misformulation in feedlot cattle	Tropical Southeast Asia	Urea/NPN supplement misformulation	Beef cattle	Sudden deaths due to acute ammonia toxicosis	Gupta (2018b)
Nitrate surge after drought–rainfall cycle	Malaysia	Nitrate accumulation in annual forage crops	Dairy cattle	Multiple cases of acute methemoglobinemia and sudden death	Daam and Van den Brink (2010)
Salt toxicosis after water deprivation	Arid/semiarid tropics (reported in swine units)	Excess sodium intake + rapid rewatering	Swine	Neurological signs; high mortality in outbreaks	Plumlee (2004)

IPM, integrated pest management; IVM, integrated vector management; LAARs, long-acting anticoagulant rodenticides; MoA, mode of action; ULV, ultra-low volume.

Ultimately, safeguarding animal health in the tropics requires bridging veterinary toxicology with agronomy, ecology, and public health. By integrating regulatory oversight, farmer and veterinarian training, and practical field diagnostics, we can reduce the burden of agrichemical toxicoses while maintaining agricultural productivity. This chapter highlights that in tropical veterinary practice, pesticides and agricultural chemicals are not merely tools of production but critical determinants of animal welfare, ecosystem resilience, and One Health outcomes.

References

Agency for Toxic Substances and Disease Registry. (n.d.). *Nitrate/nitrite toxicity: How should patients overexposed to nitrates and/or nitrites be treated?* U.S, Department of Health and Human Services. https://archive.cdc.gov/www_atsdr_cdc_gov/csem/nitrate-nitrite/patients_exposed.html

Al-Jobory, M. M., & Mohammad, F. K. (2005). Validation of an electrometric method for measurement of blood cholinesterase activity in goats. *Journal of Veterinary Science*, *6*(4), 299–303. https://doi.org/10.4142/jvs.2005.6.4.299

Andreasen, J. R., Jr. (1993). Metaldehyde toxicosis in ducklings. *Journal of Veterinary Diagnostic Investigation*, *5*(3), 500–501. https://doi.org/10.1177/104063879300500341

Assis, C. R. D., Linhares, A. G., Cabrera, M. P., Oliveira, V. M., Silva, K. C. C., Marcuschi, M., Maciel Carvalho, E. V. M., Bezerra, R. S., & Carvalho, L. B., Jr. (2018). Erythrocyte acetylcholinesterase as biomarker of pesticide exposure: new and forgotten insights. *Environmental Science and Pollution Research*, *25*, 18364–18376. https://doi.org/10.1007/s11356-018-2303-9

Bates, N. S., Sutton, N. M., & Campbell, A. (2012). Suspected metaldehyde slug bait poisoning in dogs: a retrospective analysis of cases reported to the Veterinary Poisons Information Service. *Veterinary Record*, *171*(13), 324. https://doi.org/10.1136/vr.100734

Botelho, A., Lima, J. L. F. C., & Barbosa, R. (2020). Fatal metaldehyde poisoning in a dog confirmed by gas chromatography. *BMC Veterinary Research*, *16*, 348. https://doi.org/10.1186/s12917-020-02348-w

Bus, J. S., Cagen, S. Z., Olgaard, M., & Gibson, J. E. (1976). A mechanism of paraquat toxicity in mice and rats. *Toxicology and Applied Pharmacology*, *35*(3), 501–513. https://doi.org/10.1016/0041-008X(76)90073-9

Caloni, F., Cortinovis, C., Rivolta, M., & Davanzo, F. (2016). Suspected poisoning of domestic animals by pesticides. *Science of the Total Environment*, *539*, 331–336. https://doi.org/10.1016/j.scitotenv.2015.09.005

Carson, R. (1962). *Silent spring*. Houghton Mifflin Company.

Castle, G. D., Mills, G. A., Gravell, A., Jones, L., Townsend, I., Cameron, D. G., & Fones, G. R. (2017). Review of the molluscicide metaldehyde in the environment. *Environmental Science: Water Research & Technology*, *3*, 415–428. https://doi.org/10.1039/C7EW00039A

Chang, Y. Y., Tan, J., & Tan, J. L. (2021). Knowledge and attitude of Malaysian fruit growers on integrated pest management (IPM). *ASM Science Journal*, *16*(1), 1–13. https://doi.org/10.32802/asmscj.2021.804

Corfield, G. S., McKiernan, B. C., & O'Brien, R. T. (2008). Intussusception following methiocarb toxicity in three dogs. *Journal of Small Animal Practice*, *49*(7), 335–337. https://doi.org/10.1111/j.1476-4431.2007.00271.x

Daam, M. A., & Van den Brink, P. J. (2010). Implications of differences between temperate and tropical freshwater ecosystems for the ecological risk assessment of pesticides. *Ecotoxicology*, *19*(1), 24–37. https://doi.org/10.1007/s10646-009-0402-6

Daam, M. A., Chelinho, S., Niemeyer, J. C., Owojori, O. J., De Silva, P. M. C. S., Sousa, J. P., van Gestel, C. A. M., & Römbke, J. (2019). Environmental risk assessment of pesticides in tropical terrestrial ecosystems: Test procedures, current status and future perspectives. *Ecotoxicology and Environmental Safety*, *181*, 534–547. https://doi.org/10.1016/j.ecoenv.2019.06.038

Department of Agriculture Malaysia. (2020). *Guidelines on toxicological data requirements for pesticide registration (GP 2/2020)*. Pesticides Board.

Dinis-Oliveira, R. J., Duarte, J. A., Sánchez-Navarro, A., Remião, F., Bastos, M. L., & Carvalho, F. (2008). Paraquat poisonings: Mechanisms of lung toxicity, clinical features, and treatment. *Critical Reviews in Toxicology*, *38*(1), 13–71. https://doi.org/10.1080/10408440701669959

Dutil, M., et al. (2023). 'A prospective study on clinical signs, management, outcomes, and delayed neurologic sequelae due to metaldehyde poisoning in 26 dogs', *Open. Veterinary Journal*, *13*(5). https://doi.org/10.5455/OVJ.2023.v13.i5.2

Ecobichon, D. J. (1991). Toxic effects of pesticides. In M. O. Amdur, J. Doull, & C. D. Klaassen (Eds.), *Casarett and Doull's Toxicology: The Basic Science of Poisons* (4th ed., pp. 565–622). Pergamon Press.

EFSA. (2018). Peer review of the pesticide risk assessment of the active substance methiocarb. *EFSA Journal*, *16*, e05429. https://doi.org/10.2903/j.efsa.2018.5429

European Commission. (2009). Regulation (EC) No 1107/2009 concerning the placing of plant protection products on the market. *Official Journal of the European Union*, *L309*, 1–50.

European Food Safety Authority (EFSA) Panel on Additives and Products or Substances used in Animal Feed (FEEDAP). (2012). Scientific opinion on the safety and efficacy of urea for ruminants. *EFSA Journal*, *10*(6), 2624. https://doi.org/10.2903/j.efsa.2012.2624

FAO. (2007). *Feed supplementation block technology (FAO animal production and health paper no, 164)*. Author.

FAO. (2024). *Pesticides use and trade, 1990–2022* (FAOSTAT Highlights). https://www.fao.org/statistics/highlights-archive/highlights-detail/pesticides-use-and-trade-1990-2022/en

FAO and WHO. (2014). *The international code of conduct on pesticide management*, Rome/Geneva.

FAO and WHO. (2019). *Guidelines on highly hazardous pesticides*, Rome/Geneva.

Food and Agriculture Organization of the United Nations. (2021). *Desert locust guidelines: Chapter 6–7 (Control operations, pesticides and ULV applications)*. FAO.

Food and Agriculture Organization of the United Nations & World Health Organization. (2019). *International code of conduct on pesticide management and guidance on highly hazardous pesticides* (updated ed.). FAO/WHO.

FRAC (Fungicide Resistance Action Committee). (2024). *FRAC code list: Fungicides sorted by mode of action*.

Frick, T. W., Dalo, S., O'Leary, J. F., Runge, W., Borner, J. W., Baraniewski, H., Dressel, T., Shearen, J. G., & Goodale, R. L. (1987). Effects of insecticide, diazinon, on pancreas of dog, cat and guinea pig. *Journal of Environmental Pathology, Toxicology and Oncology*, *7*(4), 1–11. PMID: 3598877

Fukuda, Y., Ferrans, V. J., Schoenberger, C. I., Rennard, S. I., & Crystal, R. G. (1985). Patterns of pulmonary structural remodeling after experimental paraquat toxicity: the morphogenesis of intraalveolar fibrosis. *American Journal of Pathology*, *118*(3), 452–475.

Fungicide Resistance Action Committee (FRAC). (2024). *FRAC code list: Fungicides sorted by mode of action*. https://www.frac.info

Gawarammana, I. B., & Buckley, N. A. (2011). Medical management of paraquat ingestion. *British Journal of Clinical Pharmacology*, *72*(5), 745–757. https://doi.org/10.1111/j.1365-2125.2011.04026.x

Gupta, R. C. (2011). *Veterinary toxicology: Basic and clinical principles* (2nd ed.). Academic Press.

Gupta, R. C. (2018a). Anticoagulant rodenticides. In *Veterinary toxicology* (3rd ed.). Academic Press.

Gupta, R. C. (Ed.). (2018b). *Veterinary toxicology: Basic and clinical principles* (3rd ed.). Academic Press.

Harputluoglu, M. M. M., et al. (2003). Acute pancreatitis: an obscure complication of organophosphate intoxication. *Human and Experimental Toxicology.* https://doi.org/10.1191/0960327103ht347cr

Hoffmann, A. A., et al. (2024). Wolbachia method field implementation in greater Kuala Lumpur / Malaysia dengue reduction. *iScience*, *27*, 108942. https://doi.org/10.1016/j.isci.2024.108942

Insecticide Resistance Action Committee (IRAC). (2024). *IRAC mode of action classification scheme.* https://www.irac-online.org

International Labour Organization (ILO). (2011). Case Study: Malaysian Information Service on Pesticide Toxicity. In *ILO Encyclopaedia of Occupational Health and Safety (web portal).* International Labour Organization. Available at: https://www.iloencyclopaedia.org/part-iii-48230/resources-information-and-osh/item/211-case-study-malaysian-information-service-on-pesticide-toxicity.

IRAC (Insecticide Resistance Action Committee). (2024). *IRAC mode of action classification scheme.*

Jokanović, M., & Prostran, M. (2009). Pyridinium oximes as cholinesterase reactivators: Structure–activity relationship and efficacy in organophosphorus poisoning. *Current Medicinal Chemistry*, *16*(17), 2177–2188. https://doi.org/10.2174/092986709788186147

Kahn, C. M., & Line, S. (Eds.). (2010). *The Merck veterinary manual* (10th ed.). Merck & Co., Whitehouse Station, NJ. Sections on pesticide and rodenticide poisoning.

Karami-Mohajeri, S., & Abdollahi, M. (2013). Mitochondrial dysfunction and organophosphorus compounds. *Toxicology and Applied Pharmacology*, *270*(1), 39–44. https://doi.org/10.1016/j.taap.2013.04.001

Klaassen, C. D. (Ed.). (2018). *Casarett and Doull's toxicology: The basic science of poisons* (9th ed.). McGraw-Hill.

Kumar, S., Gupta, S., Bansal, Y. S., Bal, A., Rastogi, P., Muthu, V., & Arora, V. (2021). Pulmonary histopathology in fatal paraquat poisoning. *Autopsy & Case Reports*, *11*, e2021342. https://doi.org/10.4322/acr.2021.342

Levi, M., Eerenberg, E., & Kamphuisen, P. W. (2011). Bleeding risk and reversal strategies for old and new anticoagulants and antiplatelet agents. *Journal of Thrombosis and Haemostasis*, *9*(9), 1705–1712. https://doi.org/10.1111/j.1538-7836.2011.04432.x

Lotti, M., & Moretto, A. (2005). Organophosphate-induced delayed polyneuropathy. *Toxicological Reviews*, *24*(1), 37–49. https://doi.org/10.2165/00139709-200524010-00003

Matsumura, F. (1975). *Toxicology of Insecticides. Plenum Press, New York.* https://doi.org/10.1007/978-1-4613-4410-0

McFarland, S. E., Mischke, R. H., Hopster-Iversen, C., von Krueger, X., Ammer, H., Potschka, H., . . . Greiner, M. (2017). Systematic account of animal poisonings in Germany, 2012–2015. *Veterinary Record*, *180*(13), 327. https://doi.org/10.1136/vr.103973

Merck Veterinary Manual. (2024a). *Urea and other NPN poisoning in ruminants.* MSD Veterinary Manual. https://www.merckvetmanual.com/

Merck Veterinary Manual. (2024b). *Nitrate and nitrite poisoning in ruminants.* MSD Veterinary Manual. https://www.merckvetmanual.com/

Merck Veterinary Manual. (2024c). *Sodium ion (salt) toxicosis.* MSD Veterinary Manual. https://www.merckvetmanual.com/

Merck Veterinary Manual 2025, 'Metaldehyde poisoning in animals', *MSD/Merck Veterinary Manual* (Professional version), modified March 2025, accessed 17 January 2026.

Ministry of Health Malaysia. (2024). *Wolbachia Malaysia – National Wolbachia Deployment Program.* https://wolbachia.nih.gov.my/

Motlagh, J. (2013). *'Palm oil casualty? 14 pygmy elephants fall prey to pesticides in Borneo', Pulitzer Center on Crisis Reporting / The Christian Science Monitor.* https://pulitzercenter.org/stories/palm-oil-casualty-14-pygmy-elephants-fall-prey-pesticides-borneo

Munday, J. S., Thompson, K. G., & Best, S. J. (2003). Brodifacoum toxicosis in two neonatal puppies. *Veterinary Pathology*, *40*(2), 216–220. https://doi.org/10.1354/vp.40-2-216

National Academies of Sciences, Engineering, and Medicine. (2016). *Nutrient requirements of beef cattle* (8th ed.). National Academies Press. https://doi.org/10.17226/19014

National Pesticide Information Center. (2018). *Metaldehyde technical fact sheet.* Oregon State University & U.S. Environmental Protection Agency. http://npic.orst.edu

North Dakota State University Extension. (2020). *Nitrate poisoning of livestock (Publication No, V839, rev.).* https://www.ndsu.edu/agriculture/extension/publications/nitrate-poisoning-livestock

Nurul-Nastasea, S., Yu, K.-X., Rohani, A., Zurainee, M. N., Tengku-Idris, T. I. N., Dianita, R., Sabrina, M. R., & Ali Wan Najdah, W. M. (2023). Insecticide resistance status of Aedes aegypti and Aedes albopictus in Malaysia (2010 to 2022): A review. Asian Pacific Journal of Tropical Medicine, https://doi.org/10.4103/1995-7645.378561

Papich, M. G. (2019). *Saunders handbook of veterinary drugs* (5th ed.). Elsevier.

Peter, J. V., Sudarsan, T., & Moran, J. (2014). Clinical features of organophosphate poisoning: A review of different classification systems and approaches. *Indian Journal of Critical Care Medicine*, *18*(11), 735–745. https://doi.org/10.4103/0972-5229.144017

Plumlee, K. H. (2004). *Clinical veterinary toxicology*. Mosby.

Radostits, O. M., Gay, C. C., Hinchcliff, K. W., & Constable, P. D. (2007). *Veterinary medicine* (10th ed.). Elsevier.

Rattner, B. A., Lazarus, R. S., Elliott, J. E., Shore, R. F., & van den Brink, N. W. (2014). Adverse outcome pathway and risks of anticoagulant rodenticides to predatory wildlife. *Environmental Science & Technology*, *48*(15), 8433–8445. https://doi.org/10.1021/es501740n

Ravindran, S., Mohd Noor, H., & Salim, H. (2022). Anticoagulant rodenticide use in oil palm plantations in Southeast Asia and hazard assessment to non-target animals. *Ecotoxicology*, *31*(6), 976–997. https://doi.org/10.1007/s10646-022-02559-x

Schlipalius, D. I., Chen, W., Collins, P. J., Nguyen, T., Reilly, P. E. B., & Ebert, P. R. (2008). Gene interactions constrain the course of evolution of phosphine resistance in the lesser grain borer, *Rhyzopertha dominica*. *Heredity*, *100*(5), 506–516. https://doi.org/10.1038/hdy.2008.4

Sivapragasam, A., & Goh, A. (2025). *Mainstreaming biopesticide use in Malaysia: Farmer and industry perspectives, Asia-Pacific Biofertilizers and Biopesticides Platform (FFTC-AP).* https://apbb.fftc.org.tw/article/715

Smith, P., & Heath, D. (1974). Paraquat lung: a reappraisal. *Thorax*, *29*(6), 643–653. https://doi.org/10.1136/thx.29.6.643

Staudacher, P., Fuhrimann, S., Farnham, A., Mora, A. M., Atuhaire, A., Niwagaba, C., . . . Winkler, M. S. (2020). Comparative analysis of pesticide use determinants among smallholder farmers from Costa Rica and Uganda. *Environmental Health Insights*, *14*, 1178630220972417. https://doi.org/10.1177/117863022097241

Stoytcheva, M., & Zlatev, R. (2018). 'Poisoning by anticoagulant rodenticides in humans and animals: Causes and consequences', in *Rodenticides. IntechOpen.* https://doi.org/10.5772/intechopen.69955

Strelitz, J., Engel, L. S., & Keifer, M. C. (2014). Blood acetylcholinesterase and butyrylcholinesterase as biomarkers of cholinesterase depression among pesticide handlers. *Occupational and Environmental Medicine*, *71*, 842–845. https://doi.org/10.1136/oemed-2014-102215

Stubbings, D. P. (1976). Cases of metaldehyde poisoning in cattle. *Veterinary Record*, *99*(23), 468. https://doi.org/10.1136/vr.99.23.468

Subbiah, R., & Tiwari, R. R. (2021). *The herbicide paraquat-induced molecular mechanisms in the development of acute lung injury and lung fibrosis. Critical Reviews in Toxicology*, *51*(1), 36–64. https://doi.org/10.1080/10408444.2020.1864721

Sutherland, C. (1983). Metaldehyde poisoning in horses. *Veterinary Record*, *112*(3), 64–65. https://doi.org/10.1136/vr.112.3.64

Tie, J.-K., & Stafford, D. W. (2016). Functional Study of the Vitamin K Cycle Enzymes in Live Cells. *Methods in Enzymology*, *584*, 349–394. https://doi.org/10.1016/bs.mie.2016.10.015

Timbrell, J. (2023). *Introduction to toxicology* (7th ed.). CRC Press.

Tinson, E., Frigerio, C., McAlees, T., & Fawcett, A. (2017). Intermediate syndrome in a dog after methiocarb toxicity. *Australian Veterinary Journal*, *95*(3), 77–80. https://doi.org/10.1111/avj.12585

Tudi, M., Ruan, H. D., Wang, L., Lyu, J., Sadler, R., Connell, D., Chu, C., & Phung, D. T. (2021). Agriculture development, pesticide application and its impact on the environment. *International Journal of Environmental Research and Public Health*, *18*(3), 1112. https://doi.org/10.3390/ijerph18031112

University of Nebraska–Lincoln Extension. (n.d.). *Nitrates in livestock feeding (G1779)*. https://extensionpubs.unl.edu/publication/g1779/na/html/view

Unsworth, J. B., Wauchope, R. D., Klein, A.-W., Dorn, E., Zeeh, B., Yeh, S. M., Akerblom, M., Racke, K. D., & Rubin, B. (1999). Significance of the long range transport of pesticides in the atmosphere. *Pure and Applied Chemistry*, *71*(7), 1359–1383. https://doi.org/10.1351/pac199971071359

Valentine, B. A., Rumbeiha, W. K., Hensley, T. S., & Halse, R. R. (2007). Arsenic and metaldehyde toxicosis in a beef herd. *Journal of Veterinary Diagnostic Investigation*, *19*(2), 212–215. https://doi.org/10.1177/104063870701900216

Wallin, R., & Martin, L. F. (1987). Warfarin poisoning and vitamin K antagonism in rat and human liver. Design of a system in vitro that mimics the situation in vivo. *Biochemical Journal*, *241*(2), 389–396. https://doi.org/10.1042/bj2410389

Wang, Q., et al. (2021). A paper-based analytical device for analysis of paraquat in urine and its validation with optical-based approaches. *Diagnostics*, *11*(1), 6. https://doi.org/10.3390/diagnostics11010006

Whitlon, D. S., Sadowski, J. A., & Suttie, J. W. (1978). Mechanism of coumarin action: significance of vitamin K epoxide reductase inhibition. *Biochemistry*, *17*(8), 1371–1377. https://doi.org/10.1021/bi00601a003

Williams, J. H., Whitehead, Z., & van Wilpe, E. (2016). Paraquat intoxication and associated pathological findings in three dogs in South Africa. *Journal of the South African Veterinary Association*, *87*(1), a1352. https://doi.org/10.4102/jsava.v87i1.135

Wilmar Sugar Australia. (2019). *Stockfeed with urea: User guide*. Author.

World Health Organization. (n.d.). Vector control. Accessed 17 January 2026.

World Mosquito Program. (2024). Annual Review 2024. *Wolbachia method – factsheet*. https://www.worldmosquitoprogram.org/sites/default/files/2024-10/2024-Jun-WMP_Wolbachia_factsheet.pdf (accessed 17 January 2026)

8

Heavy Metal Poisoning

Heavy metals are unavoidable, as they are intrinsic components of the Earth's crust and cycle continuously through air, water, soil, plants, and animals (see Figure 8.1: Heavy Metals – Sources, Pathways, Exposure, Health effects). With industrialization, urbanization, and intensified extraction of natural resources (mining, fossil fuels), environmental burdens of certain metals have increased and may rise further alongside e-waste and informal recycling – raising One Health concerns because most heavy metals are nonbiodegradable and persistent (Nordberg et al., 2014).

Certain metals are essential at trace levels. For example, copper and selenium are required for key enzyme systems, and zinc supports wound healing, hair and wool growth, immune function, and overall thriftiness; however, excess intake produces toxicity in animals (and humans) when homeostatic limits are exceeded (Suttle, 2010).

Heavy-metal poisoning occurs in domestic animals because exposures are widespread and multifactorial: agricultural chemicals and fertilizers; oils and greases used on farm machinery; waste materials discarded on pastures; feed and water contamination (including some feed additives or mineral premixes); and legacy pollutants in soils and sediments. Some plants may hyperaccumulate metals and become toxic forages. Improper burning or dumping of materials containing lead, arsenic, or mercury can contaminate premises for years, causing severe losses when livestock are later introduced. In many tropical settings, additional high-risk sources include artisanal and small-scale gold mining for mercury; phosphate fertilizers and industrial effluents for cadmium; tannery/electroplating wastewater for hexavalent chromium; and e-waste or battery recycling for lead, cadmium, and nickel – pathways summarized in Figure 8.2 (One Health Exposure Pathways Framework), which links source hotspots to plant/forage uptake, animal exposure, and food-chain transfer.

To guide the "what to do next," Figure 8.3 provides a one-page diagnostics-to-mitigation workflow tailored to tropical production systems, moving from history and examination to matrix-appropriate laboratory testing and a decision node (elevated levels?) that routes either to treatment (chelation/support, source elimination, nutritional support) and follow-up or to monitoring and periodic retesting. Use Figure 8.3 as the quick reference from clinical suspicion → choice of samples → immediate containment → longer-term remediation.

Complementing that visual, Table 8.1 serves as a bench-side quick reference for comparative clinical syndromes by metal and species, aiding triage and differentials. In practical terms: whole blood is the frontline matrix for **lead** (acute/ongoing exposure); **hair** (and sometimes feathers) trends chronic **mercury** and **arsenic** burdens; liver best reflects recent copper/selenium status; kidney cortex is most

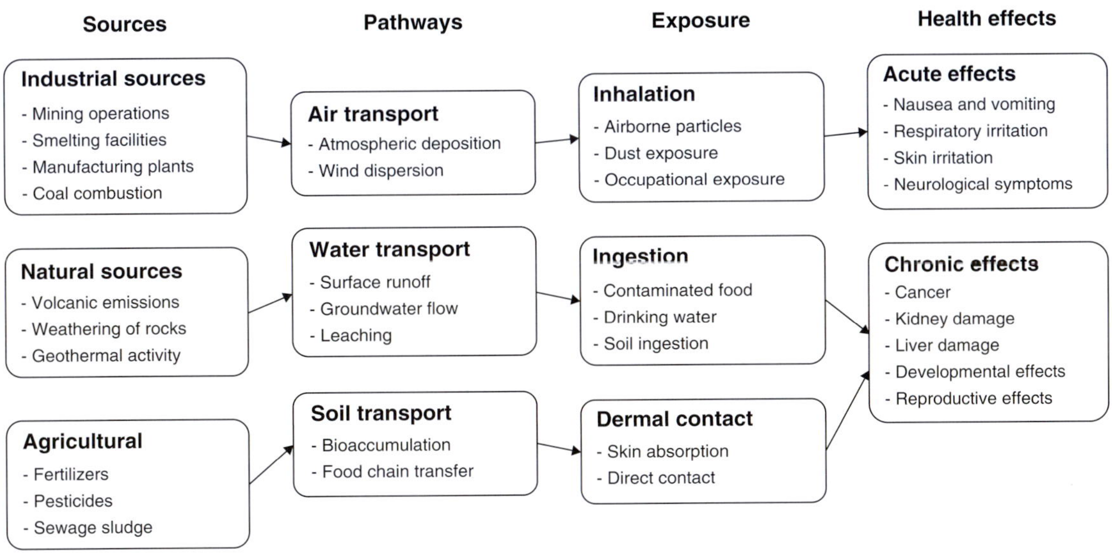

Figure 8.1 Heavy metals – sources, pathways, exposure, and health effects. Industrial, natural, and agricultural sources feed into **air, water,** and **soil** transport pathways, leading to exposure via **inhalation, ingestion, and dermal contact.** Resulting health outcomes are summarized as **acute effects** (e.g., nausea/vomiting, respiratory and skin irritation, neurological symptoms) and **chronic effects** (e.g., cancer; kidney and liver damage; developmental and reproductive effects). *Note:* Schematic overview; arrows indicate predominant flow and are not exhaustive or to scale.

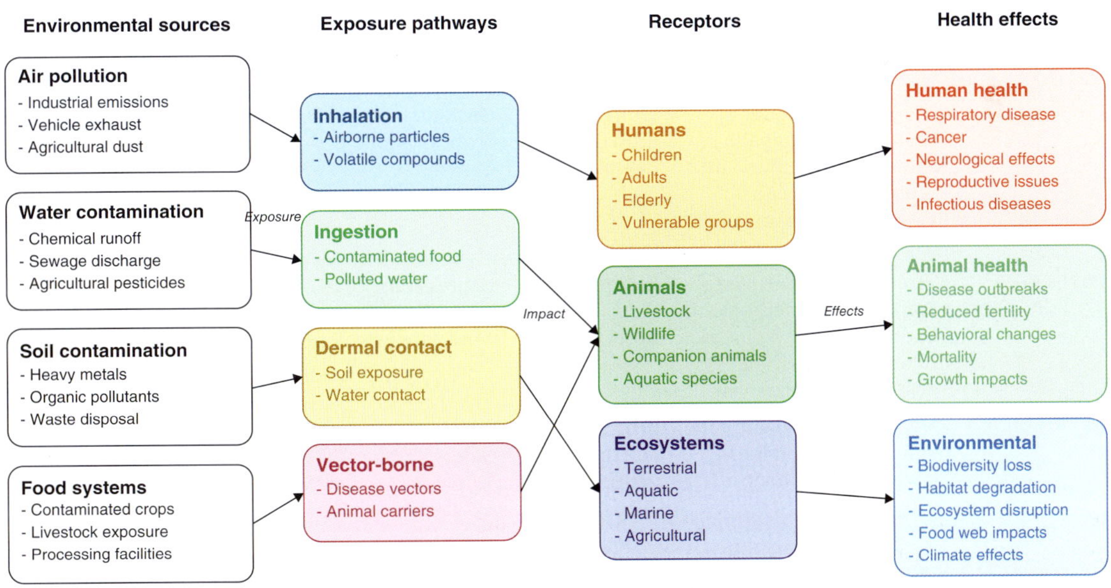

Figure 8.2 One Health exposure pathways framework. Environmental sources – **air pollution, water contamination, soil contamination, and food systems** – drive exposure via **inhalation, ingestion, dermal contact,** and **vector-borne** routes. These pathways affect **receptors** (**humans** – including vulnerable groups; **animals** – livestock, wildlife, companion animals; **ecosystems** – terrestrial, aquatic, marine, agricultural), resulting in **health effects** spanning **human health**, **animal health**, and **environmental** outcomes (e.g., respiratory disease, cancer, reduced fertility, biodiversity loss).

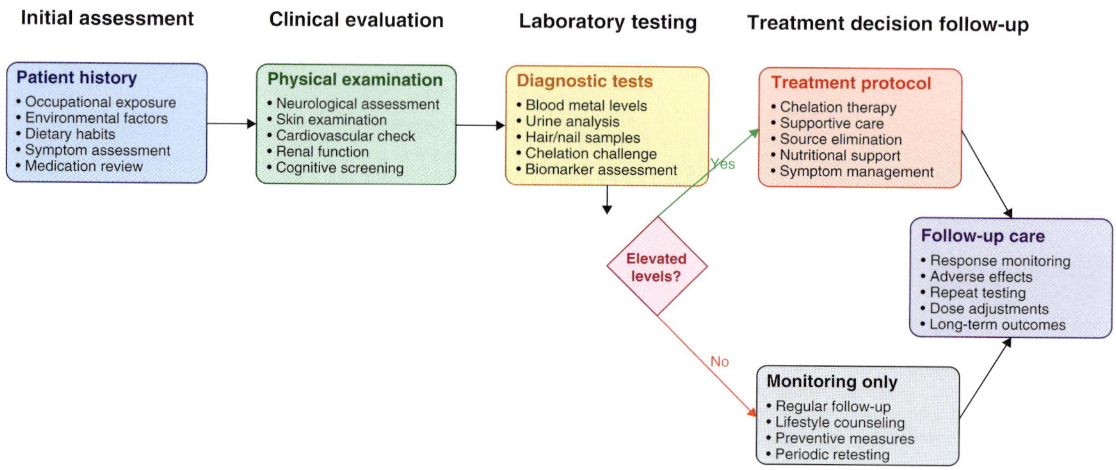

Figure 8.3 Diagnostic workflow for suspected heavy-metal exposure. Initial assessment (**patient history**) and **physical examination** lead to **laboratory testing** (e.g., blood/urine metals, hair/nail analysis, challenge tests, biomarkers). A decision node – **elevated levels?** – routes either to **treatment protocol** (chelation, supportive care, source elimination, nutritional support) with **follow-up care**, or to **monitoring only** (counseling and periodic retesting).

Table 8.1 Comparative clinical syndromes by metal and species.

Metal	Ruminants	Horses	Pigs	Poultry	Dogs/cats	Hallmark signs
Cu (Copper)	Sheep: chronic hepatic accumulation; hemolytic crisis	Rare; hepatic injury after high supplements	GI irritation; growth depression at high Cu	Gizzard erosion; poor growth	Dogs: copper-storage hepatopathy (Bedlington)	Sheep hemolysis with icterus after stress
Pb (Lead)	Calves: acute neuro, cortical blindness, bruxism	Peripheral neuropathy; dysphagia, laryngeal paralysis	Seizures, ataxia; GI upset	Depression, green diarrhea, wing paralysis	GI signs, anemia; seizures in acute	Cattle: sudden blindness, head pressing, convulsions
As (Arsenic)	Peracute hemorrhagic diarrhea, colic, dehydration	Severe colic, diarrhea, shock	Profuse diarrhea, vomiting, dehydration	Weakness, watery droppings, mortality	Vomiting, bloody diarrhea, shock	Acute hemorrhagic gastroenteritis with shock
Hg (Mercury)	Inorganic: stomatitis, renal failure	Organic: ataxia, blindness; weight loss	Inorganic nephrotoxicity; anorexia, weight loss	Embryotoxicity; poor hatchability	Methylmercury: cerebellar signs, blindness	Renal failure (inorganic) or neurological deficits (organic)

Table 8.1 (Continued)

Metal	Ruminants	Horses	Pigs	Poultry	Dogs/cats	Hallmark signs
Cd (Cadmium)	Chronic renal tubular damage; anemia	Rare; weight loss, renal lesions	Poor growth, renal lesions; anemia	Reduced egg production; shell defects	Proteinuria, renal insufficiency; vomiting	Chronic renal tubular dysfunction with proteinuria
Se (Selenium)	Alopecia, hoof sloughing; "alkali disease"	Hair loss, hoof cracks; lameness	Alopecia, hoof lesions; paresis	Poor hatchability; embryonic deformities	Vomiting, hair loss; brittle claws	Alopecia and hoof lesions; garlic odor
Cr(VI)/Ni	Contact dermatitis; respiratory irritation near industry	Nasal discharge; skin irritation	Dermatitis; poor growth near waste sites	Poor growth; reduced egg production	Allergic dermatitis; asthma-like signs	Contact dermatitis and airway irritation

Cross-species summary of frequent clinical presentations for major heavy metals in tropical agro-ecosystems. "Hallmark signs" highlight typical field patterns but **will vary with dose, chemical form, exposure duration, age, and nutritional status** (e.g., Cu–Mo–S interactions). This table supports triage and differential diagnosis; confirmatory testing should follow matrix-appropriate analytical methods.

informative for cadmium (and postmortem lead); and milk can be used for **arsenic** surveillance in dairy belts. **Pair** Figure 8.3 for the decision steps with Table 8.8 for sampling choices and interpretation in the field.

Although 52 metals are of industrial or economic importance (Nordberg et al., 2014), relatively few repeatedly cause veterinary poisoning. Classically these include copper, lead, arsenic (a metalloid allied to the heavy metals), mercury, and selenium; in tropical hotspots, cadmium and chromium (VI)/nickel may also be consequential. Accordingly, this chapter presents in-depth sections on copper, lead, and arsenic and – reflecting recent updates – adds parity sections for mercury, selenium, cadmium, and chromium (VI)/nickel, accompanied by case studies highlighting global (tropical) challenges and a practical toolbox of mitigation techniques for tropical ecosystems.

Copper Poisoning

Copper is one of the essential elements required by plants and animals. In animals, copper is necessary for iron absorption, hemoglobin formation, and the synthesis of keratin for hair and wool growth, as well as various enzyme systems. Table 8.2 shows the levels of copper per kg of diet (DM) required when diets are not high in molybdenum and/or sulfate. However, high levels of molybdenum and/or sulfate may increase the copper requirement two-to threefold (Suttle, 2010). Deficiency in this essential element in mammals leads to anemia, reduction in hematopoiesis, cardiovascular lesions, defects in pigmentation, keratinization, bone formation and reproduction, muscular incoordination, myelination of the spinal cord, connective tissue formation, reduction in growth, abnormal wool growth in sheep, and weakness at birth

Table 8.2 Recommended dietary copper concentrations (mg/kg of feed, DM basis) for major domestic species under typical conditions when dietary molybdenum and sulfate are not elevated: dairy cattle 10; beef cattle and sheep 4–5; swine 6; horses 5–8. Requirements may increase two- to threefold when molybdenum and/or sulfate are high.

Species	Level of copper (mg/kg of feed – DM)
Dairy cattle	10
Beef cattle and sheep	4–5
Swine	6
Horses	5–8

Source: Suttle, (2010)/CABI.

(Suttle, 2010). The metabolism of copper is highly complex and interrelated with other elements such as molybdenum and inorganic sulfate. Since the copper–molybdenum–sulfate interaction is more significant in ruminants than in nonruminants and copper poisoning occurs mostly in sheep, the discussion focuses on copper poisoning in sheep. Figure 8.4 provides a concise toxicokinetic schematic (chronic hepatic storage progressing to an acute hemolytic crisis under stress), highlighting sheep as the highest-risk species.

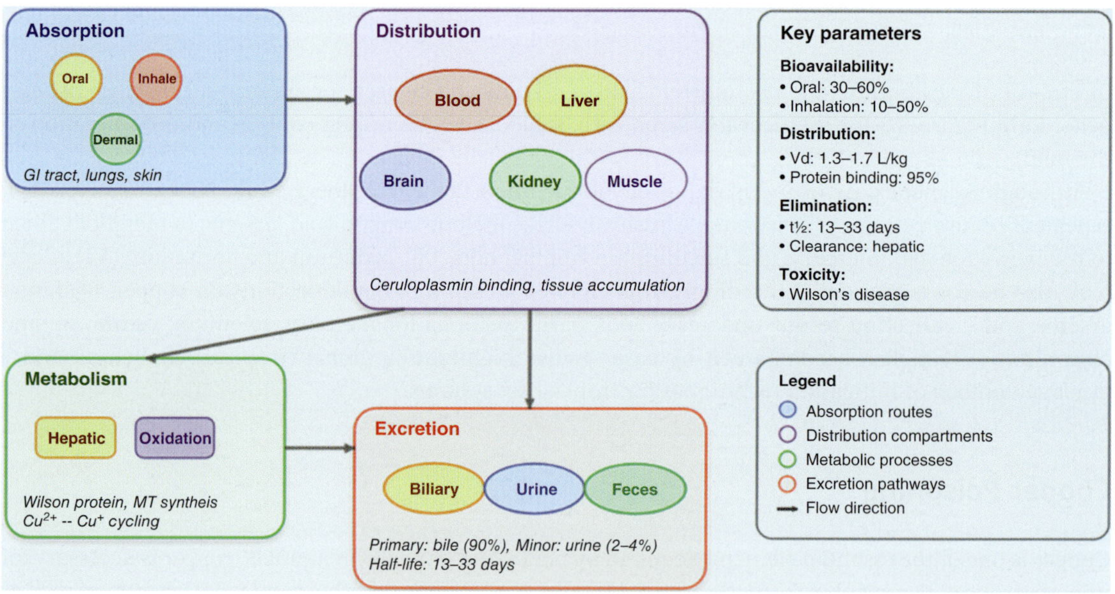

Figure 8.4 Copper (Cu) toxicokinetics – absorption, distribution, metabolism, and excretion. Cu enters via **oral**, **inhalational**, and **dermal** routes, then distributes (largely **ceruloplasmin-bound**) to **blood**, **liver**, **brain**, **kidney**, and **muscle**. Metabolism is primarily **hepatic** (oxidation; metallothionein/Wilson protein; $Cu^{2+} \rightleftarrows Cu^{+}$ cycling). Elimination is **biliary-dominant** (≈90%), with **minor urinary** loss (≈2–4%); effective **half-life** ≈**13–33 days**. Typical parameters shown: **oral bioavailability 30–60%**, **inhalation 10–50%**, **Vd 1.3–1.7 L/kg**, **protein binding ~95%**; **Wilson's disease** noted under toxicity. Arrows indicate flow; color keys correspond to the legend. *Schematic; values are representative and species-dependent.*

Source

In Malaysia, copper toxicoses in sheep and goats have been linked with the feeding of palm kernel cake (PKC) (Suttle, 2010), one of the major by-products of the oil palm industry. PKC contains high levels of copper, which is potentially toxic to sheep and goats. Another important source of copper that may cause poisoning in livestock in the tropics is copper sulfate, which is used as a footbath and molluscicide. Copper toxicosis also occurs in ruminants due to dietary trace element imbalances; ad libitum consumption of mineral mixtures or conventional feeds, which have been fortified with inappropriate mineral mixtures, has resulted in dietary imbalances of copper and molybdenum and subsequent copper toxicosis.

Clinical Signs

Copper poisoning is common in sheep and certain breeds of dogs, such as Bedlington Terriers. In sheep, copper poisoning is exhibited in two forms, either the peracute form, which is uncommon, or the common chronic copper intoxication, which is also known as copper loading disease.

In sheep or other domestic animals, the peracute form of copper poisoning is always traceable to improper use of copper compounds, e.g., $CuSO_4$ for footbath and for the control of liver fluke. The toxic single dose of $CuSO_4$ is 200–800 mg/kg (Plumlee, 2013; Suttle, 2010) and 20–100 mg/kg body weight in cattle and sheep, respectively. Copper chloride ($CuCl_2$) is more toxic than copper sulfate ($CuSO_4$). The symptoms of peracute copper poisoning include profuse salivation, violent colic, diarrhea, convulsions, paralysis, collapse, and death within 24–48 hours after exposure. The feces are deep green in color and may contain 1,000–10,000 ppm of copper (Plumlee, 2013).

Chronic copper poisoning occurs when an animal consumes small amounts of copper over a period of weeks to months through excessive mineral supplementation, especially when the copper-to-molybdenum ratio is greater than 10:1. Toxic signs are manifested when the copper level in the liver is excessively high and the organ is unable to handle more copper. Any form of stress to the liver such as physical handling of the animals or strenuous exercise will trigger the release of free copper from the liver, leading to the manifestation of clinical signs of copper poisoning. The outset of clinical signs is sudden and the course is normally within 24–48 hours.

The affected animals normally show signs of weakness, trembling, exhaustion, anorexia, and arching of the back, probably due to renal colic. On physical examination, the poisoned animals show intense generalized icterus (Figure 8.5), with all mucous membranes and secretions stained permanently yellow. Copper poisoning causes hemolysis leading to hemoglobinuria and hemoglobinemia (Figure 8.6), and bloody nasal discharge. Although the morbidity is usually low (less than 5%), the mortality is normally high (more than 75%).

Necropsy examination shows the characteristic hemolytic crisis – generalized icterus, swollen friable liver, dark-metallic ("gun-metal") kidneys (Figure 8.7), and brown-black urine in the bladder. The blood is watery and fails to clot normally.

Mechanism of Action

A considerable amount of copper may be metabolized by the liver in the presence of molybdenum and sulfate. Copper is stored more readily in the liver of sheep compared to that of other species of animals. The normal concentration of copper in the liver is 10–50 ppm on a weight-weight basis. The

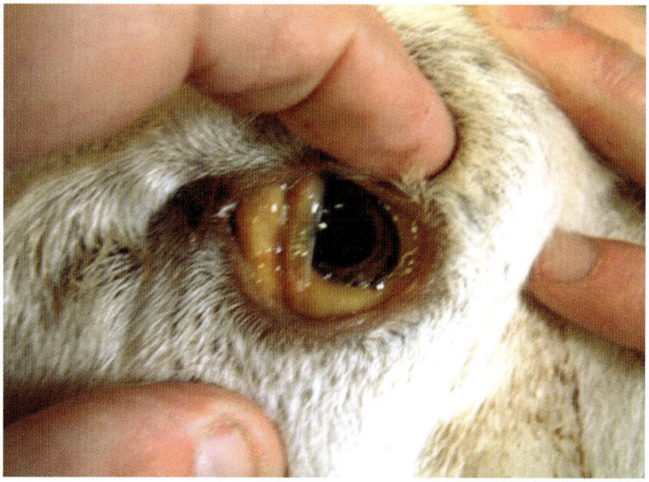

Figure 8.5 Marked scleral and conjunctival **icterus (jaundice)** in a sheep during the hemolytic crisis of chronic copper toxicosis. Mucous membranes are diffusely yellow due to hyperbilirubinemia following intravascular hemolysis. *Source:* Photo by National Animal Disease Information Service, https://www.nadis.org.uk/.

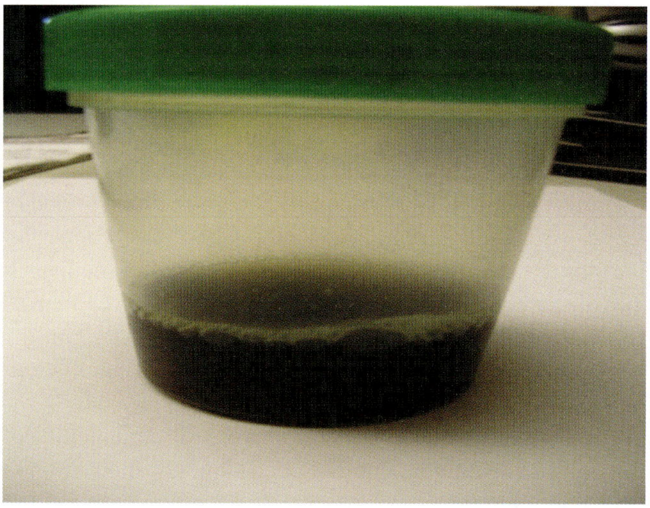

Figure 8.6 Port-wine to black urine (**hemoglobinuria**) from a sheep in the hemolytic crisis phase of chronic copper toxicosis. Free hemoglobin darkens the urine; dipstick is heme-positive with few/absent RBCs on sediment. *Source:* Jones & van der Merwe, (2008)/Kansas State University.

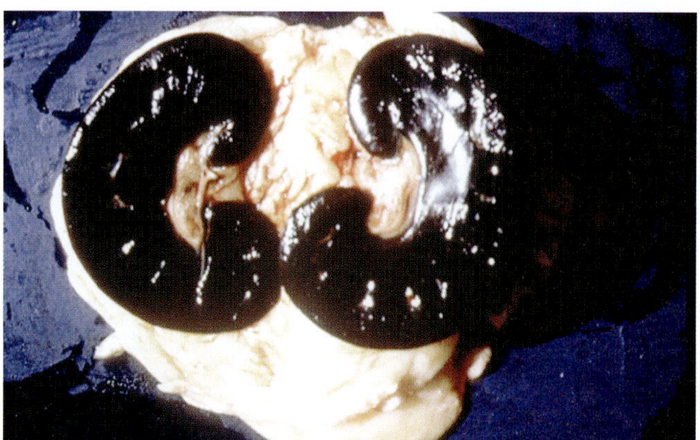

Figure 8.7 "Gun-metal" kidneys in an adult sheep with chronic copper toxicosis (enzootic icterus). Cut surfaces are **diffusely dark – almost black**, the classic gross appearance recorded for this lesion. *Source:* Cornell Veterinary Medicine / https://secure.vet.cornell.edu/nst/nst.asp?Fun=Image&imgID=10362 / last accessed on Dec 27, 2025.

characteristic hemolytic crisis of copper poisoning appears when the level is 150 ppm or more. A sudden release of copper from the liver into the bloodstream triggers the appearance of clinical signs of copper poisoning. Physically stressing the animals such as unaccustomed handling, strenuous exercise, or transportation of animals, and even extreme weather conditions, prompts the release of copper from the liver.

It has been estimated that less than 30% of the copper consumed is absorbed from the small intestine in most species of domestic animals. The absorption and retention of copper are greatly influenced by the chemical form of ingested copper, the dietary levels of other minerals and organic substances, and by the acidity of the intestinal contents. The absorbed copper binds loosely to serum albumin and is distributed widely to the tissues and the erythrocytes. However, copper in ceruloplasmin does not become readily available for exchange or transfer.

On reaching the liver, the primary organ that metabolizes copper, it is incorporated into the mitochondria, microsomes, nuclei, and soluble fraction of the parenchymal cells. The copper is either stored in the above-mentioned sites or released and incorporated into copper-containing enzymes. Copper from the liver is excreted into the intestine via the bile. Small amounts of copper in the plasma are excreted by the kidney.

In chronic copper poisoning in sheep and cattle, the animals appear normal until the sudden appearance of clinical signs. Blood copper concentrations are within the normal range of 75–130 µg/100 mL (Kahn & Line, 2016; Suttle, 2010) (0.75–1.35 ppm) during the period of accumulation of copper; however, this level increases very markedly and abruptly 24 hours prior to the onset of clinical signs. A sudden hemolytic crisis and jaundice are common clinical features of chronic copper poisoning, although these may not be the causes of death. Blood copper concentrations increase many-fold at the onset of the hemolytic crisis.

On necropsy, the carcass shows generalized icterus, enlarged, friable, and yellowish liver and distended gall bladder with thick greenish bile. The kidneys are greatly enlarged showing gun-metal gray color and hemorrhagic mottling. The spleen is also enlarged.

Histopathology: Histopathological examinations of the liver sections show cytoplasmic vacuolation and centrilobular (zone 3) hepatocellular necrosis (Figure 8.8). Clusters of necrotic cells with fragmented nuclei and acidophilic cytoplasm are found in the lobules. Sections of the kidneys show degeneration and necrosis of the tubular and glomerular cells in addition to the accumulation of hemoglobin in the tubules. The spleen is crowded with fragmented erythrocytes, and the central nervous system shows status spongiosus in the white matter.

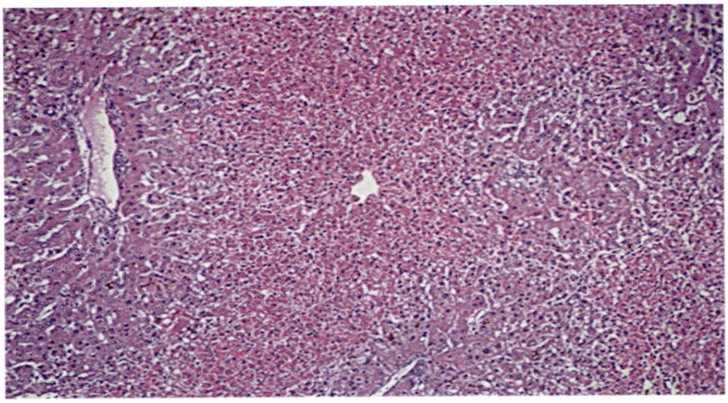

Figure 8.8 Liver, bovine – chronic copper poisoning. **Centrilobular (zone 3) hepatocellular degeneration/necrosis with sinusoidal congestion** (H&E). Lesions are typical of copper loading with periacinar injury in cattle from endemic areas. *Source:* Martins et al., 2020 (Pesquisa Veterinária Brasileira).

Morphological and histochemical changes occur in sheep during the period of accumulation of copper in the liver. Swelling and necrosis of isolated hepatic parenchymal cells appear in biopsies taken 6 months before the hemolytic crisis. Serum levels of various hepatic enzymes also increase six to 8 weeks prior to the crisis. Many studies on copper toxicity in sheep show increases in activities of serum glutamic oxaloacetic transaminase, lactic dehydrogenase, sorbitol dehydrogenase, arginase, and glutamic dehydrogenase.

Diagnosis

Chronic copper poisoning may be diagnosed using chemical analysis of the tissues, blood, and the rations, as well as clinical signs and postmortem findings. Blood concentrations higher than 1.3 ppm are indicative of copper poisoning. Liver and kidney concentrations of copper in positive cases are normally higher than 150 ppm and 15 ppm, respectively, on a weight-weight basis. Differential diagnoses include leptospirosis, babesiosis, anaplasmosis, phenothiazine poisoning, hepatitis, and *Brachiaria decumbens* poisoning (use Figures 8.7 and 8.8 as visual references for the typical gross, histologic lesions).

Treatment

Copper poisoning may be prevented by giving small amounts of molybdenum, 50–500 mg ammonium molybdate and 0.3–1 g of thiosulfate daily for 3 weeks. Alternatively, molybdenumized licks or mineral mixture can also be used. Once clinical copper toxicosis is underway, therapeutic options are limited; chelation (e.g., penicillamine or calcium disodium ethylenediaminetetraacetic acid (EDTA) has been attempted in individuals, but outcomes are often poor. Emphasis remains on prevention and flock-level mineral balancing.

Lead Poisoning

Lead poisoning is common in cattle (Gupta, 2018) and dogs and remains one of the most frequently diagnosed metal toxicoses in veterinary practice (Gupta, 2018). Acute toxicosis follows ingestion of a large dose, whereas chronic toxicosis results from repeated intake of smaller amounts over time. Figure 8.9 summarizes Pb absorption, distribution, metabolism, and excretion (ADME) and pathophysiology – exposure routes (inhalation, ingestion, limited dermal), distribution from blood to soft tissues and a dominant bone reservoir, elimination via urine and bile/feces, and major mechanisms/target systems (Central nervous system [CNS]; hematologic pathways, plus renal, gastrointestinal [GI], reproductive effects).

Source

Lead-based paints, which may contain either lead oxide (red lead, triplumbic tetroxide), white lead (basic lead carbonate), lead sulfate, or lead chromate, is the major source of lead that may cause intoxication in animals. Other sources of lead that can cause poisoning in domestic animals include the white and red lead used by plumbers, roofing materials containing lead, lead weights used by anglers, grease, used

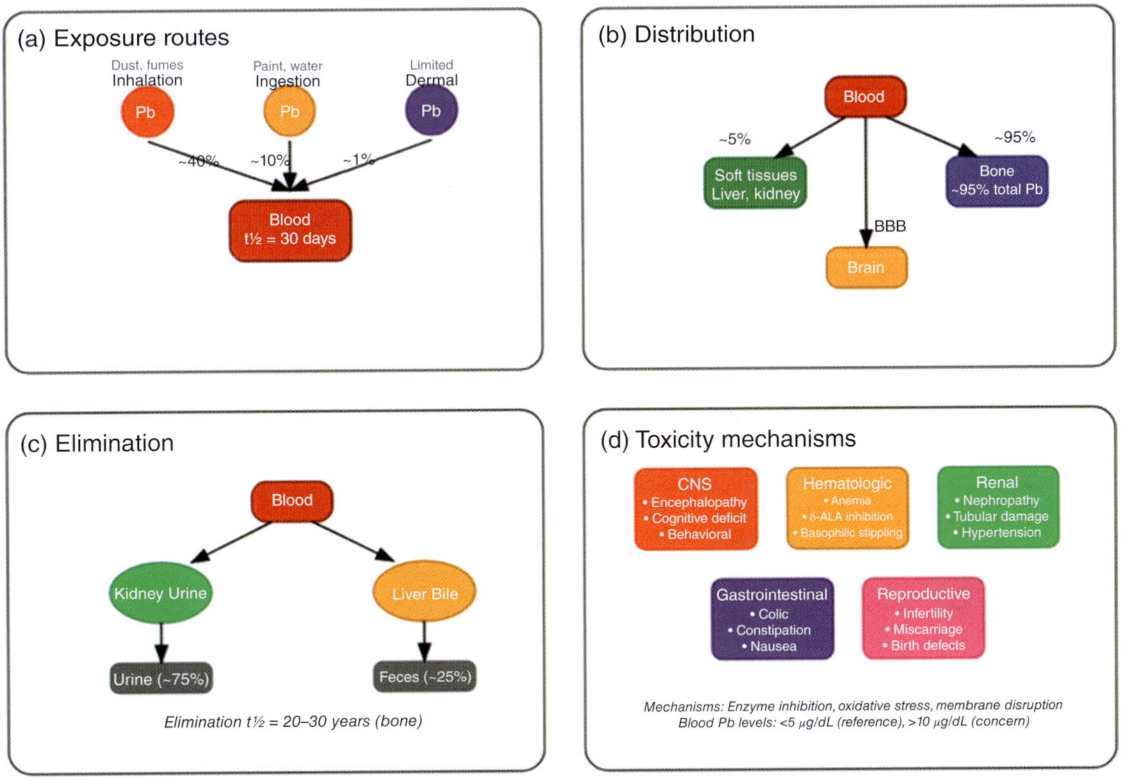

Figure 8.9 Lead (Pb) toxicokinetics – mini-panels. (a) **Exposure routes:** inhalation, ingestion, limited dermal; relative fractional absorption shown. (b) **Distribution:** blood to soft tissues and a large bone reservoir (~95% of body Pb); brain exposure indicated across the BBB; blood t½ ≈ 30 days. (c) **Elimination:** primarily kidney/urine (~75%) and liver/bile → feces (~25%); whole-body elimination prolonged by bone stores (≈20–30 years). (d) **Toxicity mechanisms/targets:** CNS, hematologic (δ-ALA dehydratase inhibition; basophilic stippling), renal, gastrointestinal, and reproductive systems. Arrows depict flow; schematic, not to scale.

lubricating oil, lead-mining waste, motor-vehicle exhaust emissions, lead pipes and sprays containing lead arsenate (Thompson, 2018), and discarded batteries. Lead toxicity in cattle may also be associated with feeding of heavily contaminated pasture or feedstuffs (Thompson, 2018). (See Figure 8.9 – panel A – for common sources; absorption modifiers such as Ca/Fe deficiency; age.)

Toxicity

The data on the acute and chronic toxicity of lead in various species are available (Thompson, 2018) and are presented in Table 8.3. All species of animals are susceptible to lead poisoning; however, susceptibility varies with age, species, and eating habits. For example, horses, which tend to eat grass closer to the ground and occasionally pull up the grass by the roots, may ingest more lead from contaminated forage and soil. This may explain why horses suffer from lead toxicosis while cattle grazing in the same area remain unaffected.

Table 8.3 Comparative lead (Pb) toxicity by species – reported acute and chronic dose ranges.

Species	Normal animal	Lead poisoned animals
Calves	0.282 ± 0.0269	0.35 or more
Cattle	0.025–0.25	
Horses	0.107–0.2	0.2–0.38
Dogs	0.053–0.28	0.22–0.6
Cats	<0.052	
Pigs	—	Up to 143
Chickens	—	About 13
Swans	—	Up to 32.9
Mallard ducks	—	10

Approximate dose ranges associated with clinical poisoning or lethality in domestic animals. Data highlight species differences (e.g., calves more susceptible than adult cattle) and routes of exposure (feed, paint, engine oil, batteries). Values are adapted primarily from Thompson (2018) with supplementary details from Cowan and Blakley (2016), Scrivens et al. (2023), and Siddiqui & Rajurkar *(2008)*. Reported doses vary with compound, solubility, age, nutritional status, and exposure duration.

Young animals are more susceptible than adults, and species such as goats, poultry, and swine are more tolerant. Diets may also affect susceptibility to lead poisoning. Calves fed a milk diet are more susceptible to lead toxicity (Thompson, 2018) because they absorb lead much faster than calves fed on grain diets (Thompson, 2018).

A single exposure to as low as 4.8 mg/kg of red oxide from lead in paint has resulted in the death of 18 of 20 dairy cattle, although the acute lethal single exposures are usually considered to be 400–600 mg/kg in calves and 600–800 mg/kg in adult cattle. The minimum daily dose that will eventually cause toxicosis in horses and cattle is estimated to be 6–7 mg/kg body weight (Hooper & Geelhoed, 2020; Thompson, 2018; Waldner et al., 2002).

Clinical Signs

Clinical signs of lead toxicity may develop within a few days to a few weeks after large exposures to this heavy metal (Thompson, 2018). Lead-poisoned animals usually show abdominal and neurological syndromes, although slight variations in clinical signs are observed among the various species of domestic animals.

In lead-poisoned cattle, the clinical signs include anorexia, rumen atony, grinding of teeth, bellowing, depression, ataxia, head pressing against the wall, blindness, circling, aggressiveness, and convulsions (Figure 8.10). The prognosis is unfavorable with the appearance of convulsive seizures because these animals normally die shortly thereafter. However, not all affected animals show evidence of lead intoxication prior to the onset of a sudden convulsive seizure and rapid death.

Lead-poisoned dogs normally develop anorexia, vomiting, colic, diarrhea or constipation. These early clinical signs usually escape the owner's attention, and the pet is presented for treatment only when the

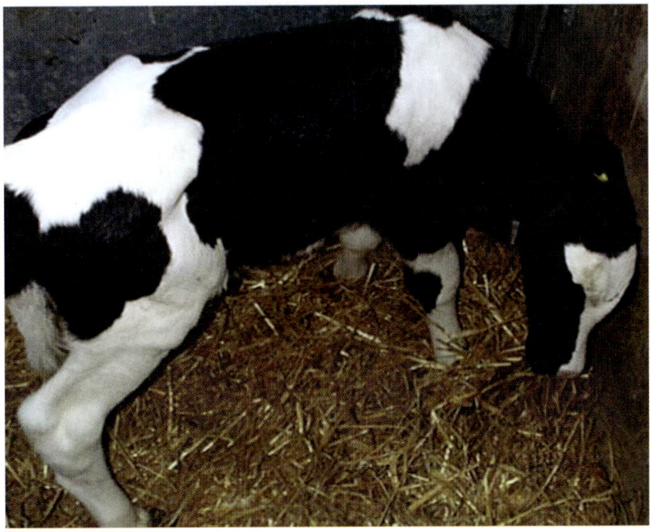

Figure 8.10 Lead poisoning in cattle – blind circling and bruxism. Representative field images of cortical blindness with compulsive circling and jaw champing (bruxism), consistent with lead toxicosis. *Source:* Author's collection (used with permission).

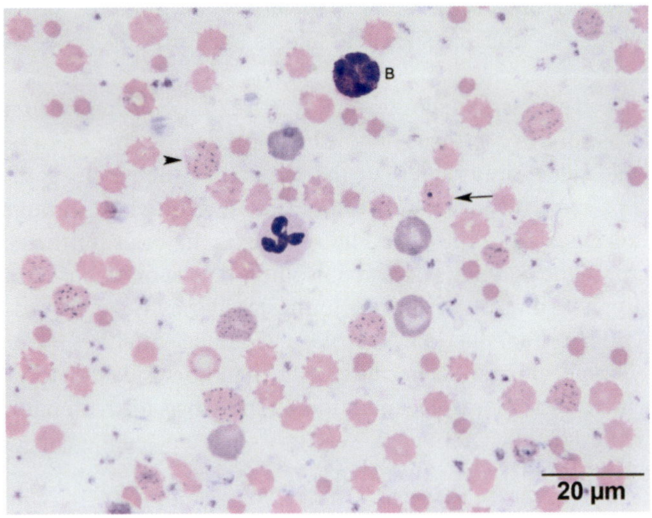

Figure 8.11 Basophilic stippling in lead toxicity (peripheral blood smear). Wright–Giemsa smear demonstrating coarse basophilic stippling; metarubricytes may be present. *Source:* Author's laboratory image (used with permission).

neurological syndromes, such as CNS depression, hyperexcitability, hysterical barking, convulsion, opisthotonus, muscular spasm, or blindness are noticed. The convulsive seizures in lead poisoning cannot be stimulated by noise as in strychnine-poisoned dogs. Reticular (basophilic) stippling (eClinpath n.d.; Harvey n.d.) of red blood cells (Figure 8.11) and the presence of 5–40 nucleated erythrocytes per 100 leukocytes differentiate lead poisoning from distemper in dogs.

Lead poisoning causes colic, diarrhea, loss of body weight, stiffness of joints, progressive arching of the back, and cachexia in the horse. In addition, lead poisoning causes roaring in the horse due to paralysis of the recurrent laryngeal nerve. Young foals are severely affected compared to older horses.

Although the kidneys are also affected by lead in all species, the effect is undetectable clinically. The reproductive and immune systems are also affected by lead.

Impaired fertility was observed for several months in lead-poisoned dairy cows (Thompson, 2018). The mechanism of reproductive infertility due to lead appears to result from enzyme dysfunction.

Exposure to low levels of lead insufficient to cause clinical symptoms of lead poisoning reduced the resistance of mice to bacterial infection by inhibiting antibody production or tying up existing antibodies (Fenga 2017).

Mechanism of Action

The absorption of ingested lead – either in soluble form (lead acetate), insoluble form (lead carbonate), or metallic lead – is small compared with that of other toxic metals such as copper and mercury (Thompson, 2018). Only 1–2% of orally administered lead is absorbed from the GI tract. However, due to its slow elimination, lead can accumulate in tissues after a prolonged exposure to low quantities and produce its toxic effect. Initially, a large fraction of absorbed lead is retained in the soft tissues and later in bone. It has been reported that the erythrocyte membranes carry 60–90% of absorbed lead and the remainder is bound to serum albumin (Thompson, 2018). Less than 1% of blood lead exists as free lead. In steady state, bone serves as the dominant reservoir for lead (the great majority of total body burden), with slow exchange back to blood over months to years; this skeletal deposition is illustrated in Figure 8.13.

Lead affects all major organs. It causes anemia due to hemolysis and bone marrow depression. Anemia is also due to decreased biosynthesis – namely heme – as a result of the action of lead at the cellular level. Lead causes impairment of the enzymes in heme biosynthesis, delta-aminolevulinic acid dehydratase, coproporphyrinogen oxidase, and heme synthetase through enzymatic inhibition. The interference in this biochemical process (Figure 8.12) is the basis for the clinical pathology changes and is also important in the diagnosis of lead poisoning. The central nervous system is edematous due to decreased blood supply as a result of damage to the capillaries. Segmental demyelination of peripheral nerves interferes with nerve conduction. Neurological damage of either the cranial nerves or the brain stem nuclei causes pharyngeal paralysis in cattle, roaring in horses, and paralysis of the masseter muscles in dogs.

Lead also causes degeneration and necrosis of the renal tubules and the liver. Acute exposure causes necrosis of the GI mucosa. Lead crosses the placental barrier and accumulates to toxic levels in the liver of the fetus. It may cause abortion, fetal resorption, and sterility.

Pathophysiology

Although lead is known as a chronic cumulative toxicant, most cases of lead poisoning in cattle show an acute onset of symptoms and rapid death with few cellular lesions (Thompson, 2018). Gross lesions are often minimal in acute or subacute lead toxicosis. Figure 8.13 illustrates the ribs (periosteum; cortical bone), emphasizing skeletal deposition – the major long-term reservoir for lead. Bone may appear grossly unremarkable; confirmation relies on exposure history and tissue-lead quantification (with histology/chemistry as indicated).

Acute lead poisoning results in hyperemia and hemorrhages of the kidneys. However, chronic exposure to lead causes degeneration and fibrosis of this organ. Examination of the histological section of

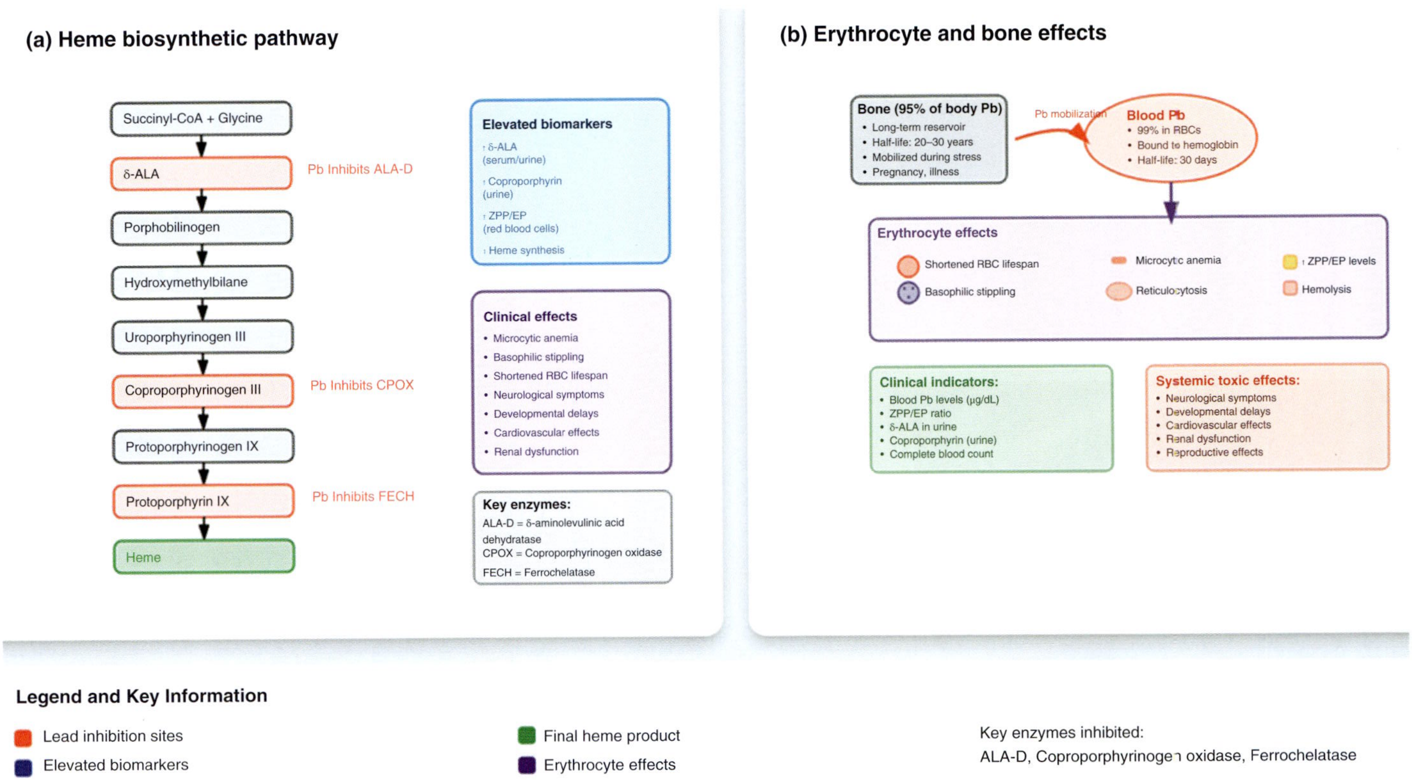

Figure 8.12 Lead (Pb) mechanistic overview – heme biosynthesis and erythrocyte effects. (a) Normal porphyrin/heme biosynthetic pathway with Pb-inhibited enzymes (δ-aminolevulinic acid dehydratase, coproporphyrinogen oxidase, and ferrochelatase), leading to elevated biomarkers (↑ δ-aminolevulinic acid in serum/urine, ↑ coproporphyrin, ↑ zinc protoporphyrin/erythrocyte protoporphyrin). (b) Pb interference with iron incorporation and globin synthesis in erythrocytes and bone marrow, resulting in anemia, basophilic stippling, and nucleated red blood cells. Bone serves as the principal long-term reservoir for Pb, with slow exchange back to blood. *Schematic; not to scale.*

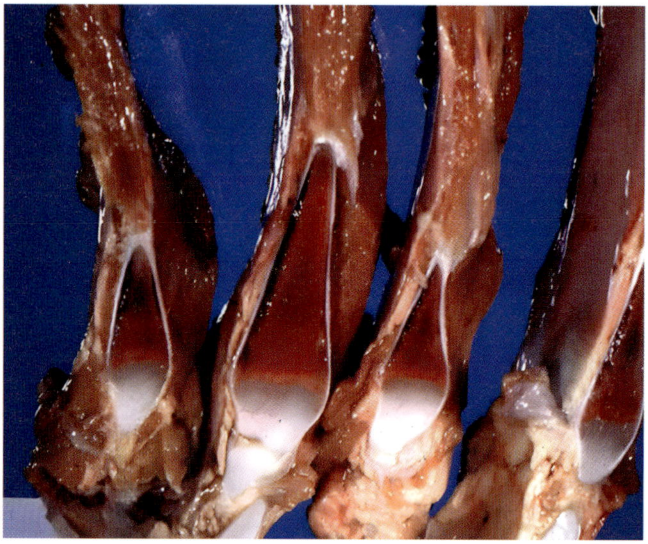

Figure 8.13 Lead toxicosis – ribs (costae), periosteum, and cortical bone. Skeletal tissues serve as the principal long-term reservoir for lead. This image highlights ribs with periosteum and cortical bone as typical sampling sites for Pb analysis. Gross appearance of bone is often unremarkable in acute/subacute cases; diagnosis relies on exposure history, tissue lead quantification, and histology/chemistry rather than pathognomonic gross lesions. *Source:* Cornell Veterinary Medicine / https://secure.vet.cornell.edu/nst/nst.asp?Fun=Display&imgID=978 / last accessed on Nov 05, 2025.

the kidney reveals a thickened glomerular capsule, degeneration, and necrosis of the proximal convoluted and descending tubules. Cerebral changes also occur in the brain, which include edema, swelling, and congestion of the cerebral cortical tissue, petechial hemorrhages, and laminar neuronal necrosis.

Diagnosis

A good history of the case, which includes the possible source of exposure to this toxic metal and the clinical symptoms, is definitely important in diagnosing lead poisoning in domestic animals. This is followed by the determination of tissue-lead levels to support the diagnosis (Table 8.3). Lead levels of the blood, liver, kidney, and the stomach content are presently employed in establishing the diagnosis of lead toxicosis. The lead levels in various tissues of normal and lead-poisoned animals are summarized in Tables 8.4 and 8.5. Diagnostically, significant tissue-lead levels in poisoning are quite difficult to establish because of wide variation in individual susceptibility. Very low levels of lead have been reported in the liver, kidney, and ingesta of lead-poisoned cattle (Thompson, 2018). Nevertheless, lead concentrations greater than 10 and 15 ppm in the liver and kidney, respectively, on a weight-weight basis are indicative of lead poisoning. Whole blood levels of at least 0.35 ppm are also considered significant in cattle and other ruminants.

Treatment

Lead poisoning is treated using complexing agents to remove the lead out of the system. The complexing agent usually used is calcium disodium EDTA, given 75 mg/kg daily by slow intravenous infusion (Plumb, 2018; Peterson & Talcott, 2013). This and other chelating substances bind the lead strongly to form a stable, soluble complex, which may be excreted (Figure 8.14).

Table 8.4 Normal background lead concentrations in animal tissues (mg/kg wet weight).

	Lead concentration in tissue (mg/kg wet weight as means ± sd or ranges)		
Species	**Liver**	**Kidney**	**Muscle**
Horses	0.0023–0.75	0.0013–1.0	0.002 – 0.05
Cattle	<5	<5	0–0.0.34
	0.5	0.45	0.46
	0.405 ± 0.365	0.573 ± 0.491	0.14 ± 0.16
	(0.1–1.6)	(0.20–2.60)	(0.03–0.40)
	1.47 ± 0.42	1.49 ± 2.27	—
	0.85–44	2–190	
	1.6	1.8	
Buffaloes	1.65 ± 0.22	1.37 ± 0.25	
Pigs	0–2 (0.20–0.60)	0.2 – 2.3 (0.20 – 1.20)	0–0.01 (0.04–0.50)
Lambs	0.537 ± 0.219	0.696 ± 0.361	0.226 ± 0.132
	(0.30–0.88)	(0.30–1.43)	(0.05–0.40)
Sheep	4.44 ± 4.11	3.92 ± 1.56	
Goats	3.23 ± 2.10	2.94 ± 1.42	
Dogs	0.09–1.22		

Reported mean values and ranges for Pb residues in liver, kidney, and muscle of horses, cattle, buffaloes, pigs, lambs, sheep, goats, and dogs. Concentrations represent background levels expected in animals not acutely poisoned. Values illustrate interspecies variation and typical tissue distribution patterns (liver > kidney > muscle).
Source: Adapted from Thompson, (2018) and supporting literature.

Table 8.5 Concentration of lead in the tissues of lead-poisoned animals (mg/kg wet weight).

	Tissue		
Species	**Liver**	**Kidney**	**Muscle**
Cattle	>10	>35 (cortex)	—
	18.9–23.2	23.2–62.8	>0.1
Calves	52.5	340	—
Horses	3.9–98	4.5–48	—
	—	40 (cortex)	—
Pigs	37–41	26–38	6–14
Chickens	>10	—	—
Mallard ducks	6–20	6 – 20	—
Bald eagle	>10	>5	—

(*Continued*)

Table 8.5 (Continued)

Species	Tissue		
	Liver	Kidney	Muscle
Swans	—	52.2–992	—
	—	135	—
	5.8	6.7	2.2
Albatross chicks	1.5–27.5	—	—
Captive birds of prey	35.7–204	4.6–33.0	—

Representative ranges and threshold concentrations of Pb in liver, kidney, and muscle from cattle, calves, horses, pigs, poultry, and selected wild birds. Values reflect diagnostic findings in confirmed cases of lead toxicosis and illustrate species- and tissue-specific accumulation (notably high in kidney cortex).
Source: Adapted from Thompson (2018) and additional literature sources.

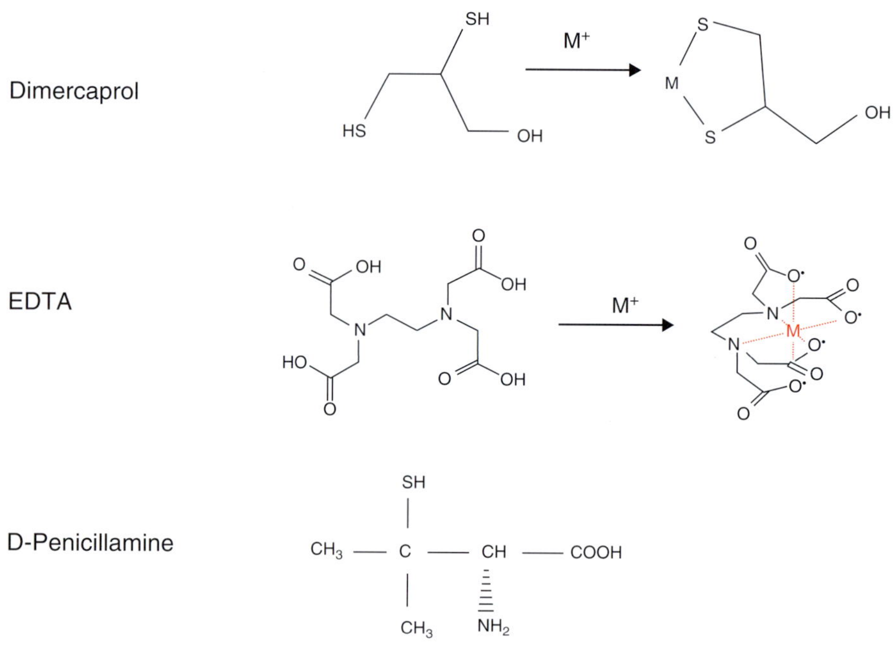

Figure 8.14 Chelation of lead (Pb) by therapeutic agents. Schematic showing the binding of lead ions (Pb^{2+}) by chelating agents, resulting in stable, water-soluble complexes that can be excreted. This mechanism underlies the use of chelators such as calcium disodium EDTA, dimercaprol (BAL), DMSA, or succimer in the treatment of lead toxicosis.

This treatment should be continued for several days. It is recommended that the daily dose be given in four divided doses for 2–5 days. Lead-poisoned cattle require about 2 weeks to recover, and several series of treatment may be instituted in severely affected animals.

As a precaution, lead should not be mobilized too rapidly to avoid fatal results (Plumb 2018; Peterson & Talcott, 2013), and calcium disodium EDTA may cause temporary toxic nephrosis.

Another chelating substance used in lead poisoning is penicillamine. In fact, penicillamine therapy is considered superior (Peterson & Talcott, 2013) to calcium disodium edetate for treatment in the dog. This was based on values of urine delta-aminolevulinic acid (UALA) following experimental lead intoxication in dogs and chelation therapy. In addition to the use of chelating agents to mobilize the lead, other therapeutic measures may also be taken during lead poisoning. Magnesium sulfate could be given orally to prevent or reduce further absorption of lead from the gut by forming an insoluble lead sulfate.

In the presence of neurological disorders, barbiturates may be given to depress the central nervous system. Mannitol may also be given to reduce cerebrospinal fluid pressure and cerebral edema.

Fluid therapy may be required if the affected animals are anorexic, emaciated, and dehydrated. However, fluids should not be given in the presence of neurological symptoms to avoid worsening of cerebral edema.

Arsenic Poisoning

Cases of arsenic poisoning in domestic animals are less common compared to lead poisoning. However, when it occurs, it is very dramatic because arsenic intoxications are usually peracute or acute with high morbidity and mortality. Arsenic poisoning is caused either by inorganic, aliphatic, and trivalent organic arsenites, or phenylarsonic feed additives. Intoxication due to inorganic or organic arsenicals produces an entirely different syndrome from that caused by phenylarsonic feed additives. A toxicokinetic overview is shown in Figure 8.15.

(a) Absorption

- Rapid absorption via GI tract (especially inorganic arsenicals)
- Dermal absorption possible (organic arsenicals, arsenical dips)
- Inhalation in mining/industrial exposures
- Absorption enhanced by poor nutrition, low protein diets

(b) Distribution

- Widely distributed to liver, kidney, lung, GI mucosa, skin, hair
- Binds to sulfhydryl groups in proteins and enzymes
- Crosses placenta and concentrates in fetal tissues
- High affinity for keratin-rich tissues (skin, hooves, hair)

(c) Metabolism

- Biotransformation via methylation in liver (to MMA, DMA)
- Inorganic As(III) (arsenite) is more toxic than As(V) (arsenate)
- Methylated metabolites somewhat less toxic but still reactive
- Arsenic interferes with oxidative phosphorylation, ATP synthesis

(d) Excretion

- Mainly urinary excretion as inorganic and methylated forms
- Biliary and fecal elimination contribute
- Hair, hoof, and skin as chronic exposure indicators
- Half-life varies: hours to days for blood, months in keratin tissues

Figure 8.15 Arsenic (As) toxicokinetics – mini-panels (4×). (a) Rapid gastrointestinal absorption with possible dermal and inhalational routes. (b) Distribution to liver, kidney, gastrointestinal mucosa, skin, and hair; high affinity for sulfhydryl groups and keratinized tissues. (c) Hepatic methylation to monomethylarsonic acid (MMA) and dimethylarsinic acid (DMA); inorganic As(III) is more toxic than As(V). (d) Predominantly urinary excretion; hair/hoof useful as biomarkers of chronic exposure. *Source:* Author illustration.

Several factors influence the toxicity of arsenic. These include:

Form: Organic arsenicals are generally less hazardous than inorganic arsenicals. Trivalent arsenic is four to 10 times more toxic than the pentavalent compound.
Finely divided: Soluble arsenic compounds are more toxic than the coarse and poorly soluble compound.
Health status: Weak, debilitated, and dehydrated animals are more susceptible to arsenic toxicosis.
Species. Cats, dogs, and herbivorous animals are susceptible. The lethal dose of sodium arsenite in cats is less than 5 mg/kg. Swine and fowl are rarely poisoned, probably due to limited exposure of these species to arsenicals.
Rate of excretion: Toxicity increases with a decrease in rate of excretion.
Tolerance: A degree of tolerance to arsenic may occur due to constant exposure.

Sources

The main sources of arsenic in domestic animals in the tropics are probably pesticides containing arsenic. Much of the inorganic arsenic is presently used in pesticide formulations. Arsenic trioxide (white arsenic), sodium arsenate, and alkaline salts of arsenic, such as potassium, calcium, lead, and sodium arsenates, are used as herbicides and defoliants. Inorganic arsenic is also present in insulation materials, wood preservatives, paint pigments (emerald green), detergents, and therapeutic preparations such as Fowler's solution. Certain herbicides also contain organic arsenicals such as monosodium methanearsonate (MSMA) and disodium methanearsonate (DSMA). These compounds can produce signs and lesions similar to those produced by inorganic arsenicals. Another organic arsenical that may cause toxicosis, especially in small animals, is thiacetarsamide sodium (Caparsolate®) (Figure 8.16), a drug used in the treatment of *Dirofilaria immitis* in dogs. Representative exposure sources are summarized in Figure 8.17.

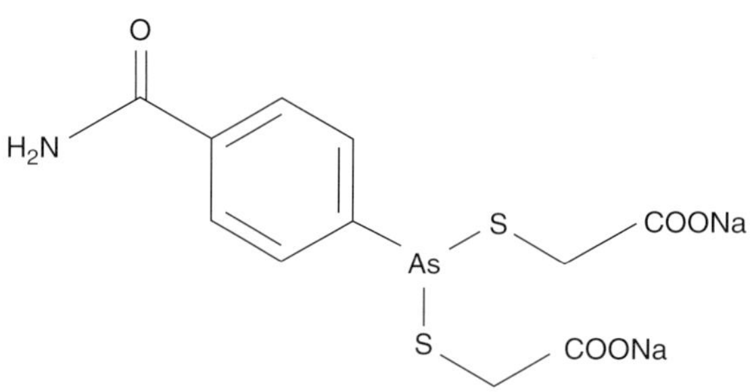

Figure 8.16 Thiacetarsamide sodium (Caparsolate®) – therapeutic arsenical for adult heartworm in dogs; misuse or overdose can result in arsenic toxicosis. *Source:* Author's image (used with permission).

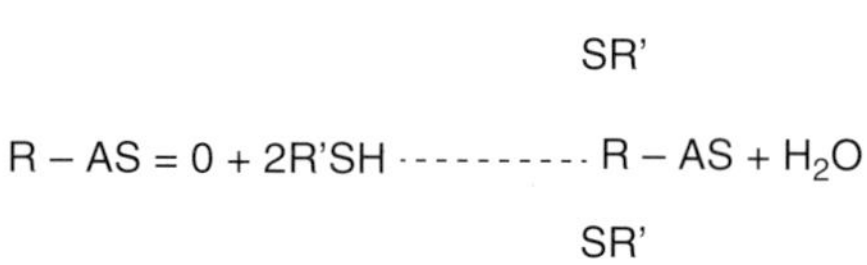

Figure 8.17 Common sources of arsenic exposure in domestic animals – examples include arsenic-containing pesticides (e.g., MSMA/DSMA), wood preservatives, paints/pigments, treated timber, and legacy insecticides. *Source:* Author schematic.

Toxicity

All species of animals and humans are susceptible to arsenic poisoning. Arsenic poisoning frequently occurs in cattle due to forage contamination and in cats following ingestion of insect baits. The average total oral lethal dose of arsenic trioxide and sodium arsenite (Peterson & Talcott (2013); Gupta (2018); Merck Veterinary Manual (2024) presented in Table 8.6. Sodium arsenite is one of the most toxic arsenicals because it is inorganic, highly water-soluble, and trivalent.

Mechanism of Action

The major actions of arsenic are attributed to the trivalent form, irrespective of whether an arsenic compound entered the body in a trivalent or pentavalent form. All arsenicals exert their effects by reacting with sulfhydryl groups in the cells. This reaction inhibits sulfhydryl enzyme systems, resulting in the blocking of fat and carbohydrate metabolism and cellular respiration. Arsenic also affects tissues with high oxidative systems such as the GI tract, liver, kidney, lung, and the epidermis. Clinical signs such as shock and severe hemorrhagic diarrhea **in** arsenic poisoning are due to the capillary damage and dilatation, which subsequently cause transudation of plasma into the intestinal tract and excessive reduction in blood volume. Severe hypotension and depression of cardiac muscle contribute to shock and circulatory failure. Capillary transudation of plasma results in edema of the GI mucosa and subsequent sloughing and discharge of the plasma into the GI tract.

Clinical Signs

Arsenic poisoning is usually peracute and acute, accompanied by high morbidity and mortality within a few days. Symptoms include severe colic, weakness, staggering gait, trembling, salivation, and vomiting in dogs, cats, and pigs. Severe diarrhea – sometimes hemorrhagic – prostration, normal to subnormal temperature, collapse, coma, and death could also occur. Illustrates a swine case showing flaccid limb paralysis and collapse during acute intoxication (Figure 8.18).

Table 8.6 The average total oral lethal dose (g) arsenic trioxide and sodium arsenite of various species.

Species	Arsenic trioxide	Sodium arsenate
Horse	10–45	1–3
Cattle	15–45	1–4
Sheep and goat	3–10	0.2–0.5
Swine	0.5–1	0.05–1
Dog	0.1–0.15	0.05–0.15
Fowl	0.05–3	0.01–0.1
Cat	—	<5 mg/kg

Source: Compiled from Peterson and Talcott (2013), Gupta (2018), and Merck Veterinary Manual (2024).

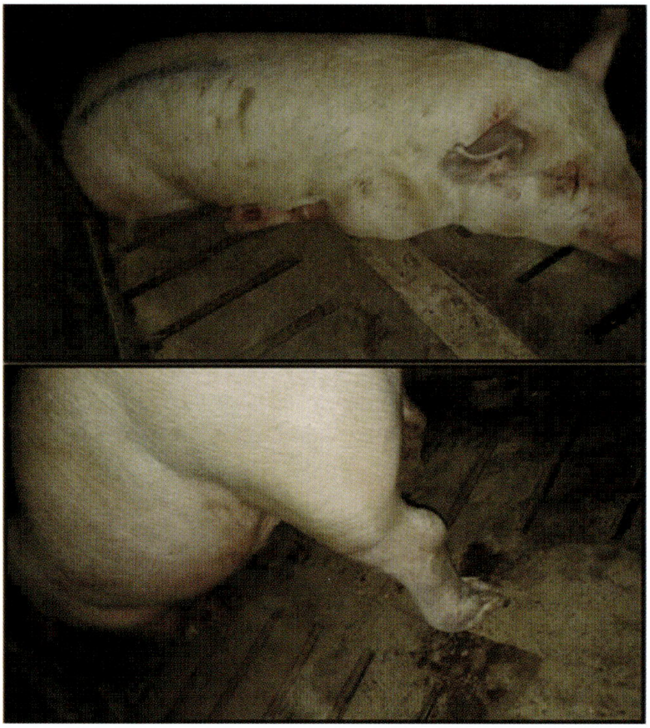

Figure 8.18 Pigs with clinical signs of arsenic poisoning – flaccid limb paralysis and collapse during acute intoxication. *Source:* Scollo et al. (2022) / John Wiley & Sons / CC BY 4.0.

However, in subacute cases the affected animals may survive for several days, exhibiting clinical signs such as anorexia, depression, diarrhea, dehydration, thirst, partial paralysis of the hind limbs, trembling, cold extremities, stupor, subnormal rectal temperature, and death. The diarrhea may be watery, blood-tinged with shreds of intestinal mucosa, and sometimes foul-smelling.

Pathophysiology

On necropsy, the animals that had died of arsenic poisoning have characteristic gross lesions in the GI tract. These include a generalized reddening of gastric (or abomasal in ruminants) and small intestinal mucosa. The liver is soft and icteric, and the lungs are red and edematous. Irritation by arsenic leads to necrosis of mucosa and submucosa and occasionally progresses to perforation of the wall of the gut. Hemorrhages sometimes appear on all surfaces of the heart as well as on the peritoneum (Figure 8.19).

Histopathologic lesions include edema of the mucosa and submucosa, necrosis and sloughing of the epithelium of the GI tract, degeneration of the renal tubule, fatty changes and necrosis of the liver, and degeneration in the vascular beds of the GI tract, skin, and other organs. The liver, kidneys, and GI contents of animals that died of peracute, acute, and subacute arsenic poisoning often contain between 2 and 100 ppm arsenic (ATSDR, 2020c; Texas A and M Veterinary Medical Diagnostic Laboratory, n.d.) on a wet-weight basis compared to less than 0.5 ppm in these tissues in unaffected animals (Figure 8.20).

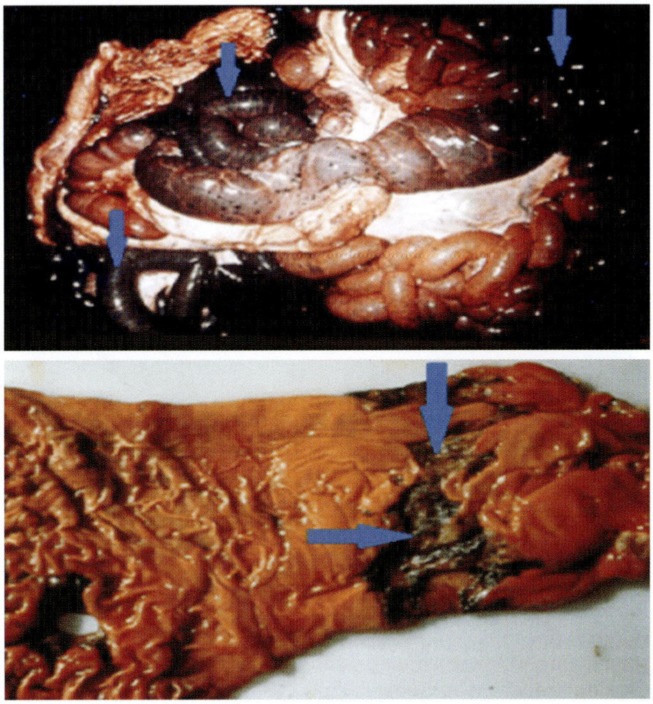

Figure 8.19 Gross postmortem lesions in arsenic poisoning – generalized reddening/erosion of gastric (abomasal) and small intestinal mucosa with necrosis and sloughing; serosal petechiae may be present. *Source:* Courtesy of Dr. Tam Garland.

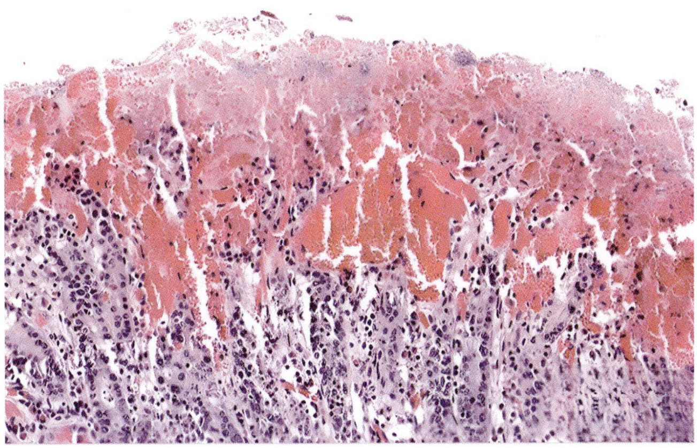

Figure 8.20 Histopathology in arsenic poisoning – abomasal/intestinal mucosal necrosis with submucosal edema; renal tubular degeneration; hepatocellular fatty change/necrosis. *Source:* Texas A&M Veterinary Medical Diagnostic Laboratory / https://tvmdl.tamu.edu/case-studies/arsenic-toxicosis-in-two-calves/ / last accessed on Nov 05, 2025.

Diagnosis

A history of a rapid onset of violent symptoms such as severe abdominal pain, hemorrhagic diarrhea, shock, and sudden death in cattle suggests that the animals have been poisoned by inorganic or aliphatic organic arsenicals. Confirmatory diagnosis may be based on necropsy findings, such as excessive fluid in the GI tract plus varying degrees of inflammation and necrosis of the GI mucosa and the arsenic content

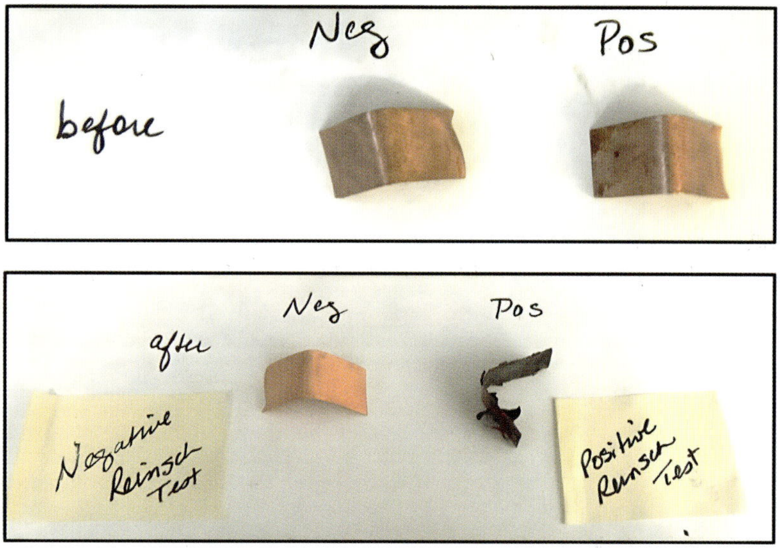

Figure 8.21 Reinsch test for arsenic – negative vs. positive. Copper strips before (top row) and after (bottom row) immersion in an acidified sample. The **positive** strip (right) develops a dark/black film from arsenic deposition (screening result), whereas the **negative** strip (left) remains unchanged. Note: the Reinsch test is a **qualitative screen** only; diagnosis requires confirmatory quantitative analysis (e.g., liver/urine arsenic by ICP-MS). *Source:* Texas A&M Veterinary Medical Diagnostic Laboratory / https://tvmdl.tamu.edu/case-studies/arsenic-toxicosis-in-two-calves/ / last accessed on Nov 05, 2025.

of the liver, kidney, stomach, and the intestine. Typical laboratory clues (e.g., tissue/urine arsenic, screening/confirmatory tests) are summarized in Figure 8.21.

In cattle, arsenic poisoning may be confused with urea poisoning, organophosphorus poisoning, and poisoning from plants containing cyanide, nitrate, and oxalate, and bovine viral diarrhea.

In dogs and cats, poisoning caused by heavy metals such as thallium, mercury, and lead may be confused with arsenic poisoning. Confusion may also occur in animals with enteric infections, which cause vomiting, diarrhea, and collapse.

Treatment

Therapeutic success in inorganic and aliphatic organic arsenical poisoning depends mainly on the speed of the diagnosis and initiation of the treatment. Nevertheless, the prognosis is still heavily guarded.

Following early diagnosis of arsenic poisoning, the therapeutic aim is mainly directed toward preventing further absorption of the poison. This may be achieved through the administration of adsorbents such as activated charcoal, especially in the species of animals that do not vomit readily such as ruminants and horses. In pet animals such as dogs and cats, absorption may also be prevented by giving emetics, provided that the affected animals have not shown signs of arsenic toxicity. Demulcents such as *Acacia, Tragacanth* and *Glycyrrhiza* syrup may be given to coat the irritated or abraded GI mucous membrane to protect the underlying cells.

Dimercaprol (BAL) is administered as a specific treatment in arsenic poisoning. It is a dithiol-containing chelating substance that can form a relatively non-toxic complex with arsenic and is excreted easily. Dimercaprol BAL should be given as a 5% mixture in a 10% solution of benzyl benzoate in arachis oil at a rate of 3 mg/kg body weight intramuscularly (Plumb, 2018). The recommended treatment with BAL is every four hours for the first 2 days, 4 times on the third day, and twice daily for the next 10 days until recovery is complete.

In addition to the administration of BAL, sodium thiosulfate should also be given. For dogs, the initial dose of thiosulfate is 40–50 mg/kg (Plumb, 2018) of body weight, in a 20% solution. It should be given intravenously and repeated 2–3 times daily until recovery.

Intensive supportive therapy is essential in arsenic poisoning. Fluid and electrolyte therapy are necessary to combat dehydration due to vomiting and diarrhea. Whole blood transfusion is also required if loss of blood is significant. In fact, antibiotic therapy is also recommended to prevent secondary bacterial infections. With arsenic covered, the next sections provide quick-reference summaries of other metal toxicants of tropical concern: mercury, cadmium, selenium, and chromium (VI)/nickel.

Mercury Poisoning

Source

Artisanal and small-scale gold mining (ASGM) is a dominant mercury source (Blakley 2024; Weinhouse et al., 2021) in many tropical belts, contaminating air, soils, and waterways. Grazing near mine sites and the use of contaminated surface water/forage are the principal livestock pathways; fishmeal and rice-based feeds can occasionally contribute (Kahn & Line, 2016).

Toxicity

Methylmercury is efficiently absorbed and distributes widely, whereas inorganic mercury salts are less well absorbed orally but cause marked local injury to GI mucosa and are nephrotoxic to proximal tubules. Chronic low-grade exposures are of greatest concern around ASGM belts.

Clinical Signs

Ruminants: Anorexia, salivation, abdominal pain, headshaking/ataxia; chronic low-grade exposure can produce subtle coordination deficits. Swine/poultry: prominent neurological signs (tremor, seizures, blindness). Dogs/cats (if exposed): vomiting, ataxia, and behavioral change (Chung et al., 2020). An example of severe neurological presentation is illustrated in Figure 8.22.

Mechanism of Action

Methylmercury crosses the blood–brain barrier and accumulates in the CNS, producing cerebellar and cortical neurotoxicity. Inorganic Hg salts are caustic and nephrotoxic (proximal tubules). Sulfhydryl

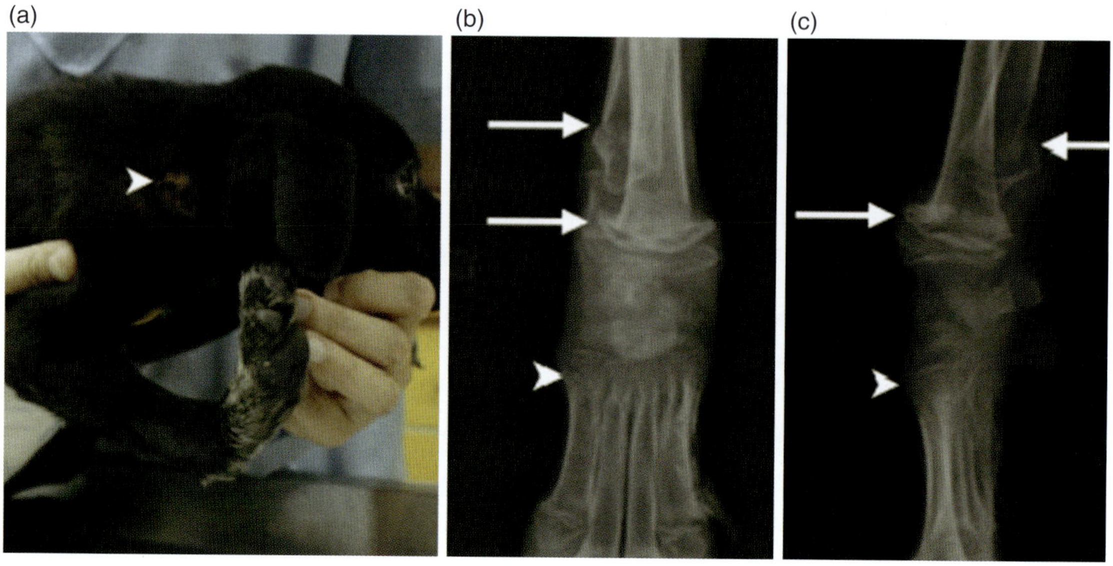

Figure 8.22 Clinical signs in mercury toxicosis – canine case with severe neurological deficits (progression to nonambulatory tetraplegia). *Source:* Chung et al. (2020)/ with permission of Elsevier. **(a)** Affected puppy with **marked mydriasis** (arrowhead) and profound weakness, consistent with **severe neurologic involvement** reported in the canine mercury toxicosis case. **(b) Dorsoplantar tarsal radiograph** showing **distal limb soft-tissue swelling** (arrowhead) and **irregularity/widening at the distal tibial metaphysis/physeal region** (arrows); **nonspecific changes noted during case evaluation. (c) Lateral tarsal radiograph** confirming **distal tibial metaphyseal/physeal irregularity** (arrows) with associated **periarticular/distal limb soft-tissue swelling** (arrowhead); **findings are nonspecific and included as part of the diagnostic work-up**.

binding and oxidative stress drive cellular injury (Chung et al., 2020). A concise visual of these contrasting pathways is shown in Figure 8.23 (Blakley, 2024).

Pathophysiology

Clinicopathology may show azotemia with tubular casts (inorganic Hg) and variable leukocytosis. Gross lesions include erosive–ulcerative abomasitis/enteritis and swollen, pale kidneys (see Figure 8.24). Histology shows acute proximal tubular necrosis and neuronal degeneration (see Figure 8.25) (Chung et al., 2020).

Diagnosis

Preferred matrices include blood (recent exposure), hair (chronic), and liver/kidney (postmortem). Typical laboratory clues – including urine sediment casts (Blakley, 2024; Kahn & Line, 2016) indicating tubular injury – and method/specimen snapshots are summarized in Figure 8.26. Consider feed/water mapping around ASGM catchments.

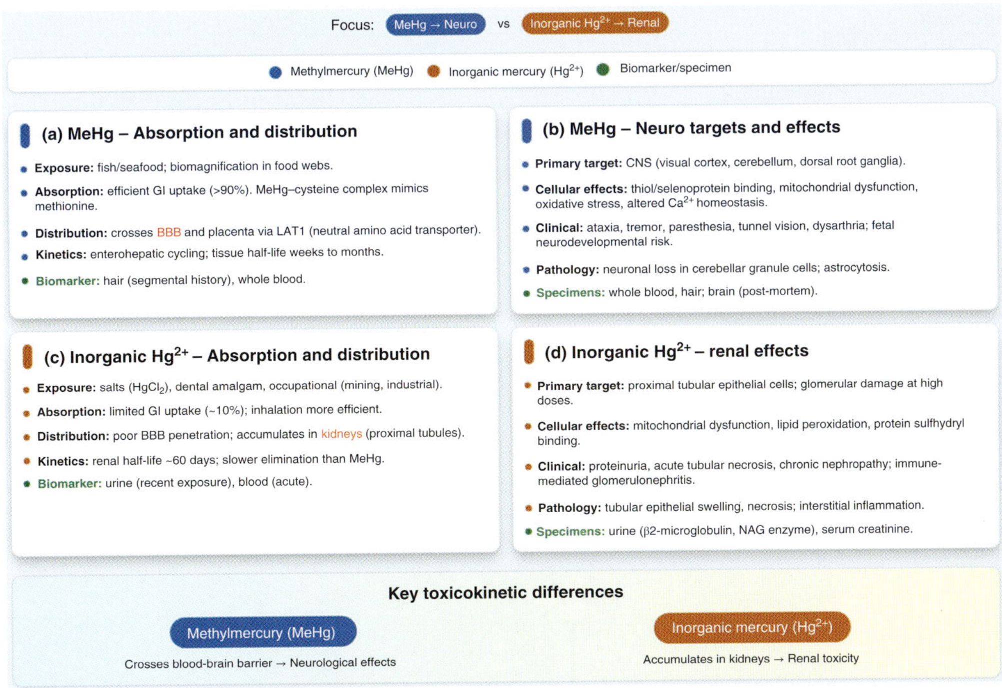

Figure 8.23 Toxicokinetics – mercury (Hg): MeHg neuro vs. inorganic Hg^{2+} renal. (a) MeHg is efficiently absorbed from the gastrointestinal tract (often via fish/seafood exposure) and distributes widely as a MeHg–cysteine complex that mimics methionine, crossing the blood–brain barrier (BBB) and placenta via the L-type amino acid transporter 1 (LAT1), with slow clearance due to tissue persistence and enterohepatic cycling. (b) MeHg preferentially targets the central nervous system (e.g., visual cortex, cerebellum, dorsal root ganglia), causing neurological and neurodevelopmental effects through thiol/selenoprotein binding, mitochondrial dysfunction, and oxidative stress; hair and whole blood are commonly used biomarkers/specimens. (c) Inorganic Hg^{2+} is less efficiently absorbed orally (with greater absorption via inhalation in some settings), has poor BBB penetration, and accumulates predominantly in renal tissue – especially proximal tubules – with a relatively prolonged renal half-life. (d) Inorganic Hg^{2+} primarily produces nephrotoxicity (proximal tubular injury and, at higher exposures, glomerular involvement), with assessment supported by urinary biomarkers (e.g., β2-microglobulin, N-acetyl-β-D-glucosaminidase [NAG]) and serum creatinine. **Key distinction:** MeHg → neurotoxicity; Hg^{2+} → renal toxicity. *Source:* Author's schematic (this chapter).

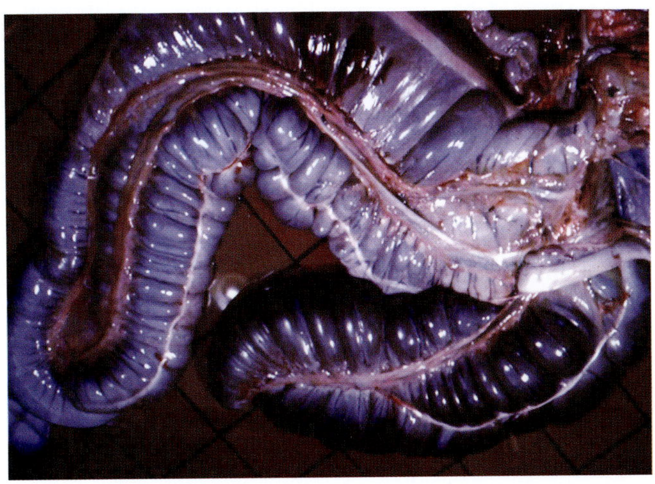

Figure 8.24 Postmortem lesions compatible with mercury exposure – equine cecum/colon, acute locally extensive colitis (uremic colitis/typhlitis). *Source:* Cornell Veterinary Medicine / https://secure.vet.cornell.edu/nst/nst.asp?Fun=Display&imgID=18 / last accessed on Nov 05, 2025.

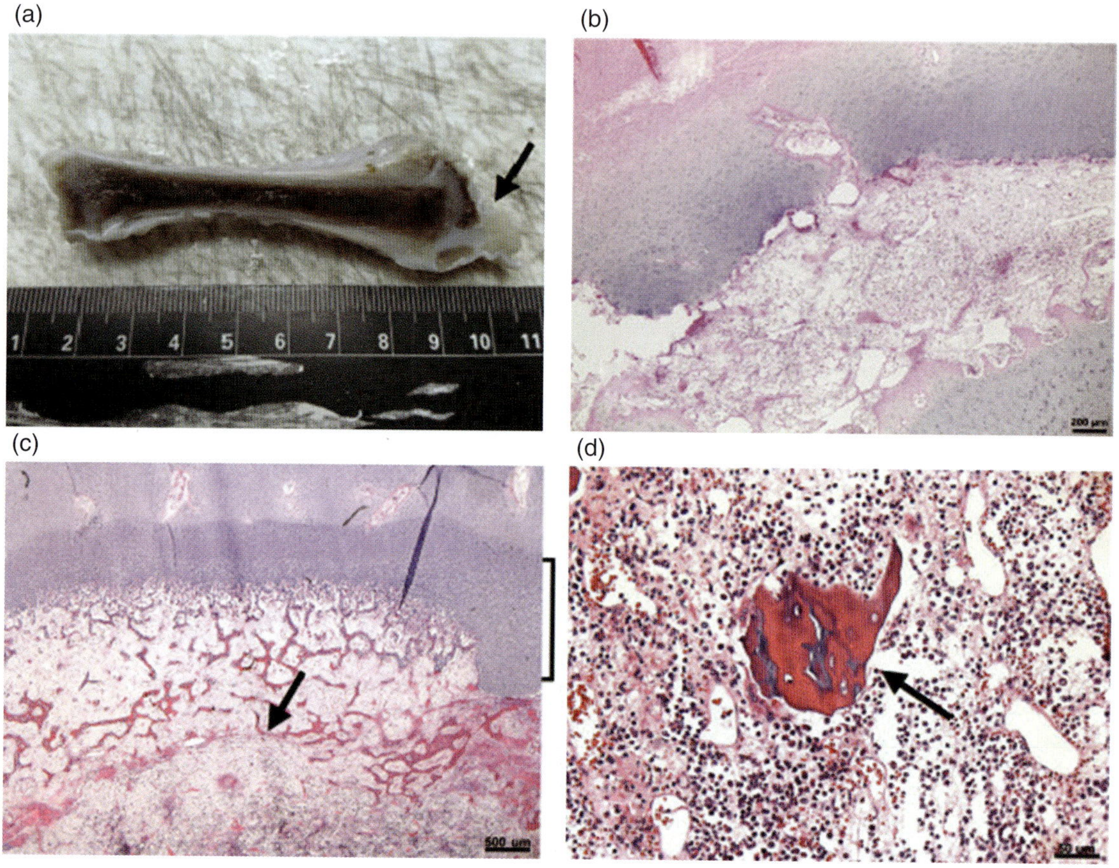

Figure 8.25 Skeletal lesions associated with mercury intoxication – physeal/metaphyseal injury. (a) **(gross):** Longitudinal section of a growing long bone. The arrow marks a dense, pale linear band paralleling the physis at the metaphyseal side, consistent with growth-plate/metaphyseal injury. A metric scale is shown. (b) **(H&E, low power):** Disruption at the chondro-osseous junction with loss of orderly columnar architecture and subphyseal trabecular injury; edema and fibrinous debris extend into the metaphysis. (c) **(H&E, lower power overview):** Broad band of osteochondral damage beneath the physis (bracket), with necrosis of primary spongiosa and reduced remodeling (arrow). (d) **(H&E, higher power):** Necrotic trabecula with empty osteocyte lacunae and irregular cement lines (arrow), surrounded by reactive marrow – features of metaphyseal osteonecrosis following toxic injury. **Interpretation:** The constellation of a metaphyseal band, disorganized/necrotic primary spongiosa, and impaired remodeling is **compatible with heavy-metal toxicosis** and, in this case, was associated with **mercury exposure** as documented in the accompanying case report. Lesions may mimic those classically described in lead poisoning; definitive etiologic assignment requires toxicological confirmation (e.g., tissue/blood Hg). *Source:* Chung et al. (2020)/ with permission of Elsevier.

Treatment

Immediate source control (keep stock off mining drainage and tailings), fluids, and GI protectants (Blakley, 2024; Kahn & Line, 2016) are cornerstones. Chelation (e.g., Sodium 2,3-dimercapto-1-propanesulfonate (DMPS)/2,3-dimercaptosuccinic acid (DMSA) may be considered in valuable individuals where permitted. Long-term mitigation emphasizes community shifts to Hg-free gold recovery and protected water points for stock.

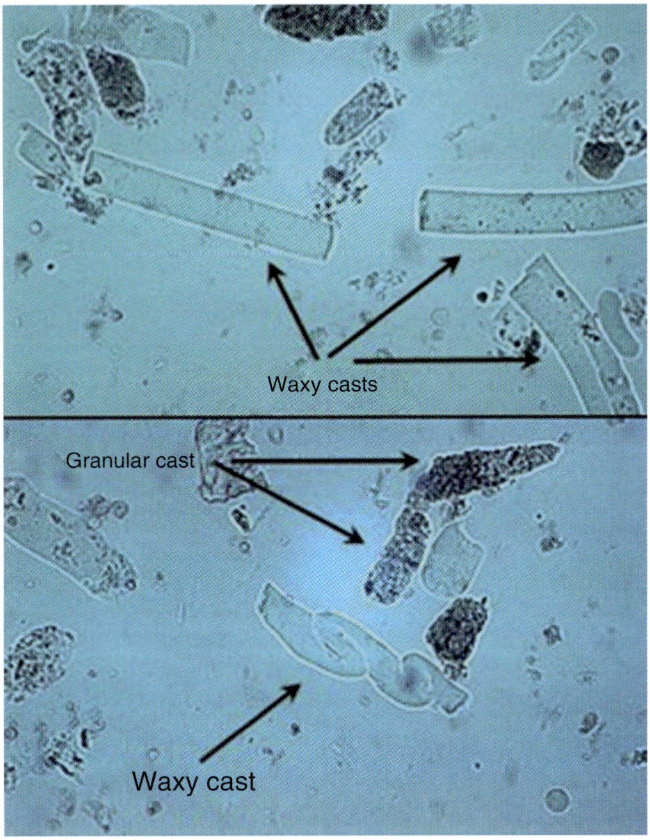

Figure 8.26 Laboratory findings in mercury poisoning – urine sediment casts (waxy/coarse granular) indicating tubular injury; specimen and method snapshots. *Source:* Photo by Tracy Stokol- https://eclinpath.com/urinalysis/cellular-constituents/waxycomp1/- Last accessed on 29 Jan,2026.

Cadmium Poisoning

Source

Phosphate fertilizers, sewage sludge, smelter fallout, e-waste (EFSA, 2009; WHO, 2017) and contaminated mineral premixes are key cadmium inputs to feed chains. Uptake is greatest on acidic soils and in leafy forages; risk concentrates around fertilizer use, industrial belts, and informal recycling (ATSDR, 2012a; Kahn & Line, 2016). Figure 8.27 summarizes the soil-to-plant-to-animal pathway.

Toxicity

Cadmium is absorbed from the gut (immature animals absorb a higher fraction), binds intracellularly (e.g., metallothionein), and accumulates first in the liver then kidney. Biological half-life is long; body burden reflects cumulative exposure (ATSDR, 2012a; Kahn & Line, 2016). A compact overview of this progression is shown in Figure 8.28.

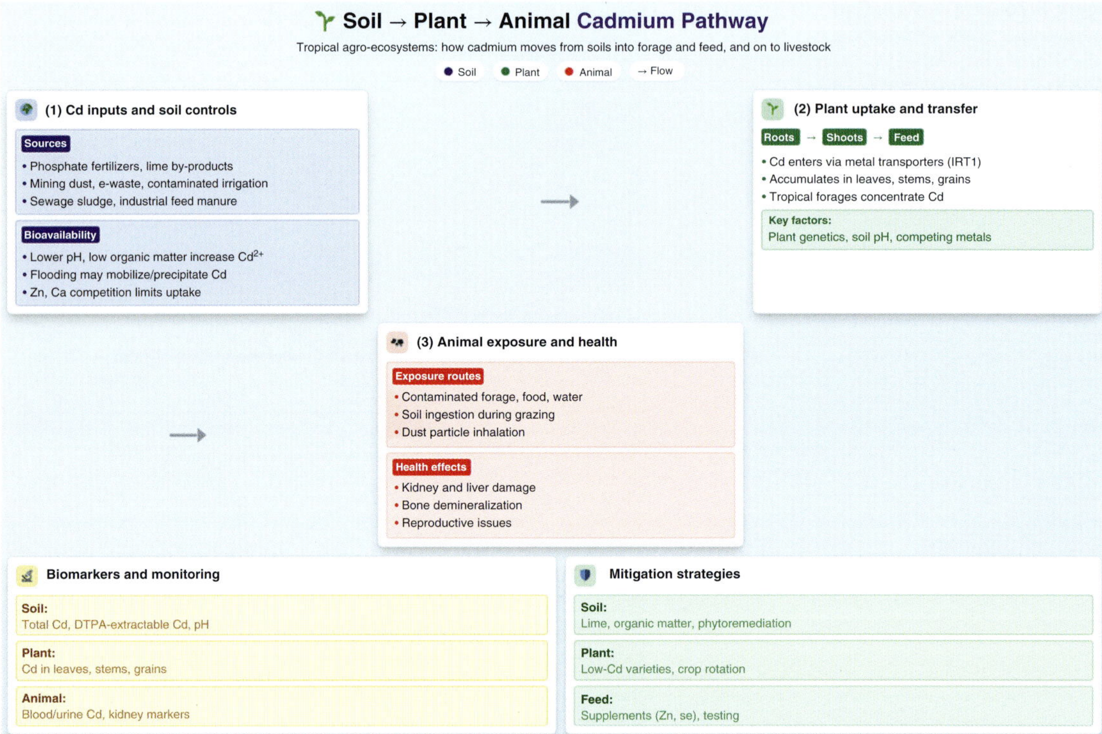

Figure 8.27 Soil–plant–animal cadmium pathway (infographic). Principal sources (phosphate fertilizers, sewage sludge, smelter/e-waste fallout, contaminated premixes) enter soils; uptake is greatest on acidic, low-Zn soils and in leafy forages; transfer occurs via forage, drinking water, and feed/mineral mixes; body burden concentrates in liver → kidney; public-health interface via offal (kidney > liver). Schematic based on ATSDR toxicology and food-chain mitigation reviews (ATSDR, 2012a; Schaefer et al., 2020; WHO, 2017).

Clinical Signs

Typically insidious: weight loss, polyuria/polydipsia, anemia, and reduced feed efficiency. Advanced cases may show osteopenia and reproductive impairment (ATSDR, 2012a; Kahn & Line, 2016).

Pathophysiology

Urinalysis reveals proteinuria and glycosuria with a bland sediment (proximal tubular leak). Gross kidneys may be pale with swollen cortices; histology shows proximal tubular degeneration/necrosis ± interstitial fibrosis (ATSDR, 2012a). The Fanconi-type pattern and lesion cues are consolidated in Figure 8.29.

Diagnosis

Prioritize matrices according to purpose and feasibility: kidney (postmortem) best indicates body burden; liver supports chronicity profiling; feed, forage, and soil sampling can help trace the exposure source – include soil pH profiling to risk-rank paddocks. Use species context (ruminant vs. monogastric) and

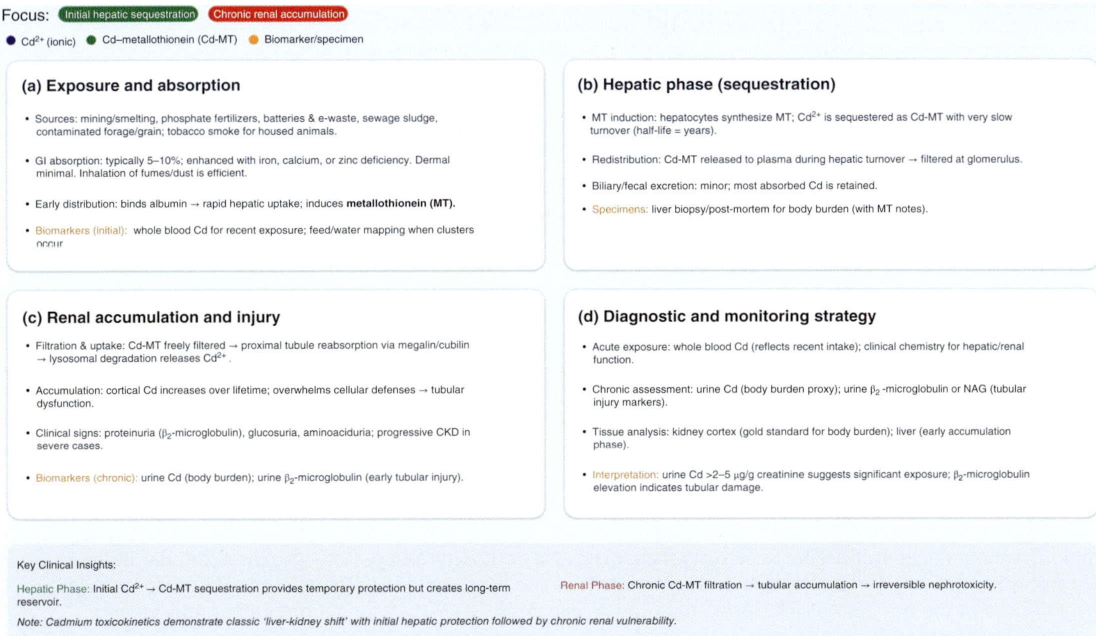

Figure 8.28 Toxicokinetics mini-panels (4×) – cadmium. Panel (a): exposure routes; Panel (b): distribution (gut → liver → kidney via metallothionein); Panel (c): long biological half-life and limited excretion; Panel (d): proximal-tubule (Fanconi-type) clinical/lab signature. Sources synthesized from ATSDR toxicology, veterinary overviews, and food-chain risk reviews (ATSDR, 2012a; Kahn and Line, 2016; Schaefer et al., 2020).

exposure history (fertilizer use, premix sourcing) to guide sampling (ATSDR, 2012a; Kahn & Line, 2016). The field workflow is laid out in Figure 8.30.

Treatment

No proven antidote for food animals. Core actions are source removal (He et al., 2021; Kong et al., 2021; Ren et al., 2021; Schaefer et al., 2020) soil liming to reduce plant Cd, organic matter/biochar additions, and dietary Zn/Fe to competitively reduce Cd uptake at plant and gut interfaces; implement tight QA on imported mineral salts/premixes to avoid contamination episodes (ATSDR, 2012a; Kahn & Line, 2016). Decision support and context-fit options are compiled in Table 8.7.

Selenium Poisoning

Source

Both deficiency and excess occur in the tropics. Toxicity follows high-Se forages (certain *Astragalus* spp., local high-Se soils) or over-supplementation (injectables, fortified blocks). The safety margin is narrow and demands locale-specific balancing (Kahn & Line, 2016; Suttle, 2010). Figure 8.31 summarizes the U-shaped intake–risk relationship with species windows.

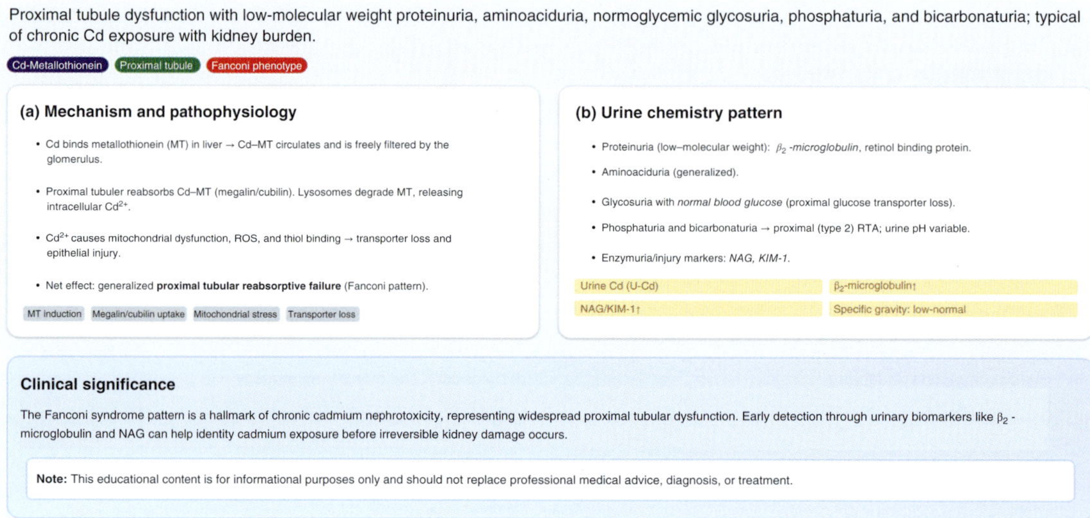

Figure 8.29 Proximal tubular injury schema with expected field findings: LMW-proteinuria, aminoaciduria, normoglycemic glycosuria, phosphaturia, ± bicarbonaturia; typical gross/histologic cues (pale swollen cortex; proximal-tubule degeneration/necrosis). **(a) Mechanism and pathophysiology (Cd – proximal tubular injury/ Fanconi pattern).** Cadmium binds metallothionein (MT) in the liver and circulates as a Cd–MT complex that is freely filtered at the glomerulus. The proximal tubule reabsorbs Cd–MT via megalin/cubilin endocytosis; lysosomal degradation releases intracellular Cd^{2+}, which induces mitochondrial dysfunction, reactive oxygen species (ROS), and thiol binding – leading to transporter loss and proximal tubular epithelial injury. Net result: **generalized proximal tubular reabsorptive failure (Fanconi phenotype). (b) Urine chemistry pattern (typical of chronic cadmium nephrotoxicity).** Characteristic findings include **low-molecular-weight proteinuria** (e.g., β2-microglobulin, retinol-binding protein), **generalized aminoaciduria**, **normoglycemic glycosuria**, **phosphaturia**, and **bicarbonaturia** (proximal/type 2 renal tubular acidosis; urine pH variable), and increased tubular injury enzymes/ markers (e.g., **NAG, KIM-1**). Urinary cadmium (U-Cd) reflects body burden/exposure and supports diagnosis.

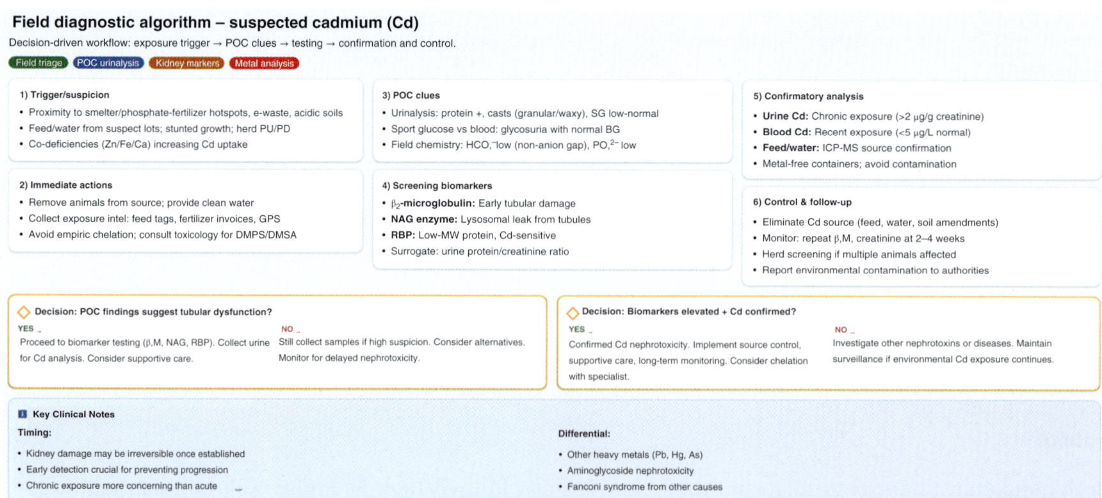

Figure 8.30 Field diagnostic algorithm – suspected cadmium. From exposure trigger → point-of-care urinalysis → targeted U-Cd/biomarkers → confirmation and source control; includes specimen handling and differentials.

Table 8.7 Mitigation toolbox vs. context (cadmium).

Measure	Mechanism	Evidence strength	Cost	Time to benefit	Field feasibility (✓/–)	Citation
Raise soil pH (agricultural lime)	Increases Cd sorption/ precipitation; lowers plant uptake	High	$$	Weeks–months	✓	He et al. (2021), Kong et al. (2021)
Add organic matter/compost (clean source)	Increases complexation/ CEC; dilutes bioavailable Cd	Moderate	$–$$	Weeks–months	✓	Schaefer et al. (2020)
Apply biochar (verified low-Cd)	Sorbs Cd; raises pH; improves CEC	Moderate	$$–$$$	Months–season	✓/–	Ren et al. (2021), Beesley et al. (2011), Woldetsadik et al. (2016)
Use low-Cd phosphate fertilizers	Reduces new Cd loading; maintains P sufficiency (limits uptake)	High	$–$$	Immediate (next application)	✓	Suciu et al. (2022)
Zinc supplementation (ration/mineral blocks)	Competitive antagonism at transporters; reduces absorption/uptake	High	$	Days–weeks	✓	Zhou et al. (2020)
Soil Zn application (zinc sulfate)	Antagonizes plant Cd uptake via transporter competition	Moderate	$–$$	Weeks–months	✓	Zhou et al. (2020)
Protected clean water points	Eliminates waterborne Cd intake	High	$–$$	Immediate	✓	WHO (2017), ATSDR (2012a)
Rotate/avoid hotspots (tailings, sludge fields)	Cuts exposure at source (forage/ water)	High	$	Immediate	✓	ATSDR (2012a)
Forage/cultivar choice (lower Cd accumulators)	Select species/ cultivars with reduced root uptake/ translocation	Moderate	$	Season (crop cycle)	✓	Schaefer et al. (2020)
Feed/forage/water screening program	Identifies contaminated lots; enables blending/ withholding	High	$–$$	Immediate (upon results)	✓	ATSDR, (2012a), Schaefer et al. (2020)
Blend/redirect high-Cd by-products (offal, certain meals)	Lowers dietary Cd concentration below action thresholds	High	$	Immediate	✓	EFSA (2009, 2011)

(*Continued*)

Table 8.7 (Continued)

Measure	Mechanism	Evidence strength	Cost	Time to benefit	Field feasibility (✓/–)	Citation
Zeolite/bentonite feed binders (targeted use)	Nonspecific GI binding (limited for Cd)	Low–Moderate	$	Immediate	✓/–	Schaefer et al. (2020)
Raise soil organic C (cover crops; vetted manures)	Long-term complexation; improves soil health	Moderate	$$	Seasons–years	✓/–	Schaefer et al. (2020)
Phytoremediation/ phytoextraction (selected plants)	Gradual removal of soil Cd via biomass harvest	Moderate	$–$$	Multi-season/ years	—	Raza et al. (2020), Suman et al. (2018)
Offal management (withhold liver/ kidney from food chain)	Interrupts human exposure via high-burden organs	High	$	Immediate	✓	EFSA (2009, 2011)
Record-keeping and exposure mapping (GPS, inputs)	Prevents re-exposure; targets interventions efficiently	High	$	Immediate	✓	ATSDR (2012a)

Summary of field-ready measures to reduce cadmium exposure in food animals, with mechanism of action, evidence strength, relative cost, expected time to benefit, and field feasibility.
Evidence strength reflects practice-oriented consensus from primary trials and reviews. Cost scale: $ = low, $$ = moderate, $$$ = high. Time to benefit is the practical interval until a measurable effect. Field feasibility: ✓ = broadly feasible; ✓/– = context-dependent; – = limited practicality without projects/grants. The rightmost column uses APA in-text citations to exemplar sources; full references appear in the chapter bibliography.

Toxicity

At supraphysiologic intakes, selenium substitutes for sulfur in amino acids and disrupts keratin and myocardial redox enzymes.

Clinical Signs

Chronic ("alkali disease"): alopecia, hoof sloughing/cracks, poor hair coat, weight loss, ill thrift ± cardiomyopathy. Acute (rare, iatrogenic): dyspnea, pulmonary edema, shock (Kahn & Line, 2016).

Pathophysiology

Clinicopathology may show low-grade anemia; creatine kinase (CK)/aspartate transaminase (AST) can be elevated with myodegeneration. Histology may show myocardial degeneration; in chronic cases, dermal/hoof matrix changes are evident (Kahn & Line, 2016). Figure 8.32 provides a schematic of these targets.

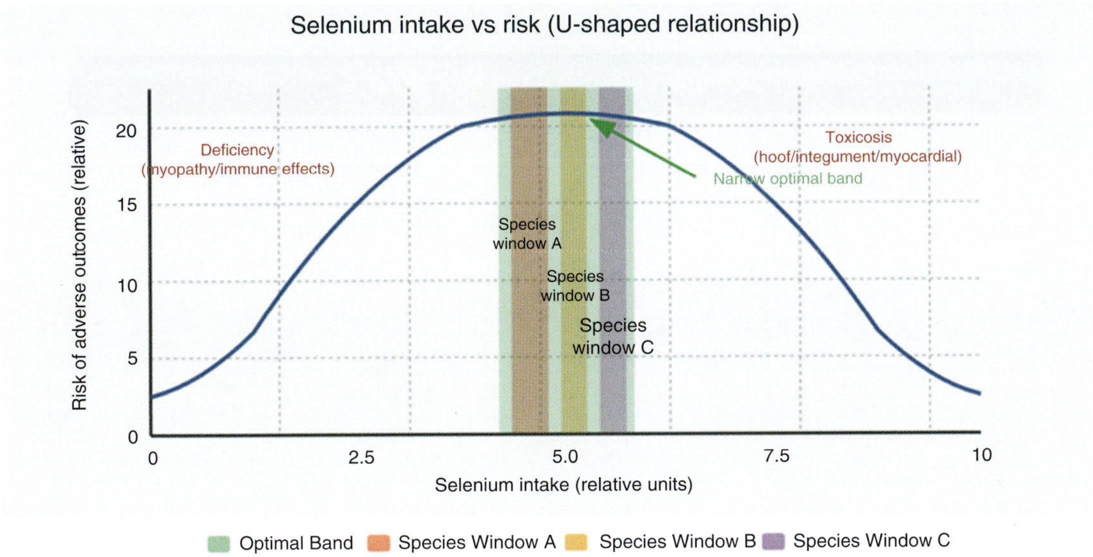

About selenium's U-shaped risk curve

Deficiency zone (left): Too little selenium leads to myopathy and compromised immune function.

Optimal zone (center): The narrow band where selenium intake provides maximum benefit with minimal risk. Different species have specific optimal windows within this range.

Toxicity zone (right): Excessive selenium intake causes toxicosis affecting hooves, integument, and myocardial function.

Key insight: The optimal range is remarkably narrow, making precise selenium supplementation critical for animal health.

Figure 8.31 Selenium intake vs. risk (U-shaped relationship). Deficiency at low intakes (myopathy/immune effects), a **narrow optimal band** in the middle, and toxicosis at high intakes (integument/hoof/myocardial injury); species "windows" indicated. *Source:* Author's illustration for this chapter; adapted from Kahn and Line, (2016) and Suttle (2010).

Diagnosis

Choose matrices according to the question (status vs. chronicity vs. recent overdose): serum/whole-blood Se (current status/over-supplementation); liver (recent intoxication profiling); hair/hoof (chronic exposure, retrospective). Optional: RBC glutathione peroxidase activity (Pavlata et al., 2012) as a functional index of status when Se measurements aren't immediately available (Kahn & Line, 2016; Suttle, 2010). Table 8.8 collates practical targets and interpretive cues by species (matrix, indicative ranges, flags, and handling notes)

Following the table, Figure 8.33 gives a field decision tree to move from forage/serum Se → classify → act → confirm → retest.

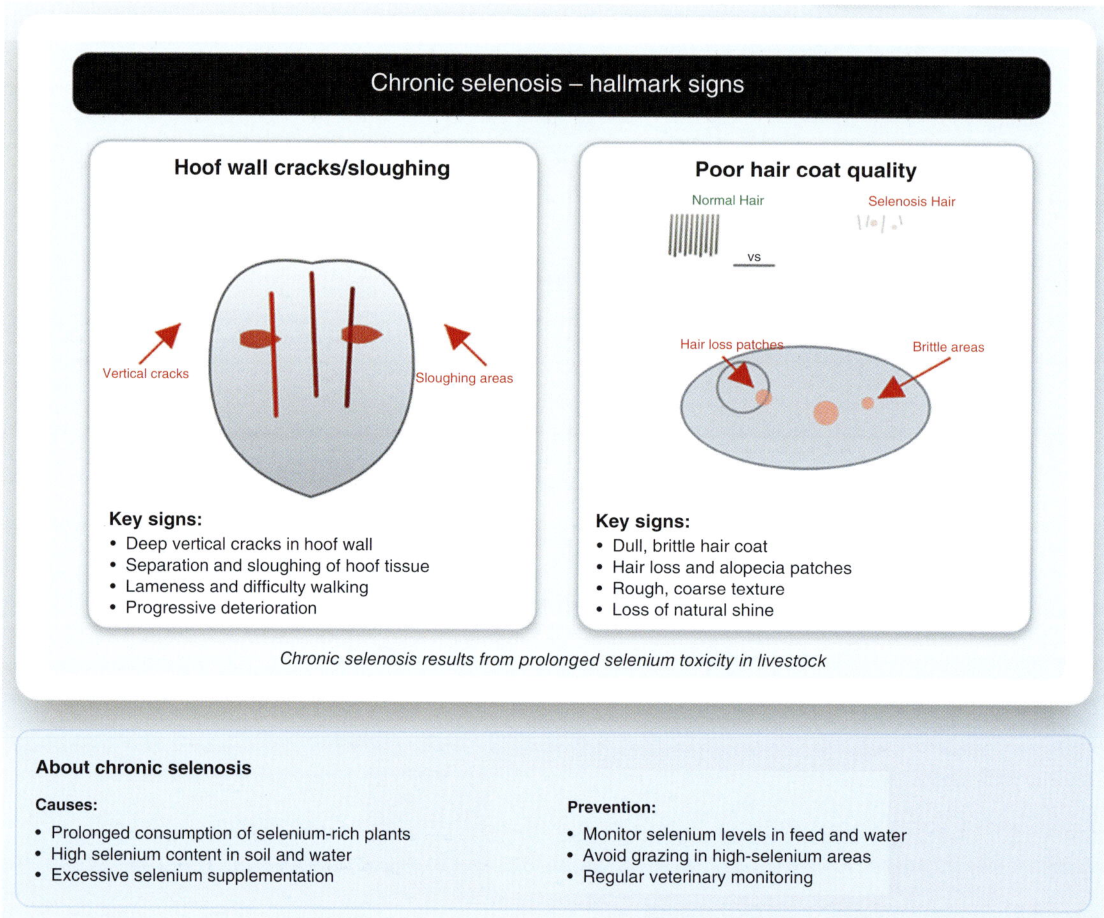

Figure 8.32 Tissue targets in selenium excess (schematic). Primary targets highlighted for chronic and acute selenosis: **integument/hoof matrix** (cracks/sloughing) and **myocardium** (degeneration/myonecrosis); includes representative histologic cues. *Source:* Author's illustration for this chapter; adapted from Kahn and Line, (2016) and Suttle (2010).

Treatment

Withdraw the source (stop Se blocks/boluses/injectables; move off suspected high-Se pastures). Correct rations and consider vitamin E as a functional antagonist. In high-Se zones, avoid additional Se in mineral mixes and use soil/forage testing to set safe supplementation windows (Kahn & Line, 2016; Suttle, 2010). Table 8.9 lists common supplementation pitfalls and safeguards with retest timing.

Table 8.8 Practical selenium targets and matrices (by species).

Species	Matrix	Indicative range	Deficiency flags	Toxicity flags	Notes (sample volume/handling, retest interval)	Citation
Cattle	Whole blood Se	≥100–300	<100	>1,000 (often with clinical signs in outbreaks)	2–3 mL EDTA whole blood; GPx preferred for herd screens; retest 4–6 weeks after ration change	Kahn & Line (2016), Davidson-York et al. (1999)
	Liver Se (postmortem, μg/g DM)	0.9–1.75	<0.8	—	Collect ~50 g; avoid surface contamination; pair with kidney for chronicity	Kahn & Line (2016)
	Hair Se (ppm, DW)	0.50–1.32	—	>1.4 (chronic selenosis range)	Clip clean flank; reflects chronic exposure; retest 2–3 months	Yaeger et al. (1998)
Sheep/goats	Whole blood Se	≈120 (mean in field herds); practical target ≥100	<100	—	2 mL EDTA; GPx tracks Se status; flock screen 4–6 weeks	Pavlata et al. (2012)
Horses	Whole blood Se	100–200	<70	>300 (risk zone reported in supplemented horses)	2–3 mL EDTA; lab RI varies; pair with diet review; retest 4–6 weeks	Kahn & Line (2016), Cornell AHDC (2021), KER (2017)
Pigs	Whole blood Se	≥100 (operational target)	<100	>1,000 (elevated in field toxicosis)	2 mL EDTA; consider feed source audit; retest 2–4 weeks	Davidson-York et al. (1999)
Poultry	Feather Se (ppm, DW)	Tracks intake (use lab's RI)	—	Elevated with dietary Se ≥7–9 mg/kg (toxic range in broilers)	Pull primary feathers; good intake biomarker; align with diet Se	Kim et al. (2020)
	Diet Se (mg/kg feed, as-fed)	0.15–0.20 (typical requirement band)	<0.1	≥7–9 (toxicity window in trials)	Verify premix specs; sample multiple lots; retest on new batch	Li et al. (2016)
All species (context)	Serum/plasma Se (equine example)	Horses: 140–240	Horses: <100	Horses: >300 caution	Serum needs trace-metal clean tubes; avoid hemolysis; interpret with species-specific RI	Cornell AHDC (2021), KER (2017)

Field-oriented reference values for key matrices (whole blood, serum/plasma, liver, hair/feather, diet) with indicative ranges, deficiency/toxicity flags, and practical sample-handling and retest notes.
Source: Merck Veterinary Manual; Davidson-York et al. (1999), Cornell AHDC; Pavlata et al. (2012), Kim et al. (2020), Li et al. (2016); KER.

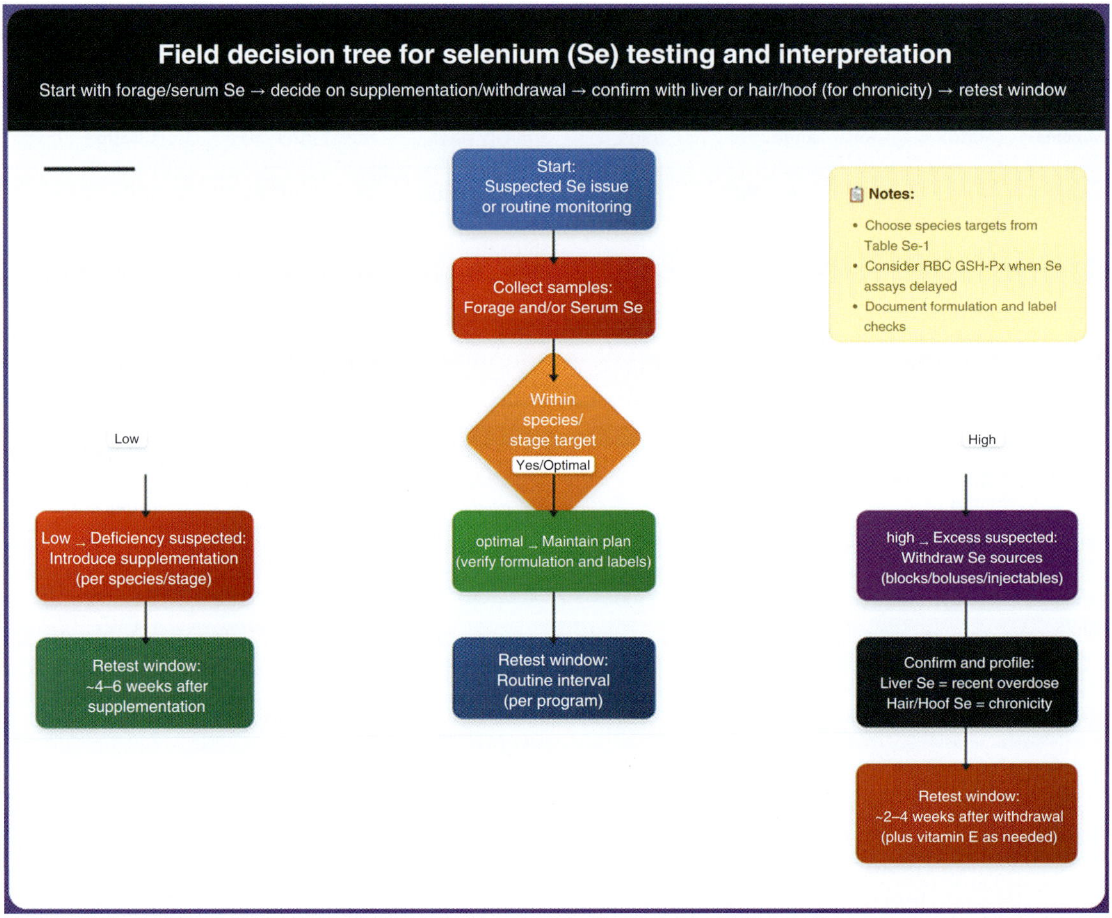

Figure 8.33 Field decision tree for Se testing and interpretation. Start with **forage/serum Se** → classify (low/optimal/high) → act (supplement, maintain, or withdraw sources) → confirm with **liver** (recent overdose) or **hair/hoof** (chronicity) → **retest window** per action/species. *Source:* Author's illustration for this chapter; integrated with chapter diagnostic workflow.

Chromium (VI) and Nickel Poisoning

Source

Tannery and electroplating effluents are important Cr(VI) sources in parts of South/Southeast Asia; irrigation with contaminated water brings chromium onto fodder. Nickel exposure clusters near refineries/e-waste – typically lower magnitude but relevant locally (ATSDR, 2012b; WHO, 2003, 2021). Figure 8.34 outlines this industrial-effluent → irrigation-canal → fodder pathway, with Ni nodes for refineries/e-waste hotspots.

Table 8.9 Supplementation pitfalls and safeguards for selenium.

Pitfall (what goes wrong)	Consequence (what happens)	Safeguard (formulation, labeling, double-check)	Retest timing*
Stacking sources (e.g., injectable + high-Se mineral block + Se in premix/TMR)	Excess intake → acute dyspnea/pulmonary edema; or chronic hoof/coat lesions	Maintain a single primary Se source; run a whole-ration Se audit; lock away extras during treatment periods	Serum/whole-blood Se at **2–4 weeks** after removing extras; repeat at **6–8 weeks** if borderline
Wrong product for species/stage (e.g., beef/cattle block used for sheep or camelids; lactation vs. dry)	Over- or under-supplementation; toxicosis in sensitive species	Species-specific products only; color-code storage shelves; add a "species" checkbox on feed sheets	Serum Se **2–3 weeks** after switch
Decimal/units error (mg vs. μg; ppm vs. mg/kg) when mixing premixes/top-dressing	10× dosing error → cluster of acute cases	Two-person calculation sign-off; calculator sheet taped to the bin; keep a "worked example" on label	Serum Se **7–10 d** post-event; liver Se if severe/iatrogenic
Confusing Se vs. sodium selenite/selenate amounts on labels	Under/over supply depending on salt basis	Convert all labels to **elemental Se** on your worksheet; keep a conversion crib	Serum Se **2–4 weeks** after correction
Bolus/injectable interval too short or repeated at shipping/vaccination	Cumulative excess → subacute signs	Record next-due dates on animal lists; hold injectables in a separate "vet-only" cabinet	Serum Se **2–3 weeks** after last dose
Using multiple Se-fortified feeds (starter + mineral + lick) without a whole-ration view	Chronic excess "creep"	Whole-diet spreadsheet; supplier spec sheets on file; one person owns the sign-off	Serum Se **4 weeks** after simplification
Assuming salt-block intake is constant (drought, palatability, hierarchy)	Unreliable Se delivery → deficiency or spikes	Prefer measured loose mineral in TMR; if blocks used, monitor disappearance and head count	Serum Se **4–6 weeks** after change; RBC GSH-Px at **6–8 weeks** if available
Not accounting for high-Se soils/forages in locality	Supplement on top of high baseline → toxicosis	Annual **forage/soil testing**; use low-/no-Se minerals in high-Se belts	Forage + serum Se at **start of season**; recheck **6–8 weeks** after adjustments
Top-dressing by hand without scales	Variable dosing between pens/animals	Use gram scales + scoop chart; pre-weighed sachets for staff	Serum Se **3–4 weeks** after standardizing
Mixing/compounding error at mill (wrong premix bag, order of magnitude error)	Herd-level outbreak	Supplier QA certificate per lot; bar-code scan at intake; retain samples for audit	Serum Se **1–2 weeks** after feed change; investigate with feed/liver if severe

(*Continued*)

Table 8.9 (Continued)

Pitfall (what goes wrong)	Consequence (what happens)	Safeguard (formulation, labeling, double-check)	Retest timing*
No retest after a change	Missed persistent deficiency/excess	Schedule retests when you write the ration; add calendar reminders	As per action: **low** = 4–6 weeks; **optimal** = routine interval; **high** = 2–4 weeks after withdrawal
Relying on a single matrix (e.g., serum only) when chronicity is suspected	Misclassification of long-term status	Pair serum with **liver** (recent overdose) or **hair/hoof** (chronic exposure)	Hair/hoof at **8–12 weeks**; liver when clinically indicated

Supplementation errors are a common cause of selenium (Se) toxicosis in tropical herds. This table lists frequent pitfalls, likely consequences, practical safeguards (formulation, labeling, double-checks), and suggested retest windows to verify correction and animal status.
Source: Adapted from Kahn and Line, (2016), Suttle (2010).

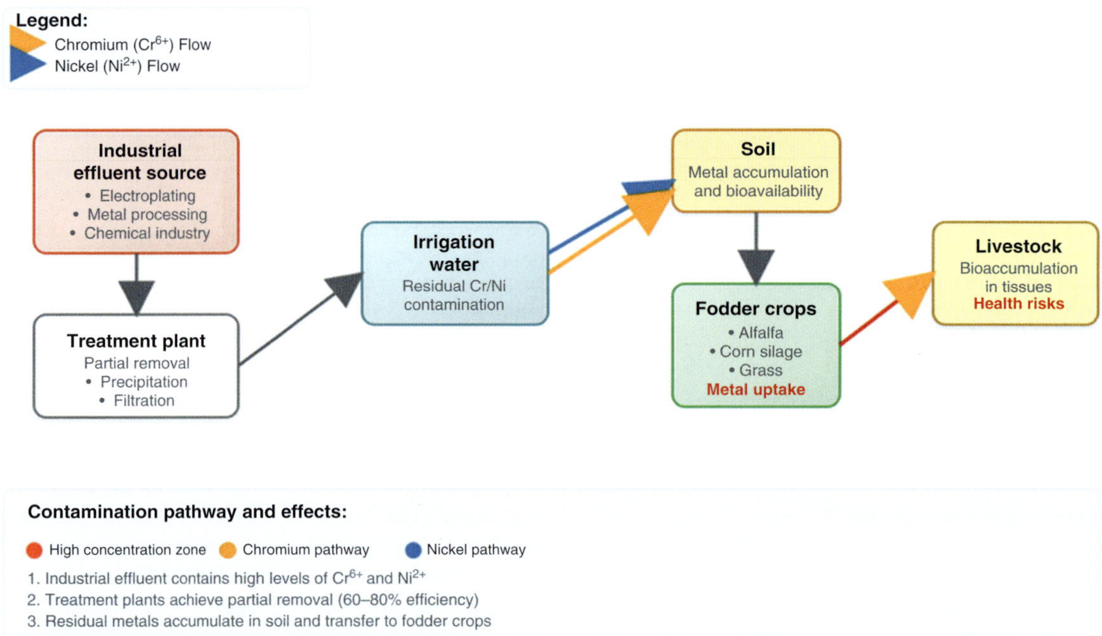

Figure 8.34 Cr(VI)/Ni exposure pathways in irrigated fodder systems. Flow map showing how **tannery/electroplating effluents** introduce **hexavalent chromium [Cr(VI)]** into irrigation canals and then onto **fodder/forage**, with parallel **nickel (Ni)** nodes from **refineries and e-waste**. Panels mark practical **sampling points** (canal/trough water for Cr(VI) speciation; forage and soil for total Cr/Ni) and note key **modifiers** (redox/pH affecting Cr(VI) stability and plant uptake). Designed for One Health triage: trace **source → transfer → animal exposure → what to sample**. *Source:* Author's schematic for this chapter; pathway emphasis adapted from Kahn and Line, (2016).

Toxicity

Cr(VI) is membrane-permeant and reduced intracellularly, generating oxidative DNA/protein damage. Cr(III) is a trace nutrient at minute doses. Nickel mainly causes GI upset and dermatitis; systemic toxicosis is uncommon in farm species (ATSDR, 2012b; Kahn & Line, 2016; WHO, 2003, 2021). Figure 8.35 contrasts Cr(III) versus Cr(VI) toxicodynamics and situates Ni as primarily a GI/dermal irritant.

Clinical Signs

In livestock, GI irritation and growth depression predominate with Cr(VI) exposure; nickel exposure is more likely to produce mucocutaneous irritation.

Diagnosis

Forage/water chromium speciation (preferably laboratory-based) is central, with animal tissue burdens added if clinical. Figure 8.36 provides a field diagnostic algorithm (history near tannery/e-waste? → test

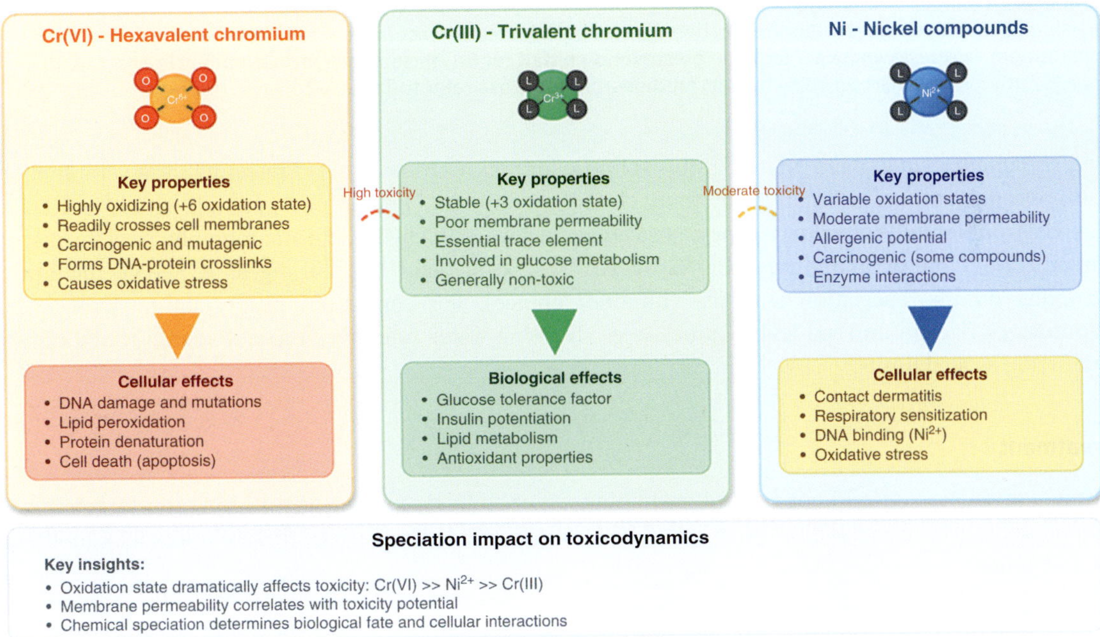

Figure 8.35 Speciation and toxicodynamics: Cr(III) vs. Cr(VI) (with Ni panel). Left: **Cr(III)** – poor membrane permeability; trace nutrient at minute doses. Center: **Cr(VI)** – membrane-permeant oxyanion; **intracellular reduction** (Cr(VI)→Cr(V)→Cr(IV)→Cr(III)) generates **reactive species** with **DNA/protein adducts** and mucosal injury; dominant veterinary syndromes are **GI irritation and growth depression**. Right: **Ni** – primarily **gastrointestinal irritant** and **dermal sensitizer** in livestock; systemic toxicosis is uncommon in field settings. *Source:* Author's schematic; aligned to mechanisms summarized in ATSDR (2012b), Kahn and Line (2016), WHO (2003, 2021).

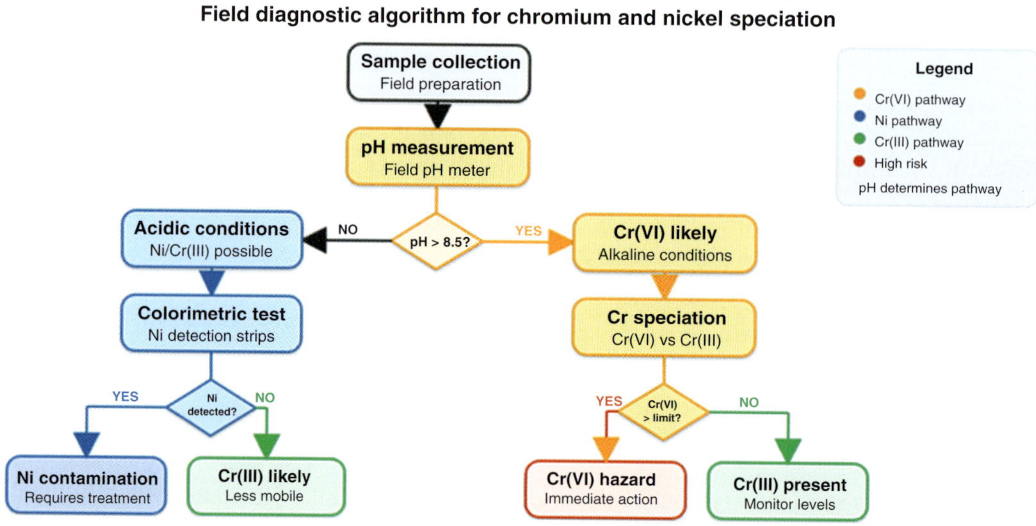

Figure 8.36 Field diagnostic algorithm for suspected Cr(VI)/Ni exposure. Start with **history/location** (tannery/electroplating belts, refineries/e-waste) → **collect source samples**: water **for Cr(VI) (speciation-preserved)** and parallel **total metals**, plus **forage/soil** → **classify** (low/optimal/high for context using Table 8.11) → if clinical/at-risk, add **animal matrices** (blood/urine; liver/kidney postmortem) → **act** (source removal, water switch, forage substitution) → **retest windows**. Flags the **preservation pitfall** for Cr(VI) (separate speciation bottle, short hold). *Source:* Author's flowchart for this chapter; methods/pitfalls cross-refer to Table 8-10.

water/forage for Cr(VI) and Ni → classify → choose animal matrices → act → retest window). Table 8.10 lists preferred matrices and analytic methods (U.S. Environmental Protection Agency, 1992, 1994a, 1994b; U.S. Environmental Protection Agency, 2025) (e.g., water Cr(VI) by ion chromatography or colorimetry under correct preservation; total Cr/Ni by ICP-MS; forage/soil by acid-digest ICP-MS), including sampling pitfalls (speciation stability, container choice). For contextual interpretation, Table 8.11 summarizes background guideline values (e.g., drinking-water references) to aid source triage rather than serve as feed limits.

Treatment

Mitigation focuses on effluent control, switching water sources, forage substitution, and targeted soil amendments/phytoremediation in irrigated belts; Figure 8.37 summarizes these choices as a toolbox/decision tree.

Less-Common Metals: Rapid Triage Pearls

Although frank field toxicoses from the following metals are uncommon in tropical production systems, brief, high-yield prompts can help clinicians not miss them in the right context. Use the sidebar for quick differentials at the crush/bench; pair with the rapid-triage table for first steps, tests, and confirmation.

Table 8.10 Preferred matrices and analytic methods (with pitfalls) for chromium (Cr) and nickel (Ni) investigations in tropical animal health.

Matrix (sample)	Purpose/what it answers	Target analyte and speciation	Preferred method (examples)	Container and preservation	Pitfalls and field notes
Irrigation/trough water (source triage near tanneries/electroplating or e-waste)	Is Cr(VI) present? Screen magnitude and need for immediate source switching	Cr(VI) (dissolved); run total Cr in parallel; include Ni (total)	Cr(VI): IC (EPA Method 218.6)[*]	Use HDPE/polypropylene bottles; for Cr(VI): filter 0.45 μm, buffer to pH 9–9.5, 4°C, analyze ≤24 h; do not acidify the Cr(VI) bottle; collect a separate acidified bottle for total metals (HNO_3, pH<2)[*]	Speciation loss (Cr(VI)→Cr(III)) with time, acidification, reducers; matrix anions can affect IC columns; avoid stainless steel contact; run blanks/spikes per method QC[*]
Canal/wastewater (effluents)	Map hotspot intensity; compliance context	Cr(VI) and total Cr/Ni	Cr(VI): IC (EPA Method 218.6); Total Cr/Ni: ICP-MS (EPA Method 200.8)[*,†]	Same as water; short hold for Cr(VI); consider on-site filtration[*]	High anions/organics can reduce Cr(VI) or overload columns – use matrix spikes and appropriate dilutions[*]
Forage/fodder (fresh, silage)	Confirms transfer from irrigation to feed	Total Cr, Ni (screening)	Acid digestion of solids (EPA Method 3050B) → ICP-MS (EPA Method 200.8) for totals[†,‡]	Clean poly bags or glass; freeze or dry; avoid metal scissors contamination; retain duplicate	Soil splash inflates values; record field soil pH and irrigation history; homogenize composite grabs
Soil/sediment (grazing pads, canal banks)	Source confirmation; risk-ranking paddocks	Total Cr, Ni	Acid digestion (EPA Method 3050B) → ICP-MS (EPA Method 200.8)[†,‡]	Poly jars; air-dry; remove stones; chain-of-custody	Heterogeneity – use composites; 3050B gives "total recoverable" (not strictly total)[†]
Whole blood/plasma (animal)	Recent/ongoing exposure (Ni); limited value for Cr(VI) speciation	Total Ni/Cr	ICP-MS (EPA Method 200.8) after validated wet-digestion (lab SOP)[†]	Trace-metal-clean tubes (no metal stoppers); refrigerate; avoid hemolysis	Use alongside source samples; interpret trends rather than a single cut-off; pair with clinical context

(Continued)

Table 8.10 (Continued)

Matrix (sample)	Purpose/what it answers	Target analyte and speciation	Preferred method (examples)	Container and preservation	Pitfalls and field notes
Urine (animal)	Renal excretion marker (Ni; total Cr)	Total Ni/Cr	ICP-MS (EPA Method 200.8) after dilution/ digestion (lab SOP)[†]	Plastic containers; chill; prompt analysis	Hydration/diuresis confounders – consider creatinine-corrected values (lab dependent)
Hair/wool (ruminants)	Chronic exposure indicator (Ni; Cr context)	Total Ni/Cr	ICP-MS after decontamination + digestion (lab SOP)	Seal in clean envelopes; document washing protocol	External contamination from dust/soil; always co-sample forage/soil for interpretation (background vs. body burden)
Liver/kidney (postmortem)	Body burden and distribution; ties to lesions	Total Ni/Cr (tissues)	Acid digestion (3050B-type) → ICP-MS (EPA Method 200.8); pathology-guided sampling[†,‡]	Fresh/frozen for chemistry (formalin not suitable); separate block for histology	Match to gross/histo; use dedicated plasticware; note any ulcerative gastritis in suspected Cr(VI) cases

* EPA Method 218.6 (ion chromatography for dissolved Cr(VI)).
† EPA Method 200.8 (ICP-MS for total Cr/Ni in waters and wastes).
‡ EPA Method 3050B (acid digestion of soils/sediments/sludges for total recoverable metals).
Field-oriented sampling and analytic choices for Cr(VI)/total Cr and Ni in livestock investigations. Speciation stability matters: collect separate bottles for Cr(VI) versus total metals, follow method-specific preservation, and interpret drinking-water values only as source-triage context, not feed limits.
Methods and toxicology context adapted from authoritative guidance (ATSDR, 2012b; U.S. Environmental Protection Agency [EPA], 1992, 1994a, 1994b, 1996; World Health Organization [WHO], 2021).

Table 8.11 Interpretation aids – contextual guideline values and veterinary notes for CrNi poisoning.

Matrix/ context	Guideline or reference value (contextual)	Veterinary interpretation notes	Suggested action/triage	Key caveats
Drinking water (human guideline, used for livestock water triage)	Nickel (Ni): **70 μg/L***; Total chromium: **50 μg/L**†; U.S. EPA MCL for total chromium: **100 μg/L**‡	Conservative triggers for **source switching** and investigation near refineries/e-waste (Ni) or tannery/ electroplating belts (Cr). Use for **triage** of livestock water when veterinary limits are absent. For chromium, interpret total Cr cautiously and prioritize **speciation (Cr(VI) vs Cr(III))** in water where feasible¶.	If ≥ WHO/EPA values: **switch/blend** water source; collect confirmatory samples (**speciation for Cr**)¶; total metals for Ni; sample forage/ soil; check animals (blood/ urine metals) if clinical signs or hotspot history.	Human guideline context only; not animal-feed limits. For chromium, **speciation matters** – Cr(VI) is the principal toxicological concern¶.
Irrigation water (protect soil resource; legacy FAO guidance)	Suggested maxima (typical): Chromium (total) **≈ 0.10 mg/L**; Nickel ≈ **0.20 mg/L**§	Use only as **context** to judge long-term soil build-up risk on fodder fields irrigated with industrially impacted water.	If ≥ suggested maxima: prioritize **source control/ blending**, adjust irrigation scheduling, and consider **phytoremediation/soil amendments**; retest and track forage metals.	Values are legacy, conservative screens; site-specific soils/crops vary. Confirm with current national/ state guidance if available.
Animal matrices (blood/ urine)	No harmonized veterinary cut-offs; interpret **trends** and compare to local lab reference intervals (if available).	Pair animal results with **source samples** (water/ forage/soil) and clinical picture; for chromium, water **speciation** is most informative¶ (animal matrices are typically **total chromium**).	Elevations with compatible exposure history → remove source; consider follow-up at **2–4 weeks** after mitigation; use postmortem liver/kidney if animals die.	Analytical method and matrix prep drive comparability; ensure validated ICP-MS methods and proper containers/ preservation.

* World Health Organization (2021). *Nickel in drinking-water: Background document...*

† World Health Organization (2003). *Chromium in drinking-water: Background document...*

‡ U.S. Environmental Protection Agency (2024). *National Primary Drinking Water Regulations (NPDWR): MCL for total chromium.*

§ Ayers & Westcot, (1985). *Water quality for agriculture (FAO Irrigation and Drainage Paper 29 Rev. 1), Table 21.*

¶ Agency for Toxic Substances and Disease Registry (2012b). *Toxicological profile for chromium* (Cr(VI) vs Cr(III) context).

Context values below are for triage and discussion (not legal limits): human drinking-water guidelines, legacy irrigation-water guidance to protect soils, and veterinary interpretation notes for field decisions. Always verify local regulations and laboratory reference intervals.

Contextual values summarized from authoritative sources: WHO drinking-water background documents (nickel; chromium), U.S. EPA National Primary Drinking Water Regulations (chromium MCL), and FAO legacy irrigation guidance (Ayers & Westcot). Use for triage only; check current local regulations and laboratory reference intervals.

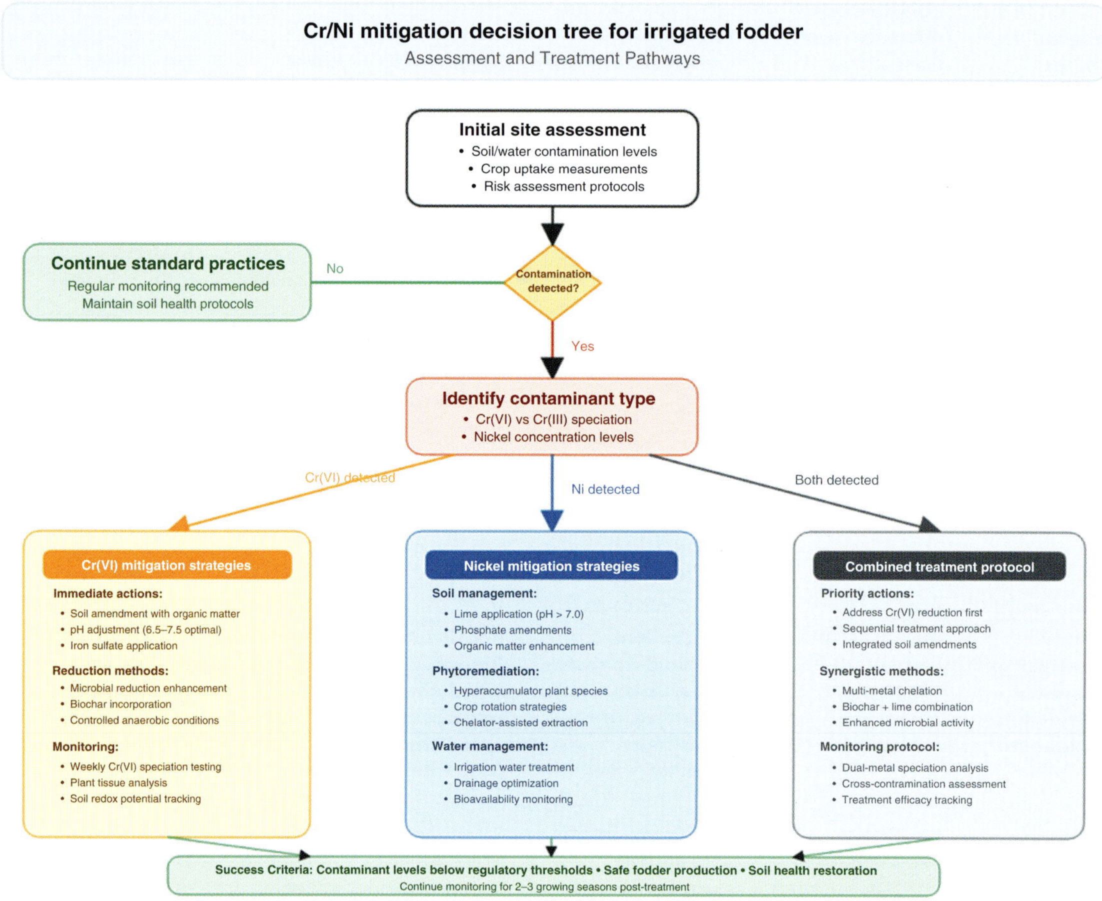

Figure 8.37 Mitigation toolbox and decision tree (Cr(VI)/Ni). If source samples are elevated: **(1)** immediate containment (**switch/blend water**, fence off canals, alternative forage), **(2) source control** with stakeholders (effluent management), **(3) field fixes** in irrigated belts (targeted **soil amendments** and **phytoremediation** where feasible), **(4) monitoring cadence** for water/forage and sentinel animals. Notes where **Cr speciation** should be rechecked after mitigation. *Source:* Author's decision tree for this chapter; aligns with diagnostic workflow.

Clinical Pearls – Less-Common Metals (Quick Triage) (Table 8.12)

Thallium (dogs/cats): Rare now, but keep in the differential for painful neuropathy, patchy alopecia, and gastrointestinal signs where legacy industrial sources exist. Consider Prussian blue; prognosis variable (see Figure 8.38).

Zinc (small animals, birds): Coin/galvanized metal ingestion → hemolytic anemia, pancreatitis; obtain radiographs and serum Zn; remove foreign body + chelation/support (see Figure 8.39).

Iron (iatrogenic/ingestions): Acute gastrointestinal corrosion → metabolic acidosis, hepatotoxicity (swine, dogs); use stage-based management; deferoxamine when indicated (see Figure 8.40).

Cobalt/Manganese (livestock – industrial hotspots): Seldom cause frank field toxicosis; treat as site-specific contaminant risks in battery/mining corridors; focus on source control and monitoring.

Table 8.12 Rapid triage – less-common metals (clinical pearls for quick field use).

Metal	Typical exposure (tropics)	Key clinical clues	Fast tests	First steps	Confirm/definitive
Thallium (dogs/cats)	Legacy industrial sites, old rodenticides/ pesticides	Painful distal neuropathy, patchy alopecia, GI signs	CBC/biochemistry; targeted toxicology (reference lab)	Supportive care; consider Prussian blue	Thallium in blood/ urine/feces or hair (reference lab)
Zinc (small animals, birds)	Coins, cages, bolts, galvanized items	Pale/icteric mucosae (hemolysis), vomiting, pancreatitis	Abdominal radiographs; serum Zn	Foreign-body removal; chelation; GI/hepatic support	Repeat serum Zn; imaging to confirm clearance
Iron (swine, dogs)	Overdose (injectables), vitamins/rodenticides	Vomiting, melena → shock; later hepatotoxicity	Serum iron, blood gases/acid–base status	Deferoxamine when indicated; fluids; timed decontamination	Trend iron with clinical course; liver enzymes
Cobalt/ Manganese (livestock)	Mining/battery corridors, dust; site-linked	Usually subclinical; reduced performance/site clusters	Forage/soil/water metals (ICP-MS)	Source control; routine monitoring	Trend matrices over time; map hotspots

Key tropical exposures, hallmark clinical clues, "fast tests," first steps, and confirmatory endpoints for thallium, zinc, iron, and cobalt/manganese. Content synthesized from standard veterinary toxicology references; intended for **triage** and bedside prompting rather than exhaustive management guidance. Compiled from Kahn and Line (2016); Peterson and Talcott (2013); Plumb (2018); ATSDR (2022d).

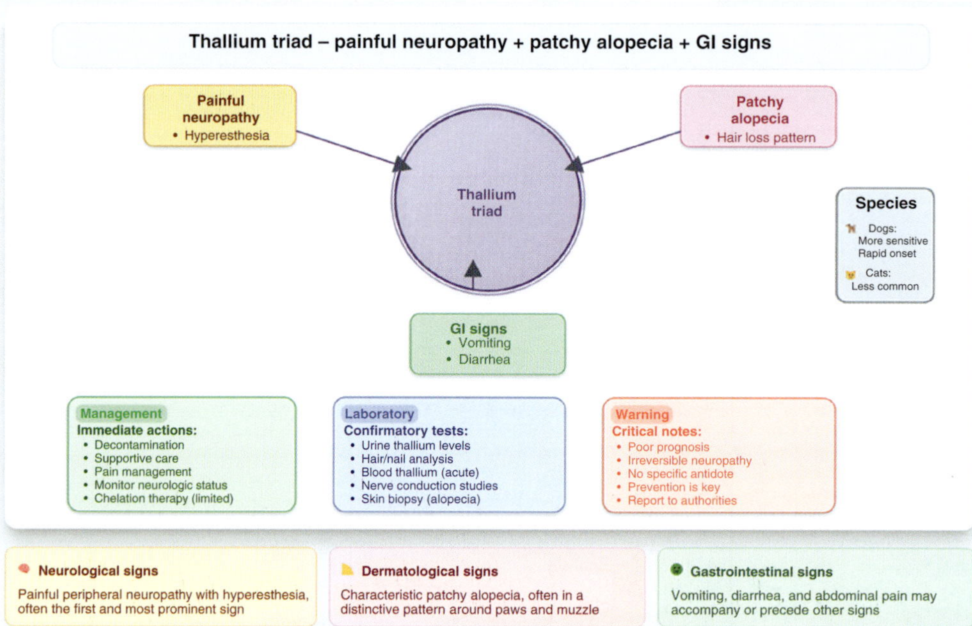

Figure 8.38 Thallium triad (dogs/cats). When **painful peripheral neuropathy** + **patchy alopecia/poor coat** + **GI signs** occur together, raise suspicion for thallium poisoning. **Initial management:** supportive care; where available and appropriate, consider **Prussian blue (ferric hexacyanoferrate)** under veterinary/toxicology guidance. **Confirmation:** submit **blood/serum** (recent exposure), **urine** (elimination phase), **feces** (especially if Prussian blue is used), and/or **hair** (chronicity). Coordinate testing with a reference laboratory that offers validated Tl methods (Agency for Toxic Substances and Disease Registry (2022d); Kahn and Line (2016).

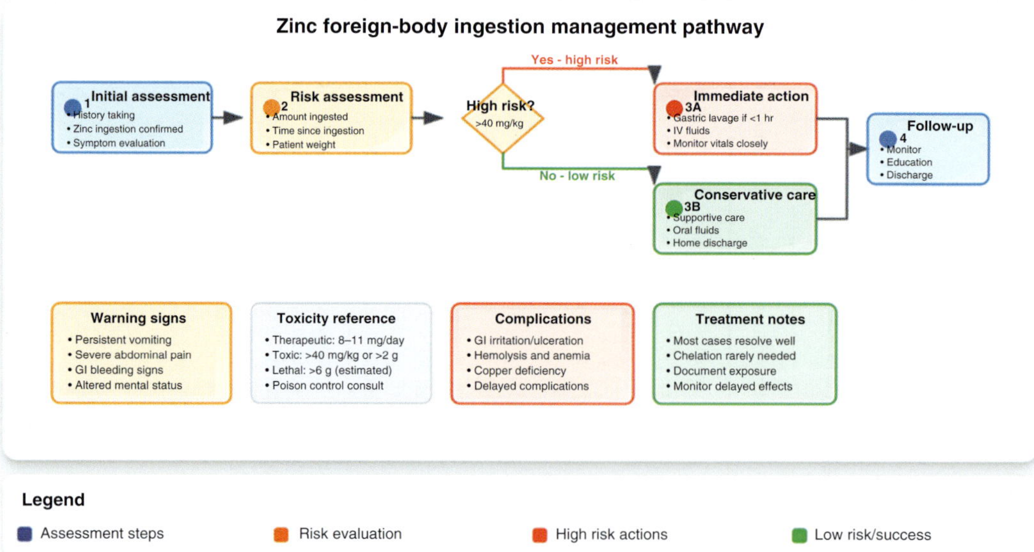

Figure 8.39 Zinc foreign-body pathway (dogs/cats). Ingestion of a zinc-containing object (e.g., post-1982 penny, zinc alloy toy) → abdominal radiographs to confirm/rule in a radiopaque foreign body → prompt removal (endoscopic or surgical) → serum zinc to document systemic burden and track decline → chelation only if zinc is markedly elevated and/or there is ongoing hemolysis → retest serum zinc and CBC/chemistry at 7–14 days. Notes: stabilize; do not induce emesis for sharp objects; address hemolysis and GI injury.

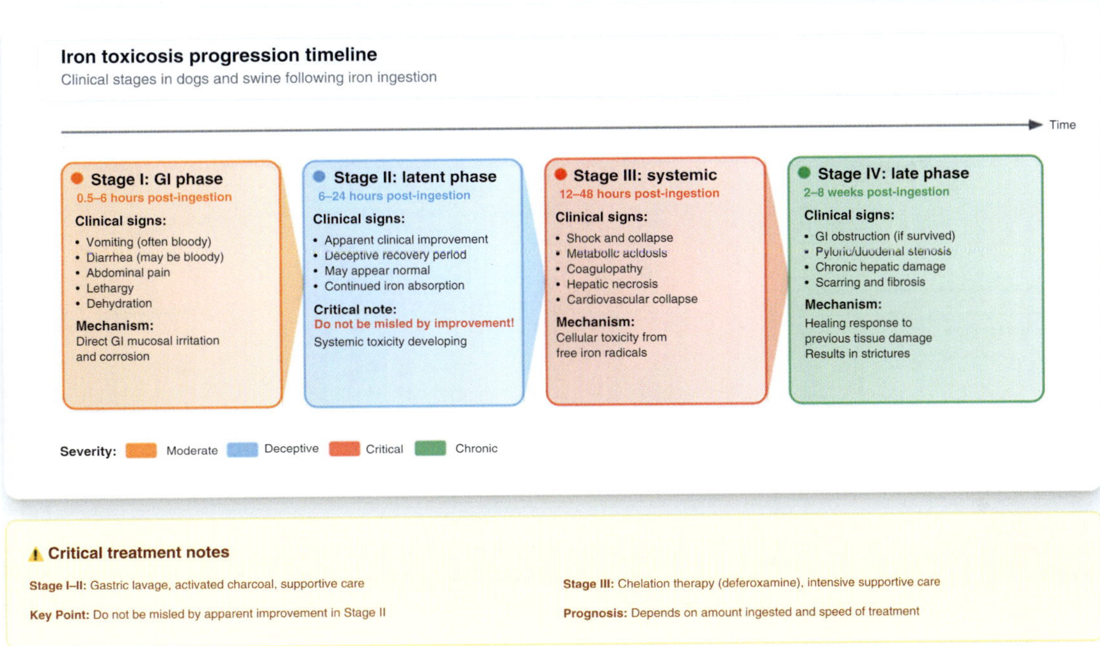

Figure 8.40 Iron toxicosis – stage ribbon (dogs/swine). Stage I (0–6 hours): Acute GI irritation – vomiting (± hematemesis/hematochezia), abdominal pain, dehydration. Stage II (6–24 hours): Apparent recovery – transient clinical improvement while mucosal and systemic injury evolve. Stage III (12–96 hours; peak 12–48 hours): Systemic toxicity – shock, metabolic acidosis, coagulopathy, hepatic injury, CNS depression/seizures; consider chelation (deferoxamine) when indicated. Stage IV (2–6 weeks): Delayed effects – GI stricture/obstruction, residual hepatic injury; recheck CBC/chemistry and manage sequelae. Species cues for dogs and swine provided beneath the ribbon.

Case Studies Highlighting Global Challenges and Mitigation Techniques in Tropical Ecosystems

Case Study: Lead Poisoning in Zamfara, Nigeria

In 2010, artisanal gold mining in Zamfara State released large amounts of lead-laden dust; hundreds of children and domestic animals died from acute lead poisoning (Centers for Disease Control & Prevention, 2024). Villagers crushed ore inside homes, contaminating soil and water; free-range livestock and poultry grazing or drinking in these areas became early indicators and vectors of exposure. For example, free-range chickens from mining villages showed extremely high tissue lead and posed risks to consumers of their meat (Oladipo et al., 2020) (see Figure 8.41).

Mitigation pointers: Source control (stop in-home ore processing; safer ore handling), environmental cleanup (soil removal/replacement), livestock management (fence off hotspots; provide clean water/feed), and community education on hazards and early animal signs (CDC, 2024).

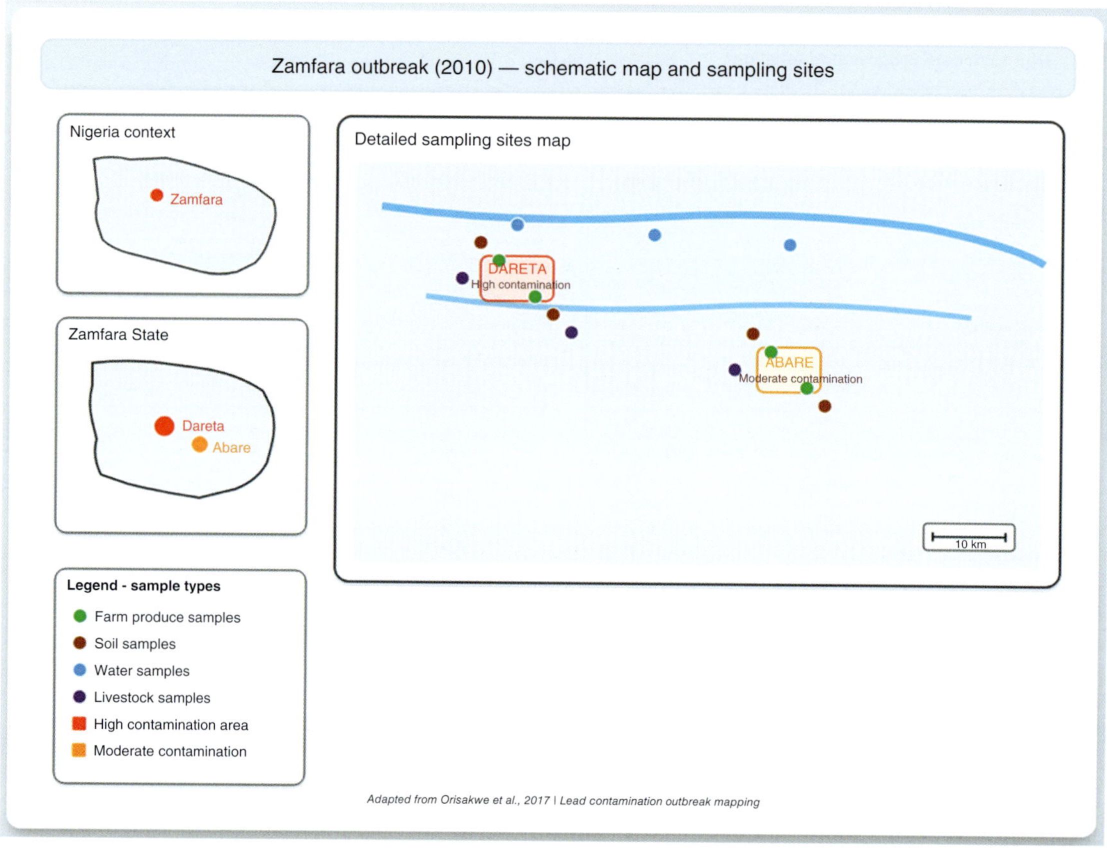

Figure 8.41 Lead outbreak in Zamfara, Nigeria – exposure pathway and hotspots. Schematic/map of Zamfara State showing artisanal mining villages, in-home ore-processing sites, and likely livestock/human exposure nodes (contaminated soil, household dust, wells, and grazing areas). Sampling points for soil, water, poultry/livestock tissues, and milk are indicated, with a One Health inset for clinical triage. *Source:* Adapted from World Health Organization (2010), Centers for Disease Control and Prevention (2024), Orisakwe et al. (2017), and Oladipo et al. (2020).

Case Study: Mercury from Artisanal/Small-Scale Gold Mining in the Peruvian Amazon

In Madre de Dios and similar tropical belts, mercury used for gold amalgamation enters rivers and sediments; microbial methylation and food-web biomagnification raise exposures far downstream (Weinhouse et al., 2021). River-dependent communities near ASGM showed hair mercury levels substantially higher than comparison populations, with associated health concerns in children (Weinhouse et al., 2021). Wildlife and fish serve as reservoirs and sentinels, linking ecosystem contamination to human and animal health (Weinhouse et al., 2021) (see Figure 8.42).

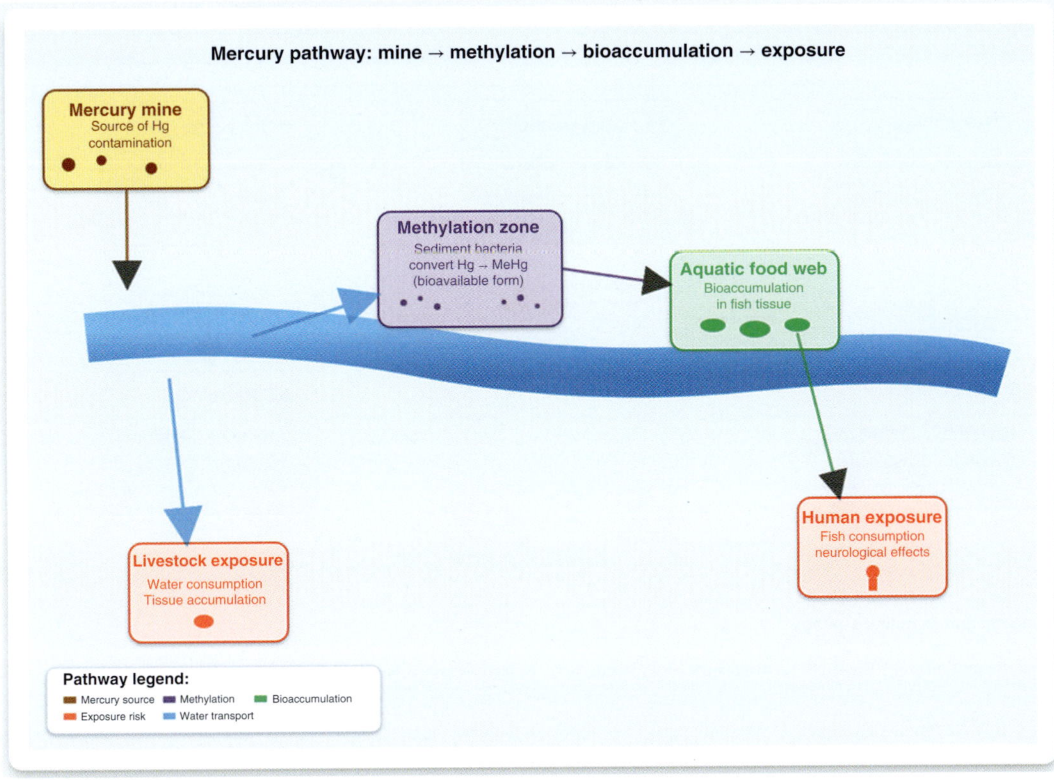

Figure 8.42 ASGM mercury in the Peruvian Amazon – riverine methylation and food-web transfer. Process diagram from mine site (elemental Hg use) → river/sediment → microbial methylation → bioaccumulation in fish (trophic ladder) → exposure of river-dependent communities, wildlife, and domestic animals. Hair sampling and fish-species advisories are annotated. *Source:* Weinhouse et al. (2021)/Springer Nature.

Mitigation pointers: Promote mercury-free or mercury-reducing technologies and retorts, formalize/regulate mining, provide dietary advisories (avoid high-trophic fish), and restore riparian habitats (Weinhouse et al., 2021).

Case Study: Arsenic in South Asian Dairy Systems (Bangladesh)

Shallow groundwater with high arsenic is used for irrigation and animal watering, driving arsenic accumulation in soils, crops (e.g., paddy straw), and cattle. In exposed dairies, arsenic moved into urine and dung (environmental cycling), whereas milk concentrations tended to be low but still relevant for cumulative dietary exposure assessment (Ghosh et al., 2013) (see Figure 8.43).

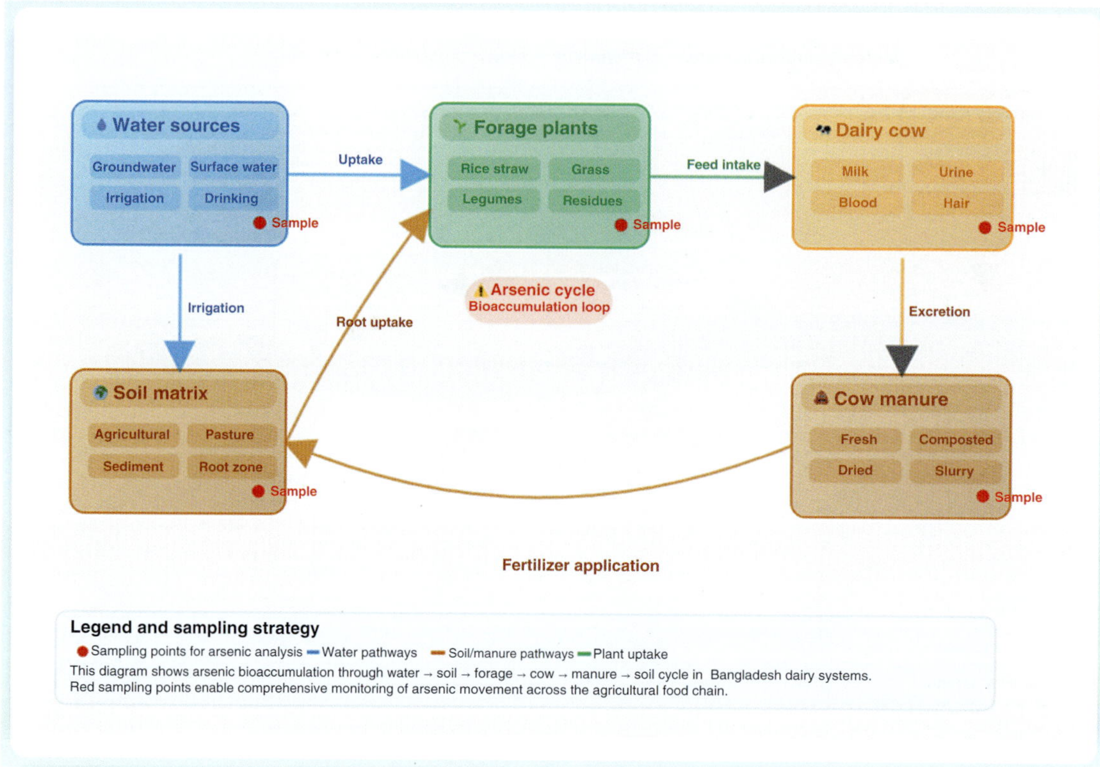

Figure 8.43 Arsenic in South Asian dairies – water → soil → paddy straw → cattle → manure loop. Flow diagram illustrating shallow tube-well water to irrigated paddy, plant uptake, feeding of arsenic-bearing straw to cattle, and excretion via urine/dung (environmental cycling). Preferred sampling matrices (water, soil, straw, urine, milk) and mitigation levers (safe wells, alternative fodder, soil amendments) are flagged. *Source:* Ghosh et al. (2013)/ Springer Nature.

Mitigation pointers: Switch to arsenic-safe water sources (deep wells/rainwater), avoid contaminated straw, adopt agronomic practices that lower plant arsenic uptake, use soil amendments or phytoremediation, and implement routine water/soil/milk testing (Ghosh et al., 2013).

Toolbox: Community-Based Mitigation for Tropical Ecosystems (One Health)

Priority actions across these scenarios include source reduction, targeted environmental monitoring, agricultural management (pasture rotation, soil amendments, safer forages), veterinary surveillance (biomarkers in livestock; wildlife), risk communication, and cross-sector coordination using a One Health framework (CDC, 2024) (see Figure 8.44).

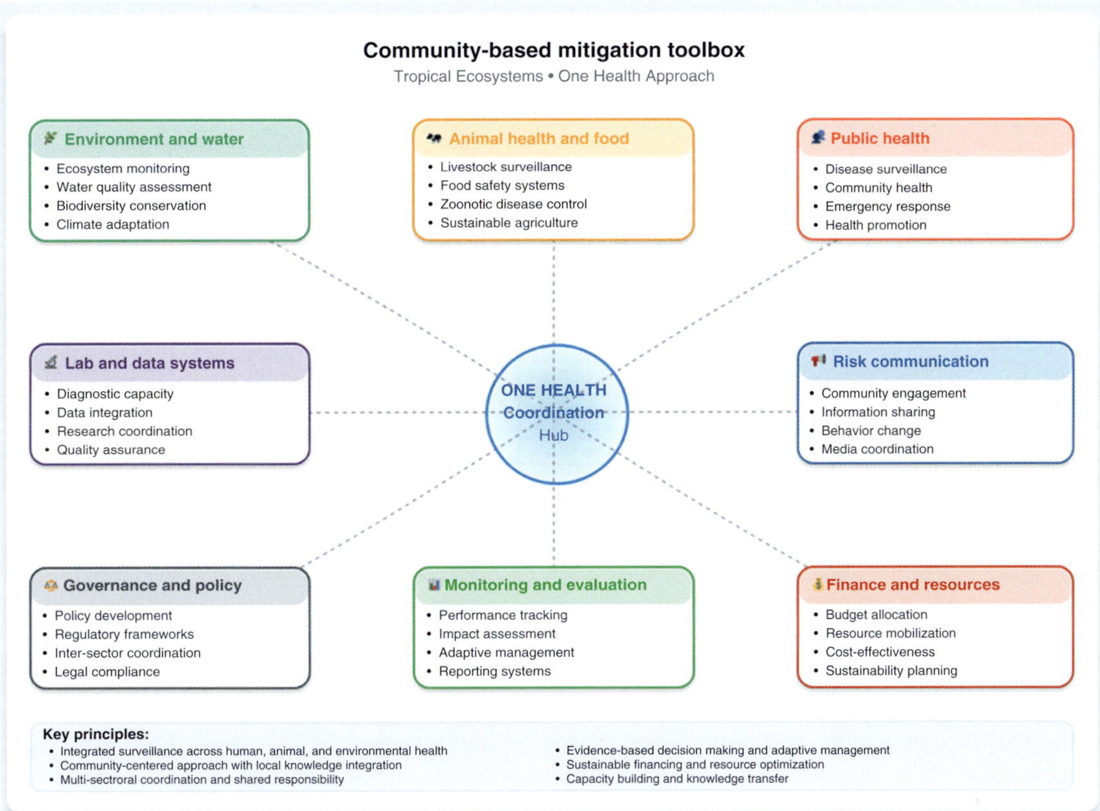

Figure 8.44 Community-based mitigation toolbox (One Health) for tropical metal hotspots. Decision tree linking source reduction (safer mining/effluent control), targeted environmental monitoring (water/soil/forage + GIS), agricultural management (pasture rotation, soil amendments, forage substitution), veterinary surveillance (biomarkers; sentinel species), and risk communication under a One Health coordination banner. *Source:* Adapted from CDC (2024) and U.S. Geological Survey One Health framework (n.d.)

References

Agency for Toxic Substances and Disease Registry. (2012a). *Toxicological profile for cadmium*. U.S. Department of Health and Human Services. https://www.atsdr.cdc.gov/toxprofiles/tp5.pdf

Agency for Toxic Substances and Disease Registry. (2012b). *Toxicological profile for chromium*. U.S. Department of Health and Human Services. https://www.atsdr.cdc.gov/toxprofiles/tp7.pdf

Agency for Toxic Substances and Disease Registry. (2020c). *Toxicological profile for arsenic. U.S. Department of Health and Human Services*. https://www.atsdr.cdc.gov/toxprofiles/tp2.pdf

Agency for Toxic Substances and Disease Registry. (2022d). *Toxicological profile for thallium. U.S. Department of Health and Human Services*. https://www.atsdr.cdc.gov/toxprofiles/tp54.pdf

Ayers, R. S., & Westcot, D. W (1985). *Water quality for agriculture (FAO Irrigation and Drainage Paper 29 Rev. 1)*. Food and Agriculture Organization of the United Nations.

Beesley, L., Moreno-Jiménez, E., Gomez-Eyles, J. L., Harris, E., Robinson, B., & Sizmur, T. (2011). A review of biochars' potential role in the remediation, revegetation and restoration of contaminated soils. *Environmental Pollution*, *159*(12), 3269–3282. https://doi.org/10.1016/j.envpol.2011.07.023

Blakley, B. R. (2024). *Mercury poisoning in animals*. MSD Veterinary Manual (Professional Version). https://www.msdvetmanual.com/toxicology/mercury-poisoning/mercury-poisoning-in-animals

Centers for Disease Control and Prevention. (2024). Lead poisoning investigation in Northern Nigeria | One Health. https://www.cdc.gov/one-health/php/stories/lead-poisoning.html

Chung, C.-S., Li, Y.-C., & Lin, L.-S. (2020). Radiographic findings and pathology of a dog with mercury toxicity. *Forensic Imaging*, *23*, 200421. https://doi.org/10.1016/j.fri.2020.200421

Cornell University College of Veterinary Medicine. (2013). *Necropsy show & tell: Gunmetal kidneys (sheep; kidney, cut surfaces) [Photograph]*.

Cornell University College of Veterinary Medicine, Animal Health Diagnostic Center 2021, 'Clinical Pathology', *viewed 30 August 2025*, https://www.vet.cornell.edu/animal-health-diagnostic-center/testing-laboratories/clinical-pathology

Cowan, V. L., & Blakley, B. R. (2016). Acute lead poisoning in western Canadian cattle—A 16-year review. *The Canadian Veterinary Journal*, *57*(4), 421–426.

Davidson-York, D., Poppenga, R. H., Thornton, J., & Evans, H. (1999). Selenium elimination in pigs after an outbreak of selenium toxicosis. *Journal of Veterinary Diagnostic Investigation*, *11*(4), 353–356. https://doi.org/10.1177/104063879901100410

eClinpath. (n.d.). *Basophilic stippling*. Cornell University. https://eclinpath.com/hematology/morphologic-features/red-blood-cells/basophilic-stippling/

EFSA. (2011). Statement on tolerable weekly intake (TWI) for cadmium. *EFSA Journal*, *9*(2), 1975.

EFSA Panel on Contaminants in the Food Chain. (2009). Cadmium in food. *EFSA Journal*, *7*(10), 980.

Fenga, C., Gangemi, S., Di Salvatore, V., Falzone, L., & Libra, M. (2017). *Immunological effects of occupational exposure to lead (Review). Molecular Medicine Reports*, *15*(5), 3355–3360. https://doi.org/10.3892/mmr.2017.6381

Garland, T. (2024). Organic arsenical toxicosis in animals. *Merck/MSD Veterinary Manual*. Available at: https://www.msdvetmanual.com/ (accessed 21 January 2026)

Ghosh, A., Majumder, S., Awal, M. A., & Rao, D. R. (2013). Arsenic exposure to dairy cows in Bangladesh. *Archives of Environmental Contamination and Toxicology*, *64*(1), 151–159. https://doi.org/10.1007/s00244-012-9810-3

Gupta, R. C. (Ed.). (2018). *Veterinary Toxicology: Basic and Clinical Principles* (3rd ed.). Academic Press.

Harvey, J. W (n.d.). *Canine blood smear—Basophilic stippling, lead toxicity*. Merck Veterinary Manual.

He, L.-L., Yin, C.-M., Chen, J.-Y., Lin, S.-S., & Sun, X.-J. (2021). Meta-analysis of liming effects on soil pH and cadmium in crops. *Process Safety and Environmental Protection*, *152*, 1–12. 10.1016/j.psep.2021.06.011

Hooper, P., & Geelhoed, E. (2020). *Lead-affected cattle (Primefact 413, 3rd ed.)*. New South Wales Department of Primary Industries.

Jones, M. L., & van der Merwe, D. (2008). *Copper toxicity and sheep (S-1536)*. Kansas State University Agricultural Experiment Station and Cooperative Extension Service.

Kahn, C. M., & Line, S. (Eds.). (2016). *The Merck Veterinary Manual* (11th ed.). Merck & Co., Inc.

KER (Kentucky Equine Research). (2017). *Selenium in horses: Requirements and testing [Technical note]*. Available at: https://ker.com

Kim, J. H., Hosseindoust, A., Lee, S. H., & Kim, Y. Y. (2020). Comparison of toxic effects of dietary organic vs. inorganic selenium in broilers. *Animals*, *10*(11), 2105. https://doi.org/10.3390/ani10112105

Kong, L., Wang, Y., Zhao, S., Wang, F., & Liu, S. (2021). Liming effectiveness on cadmium bioavailability and accumulation in rice: A field synthesis. *Science of the Total Environment*, *796*, 148949. https://doi.org/10.1016/j.scitotenv.2021.148949

Li, J. L., Sunde, R. A., Choi, Y. J., & Cheng, W. H. (2016). Selenoprotein transcript and enzyme activity as biomarkers to determine selenium requirement in broiler chicks. *PLOS ONE*, *11*(4), e0152392. https://doi.org/10.1371/journal.pone.0152392

Martins, K. P. F., Padilha, V. H. T., Damasceno, T. K., Souza, M. A., Silva, E. M. S., Ribeiro, M., Pereira, A. H. B., & Colodel, E. M. (2020). Chronic copper poisoning in beef cattle in the state of Mato Grosso, Brazil. *Pesquisa Veterinária Brasileira*, *40*(9), 651–661. https://doi.org/10.1590/1678-5150-pvb-6526

Merck Veterinary Manual. (2024). Selenium toxicosis in animals. Available at: https://www.msdvetmanual.com/ (Accessed 21 January 2026).

NADIS (National Animal Disease Information Service). (n.d.). *Copper poisoning in sheep*.

Nordberg, G. F., Fowler, B. A., & Nordberg, M. (Eds.). (2014). *Handbook on the Toxicology of Metals* (4th ed.). Academic Press/Elsevier.

Oladipo, O. O., Akanbi, O. B., Ekong, P. S., Uchendu, C., & Ajani, O. (2020). Lead toxicoses in free-range chickens in artisanal gold-mining communities, Zamfara, Nigeria. *Journal of Health & Pollution*, *10*(26), 200606. https://doi.org/10.5696/2156-9614-10.26.200606

Orisakwe, O. E., Oladipo, O. O., Ajaezi, G. C., & Udowelle, N. A. (2017). Horizontal and vertical distribution of heavy metals in farm produce and livestock around a lead-contaminated goldmine in Dareta and Abare, Zamfara State, Northern Nigeria. *Journal of Environmental and Public Health*, *2017*, 3506949. https://doi.org/10.1155/2017/3506949

Pavlata, L., Misurova, L., Pechova, A., Husakova, T., & Dvorak, R. (2012). Direct and indirect assessment of selenium status in sheep – a comparison. *Veterinární Medicína*, *57*(5), 219–223. https://doi.org/10.17221/5951-VETMED

Peterson, M. E., & Talcott, P. A. (2013). *Small animal toxicology* (3rd ed.). Elsevier.

Plumb, D. C. (2018). *Plumb's veterinary drug handbook* (9th ed.). Wiley-Blackwell.

Plumlee, K. H. (2013). *Clinical veterinary toxicology* (2nd ed.). Mosby/Elsevier.

Raza, A., Habib, M., Kakavand, S. N., Zahid, Z., Zahra, N., Sharif, R., & Hasanuzzaman, M. (2020). Phytoremediation of cadmium: Physiological, biochemical, and molecular mechanisms. *Biology*, *9*(7), 177. https://doi.org/10.3390/biology9070177

Ren, T., Chen, N., Wan Mahari, W. A., Xu, C., Feng, H., Ji, X., Yin, Q., Chen, P., Zhu, S., Liu, H., Liu, G., Li, L., & Lam, S. S. (2021). Biochar for cadmium pollution mitigation and stress resistance in tobacco growth. *Environmental Research*, *192*, 110273. https://doi.org/10.1016/j.envres.2020.110273

Schaefer, H. R., Hamer, M., & Mancini, L. (2020). Cadmium: Mitigation strategies to reduce dietary exposure. *Comprehensive Reviews in Food Science and Food Safety*, *19*(1), 313–339. https://doi.org/10.1111/1541-4337.12514

Scollo, A., Wilkinson, A., & Rogers, J. (2022). Selenium toxicity in a sheep flock due to a dietary formulation error. *Veterinary Record Case Reports*, *10*(3), e338. https://doi.org/10.1002/vrc2.338

Scrivens, S. G., Savin, K. W., Kelly, A., Fitzpatrick, J. L., & Smith, S. (2023). Lead toxicity in dairy cattle due to a contaminated mineral supplement: a case report. *Animals*, *13*(1), 174. https://doi.org/10.3390/ani13010174

Siddiqui, S., & Rajurkar, S. R. (2008). Lead—An emerging threat to livestock. *Veterinary. World*, *1*(7), 213–216.

Suciu, N. A., De Vivo, R., Rizzati, N., & Capri, E. (2022). Cd content in phosphate fertilizer: Which potential risk for the environment and human health? *Current Opinion in Environmental Science & Health*, *30*, 100392. https://doi.org/10.1016/j.coesh.2022.100392

Suman, J., Uhlik, O., Viktorova, J., & Macek, T. (2018). Phytoextraction of heavy metals: A review. *Frontiers in Plant Science*, *9*, 1476. https://doi.org/10.3389/fpls.2018.01476
Suttle, N. F. (2010). *Mineral nutrition of livestock* (4th ed.). CABI.
Texas A&M Veterinary Medical Diagnostic Laboratory. (n.d.). *Arsenic toxicosis in two calves (case study).*
Thompson, L. J. (2018). Lead. In R. C. Gupta (Ed.), *Veterinary Toxicology: Basic and Clinical Principles* (3rd ed., pp. 439–443). Academic Press. https://doi.org/10.1016/B978-0-12-811410-0.00029-5
U.S. Environmental Protection Agency. (1992). *Method 7196A: Chromium, hexavalent (colorimetric).*
U.S. Environmental Protection Agency. (1994a). *Method 218.6 (Rev. 3.3): Determination of dissolved hexavalent chromium in drinking water, groundwater, and industrial wastewater effluents by ion chromatography.*
U.S. Environmental Protection Agency. (1994b). *Method 200.8: Determination of trace elements in waters and wastes by ICP-MS.*
U.S. Environmental Protection Agency. (2024). *National primary drinking water regulations.*
U.S. EPA1996, Method 3050B: Acid Digestion of Sediments, Sludges, and Soils, Revision 2, Washington, *DC, viewed 30 August* 2026, https://www.epa.gov/sites/default/files/2015-12/documents/3050b.pdf
U.S. Geological Survey. (n.d.). *One Health conceptual diagram.*
Waldner, C., Checkley, S., Blakley, B., Pollock, C., & Mitchell, B. (2002). Managing lead exposure and toxicity in cow–calf herds to minimize the potential for food residues. *Journal of Veterinary Diagnostic Investigation*, *14*(6), 481–486. https://doi.org/10.1177/104063870201400606
Weinhouse, C., Gallis, J. A., Ortiz, E., Berky, A. J., Morales, A. M., Diringer, S. E., Harrington, J., Bullins, P., Rogers, L., Hare-Grogg, J., Hsu-Kim, H., & Pan, W. K. (2021). A population-based mercury exposure assessment near an artisanal and small-scale gold mining site in the Peruvian Amazon. *Journal of Exposure Science & Environmental Epidemiology*, *31*(1), 126–136. https://doi.org/10.1038/s41370-020-0234-2
Woldetsadik, D., Drechsel, P., Keraita, B., Marschner, B., Itanna, F., & Gebrekidan, H. (2016). Effects of biochar and alkaline amendments on cadmium immobilization, selected nutrient and cadmium concentrations of lettuce (*Lactuca sativa*) in two contaminated soils. *SpringerPlus*, *5*, 397. https://doi.org/10.1186/s40064-016-2019-6
World Health Organization. (2003). *Chromium in drinking-water: Background document for development of WHO guidelines for drinking-water quality.*
World Health Organization. (2010, July 7). *Nigeria: Mass lead poisoning from mining activities, Zamfara State (Disease Outbreak News).*
World Health Organization. (2017). *Guidelines for drinking-water quality—Cadmium fact sheet.*
World Health Organization. (2021). *Nickel in drinking-water: Background document for development of WHO guidelines for drinking-water quality (WHO/HEP/ECH/WSH/2021.6).*
Yaeger, M. J., Neiger, R. D., Holler, L., Fraser, T. L., Hurley, D. J., & Palmer, I. S. (1998). *The effect of subclinical selenium toxicosis on pregnant beef cattle. Journal of Veterinary Diagnostic Investigation*, *10*(3), 268–273. https://doi.org/10.1177/104063879801000307
Zhou, J., Zhang, C., Du, B., Cui, H., Fan, X., Zhou, D., & Zhou, J.(2020). Effects of zinc application on cadmium (Cd) accumulation and plant growth through modulation of the antioxidant system and translocation of Cd in low- and high-Cd wheat cultivars. *Environmental Pollution*, *265*, 115045. https://doi.org/10.1016/j.envpol.2020.115045

9

Natural Toxicants in Plants and Animals (Tropical Focus)

Natural toxicoses of tropical importance across Africa, Asia–Pacific, and the tropical Americas share repeating patterns that cut across species, forages, and production systems. The highest-impact problems in this chapter remain hepatogenous photosensitization from pastures (notably *Brachiaria decumbens*), plant-associated ill-thrift and neurotoxicity in leucaena-based systems (mimosine → DHP), cyanogenic crises from cassava by-products, aflatoxin contamination in feeds, and cyanobacterial hepatotoxins in warm, eutrophic waters. Risk peaks track tropical seasonality – end-of-dry/early-rains regrowth, drought-related feed gaps, and hot, still months that favor cyanoblooms. This chapter uses a pattern-based, production-first approach (source → signs → mechanism → diagnosis → control), with decision tools, sampling checklists, and case boxes that scale across regions. Core actions include immediate removal from source and shade for cholestatic injury, validated aflatoxin testing and ration reformulation, leucaena adaptation with *Synergistes jonesii* where applicable, antidote protocols for cyanide, and proactive water management for bloom-prone ponds (Allison et al., 1992).

Across the global tropics, natural toxicants arise from pastures and weeds, crop by-products, and warm, nutrient-rich waters used by livestock. While plant taxa differ by continent, the exposure mechanics are strikingly consistent. In Latin America and parts of sub-Saharan Africa and northern Australia, widespread planting or invasion of signal grasses (*Brachiaria* spp.) drives seasonal steroidal saponin cholangiohepatopathy and photosensitization – most often during early post-rain regrowth when young leaves carry higher protodioscin (Lozano et al., 2017). Cyanobacterial blooms are likewise recurrent in hot, eutrophic months and can precipitate per acute deaths or acute hepatopathy in stock and working dogs (Bischoff, 2024).

These are naturally occurring chemicals which, following ingestion in relatively small quantities, produce biochemical changes and/or physical lesions. Natural toxicants or biotoxins affecting animal health and production can be categorized as:

- Zootoxins (animal origin)
- Bacterial toxins (bacterial origin)
- Mycotoxins (fungal origin)
- Phytotoxins (plant origin)
- Phycotoxins (algae origin)

This chapter deals with poisoning caused by some of the toxicants that commonly occur in a tropical environment. For mycotoxins specifically, a concise overview of families, producer fungi, commodities, and hallmark animal effects is provided in Table 9.1, while Figure 9.1 maps where contamination typically occurs along the feed chain, and Figure 9.2 distils the temperature–humidity–time relationship that underpins risk.

Table 9.1 Core mycotoxin families at a glance – linking producer fungi, common tropical commodities, hallmark animal effects/sentinel species, and key literature anchors for quick orientation and teaching. (Families covered include aflatoxins, fumonisins, trichothecenes [A/B], zearalenone, ochratoxin A, ergot alkaloids, tremorgens, and slaframine; see in-table sources.)

Mycotoxin family (examples)	Main producer fungi (typical)	Typical commodities (tropics/global)	Hallmark animal effects/ sentinel species	Key sources (APA in-text)
Aflatoxins (AFB_1, AFB_2, AFG_1, AFG_2; AFM_1 in milk)	*Aspergillus flavus*, *A. parasiticus*	Groundnuts/ peanuts, maize, cottonseed, tree nuts, copra; warm/humid storage	Hepatotoxicity, immunosuppression; carcinogenic; AFM_1 carry-over to milk; young poultry highly susceptible	EFSA CONTAM Panel (2004), Merck Veterinary Manual, (n.d.), Pitt & Hocking, 2022
Fumonisins (FB_{1-3})	*Fusarium verticillioides*, *F. proliferatum*	Maize (grain and silage); drought–rainfall "flip" years	**Horses:** ELEM; **swine:** Porcine pulmonary edema (PPE); liver injury/ performance loss	EFSA CONTAM Panel (2018), Merck Veterinary Manual (n.d.)
Trichothecenes – Type B (DON, NIV)	*F. graminearum*, *F. culmorum*	Wheat, maize, barley, oats	Feed refusal/vomiting (pigs), diarrhea, poor gains; immunomodulation	EFSA CONTAM Panel (2017a)
Trichothecenes – Type A (T-2, HT-2)	*F. sporotrichioides*, *F. poae*	Oats, barley, maize (cool/wet harvests)	Oral/GI ulceration, dermal necrosis, hemorrhage; immunosuppression	EFSA CONTAM Panel (2011),
Zearalenone (ZEN)	*F. graminearum*, *F. culmorum*	Maize, small grains; warm–moist post-harvest	Estrogenism (vulvovaginitis, infertility), pigs most sensitive	EFSA CONTAM Panel (2017b), Merck Veterinary Manual (n.d.)
Ochratoxin A (OTA)	*Aspergillus ochraceus*, *Penicillium verrucosum*	Stored cereals (wheat/barley/ maize), coffee/ cocoa by-products	Chronic nephropathy (pigs, poultry), performance loss	EFSA CONTAM Panel (2023),
Ergot alkaloids (ergotamine, ergovaline, etc.)	*Claviceps* spp. on grains; endophyte *Epichloë* spp. in tall fescue/ryegrass	Small grains; endophyte-infected pastures	Vasoconstriction → gangrene; heat stress/agalactia ("fescue toxicosis")	EFSA CONTAM Panel (2012b, 2024),
Indole-diterpene tremorgens (e.g., lolitrem B; paspalitrems)	*Epichloë festucae* var. *lolii* (ryegrass endophyte); *Claviceps paspali*	Perennial ryegrass and paspalum pastures (seed heads)	"Staggers": intention tremors/ataxia in ruminants/ equids; recover off pasture	Merck Veterinary Manual (n.d.), Pitt and Hocking (2022)
Penitrem A/ Roquefortine C (tremorgens)	*Penicillium crustosum*, *P. roqueforti*	Moldy wastes/ garbage, spoiled dairy/meat	**Dogs:** acute tremors, seizures; GI signs	Walter (2002)
Slaframine	*Rhizoctonia leguminicola* on clovers/alfalfa	Red/white clover pastures; alfalfa hay/silage	"Slobbers syndrome": hypersalivation (horses, cattle); ± diarrhea/colic	Bennett & Klich (2003)

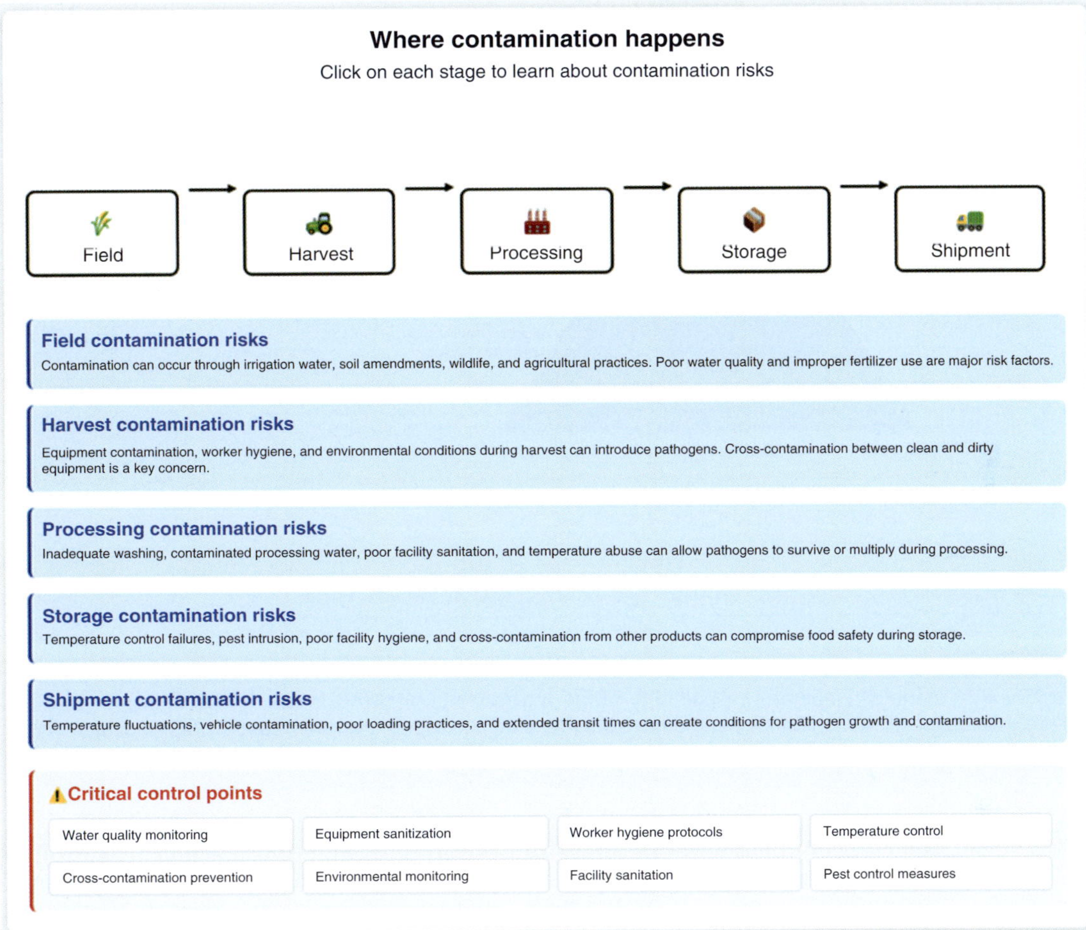

Figure 9.1 Rapid triage when forage cues don't fit (flowchart). Scene → onset → dominant signs guide toward likely causes (cyanobacterial neuro/hepatotoxins, elapid/viperid envenomation, or toad exposure), with "first samples" and immediate controls indicated (author schematic).

Leucaena-based systems (Pacific islands, northern Australia, Central America, parts of South Asia) deliver high protein but pose risk where stock are naïve or de-adapted to ruminal detoxification: mimosine → DHP toxicity persists until *S. jonesii* is established, producing classical ill-thrift, alopecia, and stomatitis (Allison et al., 1992). In mixed crop–livestock settings from West/Central Africa to South and Southeast Asia and northeast Brazil, cassava leaves/peels offered during feed gaps elevate cyanide (HCN) risk, especially when plant tissue is macerated or drought-stressed; abrupt access can convert a background hazard into per acute hypoxic collapse.

Feed substitution and storage realities add silent, cumulative threats. In many tropical countries, aflatoxins in maize, groundnuts, copra-based meals, and palm kernel cake remain a recurring issue – often clinically vague in animals – and require deliberate screening and feed management (see Table 9.1).

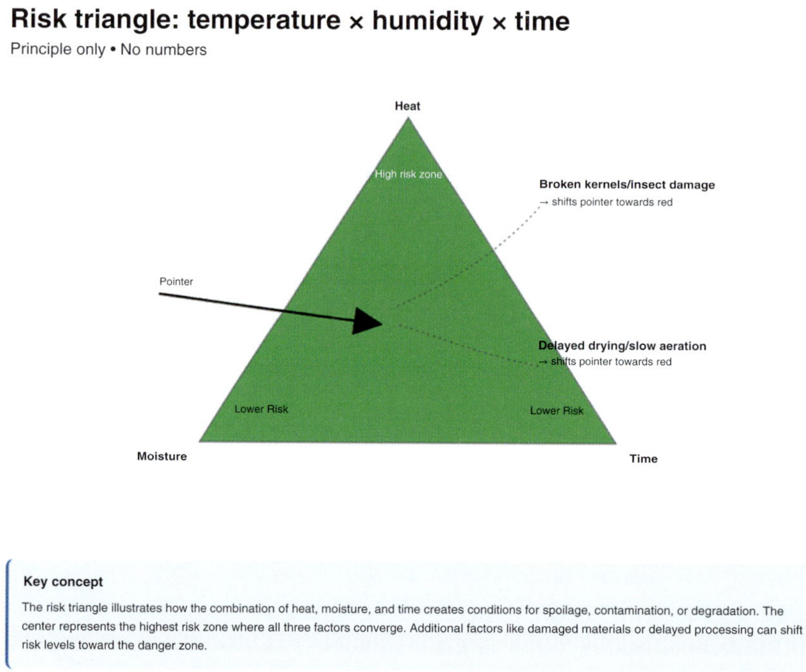

Figure 9.2 Risk triangle: temperature × humidity × time. Intrinsic mold/mycotoxin risk rises as heat, moisture, and exposure time increase; kernel damage and delayed drying shift the triangle toward higher risk (principle illustration; no numeric scale).

Water bodies – estate dams, smallholder ponds, irrigation reservoirs, aquaculture sumps – are a shared feature of tropical agriculture. In hot, eutrophic months, these favor cyanobacterial blooms (microcystins most commonly) that cause per-acute death at the waterside or acute hepatopathy, including in dogs with water access (Bischoff, 2024b).

Across regions, cases cluster in predictable scenarios:

- Regrowth windows (1–3 weeks after first rains): *Brachiaria* cholestasis/photosensitization.
- Drought/short forage: Cassava trimmings (HCN events); reliance on leucaena without adaptation.
- Hot, eutrophic months: Cyanoblooms in stock water; dog exposures at pond edges.
- Feed/ingredient substitutions and humid storage: Aflatoxin problems (see Table 9.1; Figures 9.1 and 9.2).

Under-recognition persists because clinical pictures are often nonspecific (ill-thrift, secondary infections, vague photosensitivity) and confirmatory tests are delayed. Outcomes improve when practitioners apply a simple triad: (i) Collect the right samples first time (e.g., liver fresh+formal and pasture for cholestatic cases; composite feed and milk for aflatoxin; cold, dark water and separate scum for blooms); (ii) use decision trees to separate primary vs. hepatogenous photosensitization and prioritize differentials; and (iii) implement immediate control (shade/exclusion, safe forage, antidotes where defined) while results are pending (Bookbinder 2024; EFSA CONTAM 2004; Bischoff 2024; APHL 2021).

Mycotoxins

Overview

Mycotoxins are secondary metabolites of fungi capable of producing acute or chronic toxic effects – carcinogenic, mutagenic, teratogenic, and estrogenic – in animals and humans; illnesses caused by them are termed mycotoxicoses. Although recognized since the sixteenth century, modern attention surged after the 1960 turkey outbreak in England linked to aflatoxins, and since then hundreds of mycotoxins have been identified, mainly from *Aspergillus*, *Penicillium*, and *Fusarium* species. A concise overview of families, producer fungi, commodities and hallmark animal effects is provided in Table 9.1, while Figure 9.1 maps where contamination typically occurs along the feed chain and Figure 9.2 distils the temperature–humidity–time relationship that underpins risk.

Sources and Occurrence (Field to Lab)

Mycotoxins are produced by toxigenic molds, which can grow on a variety of substrates, especially cereal grains under a wide range of environmental conditions. Figure 9.3 shows the growth of fungus *Aspergillus flavus* on an infested corn. Numerous reports on the occurrence of various mycotoxins in foods and feed have appeared since the discovery of the aflatoxins. Probably no feed commodity can now be regarded as absolutely free from mycotoxin contamination, and mycotoxin production can occur in the field, during harvesting, processing, storage, and shipment of a given commodity. It has been estimated that 1% of the

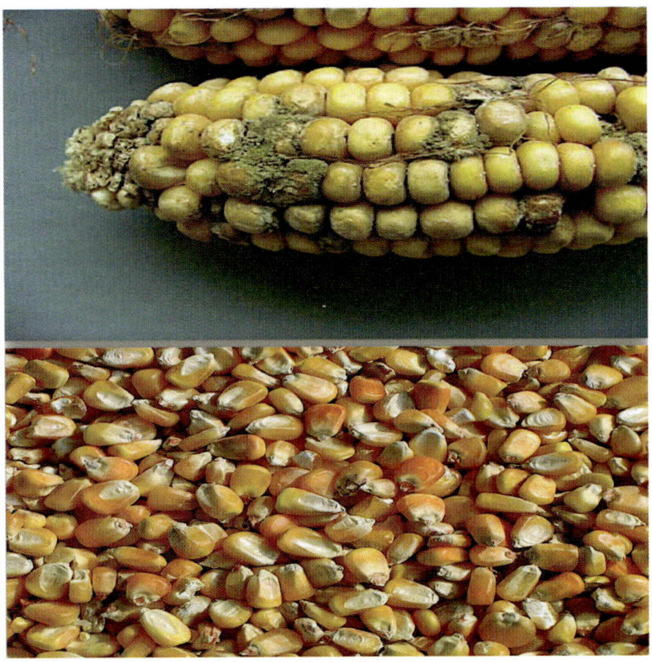

Figure 9.3 Shelled maize – moldy vs. sound kernels as a mycotoxin risk cue. Side-by-side maize kernels (seeds): a visibly mold-colonized/broken sample vs. a normal-looking sample. Warm, humid conditions and insect/mechanical damage favor *Fusarium* (fumonisins) and *Aspergillus* (aflatoxins). Visual appearance is only a screen – mycotoxins may be present even in clean-looking grain; confirm with laboratory testing.

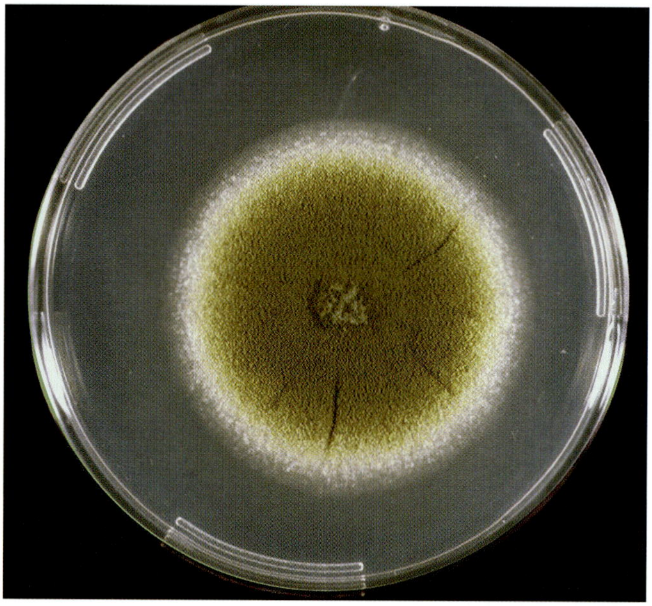

Figure 9.4 Colonies of *Aspergillus flavus* on Czapek–Dox agar (CZA). On CZA, *A. flavus* typically forms granular, flat colonies with radial grooves that start yellow and become bright to dark yellow-green as they age; conidial heads are radiate and may split into loose columns, and some strains form sclerotia (University of Adelaide Mycology, 2025). The CZA medium (sucrose + nitrate) is widely used for cultivating saprophytic *Aspergillus* spp., supporting abundant growth and sporulation (Merck KGaA/Sigma-Aldrich, 2018). *A. flavus* is a principal aflatoxin-producing species (Bennett & Klich, 2003).

world supply of grain and oil seed is rendered unfit due to fungal invasion (Alshannaq & Yu, 2017). A study in India showed that none of 240 samples of compound poultry feeds collected at random from various poultry farms were free from aflatoxins. The toxigenic fungi may also be grown in laboratories on a number of culture media (Figure 9.4).

Conditions Favorable for Fungal Growth

Fungal invasion of foods and feedstuffs may produce either toxic or nontoxic effects. The following storage factors are favorable in the initiation and development of fungal growth.

- A proper substrate (carbohydrate in readily available form).
- Moisture in grain (10 to 18%).
- Relative humidity (10%) in storage atmosphere.
- Adequate temperature for growth. It varies with the fungi, i.e., *A. flavus* can elaborate toxins between 12 and 47°C, and some Fusaria may be active at or near freezing temperatures.
- A supply of oxygen.

The effects of different storage conditions on the productions of aflatoxins in compound poultry feed are tabulated as in Table 9.2.

The duration of storage and aflatoxin production was directly proportional. Level of aflatoxin was higher in the temperature range of 22–24°C and the humidity range of 76–80%. Work by Mannaa and Kim (2017) has shown that the optimal temperature for fungal growth was not identical with that required for maximum aflatoxin production, and that the period of storage influencing aflatoxin production may be different for different strains of *A. flavus*.

Table 9.2 Effect of storage conditions on aflatoxin levels in feed samples.

Factors	Mean aflatoxin content (ppb)
Period of storage (days)	
1–10	291.70 (142)*
11–20	557.47 (78)
21 30	827.55 (14)
31–40	908.28 (6)
Temperature (°C)	
19–21	596.18 (9)
22–24	840.06 (124)
25–27	809.81 (33)
28–30	658.67 (12)
31–33	588.43 (25)
34–36	528.35 (21)
37–39	502.25 (16)
Humidity (%)	
56–60	350.42 (25)
61–65	580.65 (98)
66–70	698.18 (89)
71–75	793.25 (16)
76–80	808.75 (12)
Floor condition	
Pucca	528.76 (196)
Kacha	863.74 (44)
Ventilation	
Ventilated	564.42 (167)
Non-ventilated	

* Number in parentheses indicate number of samples in each category.
Mean aflatoxin concentrations (ppb; *n* in parentheses) increased with longer storage (1–10 d ≈ 292; 11–20 d ≈ 557; 21–30 d ≈ 828; 31–40 d ≈ 908), higher relative humidity (56–60% ≈ 350 → 76–80% ≈ 809), and poorer storage conditions (earthen kacha floors and non-ventilated lots) compared with pucca floors and ventilated stores. Temperature effects peaked in the mid-20s °C range.
Source: Adapted from Abdullah (1994).

Naturally Occurring Mycotoxins in Feedstuffs and Foods

The most encountered mycotoxins in feedstuffs and foods are aflatoxins, zearalenone deoxynivelenol (vomitoxin) and fumonisins (Alshannaq & Yu (2017). These mycotoxins have been proven as causes of, or implicated in, mycotoxicoses of either animals or humans. Table 9.3 shows some of the important mycotoxins in veterinary medicine and their chemical structures.

Table 9.3 Core mycotoxins and producing fungi (with representative chemical structures).

Toxins	Fungus	Chemical structure
Aflatoxins	*Aspergillus flavus, Aspergillus parasiticus*	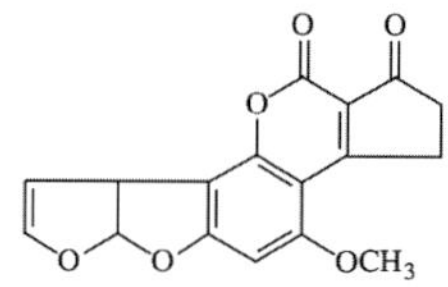
Ochratoxin A	*Aspergillus ochraceus, Penicullium viridicatum*	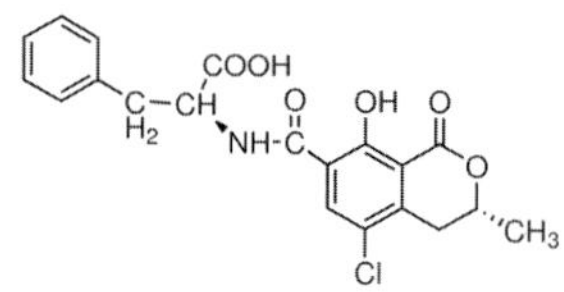
Sporidesmin	*Pithomyces chartarum*	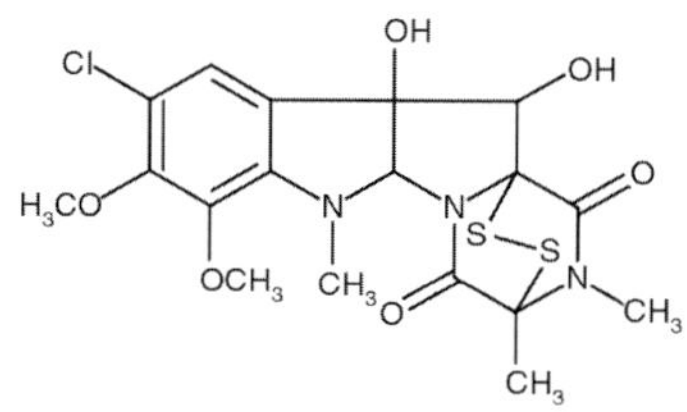
Zearalenone	*Fusarium graminearum*	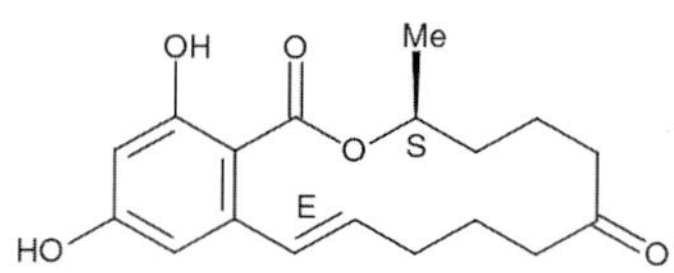
Ergot, lysergic acid	*Claviceps paspali, Claviceps purpurea*	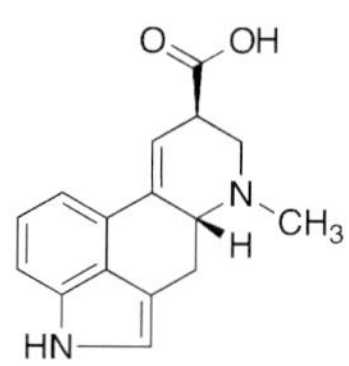
Rubratoxin	*Penicullium rubrum*	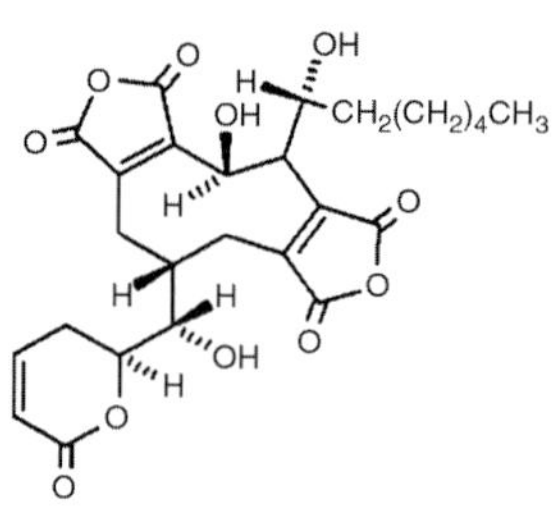
Trichothecene T-2 toxin	*Fusarium tricinctum*	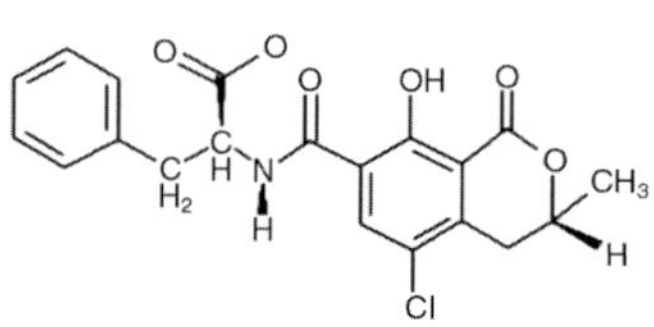

Table 9.3 (Continued)

Toxins	Fungus	Chemical structure
Fumonisins	*Fusarium moniliforme*	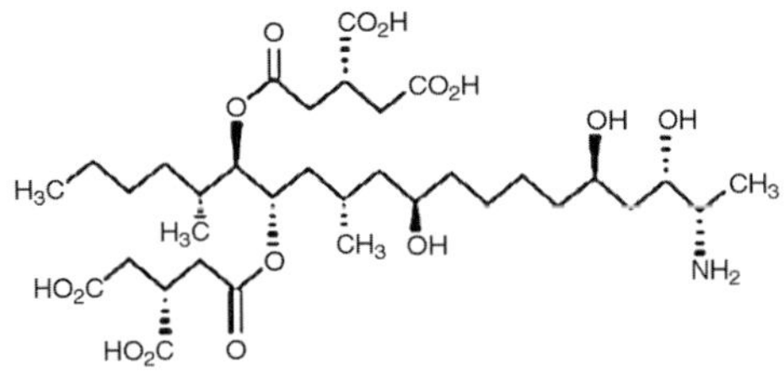

Mapping of major toxin families to principal producers – aflatoxins (*Aspergillus flavus/parasiticus*), ochratoxin A (*Aspergillus/Penicillium*), sporidesmin (*Pithomyces chartarum*), zearalenone (*Fusarium graminearum* complex), ergot alkaloids (*Claviceps* spp.), rubratoxin (*Penicillium rubrum*), T-2 (type A trichothecene; *Fusarium tricinctum*), and fumonisins (*Fusarium moniliforme/F. verticillioides*) – with structures shown to emphasize shared scaffolds underpinning toxicodynamic themes (Bennett & Klich, 2003; EFSA CONTAM Panel, 2018);

Mycotoxicoses

Mycotoxins cause acute to chronic toxicity in most species of domestic animals. Practically almost every organs system of the animal is affected. Table 9.4 summarizes the major toxic effects of mycotoxins in veterinary medicine. Figure 9.5 shows the effect of aflatoxins on the liver of chicken fed diets containing aflatoxin.

Aflatoxicosis is quite common in warm, humid settings where storage is suboptimal (Alshannaq & Yu (2017); Gupta (2018). From a number of field outbreaks in domestic animals, mycotoxicosis can be characterized as a disease:

- Whose true cause is not really identified
- Which is neither infectious nor contagious, not responding to the treatments with antibiotics or any other drugs
- Which is always linked with the consumption of certain feedstuffs with signs of fungal growth

Pathophysiology

Many of the clinical signs and postmortem lesions in aflatoxicosis, such as hepatic necrosis and fatty changes, have been linked with the impairment of protein synthesis and the ability to mobilize fat due to the depression of messenger-RNA synthesis (Bailey et al. 1996). The carcinogenic effect of aflatoxin B1 is due to the metabolic activation of the mycotoxin. Aflatoxin B1, like most environmental carcinogens, is lipophilic and a stable compound that is difficult to be excreted by the body. The oxidative enzyme, cytochrome P450 monooxygenase isozymes bound to the endoplasmic membrane of the liver play a critical role in the metabolic activation of aflatoxin B1. When an atom of oxygen is added to the aflatoxin B1, an electron is lost from one of the carbon atoms in aflatoxin B1, converting it to an electrophilic carcinogen; reaction of this electrophile with protein and nucleic acid also inactivates the electrophile and is detrimental to the survival of the cell. At the molecular level, bioactivated aflatoxin B1 forms DNA adducts that distort the helix and can trigger frame-shift mutations (Bailey et al. 1996) (Figure 9.6). The estrogenic

Table 9.4 Major toxic effects of veterinary-relevant mycotoxins (concise clinical summary).

Mycotoxins	Toxic effect	References
Aflatoxins	Aflatoxin B_1 is a very potent hepatocarcinogen. Causes hepatic lipidosis, cysts, necrosis, hepatocellular degeneration and portal lymphocytic infiltration. Acute congestion of kidneys. Retards growth and development of acquired – immunity. Decreased egg production in poultry.	Jerry (2024) Sandu (2024)
Ochratoxin A	A potent nephrotoxin. It can cause renal tubular injury and necrosis in many animal species, including fish, birds, and mammals. It is also embryotoxic/teratogenic in some species (e.g., chickens/avian embryos and rodents), and the developing central nervous system is among the important targets.	Ringot et al., (2006) Diab et al., (2018) Malir et al., (2013) Wilk-Zasadna & Minta (2009)
Zearalenone	Possesses estrogenic and anabolic properties. Pigs are most sensitive species of animals. Causes vulvovaginitis, swelling of vulva, mammary enlargement, prolonged oestrus and abortion	EFSA CONTAM (2017b)
Trichothe-cene	Generalized hemorrhage, gastroenteritis and hematopoietic depression. Reproductive disorders in pigs.	EFSA CONTAM (2011) Alshannaq & Yu (2017)
Rubratoxin	Hepatoxicity similar to aflatoxin but not carcinogenic. Generalized hemorrhage, immunosuppression may increase susceptibility to infection.	Wilson & Harbison (1973)
Sporidesmin	Pithomycotoxicosis (facial eczema) characterized by hepatogenous photo-sensitization in ruminants.	Fernández et al. (2021) Bookbinder (2024)
Ergot	Gangrene of extremities, abortion, colic, constipation or diarrhea.	Burrows & Way (1979)

Aflatoxins (*Aspergillus flavus/A. parasiticus*) primarily cause hepatotoxicity with carcinogenic potential and productivity loss; Ochratoxin A (*Aspergillus ochraceus/Penicillium viridicatum*) is a potent nephrotoxin across species; Zearalenone (*Fusarium* spp.) exerts estrogenic/anabolic effects, especially in swine; Trichothecenes (e.g., T-2, DON; *Fusarium* spp.) produce radiomimetic cytotoxicity with GI and hematopoietic effects; Rubratoxins (*Penicillium rubrum/P. purpurogenum*) are hepatotoxic and hemorrhagic; Sporidesmin (*Pithomyces chartarum*) causes hepatogenous photosensitisation ("facial eczema") in ruminants; and ergot alkaloids (*Claviceps* spp.) are vasoconstrictive with gangrene/abortifacient risks. (Key sources listed in References.)

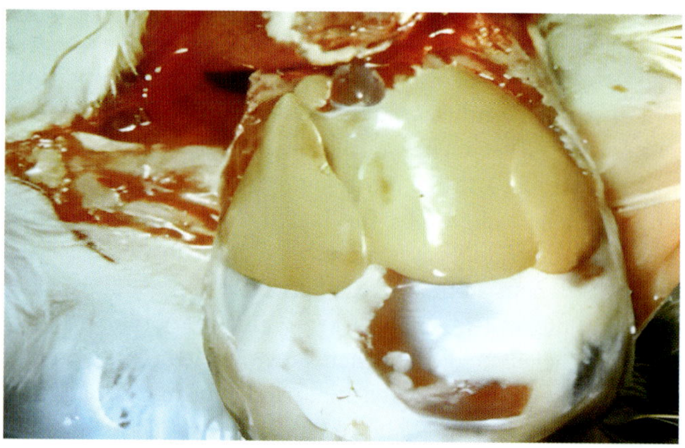

Figure 9.5 Aflatoxicosis in poultry – representative clinical and pathologic impacts. Reference images and key features (notably hepatic injury and performance losses) as summarized in the section "Aflatoxicosis in Poultry". *Source:* Sandu (2024)/The American Phytopathological Society/CC BY 4.0.

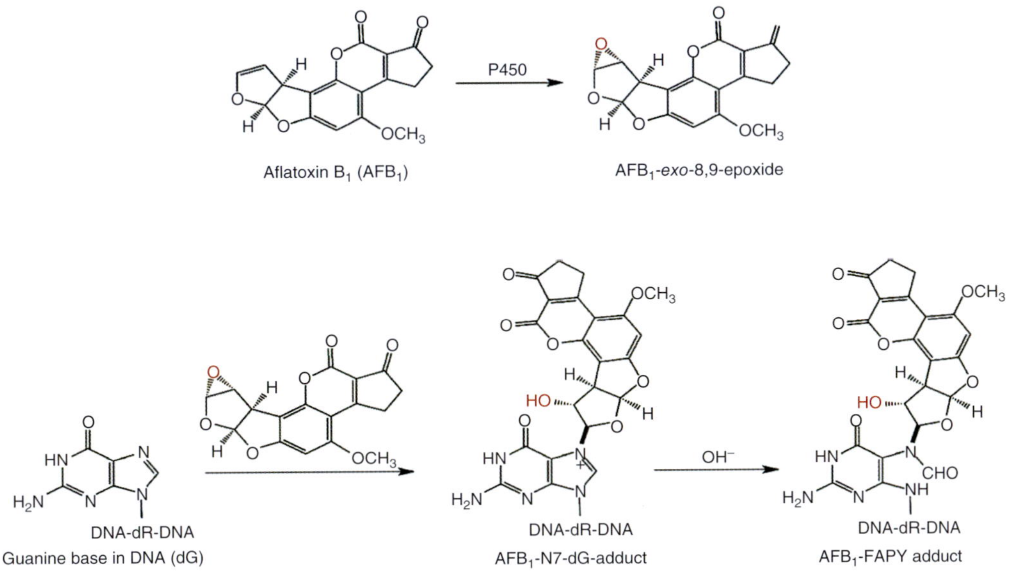

Figure 9.6 Aflatoxin–DNA adducts distort the helix and can trigger frameshift errors. Bioactivated aflatoxin B_1 forms N7-guanine and ring-opened formamidopyrimidine (FAPY) adducts that intercalate into DNA and alter local conformation; during replication these lesions can stabilize slipped-strand intermediates (especially at G·C runs), producing −1/+1 frameshift mutations (Gupta, 2018).

and anabolic effects of zearalenone are due to the increase in weight and activity of the uterus (Mostrom, 2024). Trichothecene produces its effects by inhibiting amino acid incorporation into protein and inhibits thymidine incorporation into DNA, as well as marked disaggregation of polysomes.

Evidence of acute to chronic liver diseases, such as increase in serum transaminases and alkaline phosphatase, icterus index, and decreased bromosulphalein (BSP) clearance, is shown by affected animals. Aflatoxicosis causes varying degrees of liver damage in ducks (Jerry, 2024; Sandu, 2024). All the affected ducks autopsied showed a yellow discoloration of the liver with solid, yellow-colored nodules about 1–3 cm in diameter. Microscopic examination of the liver sections showed a distorted hepatic structure by regenerative nodules of hepatocytes, which were surrounded by thin bands of fibrous tissue and bile duct hyperplasia. Sections of liver also showed multiple foci of hepatic lipidosis, hepatocellular degeneration, cysts, necrosis, and portal lymphocytic infiltration. Acute congestion of kidneys, with accompanying nephrosis, was also observed. Ducks with signs of nervous system involvement showed an acute generalized congestion of the brain and mild demyelination of the cerebellum.

Diagnosis

Several factors must be considered in diagnosing aflatoxicosis in domestic animals. The history of feeding moldy feed is pertinent and important for the diagnosis. Symptoms such as reduced growth – particularly in broiler chickens and ducks – and decreased egg production in layers are suggestive of aflatoxicosis. In addition, characteristic lesions and clinical-pathological changes are helpful in diagnosing the disease.

The presence of even low levels of aflatoxin in the feed following chemical analysis is helpful in confirming the diagnosis. Chemical analysis may be carried out using a mini-column technique high-performance liquid chromatography (HPLC), or thin-layer chromatography (TLC) immunoaffinity cleanup with liquid chromatography/liquid chromatography–mass spectrometry (LC/LC–MS) or enzyme-linked immunosorbent assay (ELISA) may be used for confirmation where available. The step-by-step analytical workflow used in this chapter – from sample intake and pre-processing to aflatoxin cleanup and chromatographic confirmation – is outlined in Figure 9.7. Final

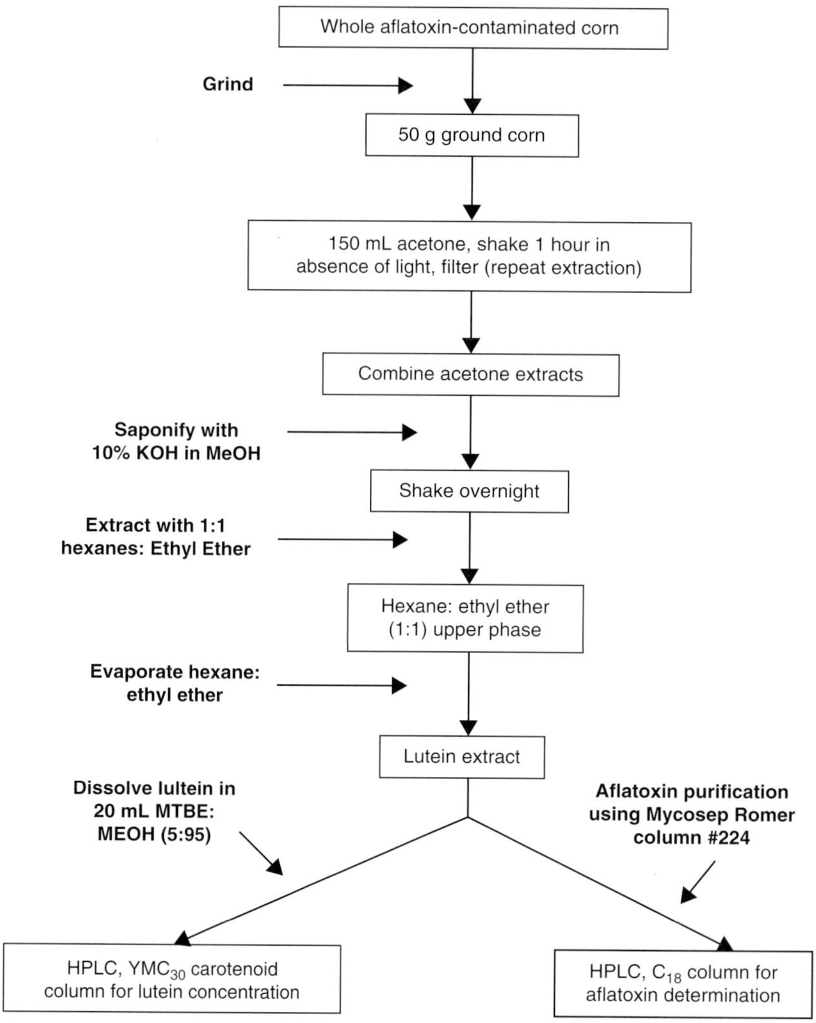

Figure 9.7 Diagrammatic procedure for isolating aflatoxin-free lutein from aflatoxin-contaminated plants and plant products. Intake and rapid aflatoxin screen → pre-processing (remove fines/size reduction; optional defatting) → carotenoid extraction under low-light/inert conditions → aflatoxin cleanup (e.g., adsorbent/solid-phase or immunoaffinity step) → lutein release by saponification (if esterified) → chromatographic enrichment (e.g., C30 prep/HPLC) → QA/QC verification of "aflatoxin < LOD/LOQ" and lutein identity/purity; toxin-bearing fractions routed to hazardous-waste handling (Weaver & Trucksess, 2010).

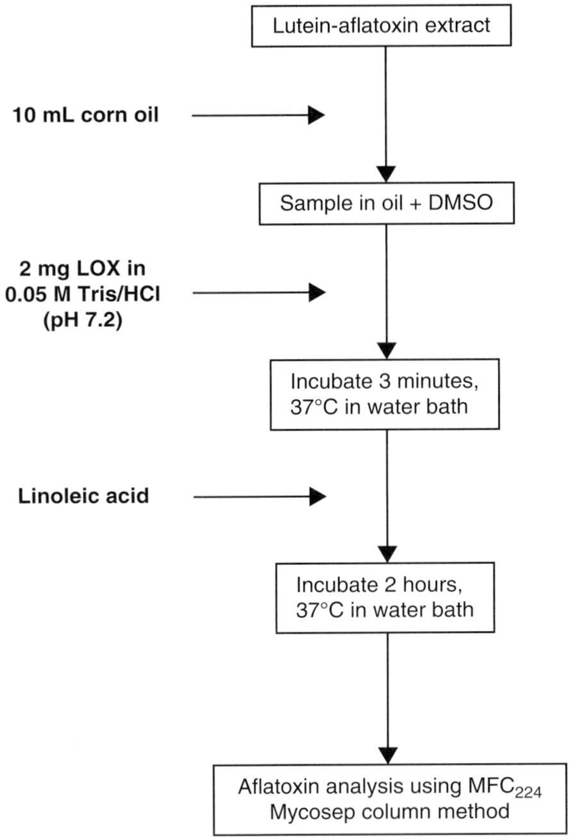

Figure 9.8 Quality verification and compliance endpoints for aflatoxin-free lutein. Representative verification outputs and control points: (i) aflatoxin confirmation by validated methods (e.g., immunoaffinity column [IAC]-cleanup with LC or ELISA/LC-MS) – target below LOQ; (ii) lutein identification and purity by chromatographic/spectroscopic profiling; (iii) documentation that detoxified/toxin-holding streams are captured and disposed per regulatory criteria (Weaver & Trucksess, 2010).

quality-verification and compliance endpoints (e.g., aflatoxin below limit of quantification (LOQ), lutein identity/purity, and documentation of proper handling of toxin-bearing fractions) are summarized in Figure 9.8.

Treatment

No specific treatment is available. Affected animals should be given easily digested low fat diets and lipotropic agents and managed without any stress. The moldy feed involved should be withdrawn. Since there is no practical way of destroying aflatoxins in contaminated feeds, once they are produced, one should adopt the "prevention is better than cure" policy.

Phytotoxins

Overview

Plant-derived toxicants drive much of the morbidity in tropical production systems, especially where pasture species, browse trees, and crop by-products fill feed gaps. This section focuses on: (i) *B. decumbens* (steroidal-saponin hepatopathy), (ii) *Leucaena leucocephala* (mimosine/DHP), (iii) cyanide (cassava and other cyanogenic plants), (iv) bracken fern (*Pteridium spp.*) syndromes, and (v) nitrate/nitrite toxicosis. We retain a pattern-based, production-first format with quick sampling checklists and decision aids. For a side-by-side quick reference to additional tropical toxicants – with hallmark syndromes, rapid field clues, and "first samples to collect" – see Table 9.5 and use it alongside each subsection to guide triage in the field.

Table 9.5 Cross-system quick reference – plants and other natural toxicants of tropical importance (clinical syndromes, rapid tests, and first actions).

Source (examples)	Key toxin(s)	Hallmark syndrome	Rapid field clues	First samples to collect
Cyanogenic plants (cassava/manioc, sorghum, young johnsongrass, laurel, stone-fruit leaves)	Cyanogenic glycosides → HCN	Peracute hypoxia; "bright-cherry" venous blood; sudden death (ruminants) (Cope, 2025).	Lush regrowth/ frosted forage; agitation → collapse; bitter-almond odor possible (Cope, 2025).	Antemortem: heparinized whole blood. Postmortem (≤4 h): rumen gas-cap and contents, suspected forage; liver, skeletal muscle. Seal airtight and chill (Cope, 2025a).
Nitrate accumulators (sorghums, Amaranthus/ pigweed, oat/millet, water run-off)	Nitrate/nitrite	Methemoglobinemia; "chocolate-brown" blood; dyspnea; abortions (Thompson, 2024a).	Stressed/droughted forage, heavy N fertilizer; stacked round bales; affected group (Thompson, 2024a).	Antemortem: plasma (preferred). Postmortem: ocular (aqueous) fluid (stable up to ~60 h). Also test suspected forage/water (Thompson, 2024a).
Oxalate-rich forbs (Amaranthus, Oxalis, some Aroids)	Soluble oxalates	Acute hypocalcemia ± renal tubular damage/ crystals (Avellaneda-Cáceres et al., 2025, Cope, 2024).	"Colic," tremors, recumbency; azotemia; high-oxalate weeds in fodder (Cope, 2024).	Kidney (histology), rumen contents, urine (calcium oxalate crystals), plant sample (Cope, 2024).

Table 9.5 (Continued)

Source (examples)	Key toxin(s)	Hallmark syndrome	Rapid field clues	First samples to collect
Pyrrolizidine-alkaloid weeds (*Senecio*/ Ragwort, *Crotalaria*, *Heliotropium*)	PA mix (e.g., senecionine, monocrotaline)	Chronic hepatopathy: megalocytosis, fibrosis, biliary hyperplasia; photosensitization (Bildfell, 2024).	Weight loss, poor thrift, sunburn on white areas; contaminated hay (Bildfell, 2024).	Liver (histology/ chem), feed/plant ID (Bildfell, 2024).
Lantana camara (ornamental hedge)	Lantadenes A/B (triterpenes)	Cholestatic hepatotoxicity → hepatogenous photosensitization (Bookbinder 2024; Sharma et al., 2007).	Sunburn/ photophobia a few days after access; icterus; bitter shrub present (Bookbinder 2024; Sharma et al., 2007).	Serum chemistry (GGT, bilirubin), liver biopsy if needed, plant sample (Bookbinder 2024; Sharma et al., 2007).
Leucaena leucocephala (forage tree)	Mimosine → 3,4-DHP	Alopecia, poor growth; goiter/low thyroid in non-adapted ruminants (Hammond, 1995).	Hair loss around eyes/face, salivation, jaw lesions; heavy leucaena diet (Hammond, 1995).	Forage sample; serum T4/T3; rumen liquor (adaptation to *Synergistes jonesii*) (Hammond, 1995).
Cardiac-glycoside ornamentals (*Nerium oleander*, yellow oleander *Cascabela thevetia*)	Cardenolides (oleandrin; peruvoside/ neriifolin)	GI upset → arrhythmias, sudden death (Sykes et al., 2023).	Yard clippings fed/ mixed with hay; brady-/ tachyarrhythmia; hyperkalemia possible (Sykes et al., 2023).	Rumen/ingesta for LC-MS/MS of glycosides; plant fragments; serum electrolytes (Sykes et al., 2023).
Castor bean (*Ricinus communis*)	Ricin (*type* II RIP); ricinine biomarker	Severe GI (hemorrhagic), hypovolemia → organ failure (CDC, 2024; Worbs et al., 2011).	Seeds/pods in pen or feed; rapid dehydration; multi-animal exposure (Worbs et al., 2011).	GI contents with seeds; feed; urine for ricinine; tissues for toxin testing (CDC, 2024; Worbs et al., 2011;).
Bracken fern (*Pteridium aquilinum*)	Ptaquiloside; thiaminase	Cattle: hemorrhagic syndrome or enzootic hematuria ()Xu, 1992; Cope, 2025b); Horses: "bracken staggers" (Cope 2025b)	Red/bloody urine in older cattle; pancytopenia in calves; neuro-cardiac signs in horses (Cope 2025b)	Whole blood/CBC; urine; suspect hay/ pasture; tissues for histo (Cope 2025b)
Coffee senna (*Senna occidentalis*)	Anthraquinones, toxalbumins	Myonecrosis and myoglobinuria; weakness → recumbency (Barth et al. 1994, TVMDL, 2024).	Seed-contaminated grain/hay after storms; dark urine; high CK (TVMDL, 2024).	Serum CK/AST; urine (myoglobin); GI contents and seed ID; feed (TVMDL, 2024).

(*Continued*)

Table 9.5 (Continued)

Source (examples)	Key toxin(s)	Hallmark syndrome	Rapid field clues	First samples to collect
Fluoroacetate plants (e.g., *Dichapetalum* "gifblaar" in Africa; *Gastrolobium*/*Acacia georginae* in Aus.)	Monofluoroacetate	Sudden death (cardiotoxic); exertion-triggered collapse (Leong et al., 2017)	Endemic shrubs present; deaths in otherwise well stock; few prodromes (Leong et al., 2017).	Freeze rumen contents, liver, and kidney for fluoroacetate analysis; submit suspected plant material (Adaska et al., 2018).
Cottonseed products (feeds, by-products)	Gossypol (free form)	Chronic cardiomyopathy (young ruminants, pigs), anemia; male infertility (Garland, 2024).	Diet includes cottonseed meal/ whole cottonseed; poor growth; dyspnea (Garland, 2024).	Retain feed for free-gossypol assay; necropsy heart/ liver; herd screen (Garland, 2024).

Examples focus on high-yield, field-relevant hazards in the tropics. "Key tests" highlight practical confirmation (where available). Always remove animals from source and institute supportive care while awaiting results. Sources for each toxicant summarized below in the reference list.

Sources and Occurrence

The major environmental and management drivers of plant toxicoses in tropical systems are summarized in Figure 9.9.

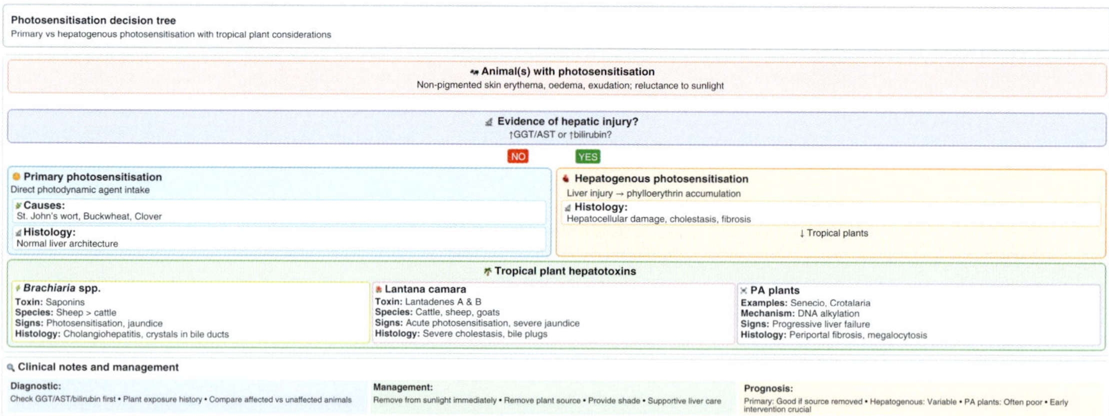

Figure 9.9 Conditions favorable for plant toxicoses in tropical systems – typical field triggers. Early post-rain regrowth elevates steroidal saponins in signal grasses (*Brachiaria* spp.), aligning with outbreaks of cholestasis and hepatogenous photosensitization (Low, 2015). Drought/frost stress and maceration of cyanogenic plants (e.g., cassava, sorghums) enhance HCN release (MSD Veterinary Manual, 2025 – Cyanide poisoning). Chronic exposure on bracken-infested pastures drives ptaquiloside-associated syndromes in cattle and thiaminase-related neurologic disease in horses (Cope 2025b– Bracken fern poisoning). High nitrogen fertilization combined with cloudy weather or a drought→rain transition predisposes forages to nitrate accumulation (Thompson 2024b– Nitrate/nitrite poisoning). Schematic created for this chapter.

Conditions Favorable for Plant Toxicoses (Drivers)

As summarized in Figure 9.10, risk clusters around early post-rain regrowth, drought/yarding, fodder gaps (reliance on browse/by-products), and intensive fertilizer use. Pasture composition and plant phenology matter: Young regrowth and stressed tissues often carry higher toxin precursors – e.g., steroidal saponins in *Brachiaria* (photosensitization outbreaks), cyanogenic glycosides that liberate HCN when plants are damaged or drought-stressed, and nitrates that accumulate under high N inputs and low photosynthesis (cool/cloudy weather or drought → rain transitions) (Bookbinder 2024; Low, 2015).

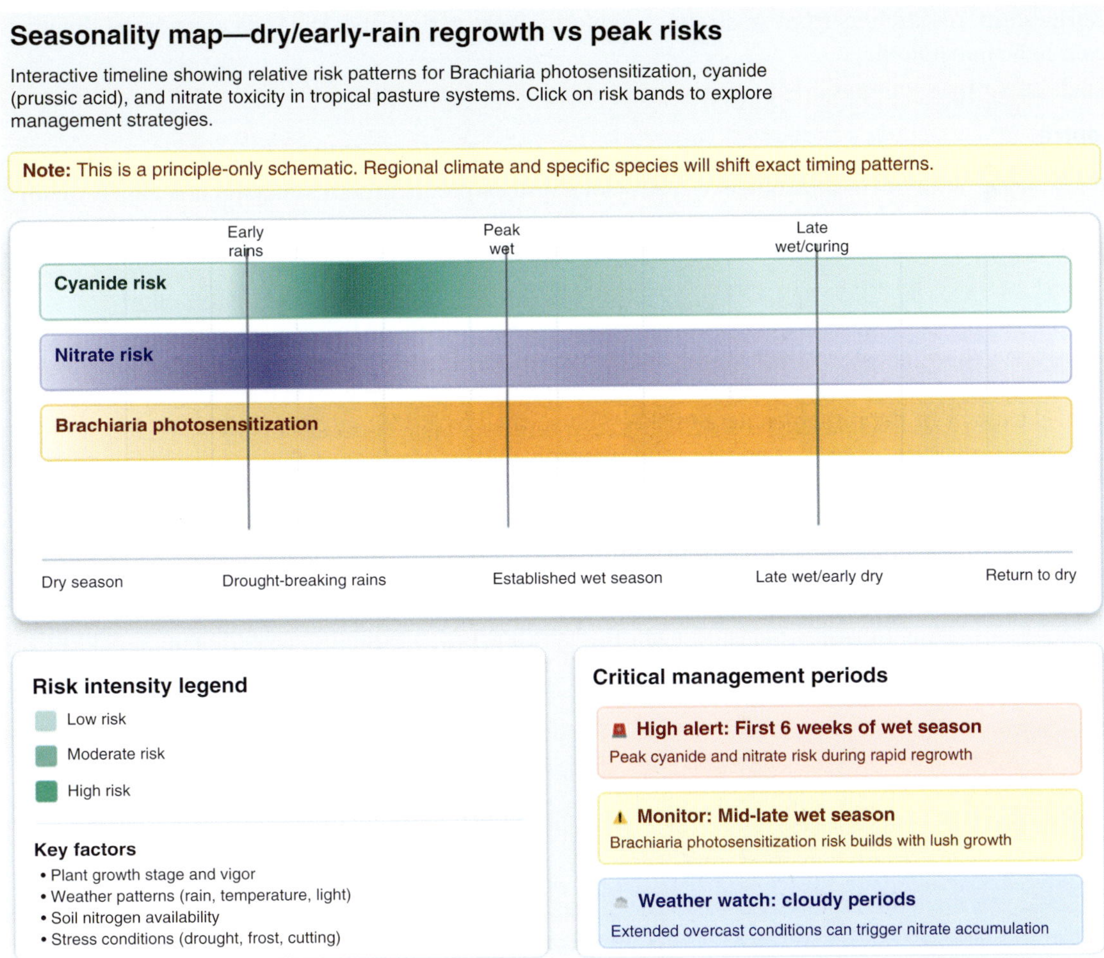

Figure 9.10 Seasonality and management drivers of phytotoxin risk in tropical systems. Early post-rain regrowth elevates steroidal **saponins** in signal grasses (*Brachiaria* spp.), predisposing to cholestasis and hepatogenous photosensitization; drought/frost/insect damage and maceration of cyanogenic plants (e.g., cassava, sorghums) increase HCN release; and high nitrogen fertilization with drought→rain or cloudy spells favors nitrate accumulation in forages. Schematic created for this chapter.

Signal Grass *(B. decumbens)* Poisoning

Signal grass (*B decumbens*) toxicosis is a well-recognized problem in tropical and subtropical grazing systems, where it causes hepatobiliary injury with secondary (hepatogenous) photosensitization and jaundice in small ruminants. Outbreaks and field cases have been widely reported from warm-climate regions, including South America, particularly Brazil (Low, 2015; Riet-Correa et al., 2011; Lozano et al., 2017). A representative pasture stand is shown in Figure 9.11, underscoring how commonly stock encounter this grass in production settings. Although reports from Colombia and Brazil suggested the involvement of the fungus *Pithomyces chartarum*, which produces the hepatotoxin sporidesmin, researchers from Australia, Indonesia, West Africa, and Malaysia considered the grass itself to be hepatotoxic.

Source

B. decumbens is an important source of fodder for livestock production in Malaysia. It is a high-yielding grass, very well adapted to tropical climatic conditions and is much preferred to other species of grass by sheep and goats. Consistent with this, Table 9.6 shows *B. decumbens* out-yielding other commonly planted tropical grasses, explaining why this species is planted in almost all livestock farms in Malaysia. It has been postulated B. decumbens per se is nontoxic but is converted into a hepatotoxic product in the rumen of sheep and goats. Ethanol extracts of the rumen content of intoxicated sheep proved hepatotoxic to rats, unlike ethanol extracts of fresh *B. decumbens*, which caused no ill effects. Spectroscopic examinations of purified extracts of the rumen content of sheep intoxicated by *B. decumbens* revealed the presence of a mixture of sapogenins identified as epi-sarasasapogenin and epi-smilagenin (Lajis et al., 1993).

Mechanism of Action

The mechanism of action of *B. decumbens* is still not clear. It is also difficult to explain why this grass is less or not toxic to other ruminants like the cattle. However, current evidence suggests ruminal biotransformation of plant saponins to hepatotoxic sapogenins, with biliary crystal formation leading to cholestasis and photosensitization – consistent with the rumen extract profiles shown in Figure 9.12.

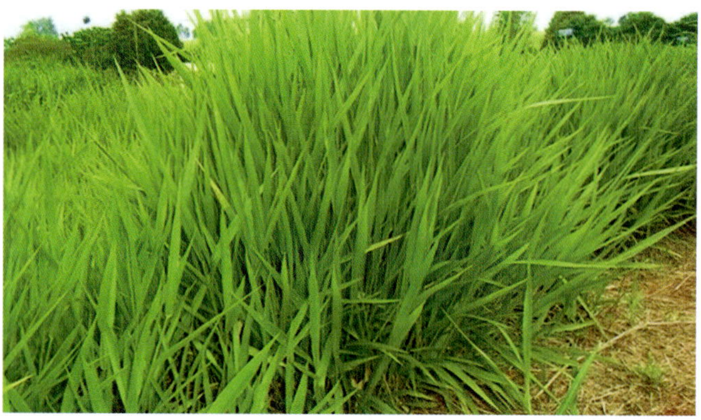

Figure 9.11 Signal grass (*Brachiaria decumbens*) in pasture. Representative field image of *B. decumbens*, a widely planted tropical grass implicated in seasonal steroidal-saponin hepatopathy and photosensitization outbreaks in small ruminants and cattle.

Table 9.6 Mean dry-matter yield of common tropical pasture/fodder species (t/ha/yr).

Pasture	Mean dry-matter yield (tonne/hectare/year)
Brachiaria decumbens	25.5
Brachiaria mutica	12.1
Panicum maximum	
cv. Colonio	18.6
Hamil	17.6
Pennisetum purpureum	
Local	13.2
Uganda	16.9
Setaria sphacelata	
cv. splendida	17.6
Setaria sphacelata	18.2

Because several of these grasses are high-biomass and broadly adapted, they tend to be favored in pasture development programs and by farmers, which can increase herd-level exposure to any pasture-associated hazards in systems where they dominate. For example, **signal grass** *(Urochloa/Brachiaria decumbens)* is often selected for its productivity and adaptability, helping explain why small ruminants may experience frequent exposure in areas where it is widely planted.
Source:

- ILRI/Feedipedia (2013). *Forage factsheet: Signal grass (Urochloa/Brachiaria decumbens).* Feedipedia, a programme by INRAE/CIRAD/AFZ/FAO.
- ILRI/Feedipedia (2013). *Forage factsheet: Para grass (Urochloa/Brachiaria mutica).* Feedipedia, a programme by INRAE/CIRAD/AFZ/FAO.
- ILRI/Feedipedia (2013). *Forage factsheet: Setaria sphacelata (Golden millet/setaria).* Feedipedia, a programme by INRAE/CIRAD/AFZ/FAO.
- Tropical Forages (n.d.). *Megathyrsus maximus × M. infestus (fine-leafed guinea grass hybrid): production potential and management notes.* Tropical Forages (CSIRO/partners).

Clinical Signs

Clinical signs normally develop in sheep as early as 2 weeks after grazing on *B. decumbens* pasture. The affected sheep exhibit signs of jaundice, emaciation, hepatogenous photosensitization, and edema of the ears, submandibular area, and the eyelids (Figure 9.13; Low, 2015; Bookbinder 2024). Photosensitization occurs in all intoxicated sheep as erythema and edema of the affected parts (Figure 9.14). In severe cases, there is exudation and necrosis of the affected parts, and the animals usually die within four to 6 weeks after grazing on this grass. In addition, the affected sheep also show neurological disorders such as stamping of forelegs, stargazing, incoordination, head pressing against the wall, and circling movement. The neurological dysfunction corresponds with the pathological changes observed in the brain, particularly in the white matter.

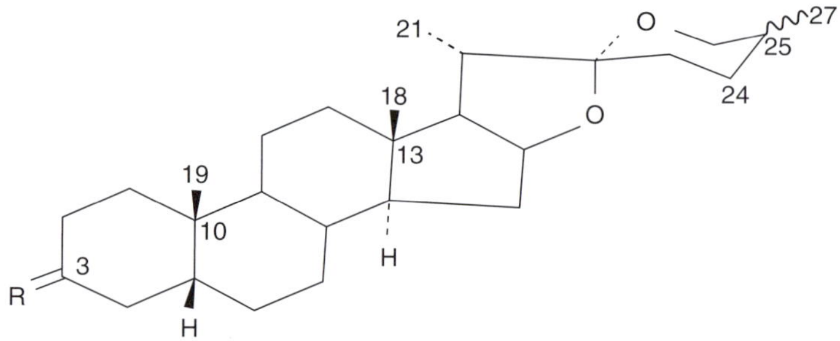

Structures of spirostane and its derivatives:

1, R = OH / H ; (25*S*)-5β-spirostan-3β-ol (sarsasapogenin);

2, R = 0; (25*S*)-5β-spirostan-3-one (sarsasapogenone);

3, R = H / OH ; (25*S*)-5β-spirostan-3α-ol (*epi*-sarsasapogenin);

4, R = H / OH ; (25*R*)-5β-spirostan-3α-ol (*epi*-smilagenin);

5, R = OH / H ; (25*R*)-5β-spirostan-3β-ol (smilagenin);

6, R = H / H ; (25*R*)-5β-spirostane.

Figure 9.12 Toxic compounds in rumen content of *Brachiaria decumbens*–intoxicated sheep. Representative analytical profile of rumen extracts from affected sheep showing sapogenin fractions implicated in cholestatic hepatopathy (e.g., epi-sarsasapogenin, epi-smilagenin). *Source:* Lajis et al. (1993).

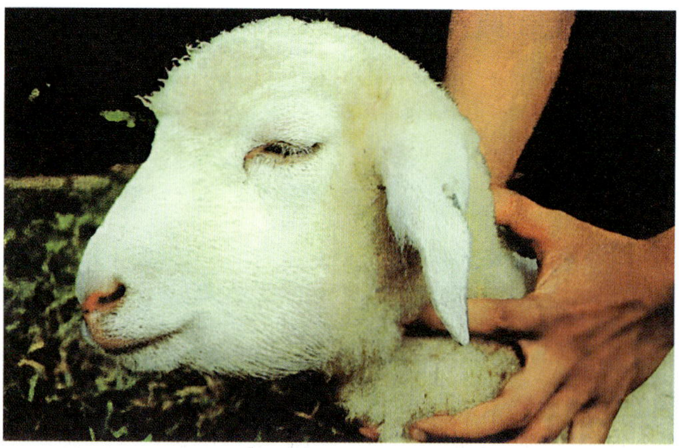

Figure 9.13 Hepatogenous photosensitization with soft-tissue edema in sheep grazing *Brachiaria decumbens*. Marked edema of the ears, peri-orbital and submandibular regions, consistent with cholestatic photosensitization in small ruminants exposed to *Brachiaria* pastures (Bookbinder 2024; Low, 2015). *Source:* chapter clinical photograph (this work).

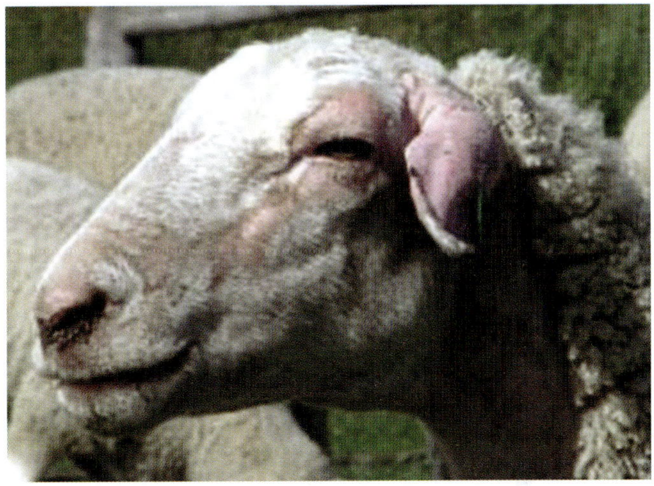

Figure 9.14 Photosensitization lesions on unpigmented skin in *Brachiaria*-affected sheep. Erythema and edema of nonpigmented areas, with potential progression to exudation/necrosis in severe cases, typical of hepatogenous photosensitization following *Brachiaria* exposure (Low, 2015). *Source:* Pipestone Veterinary Services / https://www.ovinopar.com.br/wp-content/uploads/2021/05/almanaque-1-2-2015.pdf / last accessed on Dec 27, 2025.

Pathophysiology

Necropsy revealed varying degrees of jaundice of the subcutaneous, omental, and mesenteric fat as well as serous and mucous membranes. The livers were enlarged and firm, mottled, and icteric with distended gall bladders (Figure 9.15). Histologically, individual hepatocytic necrosis was observed in almost all cases; occasionally, some necrotic changes tended to be distributed centrilobularly. The hepatocytes were hyperchromic, showing slight megalocytosis and disarray of the hepatic arrangement. The affected hepatocyte nuclei were either pyknotic or karyolytic. Kidneys were also enlarged and congested. Striking changes were also observed in the brain, particularly in the white matter, with numerous vacillations' of various sizes giving a spongy appearance.

B. decumbens toxicity also affects reticulo-rumen motility and microbial activity of sheep. Ruminal stasis (Figure 9.16) occurred within 3 weeks of grazing on this grass, and the rumen microbial population (Figure 9.17) together with the levels of volatile fatty acids (Table 9.7) were reduced, resulting in anorexia and emaciation (Salam Abdullah & Rajion, 1990).

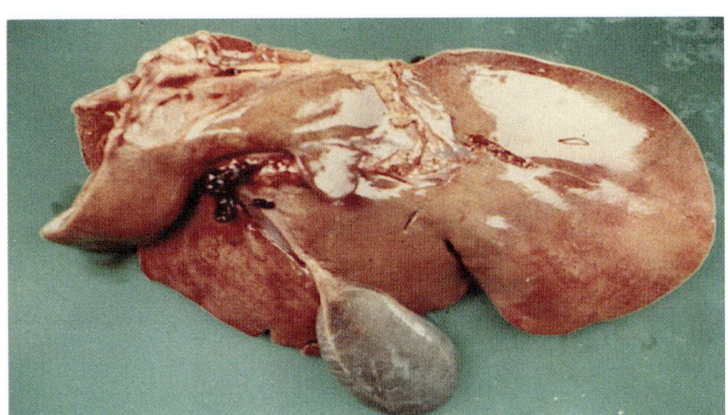

Figure 9.15 Enlarged, icteric liver with distended gall bladder in *Brachiaria*-affected sheep. Gross lesions are consistent with cholestatic cholangiohepatopathy reported in *Brachiaria* outbreaks. *Source:* Low (2015)/MDPI/CC BY 4.0.

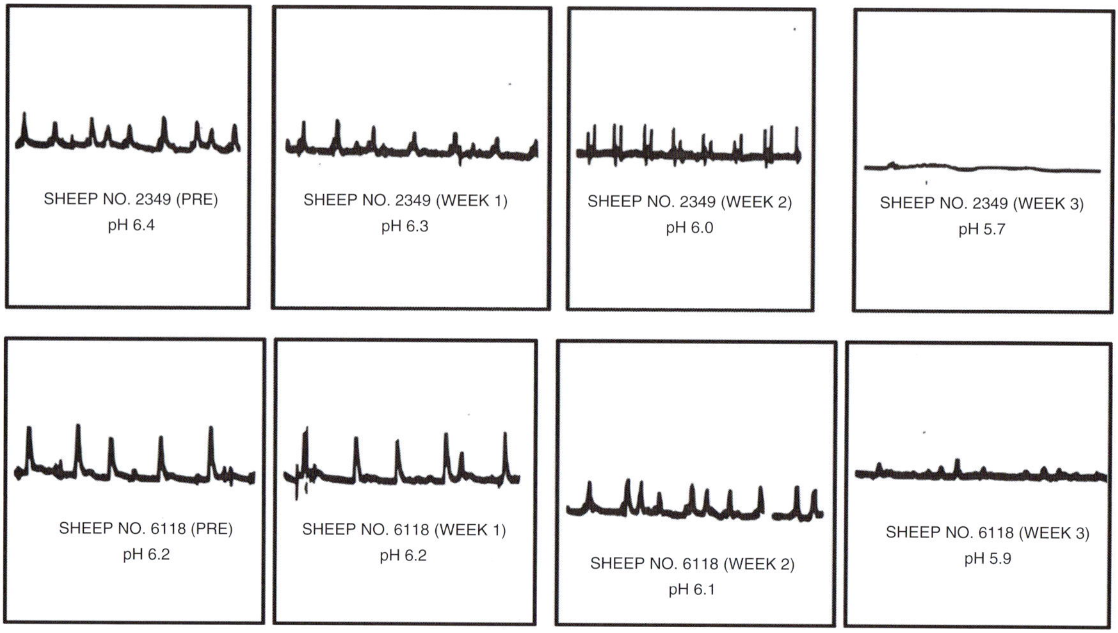

Figure 9.16 Physiograph tracing showing decreased rumen contractions in two sheep with *B. decumbens* poisoning. Reduction in reticulo-rumen motility is compatible with field observations of ruminal stasis in affected small ruminants (Salam Abdullah & Rajion, 1990).

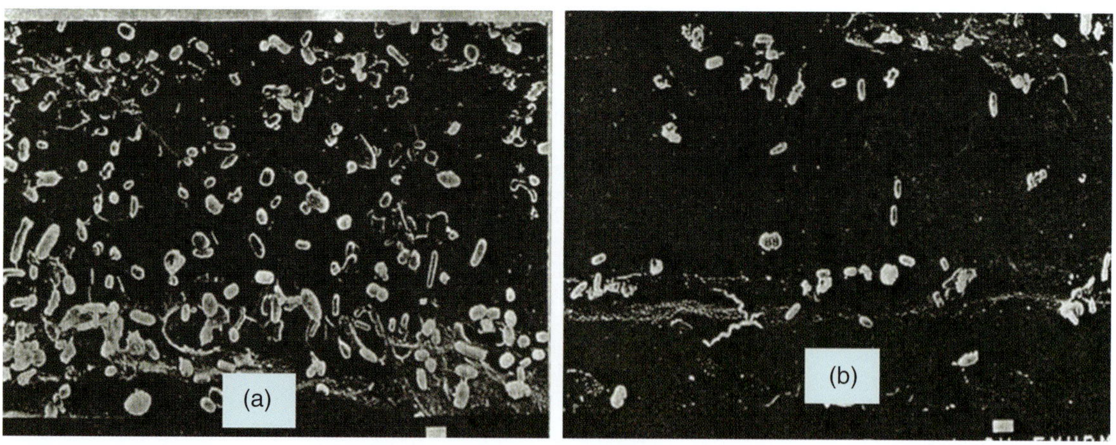

Figure 9.17 Electron micrograph of rumen microbiota in sheep feeding (a) and not feeding (b) on *B. decumbens*. Lower microbial density and altered community structure accompany clinical ruminal stasis in intoxicated sheep (Salam Abdullah & Rajion, 1990).

Table 9.7 Concentrations of volatile fatty acids (μmol/mL) in control vs. *Brachiaria decumbens*-intoxicated sheep.

Volatile fatty acids (VFA)	Control sheep $n = 6$	Treated sheep $n = 6$	Level of significance
Acetic acid	31.60 ± 4.50	9.08 ± 3.90	$P < 0.05$
Propionic acid	10.47 ± 1.82	3.37 ± 1.03	$P < 0.05$
Butyric acid	7.24 ± 1.54	3.10 ± 0.67	$P < 0.05$
Isobutyric acid	0.77 ± 0.14	0.87 ± 0.21	NS
Isovaleric acid	1.38 ± 0.14	1.23 ± 0.65	NS
Valeric acid	0.79 ± 0.20	0.83 ± 0.28	NS

Significant reductions in acetic, propionic, and butyric acids ($P < 0.05$) are consistent with depressed fermentation in affected animals (Salam Abdullah & Rajion, 1990).

Diagnosis

B. decumbens poisoning in sheep is diagnosed based on the clinical signs and history of grazing on this pasture. It may be confused with copper poisoning in sheep, but on analysis, copper levels in the liver and serum of *B. decumbens*-affected sheep were low.

Treatment

Sheep should be removed from further access to *B. decumbens*. Fluid therapy must be administered to correct the dehydration and acidosis. Rumen motility may be stimulated using oils or ruminotorics. Chelating agents such as activated charcoal may be given to absorb the toxin.

The addition of zinc sulfate to the drinking water at 1 gm/L reduced the incidence of the poisoning. The authors postulated that the effectiveness of zinc sulfate added to the drinking water in preventing *B. decumbens* toxicity in sheep might be due the binding of zinc with the toxic compound from *B. decumbens* in the rumen of sheep.

Leucaena Leucocephala (Leucaena) Poisoning

L. leucocephala is a widely used perennial tree legume in the tropics for protein browse and cut-and-carry feeding. Poisoning is most likely in naïve or de-adapted cattle and goats when leucaena constitutes a large proportion of the diet for prolonged periods.

Source

The shrub or small tree is commonly planted in hedgerows and fodder banks; young tips and pods are highly palatable and may form a high fraction of intake in feed-scarce periods (Figure 9.18; Dalzell et al., 2006).

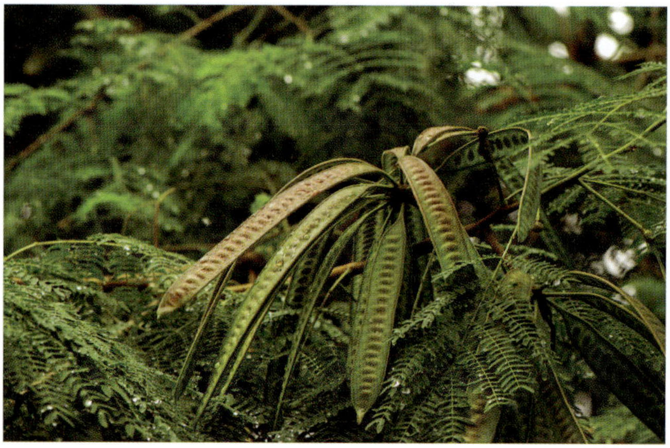

Figure 9.18 *Leucaena leucocephala* – hedgerow browse (foliage and pods). Representative field image of a leucaena fodder hedge used for cut-and-carry and strip grazing; young tips/pods are highly palatable and can dominate intake in feed-gap periods (Dalzell et al., 2006). *Source:* JakaSuryanta/Adobe Stock Photos.

Epidemiology and Risk Windows

- Naïve herds or herds turned back onto leucaena after a long break are over-represented.
- High dietary inclusion, especially sudden jumps, increases risk; mixed swards dilute exposure.
- Management signals: feed gaps, yarding moves, and "green pick" of young tips/pods.
- Cross-protection depends on *S. jonesii*; loss of this flora after time off leucaena ("de-adaptation") is common (Jones & Megarrity, 1986; Shelton et al., 2019) (Figure 9.19).

Toxic Principle and Mechanism of Action

The amino acid mimosine is converted in the rumen to 3,4- and 2,3-dihydroxypyridone (DHP), which are antimitotic and goitrogenic. The rumen bacterium *S. jonesii* normally detoxifies DHP; absence or loss of this flora predisposes to disease (Allison et al., 1992; CSIRO, 2015). Figure 9.20 summarizes the mimosine → DHP pathway and *S. jonesii* detoxification.

Mechanistic notes for clinicians (why the signs look the way they do). – Antimitotic effects impair rapidly dividing cells (hair follicles, oral mucosa, hoof/germinal epithelium) → alopecia, stomatitis/ptyalism, coronary-band lesions. – Goitrogenic effects can suppress thyroid function; overt farm-side goiter is uncommon but contributes to ill-thrift when intake is extreme (Dalzell et al., 2012; Shelton et al., 2019) – Detox ecology matters: established *S. jonesii* allows higher safe inclusion; loss after time off leucaena explains "same paddock, different outcome" cases (Allison et al., 1992; Jones & Megarrity, 1986).

Clinical Signs

Ill-thrift with rough coat; alopecia – often diffuse over the trunk/back (Figure 9.21); stomatitis with ptyalism; decreased feed intake; and lameness with coronary-band lesions are common. Fertility may be reduced with prolonged high intakes (Dalzell et al., 2012; Hatzade et al., 2020; Shelton et al., 2019).

Time course: In naïve/de-adapted cattle or goats on high intakes, signs can appear within 7–21 days; milder, subclinical forms (poor coat, "doing poorly") are easy to miss without a diet history.

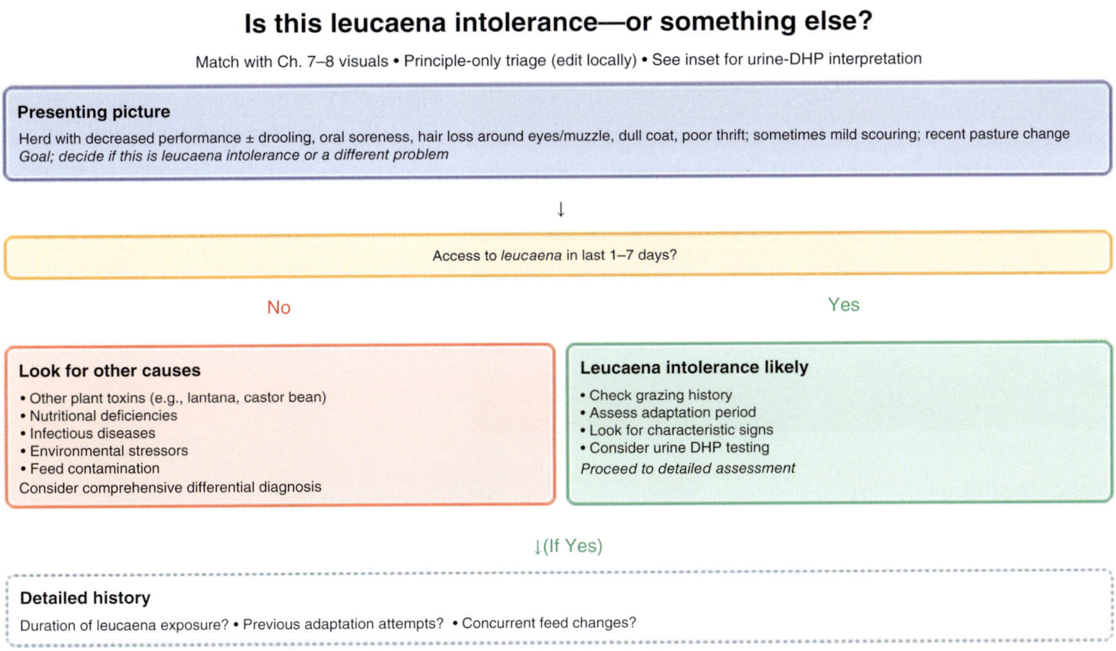

Figure 9.19 Leucaena intolerance – clinical spectrum and first-response actions. Decision aid summarizing key risk factors (naïve or de-adapted herds; high dietary inclusion; sudden jumps), core signs (alopecia, stomatitis/ptyalism, coronary-band lesions, ill-thrift), and immediate actions (dilute leucaena, mixed forage, treat lesions, inoculate with *Synergistes jonesii*, step back then readapt). Content aligned with field guidance and adaptation literature (Dalzell et al., 2012; Jones & Megarrity, 1986; Shelton et al., 2019).

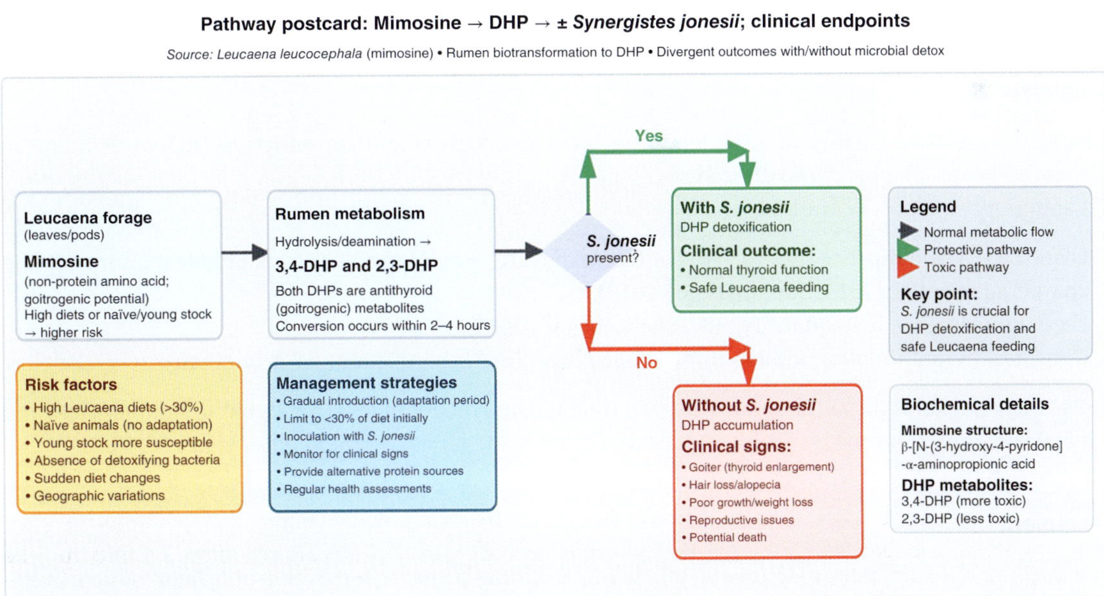

Figure 9.20 Ruminal biotransformation of mimosine and detoxification by *Synergistes jonesii*. Schematic of the mimosine → 3,4-DHP/2,3-DHP pathway (antimitotic, goitrogenic) and the detoxification step catalyzed by the rumen bacterium *S. jonesii*, which underpins adaptation and clinical tolerance to leucaena (Allison et al., 1992; Dalzell et al., 2012; Jones & Megarrity, 1986; Shelton et al., 2019).

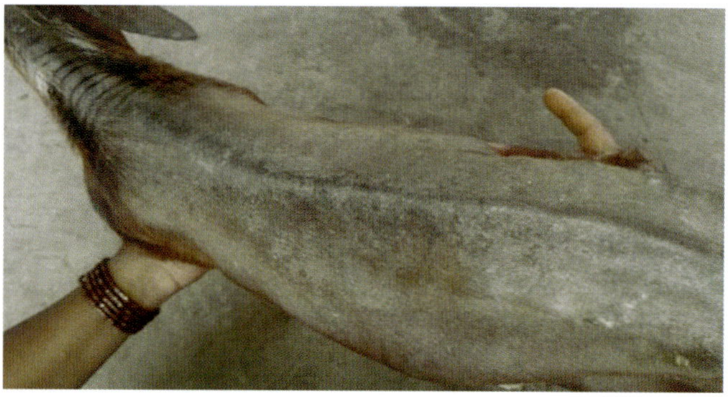

Figure 9.21 Clinical sign – generalized trunk/back alopecia in leucaena-affected small ruminant (pre-treatment). Diffuse hair loss with dry, scaly skin and lethargy typical of leucaena toxicosis; improvement follows withdrawal and supportive management. *Source:* Hatzade et.al. (2020) / The Pharma Innovation.

Pathophysiology

Antimitotic DHP effects underlie hair-cycle disruption and mucosal lesions; goitrogenic effects may be subtle unless intake is extreme. Clinical expression depends on dose and on presence/absence of rumen detoxifying flora (*S. jonesii*) (Allison et al., 1992; Jones & Megarrity, 1986).

Differential Diagnosis

- Alopecia/rough coat: Ectoparasites; trace mineral issues (Cu, Zn); photosensitization (distribution differs).
- Stomatitis/ptyalism: Vesicular diseases (jurisdictional rule-outs), caustic plants, mycotoxins.
- Lameness/coronitis: Foot rot/streptococcal dermatitis, irritant pastures.
- Ill-thrift in browse systems: Tannin-rich forages; protein–energy mismatch.

Diagnosis

Strongly suggestive: History of high leucaena inclusion with recent introduction (naïve) or break in access (de-adapted), plus compatible signs.

Laboratory support (as available):

- Urine DHP (field dipstick/LC–MS) to confirm exposure – see Figure 9.22 for a practical interpretation chart (Dalzell et al., 2012; Shelton et al., 2019).
- Feed mimosine assay to quantify risk (Shelton et al., 2019).
- Consider thyroid function indices in prolonged high-intake herds (context-dependent).

Turn-key field aids in this chapter: Table 9.8 (recognizing de-adaptation and what to sample/save) and Table 9.9 (troubleshooting by problem pattern) (Jones & Megarrity, 1986; Shelton et al., 2019).

Treatment

- Immediate: Reduce/remove leucaena, provide mixed forages, and treat lesions (oral/hoof) supportively.
- Restore detox capacity: Inoculate naïve herds with rumen fluid or cultured *S. jonesii* where available; reintroduce gradually (Allison et al., 1992; Dalzell et al., 2012; Shelton et al., 2019).
- Avoid "yo-yo" feeding: After time off leucaena, do not resume at prior high levels – step back through adaptation.

Urine–DHP interpretation chart

Field strip vs LC–MS/HPLC reporting guide. Pair results with clinical signs and recent leucaena access.

Field strip (qualitative)

ND/0

No color: DHP not detected. Re-test if suspicion remains (new exposure may lag).

trace/+

Low color: Recent/low exposure likely. Manage intake, re-check in 24–48 h.

++

Moderate color: Active intake. Initiate adaptation (buffer with hay, gradual re-intro, consider *S. jonesii*).

+++

Strong color: Significant intake. Treat as de-adaptation/over-consumption. Confirm by lab.

Field Tip: Collect paired forage sample (estimate % leucaena) and note time since last access.

LC-MS/HPLC (quantitative)

Units: µmol/L or mg/L (lab-specific)

< LOQ

Below limit of quantification. DHP not detected or trace amounts.

LOQ – X µmol/L

Low levels: Recent/minimal exposure. Monitor and manage access.

X – Y µmol/L

Moderate levels: Active consumption. Implement adaptation protocol.

> Y µmol/L

High levels: Significant intake. Risk of toxicity. Immediate intervention required.

Lab Note: Replace LOQ/X/Y with your cut-points. Correlation with clinical signs strengthens interpretation.

Clinical context and management

Clinical signs of DHP toxicity:

- Poor growth rate, weight loss
- Hair loss (especially around mouth)
- Excessive drooling, mouth ulcers
- Goiter, thyroid enlargement
- Reduced fertility

Management Strategies:

- Gradual introduction (10–14 days)
- Buffer with grass/hay (50:50 ratio)
- Consider *Synergistes jonesii* inoculation
- Monitor seasonal DHP variation
- Regular urine monitoring during adaptation

Important: This chart provides general guidance. Always consider individual animal factors, local conditions, and consult veterinary advice for clinical decisions.

Customize thresholds (LOQ, X, Y) based on your laboratory's validation data and local leucaena varieties.

Figure 9.22 Urine DHP interpretation chart. Quick field guide to urinary 3,4-dihydroxypyridine (DHP) – the principal mimosine metabolite of *Leucaena leucocephala* – to gauge adaptation status and risk: None/trace: little or no leucaena intake or well-adapted rumen (likely *Synergistes jonesii* present). Low–moderate: recent/ongoing leucaena intake with partial adaptation; monitor diet and animals. High–very high: de-adaptation or heavy intake → increased risk of leucaena toxicity (weight loss, alopecia, poor thrift). Immediate actions: confirm intake history; dilute with safe forage, ensure mixed pastures; (re)inoculate with *Synergistes jonesii* if naïve/de-adapted; address stressors; retest in 7–10 days. Sampling notes: mid-stream urine; avoid excessive dilution; chill/freeze promptly; where available, interpret colorimetric bands alongside LC–MS values and/or creatinine-corrected DHP.

Table 9.8 "Clues to de-adaptation."

Field clue/ situation	Why it flags de-adaptation	Rapid signs to watch (24–72 h)	First actions (same day)	Samples to save (for lab/records)
Purchase/ arrival of naïve stock (no known leucaena history)	Rumen likely lacks *S. jonesii*, so mimosine → DHP persists (Jones & Megarrity, 1986; Allison et al., 1992).	Reduced intake, drooling, oral soreness/lesions; dull coat (Dalzell et al., 2012).	Hold on grass/hay; inoculate *S. jonesii*; reintroduce leucaena slowly* (Shelton et al., 2021; FutureBeef, 2017/2025).	Forage (confirm % leucaena), rumen liquor (*S. jonesii* status), photos; optional sentinel serum T4/T3 (Dalzell et al., 2012).
Long period off leucaena (>4–6 weeks; drought, confinement, different pasture; recent antibiotics)	*S. jonesii* numbers can wane; previously protected mobs may lose tolerance (Dalzell et al., 2012; Graham et al., 2013).	On return to leucaena: drool/ poor thrift reappears (Graham et al., 2013).	Re-inoculate; reset adaptation steps; cap leucaena ≤10–20% DM for 3–5 d, add quality hay** (Shelton et al., 2021).	Rumen liquor (culture/polymerase chain reaction [PCR] for *S. jonesii*), feed samples; note recent medications (Graham et al., 2013).
Sudden diet switch/jump in leucaena** (storm regrowth, heavy pod zones, lot-fed silage)	Acute DHP load can overwhelm current detox capacity; hungry gorging increases risk (Dalzell et al., 2012; Shelton et al., 2021).	Off-feed, drool, oral ulcers; periocular/ muzzle hair loss, poor thrift – often multiple animals (Dalzell et al., 2012).	Remove to grass; drop to last well-tolerated level; buffer with hay/ water/shade; consider reinoculation if signs persist (Graham et al., 2013; Shelton et al., 2021).	Forage from affected areas; water sample; case notes (timing, weather, mob IDs) (Shelton et al., 2021).

* Green light to resume step-up: symptom-free ≥48 h with normal intake/rumen fill and clean muzzle/coat; then increase leucaena slowly over 7–10 days (Shelton et al., 2021).
** Important: Iodine or thyroxine therapy alone does not solve leucaena/DHP toxicity – detox microbes are required (CSIRO, 2015).
*** Field situations that flag loss/absence of effective *S. jonesii* detox (naïve arrivals, long periods off leucaena, sudden diet jumps), fast signs to watch, first actions, and samples to save; with a green-light criterion to resume step-up (Jones & Megarrity, 1986; Shelton et al., 2019).

How to implement (day-by-day). Use Table 9.10 (7–21-day adaptation plan) for targets, green/amber/ red flags, and actions; then follow the adaptation protocol flow (Figure 9.23) for when to pause, roll back, or re-inoculate (Dalzell et al., 2012; Shelton et al., 2019).

Prevention and Feeding Guidelines

Diversify the diet: During adaptation, avoid leucaena dominating > ~30% DM (adapted herds can tolerate more – monitor coat, intake, oral health, gait) (Dalzell et al., 2012; Shelton et al., 2019).

Keep the bugs alive: Avoid long periods off leucaena or plan reinoculation. Introduce youngstock with adapted companions or inoculum; train staff to spot early red flags (ptyalism, oral soreness, rubbing/coat loss, reluctance to move).

Table 9.9 Troubleshooting and quick fixes. Inoculation and gradual step-up adaptation strategies for *Leucaena* feeding, including the role of *Synergistes jonesii* in DHP detoxification and situations where adapted herds may cope without deliberate inoculation, are documented in Graham et al. (2013), Jones & Megarrity (1986), Allison et al. (1992), Shelton et al. (2019, 2021), and De Angelis et al. (2021).

Problem pattern	Likely cause	First fixes (same day)	Next steps (48–72 h)	What to sample/ save
Drooling, jaw/ tongue soreness, mouth lesions***	High mimosine/DHP exposure in naïve rumen (Hammond, 1995).	Pull back to grass/ hay; oral exam; soft hay + water.	Resume at half prior level after 48 h symptom-free; consider *S. jonesii*** (Allison et al., 1992; Jones & Megarrity, 1986).	Forage ID; photos; oral lesion notes.
Periocular/ muzzle alopecia, poor thrift	DHP intolerance; inadequate detox (Dalzell et al., 2012; Hammond, 1995).	Cut leucaena to ≤10–20% DM; add good hay; shelter.	Inoculate or re-inoculate *S. jonesii*; slow rechallenge 7–10 d* (FutureBeef, 2017/2025; Graham et al., 2013).	Forage; rumen liquor for micro status; sentinel serum T4/T3 (Dalzell et al., 2012).
Herd eats poorly after turnout	Empty-belly gorging/ unpalatable stands (Shelton et al., 2021).	Feed hay before turnout; shorten access; offer mixed pasture.	Gradually lengthen access; ensure water/ mineral; avoid heavy pod zones (Shelton et al., 2021).	Forage (eaten vs. uneaten); water sample.
Ongoing signs despite gradual plan	Missing/insufficient *S. jonesii* or diet too leucaena-heavy (Dalzell et al., 2012; Graham et al., 2013).	Cap leucaena ≤30–40% DM; add grass/legume.	Confirm *S. jonesii* presence; adjust ration; note that iodine/thyroxine therapy is not a cure** (CSIRO, 2015, Shelton et al., 2019)).	Rumen liquor (culture/PCR); feed; mineral label; blood (T4/T3).
Youngstock worse than adults	Naïve rumen; proportionally higher intake (Hammond, 1995).	Keep young on lowest step longer; pair with adapted leaders.	Extend each step by 3–5 d; track weights (Shelton et al., 2021).	

* Introduce "slowly" and adapt over days → weeks; inoculation protocols exist (e.g., 100 mL culture to 10% of herd; see local guidance) (Shelton et al., 2021; Graham et al., 2013).
** ***S. jonesii*** detoxifies DHP; classic transfer/inoculation success is documented (Jones & Megarrity, 1986; Allison et al., 1992).
*** In some settings, adapted herds may cope without deliberate inoculation; management still emphasizes gradual exposure and monitoring (De Angelis et al., 2021; Shelton et al., 2019; Shelton et al., 2021).
Common patterns (drooling/oral soreness; periocular or trunk alopecia; poor intake after turnout; persistent signs; youngstock sensitivity), likely causes, same-day fixes, 48–72 h next steps, and "what to sample/save" (Shelton et al., 2019)/ Tropical Grasslands-Forrajes Tropicales / CC BY 4.0.

Cyanide Poisoning

Cyanide (hydrocyanic acid), also known as prussic acid, is one of the most rapid-acting poisons to mammals. All species of animals, including man, are susceptible. However, ruminants appear to be more susceptible to cyanide poisoning from plants of equal cyanogenetic potential than are monogastric

Table 9.10 Practical leucaena adaptation plan (7–21 days).

Day(s)	Leucaena in diet*	What to do (daily routine)	Monitor (quick checks)	Green flags (tolerance)	Amber/red flags (intolerance)	If flags appear (immediate actions)
0 (baseline)	0%	Record baseline body condition score (BCS), heart rate (HR)/respiratory rate (RR), appetite; line up hay/grass buffer; confirm mineral program (note: iodine or thyroxine alone does **not** fix leucaena toxicity) (Hammond, 1995; CSIRO, 2015).	Appetite, feces, periocular/muzzle coat, rumen fill.	Bright, eating, normal dung.	—	—
1–3	5–10% DM	Offer leucaena **after** hay/grass; short sessions (avoid empty-belly gorging); shade + water. "Introduce slowly to allow mimosine → DHP and microbial adaptation." (Shelton et al., 2021; FutureBeef, 2017/2025).	Intake, drool/oral lesions, behavior.	Normal intake, calm rumination.	Reduced intake, drool, oral soreness.	Cut to prior safe level; add hay; observe 24–48 h (Shelton et al., 2021).
4–7	15–25% DM	Extend access time; keep roughage available; avoid heavy pod fall zones for naïve mobs (Shelton et al., 2021).	Add weight tape; manure; coat.	Holding weight, normal demeanor.	Early periocular hair loss, mild scouring.	Drop to ≤10% DM; move to grass; consider ***S. jonesii*** if naïve (Graham et al., 2013; Jones & Megarrity, 1986).
8–14	30–40% DM	Rotate through mixed swards; maintain mineral; sentinel T4/T3 in high-value animals if concerned (Dalzell et al., 2012; Hammond, 1995).	Intake, rumen motility, coat/skin, mouth.	Steady weight, clean muzzle, normal dung.	Persistent drool, oral ulcers, coat thinning.	Reduce to prior tolerated level; **inoculate** with ***S. jonesii*** or re-dose; add quality hay; reassess 3–5 d (Allison et al., 1992; FutureBeef, 2017/2025).
15–21	40–60% DM (ceiling for naïve cattle)**	Full mixed grazing; avoid sudden jumps (storms/regrowth); keep hay buffer (Shelton et al., 2021).	As above + breeding stock performance.	Normal performance on mixed pasture.	Ongoing intolerance; heat stress worsens signs.	Cap at ≤40% DM; extend adaptation; split mobs; lab support (urine DHP, rumen liquor for ***S. jonesii*** status) (Dalzell et al., 2012; Graham et al., 2013).

* Percentages are of total dry-matter intake; adjust by species/class.
** Some adapted herds exceed 60% with proven *S. jonesii* and balanced ration; do not push naïve mobs beyond ~50–60% in first 3 weeks (Shelton et al., 2021; Stifkens et al., 2022).
Daily DM % targets, simple yard/field checks, green/amber/red flags, and immediate actions if intolerance appears; note that iodine/thyroxine alone do not solve DHP toxicity (Dalzell et al., 2012; Shelton et al., 2019).

Leucaena adaptation protocol

Management of *Leucaena leucocephala* poisoning through systematic adaptation

1 Inoculate — 2 Re-introduce — 3 Maintain

Step 1: inoculate
with *Synergistes jonesii*

- Deliver approved culture per local protocol
- Hold on grass/hay for **7–10 days**
- Ensure **iodine adequate** mineral program

Tip: Re-inoculate after long breaks or if signs recur

Step 2: Gradual Re-introduction
of leucaena

- Start with **5–10% of diet**
- Increase gradually over **2–3 weeks**
- Monitor for adverse reactions

Warning: Stop if hair loss or weight loss occurs

Step 3: Mixed forage
maintenance and monitoring

- Maintain **balanced diet** with multiple sources
- Regular health monitoring
- Leucaena ≤ **50% of diet**

Success: Safe long-term leucaena consumption

Timeline overview

Days 1–10	**Inoculation and stabilization**	Hold animals on grass/hay to establish beneficial microbes
Days 11–35	**Gradual re-introduction**	Careful introduction with monitoring for adverse reactions
Days 35+	**Long-term management**	Ongoing mixed forage diet with regular health monitoring

Critical success factors

- Proper inoculation with approved *S. jonesii* culture
- Adequate iodine supplementation throughout
- Gradual introduction over 2–3 weeks minimum
- Continuous health monitoring

Warning signs

- Hair loss (especially around neck/head)
- Unexplained weight loss
- Reduced feed intake
- Lethargy or behavioral changes

Figure 9.23 Leucaena adaptation protocol (flow). Stepwise introduction (≈7–21 days), monitoring checkpoints (salivation/oral soreness, alopecia, intake), decision "pause/rollback" nodes, and *S. jonesii* inoculation points; includes red-flag criteria for reinoculation or diet dilution (Dalzell et al., 2012; Shelton et al., 2019).

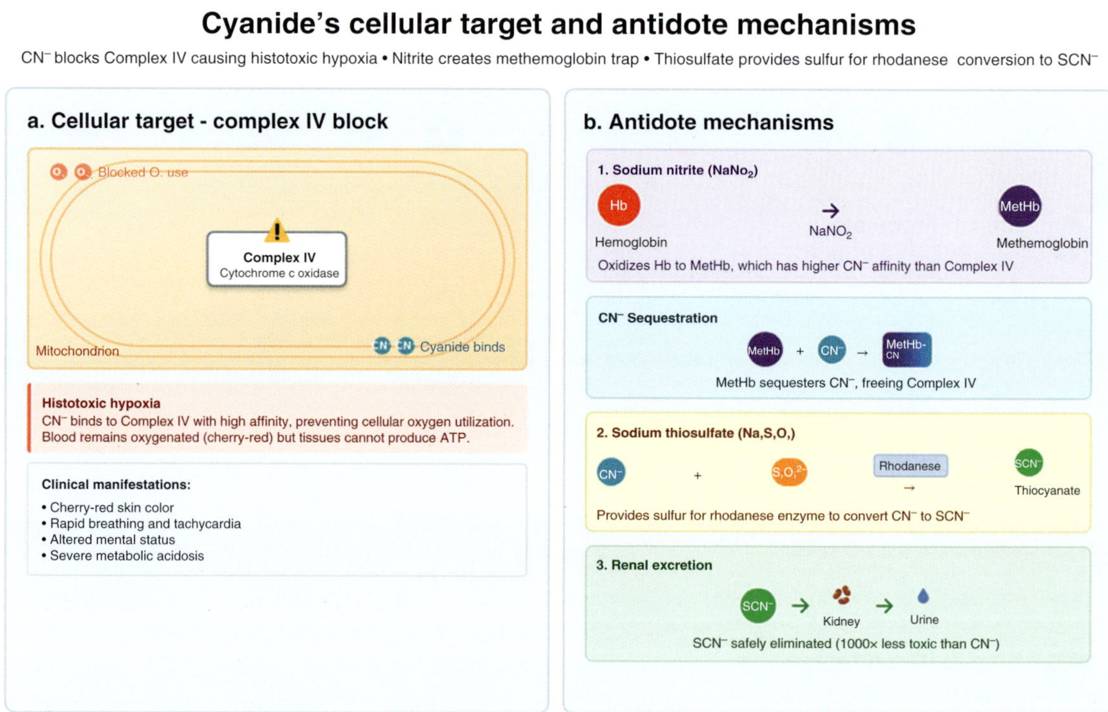

Figure 9.24 Cyanide cellular target and antidote mechanism. Schematic showing CN^- binding to mitochondrial cytochrome c oxidase (Complex IV) → histotoxic hypoxia, and the antidote sequence: sodium nitrite (controlled methemoglobinemia) then sodium thiosulfate (rhodanese substrate to form thiocyanate) (Cope (2025a); Burrows & Way (1979); Petrikovics et al. (2015).

animals and man. This may be because the microflora in the rumen provokes, and the ruminal pH stimulates a greater enzymatic breakdown compared to those in the nonruminants and man. Hydrocyanic acid is a small molecule that is rapidly absorbed into the bloodstream directly from the rumen. For a concise visual of the cellular target and why the antidotes work, see Figure 9.24 (Buonvino et al., 2022; Cope, 2025a; Petrikovics et al., 2015).

Source

Cyanide is available in a few different forms. It may be in the forms of inorganic salts, naturally occurring glycosides in cyanogenetic plants, or free HCN. Cyanide in an organic form is very toxic. Complex forms such as ferrocyanate and thiocyanate are relatively nontoxic. In the industry, cyanides are used for cleaning and electroplating metals and chemical synthesis. Inorganic cyanide compounds are used as rodenticides and vermicides. Free HCN is also used for fumigation. Another source of cyanide which may cause acute poisoning in domestic animals, particularly in ruminants, is cyanogenic glycosides. These compounds contain a nitrile group and a glycoside, which, upon hydrolysis by acid or enzyme,

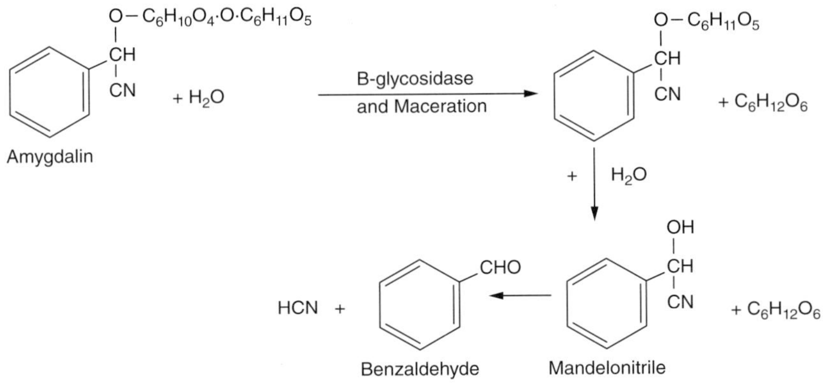

Figure 9.25 Schematic release of hydrocyanic acid from cyanogenic plants. Tissue disruption brings cyanogenic glycosides (e.g., linamarin, dhurrin) into contact with β-glucosidases/linamarase, generating HCN; risk increases with wilting, maceration, drought, frost, and ensiling errors (Cope (2025a); Burrows & Way (1979); Petrikovics et al. (2015). *Source:* Dzombak et al. (2006).

produce an aldehyde and HCN. Certain plants accumulate large quantities of cyanide in the form of cyanogenic glycoside, which liberate free cyanide upon hydrolysis (Figure 9.25).

One example is amygdalin, which is found in a number of plants, especially the seeds and leaves of cherry, almond, and peach. Chemically it is the β-glycoside (gentiobioside) of mandelonitrile, which is nontoxic, but contact with rumen or plant enzymes releases HCN. The glycoside itself is relatively nontoxic, but contact with the rumen or plant enzymes brought about by mastication and disruption of plant integrity results in the release of cyanide.

Some examples of cyanogenic plants found in the tropics are cassava (*Manihot esculenta*) and young rubber shoots (*Hevea brasiliensis*). Other cyanogenic plants of agricultural importance include sorghums and certain clovers; bamboo shoots are also notable (Figure 9.26). Figure 9.27 summarizes internationally used safety benchmarks for cassava products and the core processing steps that lower cyanide risk (CCCF, 2019; FSANZ, 2005). Cyanogenic plants may vary in their cyanide content. Young shoots are highly toxic due to high cyanogenic potential, whereas mature plants are often safer (e.g., johnsongrass). Figure 9.28 illustrates risk windows related to plant stage and stress. Practical thresholds for grazing/feeding decisions are summarized in Table 9.11 (Holman et al. 2012; SDSU Extension 2022).

Degradative enzymes of cyanogenic β-glycoside which can react to liberate cyanide from the glycoside are separated from the glycoside in intact plant cells. Thus, under normal conditions the hydrolysis of cyanogenic glycoside does not occur in plants. Enzymatic degradation and release of cyanide occur only upon wilting, cutting or trimming of the plants, chewing and maceration in the gastrointestinal tract of the animals, drought and decay of the plant itself

Toxicity

Cyanide is readily absorbed following ingestion, parenteral, and prolonged cutaneous exposure. Air containing more than 50–60 ppm of HCN gas may be absorbed in sufficient quantities to cause poisoning. The ability of the body to detoxify and excrete cyanide enables animals to tolerate small quantities of

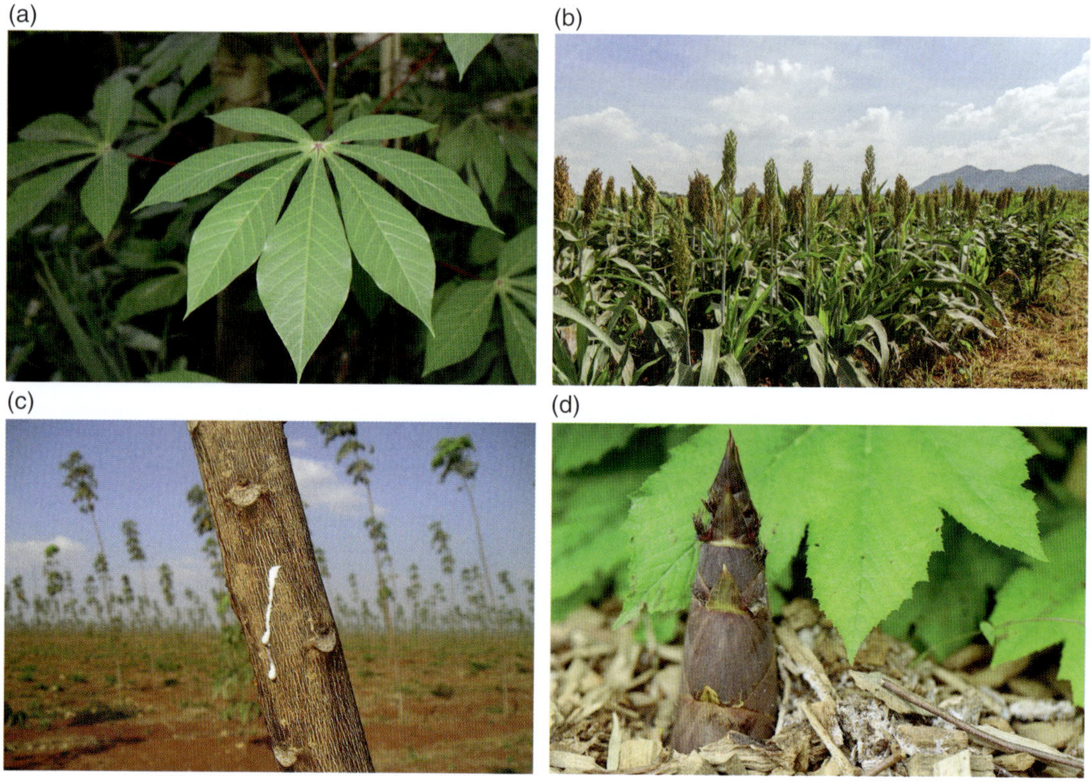

Figure 9.26 Cyanogenic plants of tropical importance (a–d). (a) Cassava (*Manihot esculenta*) leaves/peels. *Source:* mayapujiati / Pixabay; (b) Sorghum (e.g., Sorghum bicolor/johnsongrass *S. halepense*) post-rain regrowth. *Source:* Sorghum field / Freepik; (c) Young rubber shoots (*Hevea brasiliensis*). *Source:* Simon / Pixabay; (d) Bamboo shoots (culinary). Cyanogenic potential is greatest in young or stressed tissues and when plant integrity is disrupted (cutting, wilting, maceration) (OSU Extension 2017; SDSU Extension 2022; CCCF 2019; FSANZ 2005). *Source:* Nennieinszweidrei / Pixabay / CC0.

cyanide. Sheep are capable of metabolizing about 22 mg/50 kg body weight per hour (Peterson & Talcott, 2013). Cyanide toxicity in animals is influenced by several factors which include species and size of animals, the rate of ingestion, the type of food eaten together with the cyanide, the availability of active degradative enzymes in plants and in the digestive tract of the animals, the inherent ability of the animals to detoxify cyanide, the amount of plant material ingested, and the stage of growth of the plant.

Figure 9.29 provides a visual guide to threshold levels and risk spikes.

Mechanism of Action

Cyanide has high affinity for cytochrome oxidase, the enzyme responsible for regulating tissue oxygen. This enzyme is present in abundance in tissues with a high rate of oxidative metabolism such as the central nervous system and the cardiac muscle. When cyanide combines with cytochrome oxidase and

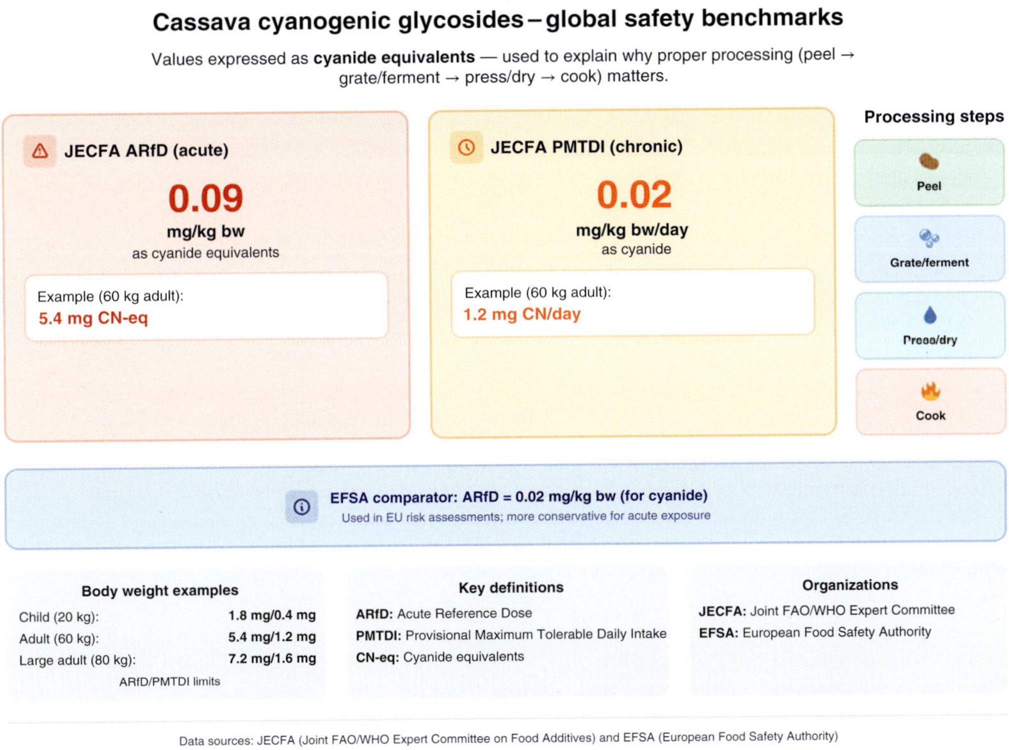

Figure 9.27 Cassava cyanogenic glycosides – safety benchmarks and processing checks. Benchmarks from international guidance (e.g.; FSANZ 2005) and key processing steps (soak/ferment/dry) that reduce cyanogens; use as a practical screen for feed/food inputs (CCCF 2019; FSANZ 2005).

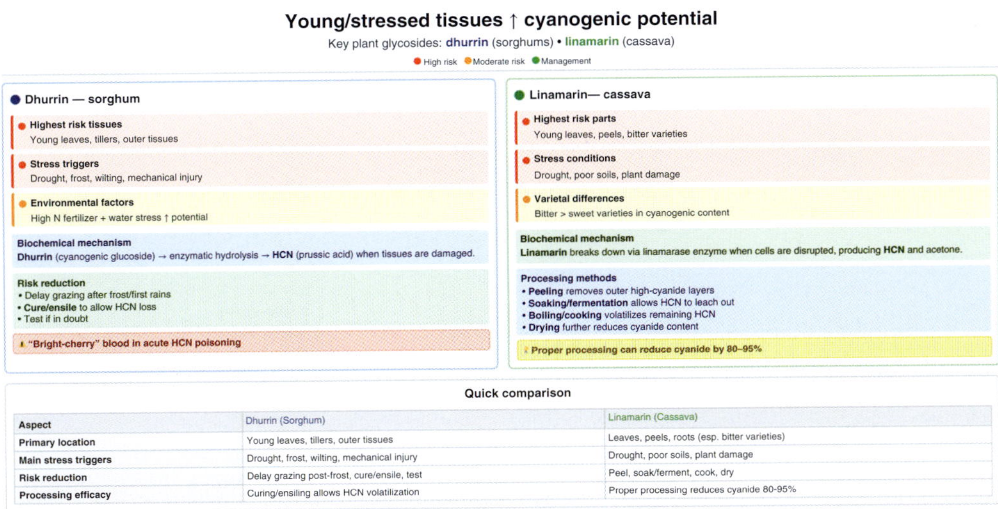

Figure 9.28 Young/stressed tissues and cyanogenic potential in plants. Cyanogenic glycosides (e.g., linamarin in cassava; dhurrin in sorghum) are typically highest in seedlings, apical leaves, and early regrowth, and they increase with stress (drought/frost injury, nutrient or pest stress). Tissue disruption (wilting, cutting, maceration/chewing) brings β-glucosidases into contact with glycosides, accelerating HCN release. Field risk therefore peaks with young regrowth and stressed plant material, especially when fed fresh or poorly processed CCCF 2019; FSANZ 2005; Gleadow & Møller 2014; OSU Extension 2017; SDSU Extension, 2022).

Table 9.11 HCN in forage (ppm, dry-matter basis) and action guidance.

HCN (ppm, DM)	Interpretation	Action guidance
0–500	Generally safe (Holman et al. 2012; SDSU Extension, 2022).	Graze/feed as part of a balanced ration; avoid turning in hungry stock; keep an eye on young regrowth and stressed plants (Holman et al. 2012).
600–1,000	Potentially toxic – do not use as the sole feed (Holman et al. 2012; SDSU Extension, 2022).	Dilute with low-risk forage; limit access/time; retest before increasing reliance (SDSU Extension, 2022).
>1,000	Dangerous – do not feed (SDSU Extension, 2022; Holman et al. 2012).	Remove animals; provide hay and clean water; seek local veterinary/extension advice; retest prior to any future use (SDSU Extension, 2022).

Actionable thresholds for grazing/feeding decisions: 0–500 ppm = generally safe; 600–1,000 ppm = potentially toxic – do not use as sole feed (dilute/limit, retest); >1,000 ppm = dangerous – do not feed. Field notes: risk rises with young regrowth after drought/frost, and fresh forage > hay/silage; allow full fermentation before feeding silage; grain sorghum types can run higher cyanogenic potential, but stage/stress drive risk. Sources summarized from Holman et al. 2012; SDSU Extension, 2022).

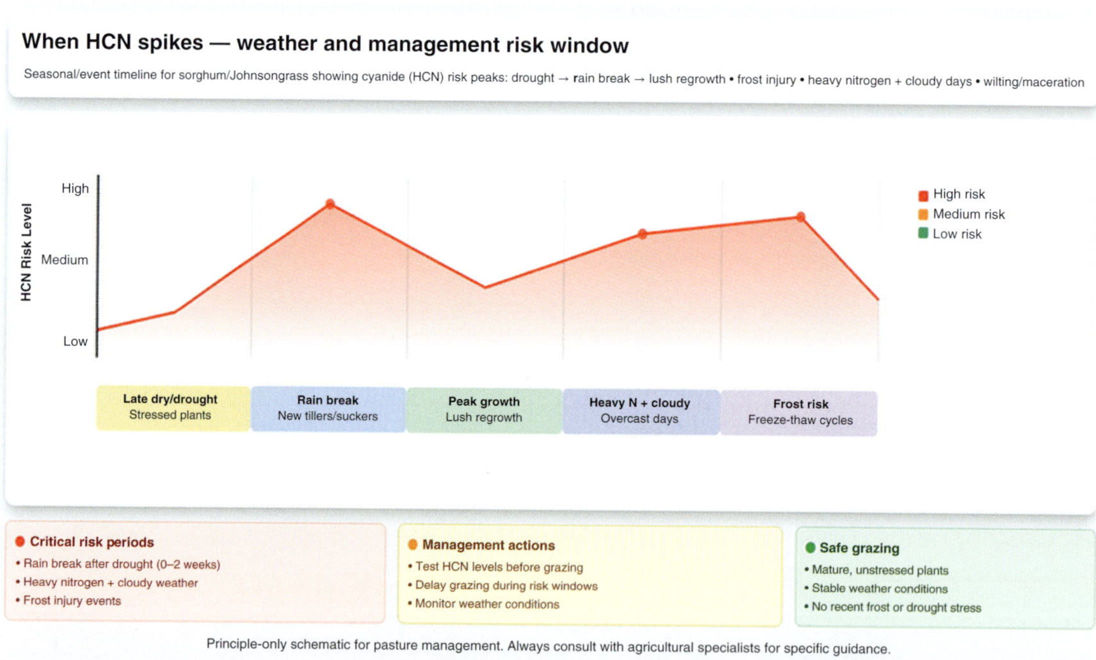

Figure 9.29 When HCN spikes—weather and management risk window for cyanogenic forages. Seasonal/event timeline for sorghum and johnsongrass showing typical peaks in hydrocyanic acid (HCN; prussic acid) risk associated with late drought stress, drought-breaking rains with lush regrowth/new tillers, rapid growth phases, heavy nitrogen with overcast or cloudy weather, frost/freeze–thaw injury, and wilting or maceration. The schematic highlights practical field actions, including delaying grazing during high-risk windows, testing suspect forage, and monitoring weather, as well as conditions consistent with safer grazing, such as mature unstressed plants, stable weather, and no recent frost or drought stress. Author-created schematic based on Richards et al. (2017), Gruss et al. (2022), and Arnold (2021).

forms a cyanide–cytochrome oxidase complex which is quite stable, the iron is maintained in trivalent form (ferric). In this form, electron transport ceases, and the chain of cellular respiration does not occur, resulting in cellular hypoxia (histotoxic anoxia). Consequently, oxygen from hemoglobin cannot be released to the electron transport system. Thus, blood remains bright red and oxygenated but cannot be utilized by the cells. Figure 9.24 (above) links this mechanism to the antidote targets (methemoglobin formation; sulfur donation to rhodanese).

Clinical Signs

Since cyanide is a very potent and rapidly acting poison, clinical signs appear immediately after ingestion and remain only for a few minutes. Thus, affected animals will commonly be found dead. Clinical signs occur in rapid succession, beginning with excitement and generalized muscle tremors. These will be followed by pronounced polypnea and dyspnea. Poisoned animals may be salivating, lacrimating, defecating, and urinating; recumbent and gasping for breath. Blood-tinged froth may be seen coming out from the nostrils and the mouth. Clonic convulsions due to hypoxia also occur. Affected animals also exhibit pupil dilation, bright red mucous membranes, and the characteristic bright-red “cherry” blood color.

A condition in the horse known as Equine Sorghum Cystitis–Ataxia Syndrome is being attributed to either a chronic low-level exposure to cyanide resulting in degeneration of the central nervous system or production of a lathyrogenic principle (nitrile-related amino acid). This condition appears in horses grazing on sorghum species or hybrid Sudan grass (Adams et al. 1969). This condition exhibits clinical signs such as urinary incontinence, posterior incoordination, and cystitis. Pregnant mares may abort and the aborted foals may have musculoskeletal disorders such as articular ankylosis. The proposed pathways for Equine Sorghum Cystitis–Ataxia and its clinical spectrum are synthesized in Figure 9.30 (Adams et al., 1969).

Pathophysiology

On necropsy, mucous membranes appear pink and the blood is colored bright cherry red and is difficult to clot. In view of terminal anoxia and violent death, subendocardial and subepicardial hemorrhages are observed. Petechial hemorrhages and congestion are also seen in the gastrointestinal tract. Fresh rumen content may liberate a bitter-almond smell. Congestion also occurs in the lung and trachea.

Diagnosis

Cyanide poisoning may be diagnosed based on the history of ingestion of cyanogenic plants or cyanide salts and the rapid onset of clinical signs relating to cellular hypoxia and sudden death. Postmortem findings such as bright cherry-red blood or pink mucous membrane also support the diagnosis.

Cyanide poisoning may be confirmed by the results of chemical analyses for cyanide in samples of plant materials ingested by the poisoned animals and in the blood, rumen contents, liver and muscle tissue of affected animals. All samples for laboratory analysis must be quick-frozen immediately and kept frozen until analysis to prevent HCN loss; hydrolysis may also be prevented by immersing the samples in 1–3% mercuric chloride where permitted (Peterson & Talcott, 2013). Figure 9.31 summarizes what to sample and how to preserve.

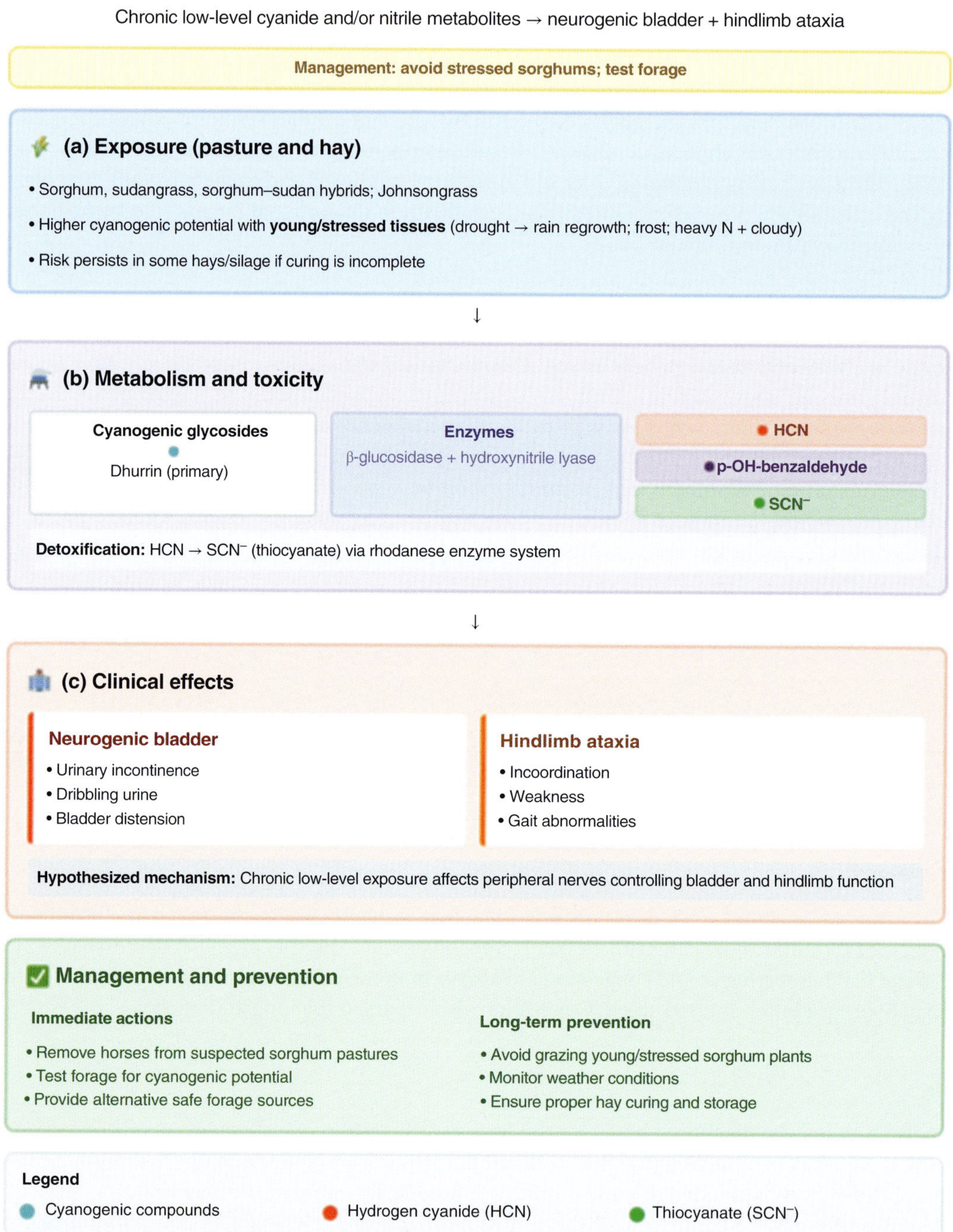

Figure 9.30 Proposed pathways and clinical spectrum of equine sorghum cystitis–ataxia syndrome. Author-created schematic summarising chronic low-level exposure to cyanogenic and/or nitrile-related compounds in sorghum, sudangrass, sorghum–sudan hybrids, and johnsongrass. The diagram links exposure to cyanogenic glycosides, enzymatic release of HCN and related metabolites, detoxification to thiocyanate, and the clinical pattern of neurogenic bladder, urinary incontinence, hindlimb ataxia, weakness, and gait abnormalities in affected horses. Management emphasis is placed on avoiding stressed sorghum forage, testing suspect forage, removing affected horses from exposure, and providing alternative safe forage. Based on Adams et al. (1969).

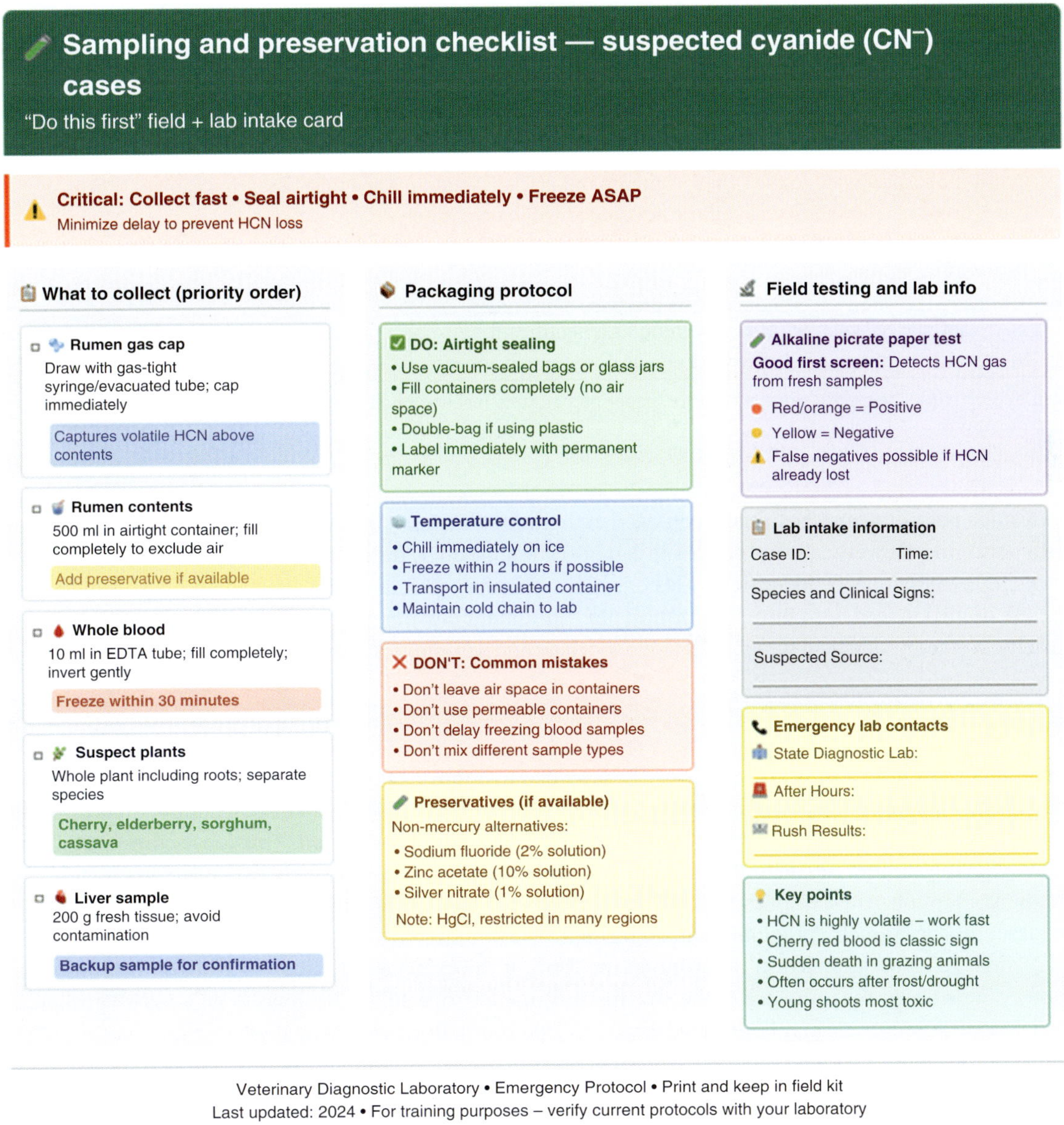

Figure 9.31 Sampling and preservation checklist – suspected cyanide cases. Collect suspect plants, rumen contents, whole blood, liver/muscle; freeze immediately or keep airtight/cold to prevent HCN loss; barn-side picrate paper can screen; note restrictions on $HgCl_2$ use (Peterson & Talcott 2013).

Cyanide levels above 20 mg/100 mL (200 ppm) in plant materials are considered significant. Nevertheless, low levels of cyanide detected in animal tissues are sufficient to suspect cyanide poisoning. A simple experiment to detect the presence of cyanide in plant materials may be carried out, as outlined in Table 9.12. Figure 9.32 shows the picrate-paper flow to accompany this test (Peterson & Talcott, 2013).

Table 9.12 Test for cyanogenic material in plants (alkaline picrate method).

1) Prepare "picrate paper" by wetting filter paper with a solution of 5.0 g sodium bicarbonate and 0.5 g picric acid in 100 mL water.
   a) Solution keeps indefinitely
   b) Dried paper can keep for a few days
2) Crush the suspect plant in the rumen contents and place in water in a test tube or jar that can be corked.
3) A few drops of chloroform and sulfuric acid added will hasten autolysis.
4) Suspend strips in a bottle after moistening them.
5) Heat to 30–35°C (86–95F)
6) A brick red color on paper indicates the presence of cyanide:
   a) A well-marked color within a few minutes is significant.
   b) A mild reaction in one to several hours is not of much concern.

Step-by-step barn-side picrate paper procedure (paper preparation, maceration in closed vessel, warming, color change interpretation).
Source: Peterson et al. (2013) / with permission of Elsevier.

Cyanide poisoning may be initially confused with nitrate poisoning in cattle, pulmonary emphysema, and urea poisoning. However, nitrate poisoning can be distinguished by the chocolate-colored blood, and pulmonary emphysema may be identified by lesions and respiratory sounds of the affected animals. A history of the use of urea in feed or pasture fertilization plus prominent nervous signs and bloat are suggestive of urea toxicity. A side-by-side field differential to guide triage and sampling is shown in Table 9.13 (Cope 2025a).

Treatment

At-a-glance antidote dosing and cautions are provided in Table 9.14 (Cope 2025a; Burrows & Way, 1979). The treatment of cyanide poisoning is extremely effective if it can be instituted soon enough. It is directed toward splitting the cytochrome oxidase–cyanide complex and its excretion. This loose complex may be split by giving sodium nitrite to the animals. The objective of sodium nitrite is to convert hemoglobin to methemoglobin because cyanide has a higher affinity for methemoglobin than the enzyme cytochrome oxidase; thus, cyanmethemoglobin will be formed.

Cyanide is readily excreted in the urine in the form of thiocyanate following the reaction of thiosulfate with cyanide under the influence of the enzyme rhodanese (Cope 2025a; Burrows & Way 1979; Petrikovics et al. 2015). Little cyanide may be excreted directly (Cope 2025a; Burrows & Way 1979; Petrikovics et al. 2015). Thus, an intravenous administration of a mixture of 1.0 mL of 20% sodium nitrite and 3.0 mL of 20% sodium thiosulfate is recommended. The above mixture (commercially as thionitrosa-H®) must be given at 4 mL/45 kg body weight. The dose recommended is 30–40 mL/1000 lb body weight.

Bracken Fern Poisoning

The bracken fern is one of the most successful weeds in the world. It has a wide geographical distribution, occurring across temperate, subtropical, and tropical regions, including parts of Asia and Malaysia (Vetter, 2009; Salim et al., 2020). A few species of bracken fern are known to cause poisoning in domestic

Picrate-paper field test (flowchart)

Prepare paper → set up sealed headspace over macerated plant/rumen → warm → read brick-red intensity vs time • Optional whole-blood adaptation

1) Prepare alkaline picrate paper

Use validated strips **or** make by soaking filter paper in alkaline picrate; dry; store airtight and dark.

Follow chemical safety/PPE; keep strips sealed until use (volatile sensitivity).

2) Prepare sample

Plants: chop/macerate **young/stressed** tissue (10–20 g) with a few mL water.
Rumen fluid: collect fresh sample, filter if needed.

Optional: For whole-blood (goat) adaptation, collect fresh blood in heparinized tube.

3) Assemble test system

- Place macerated sample (or rumen fluid/blood) in a small jar or vial.
- Suspend picrate paper strip above sample, avoiding direct contact.
- Seal container tightly to create a headspace.

4) Incubate

- Keep sealed system warm (35–40°C) for 1–2 hours.
- Use a water bath, incubator, or warm environment.
- Monitor for color change on picrate paper.

5) Interpret results

- Observe picrate paper for **brick-red** color development.
- Compare intensity to a reference color chart or time scale.
- Strong/rapid color change = high cyanogenic potential.
- Weak/slow/no change = low or absent cyanide.

Notes

- Always use proper PPE and chemical safety protocols.
- Dispose of used strips and samples according to local hazardous waste guidelines.

Figure 9.32 Alkaline picrate paper test – barn-side flow. Prepare picrate paper, macerate plant/rumen material in a closed jar, warm (30–35°C), interpret brick-red intensity vs. time as semiquantitative evidence of cyanide. Adapted from Haque et al. (2002).

Table 9.13 Cyanide vs. nitrate/nitrite vs. urea (NPN) toxicity – key one-look differences.

Feature	Cyanide (HCN)	Nitrate/nitrite	Urea/NPN (ammonia)
Onset after exposure	Very rapid: signs in 15–20 min to a few hours; survival after onset rarely >2 h (Cope, 2025).	Acute, minutes–hours; course may extend 12–24 h; abortions can follow significant methemoglobinemia in pregnant cattle (Thompson, 2024a).	Rapid: typically 20–60 min in cattle, 30–90 min in sheep; often fatal within hours (Thompson, 2024a).
Blood/ mucous membranes	Bright "cherry-red" venous blood; mucous membranes pink early, cyanotic terminally (Cope, 2025).	Chocolate-brown blood from methemoglobinemia; cyanotic mucosae (Thompson, 2024a).	No pathognomonic color; severe hyperammonemia → terminal cyanosis (Thompson, 2024a).
Rumen/ breath odor	Bitter-almond odor may be present (not always) (Cope, 2025).	No characteristic odor; blood color is the key clue (Thompson, 2024a).	Ammonia (NH_3) odor of rumen/cecum may or may not be evident (Thompson, 2024a).
Typical gross lesions	Often minimal; bright-red blood; congestion ± froth in airways; rumen gas distension; picrate-positive rumen contents possible (Cope, 2025).	Chocolate-brown blood; petechiae/ecchymoses on serosa; pulmonary and GI edema may occur (Thompson, 2024a).	No pathognomonic lesions; rapid bloat/decomposition; rumen pH ≥7.5 supportive (Thompson, 2024a)
Quick field tests/screens	Alkaline picrate paper for suspect plants/rumen; rumen gas-cap HCN detection tubes; confirm in lab (Cope, 2025).	Nitrate screens on forage/ water (diphenylamine, nitrate dipsticks); blood methemoglobin testing supports diagnosis in acute cases (Thompson, 2024a).	Rumen pH (≥7.5) and NH_3-N; freeze/preserve immediately for lab confirmation (Thompson, 2024a).
Preferred diagnostic specimens	Antemortem whole blood; postmortem rumen contents/gas-cap, liver, muscle – seal airtight, chill/freeze ASAP (Cope, 2025).	Plasma (premortem); ocular fluid (postmortem); suspect feed/water; freeze promptly (Thompson, 2024a).	Rumen fluid, serum, whole blood, urine for NH_3-N; measure rumen pH; freeze immediately (Thompson, 2024a).

Rapid comparison of onset, blood/mucosa color, odor/field clues, gross lesions, barn-side screens, and preferred specimens. Cyanide: bright "cherry-red" blood with peracute course; nitrate/nitrite: chocolate-brown blood (methemoglobinemia); urea/NPN: hyperammonemia pattern with rumen pH ≥7.5 supportive. Summarized from Merck Veterinary Manual toxicology sections.

animals. In Australia, *Pteridium esculentum*, a bracken fern closely related to *Pteridium aquilinum*, causes the same acute toxicity syndrome as *P. aquilinum* (Cope 2025b). The epidemiological survey of bracken ferns indicates that *P. aquilinum* and *P. revolutum* are toxic (Vetter, 2009; Bajracharya & Bajracharya, 2022). These weeds spread by extending their rhizomes and releasing their spores. A concise view of global/tropical spread and pasture ecology is shown in Figure 9.33 (Cope 2025b).

The toxicity and carcinogenicity of bracken fern in livestock – especially cattle – have been of particular interest, and research has demonstrated that consumption can cause acute bracken fern poisoning,

Table 9.14 Antidote doses and cautions (livestock) – cyanide (HCN).

Species	Sodium nitrite (IV)	Sodium thiosulfate (IV)	Repeat guidance	Oral thiosulfate (rumen/stomach)	Cautions/monitoring
Cattle	5 mg/kg IV, slow (use lower ruminant doses to limit methemoglobinemia) (Burrows & Way, 1979).	25–50 mg/kg IV, slow (Burrows & Way, 1979).	Reassess in 10–30 min; may repeat thiosulfate if signs persist. Repeat nitrite only with evidence of ongoing toxicosis and acceptable metHb (Cope, 2025a).	Consider as adjunct to trap CN^- in rumen; used when IV access is delayed. Evidence (large-animal models) supports survival benefit; confirm locally (Cope, 2025a; Ng et al., 2021).	Oxygen; monitor SpO_2/PaO_2, heart rate, BP. Watch for nitrite-induced methemoglobinemia (chocolate blood, hypoxia). If metHb excessive from therapy, reversal with methylene blue follows nitrate protocols – specialist guidance required (Cope, 2025a; Merck – Nitrate/Nitrite).
Sheep/goats	5 mg/kg IV, slow (ruminants are more susceptible to nitrite; keep to lower end) (Burrows & Way, 1979).	25–50 mg/kg IV, slow (Burrows & Way, 1979; Burrows, 1981).	Prefer repeat thiosulfate if needed; avoid repeated nitrite unless guided by metHb/response (Cope, 2025a).	Useful when plant/rumen CN^- production is ongoing; give promptly if IV delayed; confirm with your lab/vet (Burrows, 1981; Cope, 2025a).	Small ruminants: higher risk of over-methemoglobinemia; monitor closely; pregnancy and severe anemia increase risk. Oxygen if available (Cope, 2025a).
Nonruminants (e.g., horses, swine)	Up to 20 mg/kg IV over 3–4 min as per general animal guidance; consider alternatives if available (Cope, 2025a).	≥500 mg/kg IV (20% w/w), slow; may repeat (Cope, 2025a).	Nitrite may be carefully repeated at ~10 mg/kg every 2–4 h based on clinical response/metHb (Cope, 2025a).	Not a rumen species; oral thiosulfate is generally less relevant except for gastric exposures – follow specialist guidance (Cope, 2025a).	Consider hydroxocobalamin (70 mg/kg IV) + oxygen when available (does not worsen tissue hypoxia). Monitor for hypotension with nitrites (Cope, 2025a).

How to use this table (quick notes).

- Remove animals from source and start oxygen if available. 2) For ruminants, start with lower nitrite (≈5 mg/kg) then thiosulfate (25–50 mg/kg); prioritize repeat thiosulfate over repeat nitrite if ongoing signs and metHb limits are a concern (Burrows & Way, 1979; Cope, 2025a).
- Oral thiosulfate may help convert residual CN^- to SCN^- in the rumen/stomach; experimental large-animal work supports its potential, but follow local protocols (Cope, 2025a; Ng et al., 2021).

Ruminants: sodium nitrite ~5 mg/kg IV (slow) followed by sodium thiosulfate 25–50 mg/kg IV (slow); prioritize repeating thiosulfate if needed; repeat nitrite only with metHb/clinical justification. Nonruminants: higher nitrite upper bounds appear in general guidance but require close monitoring. Consider oxygen, watch for nitrite-induced methemoglobinemia; reversal strategies follow nitrate/nitrite protocols. Summarized from classic dosing studies and the Merck Veterinary Manual.

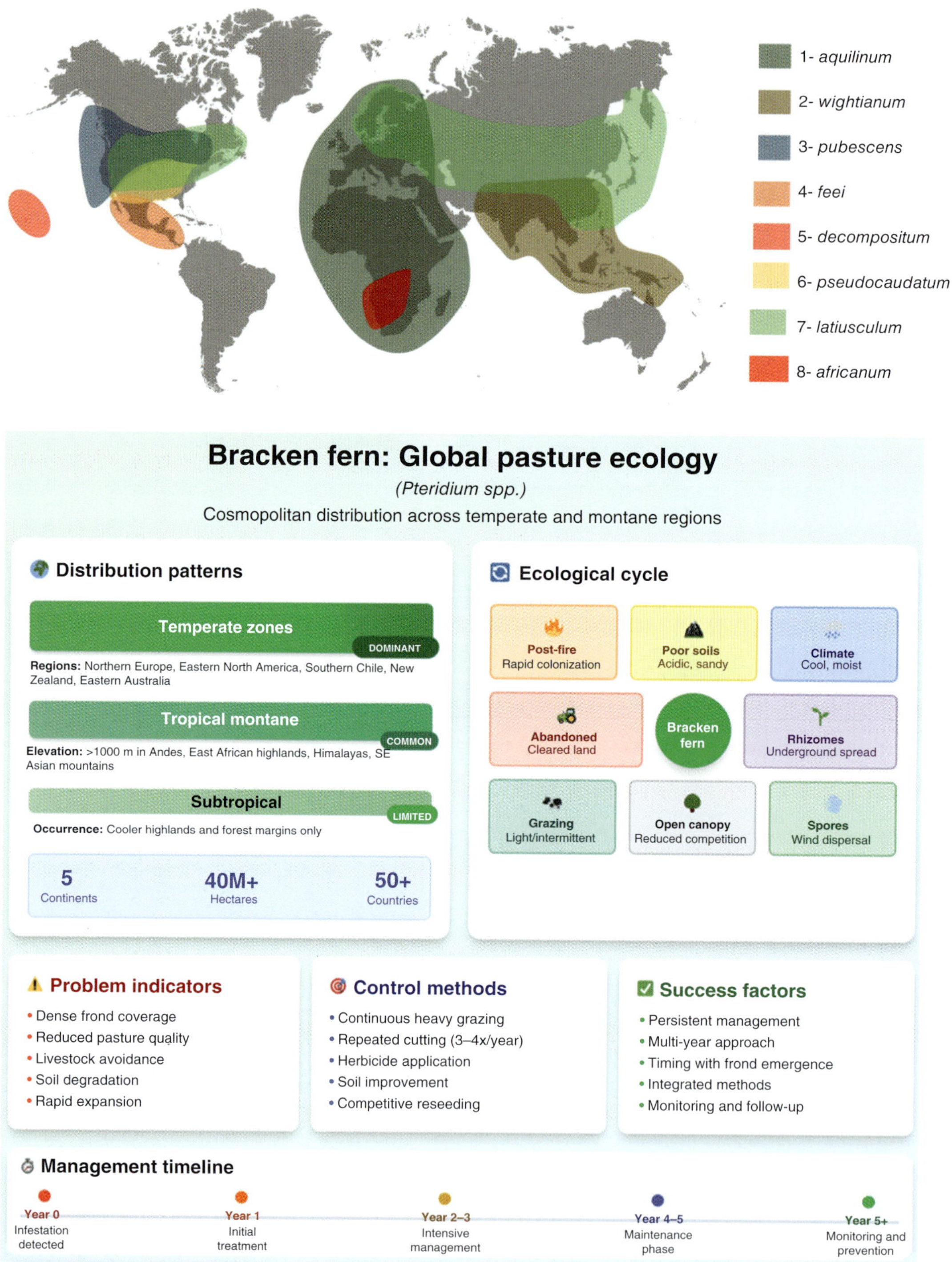

Figure 9.33 Global–tropical context and spread of bracken (*Pteridium* spp.). Distribution and ecology summary: expansion via long-lived rhizomes and airborne spores; growth favored by canopy opening, fire history, and intermittent grazing pressure (McGlone et al. 2005).

enzootic hematuria, and urinary bladder tumors (Carvalho et al. 2006; Xu 1992). Bracken fern poisoning has also been reported in sheep. However, goats, rabbits, and possibly sheep have been considered more resistant to bracken carcinogens than other species (Xu 1992; Cope 2025b).

Description

Bracken fern is common in recently cleared lands or abandoned fields, where the soil is sandy and dry. It is an herbaceous perennial with a stout, blackish, horizontal rhizome. The leaves are scattered, erect, coarse, and normally triangular in shape (Figure 9.34). Figure 9.35 complements Figure 9.34 by illustrating the diagnostic frond and rhizome features used in the field.

Clinical Signs

Table 9.15 provides a one-look matrix for species × syndrome patterns (acute hemorrhagic, enzootic hematuria, bright blindness, thiaminase neurologic) (Cope, 2025b; Hirono et al., 1984, Xu 1992).

In cattle, clinical manifestations include higher fever (40.5–42.5°C), dullness, profuse salivation, petechial spots, or hemorrhages on visible mucous membranes (conjunctiva and vagina) and the skin, bloody sweat, epistaxis, hematuria, and hemorrhagic diarrhea. Pale mucous membranes, anorexia, cessation of rumination, and cardiac arrest may be observed toward the terminal stage of acute bracken

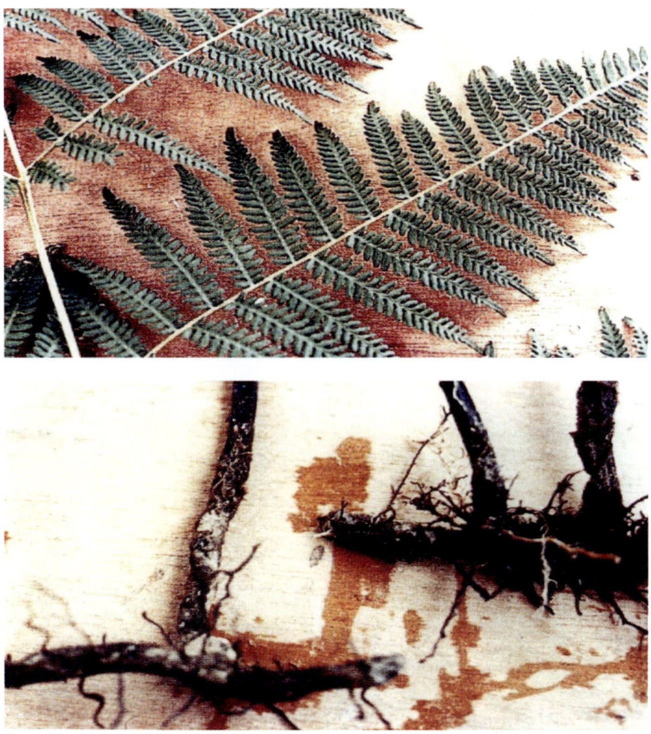

Figure 9.34 Leaves and rhizome of bracken fern (*Pteridium esculentum*). Field identification plate showing a triangular frond (bipinnate–tripinnate) and a black, creeping rhizome typical of bracken species; common on recently cleared/abandoned land and sandy soils (Flora of Pennsylvania n.d.)

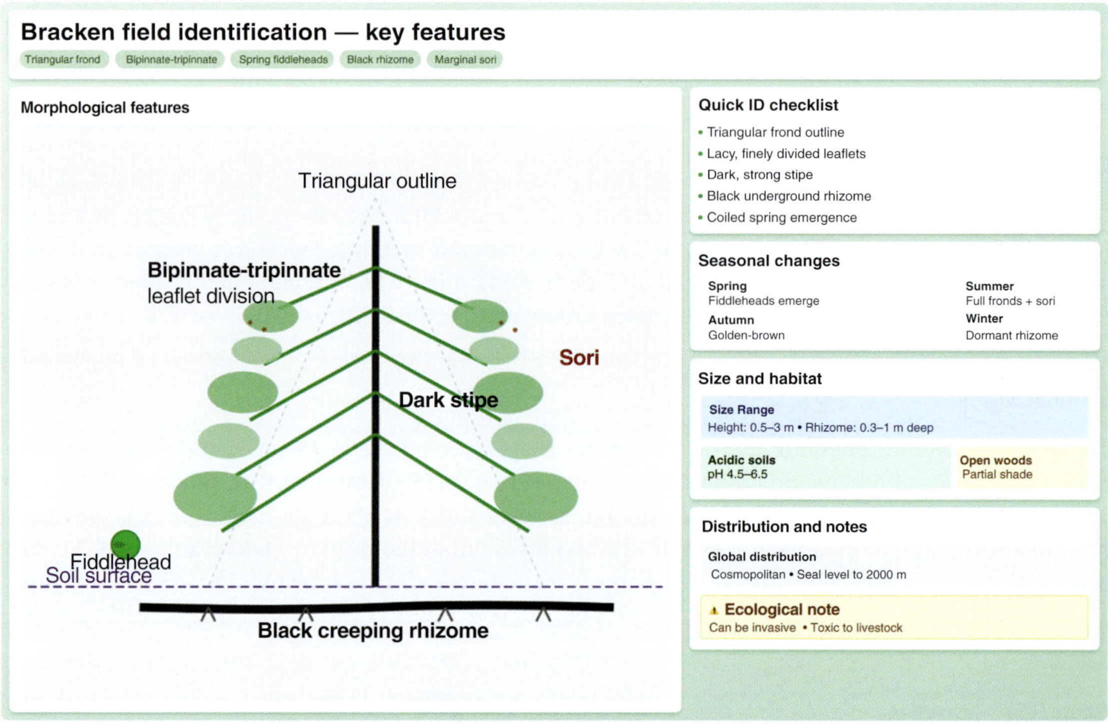

Figure 9.35 Bracken fern identification – key features. Field ID plate highlighting the triangular, bipinnate–tripinnate frond; coarse, erect petiole; and black, creeping rhizome typical of *Pteridium* spp.; common on recently cleared/abandoned land with sandy soils (Cope 2025b).

fern poisoning. Clinical signs involving the central nervous system such as convulsions may also be seen in cattle toward the terminal stage but are not prominent. Representative field images and lesions are collated in Figure 9.36 (kll University College of Veterinary Medicine, n.d.-a; Cope, 2025b; National Toxicology Program, 2024).

Young cattle may develop edematous swellings in the throat region, resulting in difficult breathing and eventual death (Cope 2025b). The clinical signs described above have been observed in both field and experimental cases of bracken fern poisoning (Cope 2025b).

Mechanism of Action

According to Cope (2025b), bracken fern (*P. aquilinum*) contains thiaminase and another more slowly acting poison, which affects the bone marrow. Therefore, a steady ingestion of bracken fern for many weeks by ruminants causes severe destruction of the bone marrow. This is manifested as blood dyscrasia, characterized mainly by diminished leukocyte and platelet counts. This toxicosis is similar in clinical signs and therapeutic response to radiation toxicity (Gupta, 2018). Figure 9.37 visualizes the parallel thiaminase pathway (monogastrics/equids) and the ptaquiloside-driven marrow/urothelial pathway (ruminants) (Cope 2025b).

Table 9.15 Bracken fern syndromes by species, exposure, and hallmarks.

Species	Typical exposure window	Dominant syndrome	Hallmark clinical/lab clues	Signature lesions	Key differentials
Cattle (acute)	Weeks on heavy bracken (young fronds or contaminated hay) (Cope, 2025b).	Acute hemorrhagic syndrome from bone-marrow aplasia due to ptaquiloside (Cope, 2025b; Hirono et al., 1984).	Fever, petechiation, hemorrhagic diarrhea; severe pancytopenia (thrombocytopenia → leukopenia) (Cope, 2025b).	Hypocellular/aplastic bone marrow; diffuse hemorrhages, GI ulceration; marrow may appear "gelatinous/serous" in severe atrophy (Cope, 2025; National Toxicology Program, 2024b).	Anticoagulant rodenticide (warfarin) toxicosis; septicemias/vasculitis; BVDV/BNP context as appropriate (Cope, 2025b).
Cattle (chronic)	Months–years of intermittent intake (often >3-year-old cattle) (Cope, 2025).	Enzootic hematuria ± GI cancers; BPV synergy implicated (Xu 1992, Cope, 2025b).	Recurrent hematuria, anemia, poor thrift (Cope, 2025b).	Bladder tumors (epithelial/mesenchymal), mucosal hemorrhages and dilated vessels (Cope, 2025b).	Urolithiasis; leptospirosis-associated hematuria (context) (Cope, 2025b).
Sheep	Chronic exposure on bracken-infested ranges (Cope, 2025).	"Bright blindness" (progressive retinal degeneration); bracken/ptaquiloside-associated (Cope, 2025b; Hirono et al., 1993).	Daytime blindness, retinal atrophy on ophthalmoscopy; ± PEM episodes where thiaminases are high (Cope, 2025)b.	Retinal degeneration; ± lesions consistent with PEM in some outbreaks (Cope, 2025b).	Other retinal degenerations/retinopathies; trace element or infectious retinopathies as regionally appropriate.
Horses/monogastrics	Weeks–months on bracken or bracken-contaminated hay (Cope, 2025b).	Thiaminase-mediated thiamine deficiency ("bracken staggers") (Cope, 2025b).	Ataxia, tremors, wide-based stance; seizures in severe cases; response to parenteral thiamine (Cope, 2025b).	Lesions consistent with thiamine deficiency; ± myocardial changes reported (Cope, 2025b).	Polioencephalomalacia from other causes (sulfur, lead, thiamine antagonists), equine neurodifferentials (Cope, 2025b).

Species × exposure window × dominant syndrome × hallmark clinical/lab clues × signature lesions × key differentials; includes acute hemorrhagic syndrome (cattle), enzootic hematuria (cattle), "bright blindness" (sheep), and thiaminase-mediated neurologic disease (equids/monogastrics) (Cope, 2025b; Hirono et al., 1984, Xu 1992; National Toxicology Program, 2024).

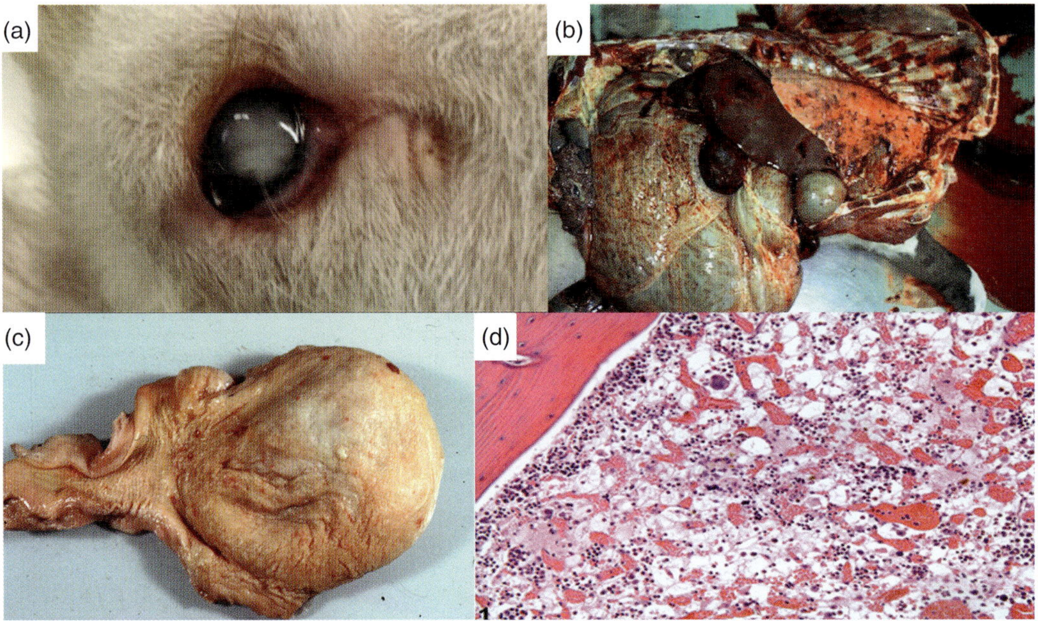

Figure 9.36 Bracken fern – clinical signs and lesions (author composite). (a) Cattle with **acute bracken poisoning**: depression/weakness, fever, mucosal petechiation/ecchymoses, and bleeding tendency consistent with **bone-marrow aplasia**, where **thrombocytopenic hemorrhage precedes leukopenia** (Silva et al., 2023). *Source:* Cope (2025) / MDPI / CC BY 4.0. (b) Acute cases may show widespread petechial/ecchymotic to suffusive hemorrhages at necropsy (example image from teaching archive). *Source:* Cornell University College of Veterinary Medicine (2014). (c) Chronic bracken exposure (enzootic hematuria) – representative urinary bladder histopathology (teaching archive image). *Source:* Cornell University Medicine / https://secure.vet.cornell.edu/nst/nst.asp?Fun=Display&imgID=12385 / last accessed on Nov 05, 2025. (d) Bone marrow hypoplasia/aplasia may be accompanied by gelatinous transformation (serous atrophy) in severe cases; image shown is an illustrative example of this lesion pattern (not disease-specific). *Source:* U.S. Department of Health and Human Services (2024) / National Toxicology Program / Public domain.

Pathophysiology

Hematological analysis shows leucopenia and thrombocytopenia in all cases of bracken fern poisoning. At the same time, all the white blood cell components except the lymphocytes completely disappear from the blood of affected animals. In some cases, there is an increase in capillary fragility, bleeding time, and blood coagulation time.

Necropsy shows incomplete blood coagulation, hemorrhages, and edema in almost all organs and tissues. The connective and adipose tissues become gelatinous, and degeneration of liver, atrophy of spleen, and ulcerations of the mucosa are observed in some cases. Postmortem examination also shows marked changes in the bone marrow, with yellow marrow becoming gelatinous and red marrow infiltrated with fat. Histopathological and cytological examinations show aplasia of the hematopoietic tissues – especially the granulocytic and thrombocytic series – suggesting depression of bone marrow activity leading to blood dyscrasia. Figure 9.38 illustrates the field decision process that helps clinicians connect these patterns to likely bracken exposure at the paddock level (Cope, 2025b).

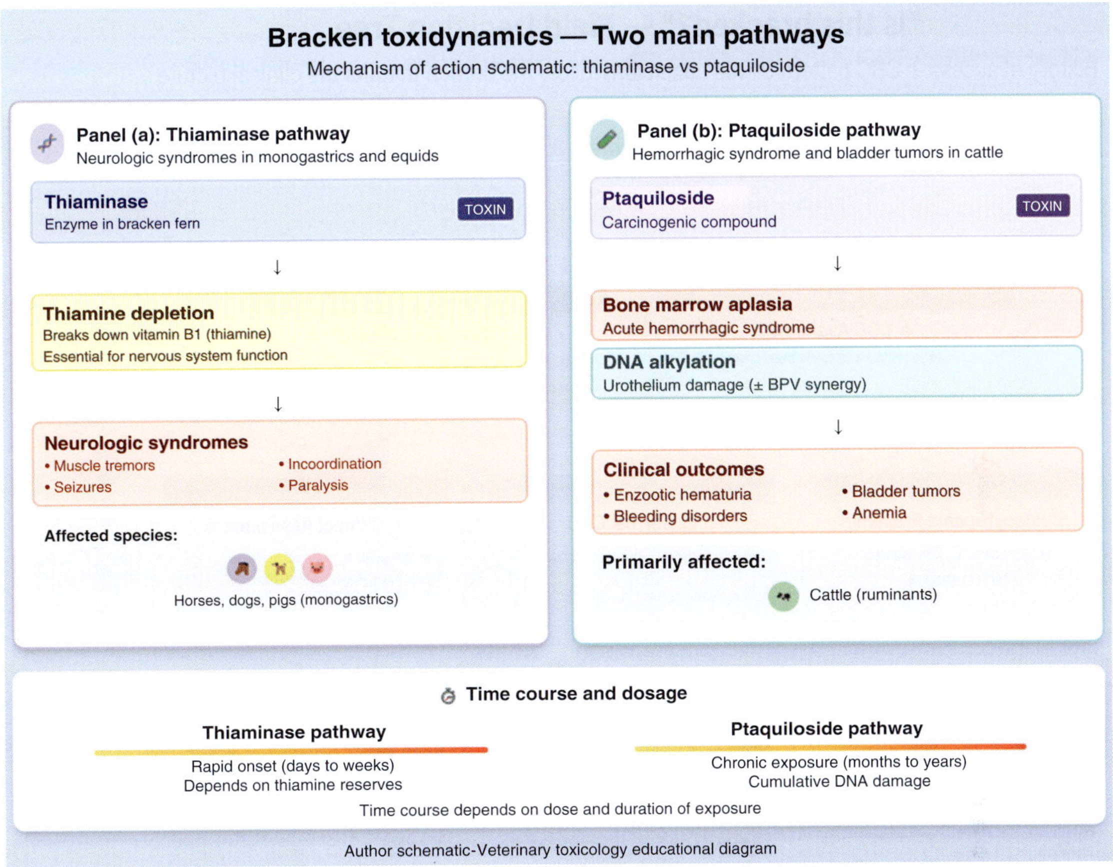

Figure 9.37 Bracken toxicodynamics. Dual pathways: (a) thiaminase → thiamine depletion → neurologic disease in monogastrics/equids; (b) ptaquiloside (norsesquiterpene glycoside) → bone-marrow aplasia (acute hemorrhagic syndrome) and urothelial DNA damage (± bovine papilloma virus [BPV] synergy) → enzootic hematuria/bladder tumors in cattle (Cope 2025b, Gupta, 2018).

Enzootic hematuria of cattle associated with bracken fern poisoning is characterized by hematuria, tumors in the urinary bladder, and hemorrhages in the bladder mucosa (Carvalho et al., 2006; Xu, 1992).

Diagnosis

The availability of bracken fern in surrounding areas, typical clinical signs, and the detection of urinary bladder tumors on necropsy are sufficient evidence to conclude the diagnosis of bracken fern poisoning. For a rapid field work-up, Figure 9.38 provides a decision tree, and Table 9.16 lists the minimum diagnostic panel and what to sample first (Cope, 2025b).

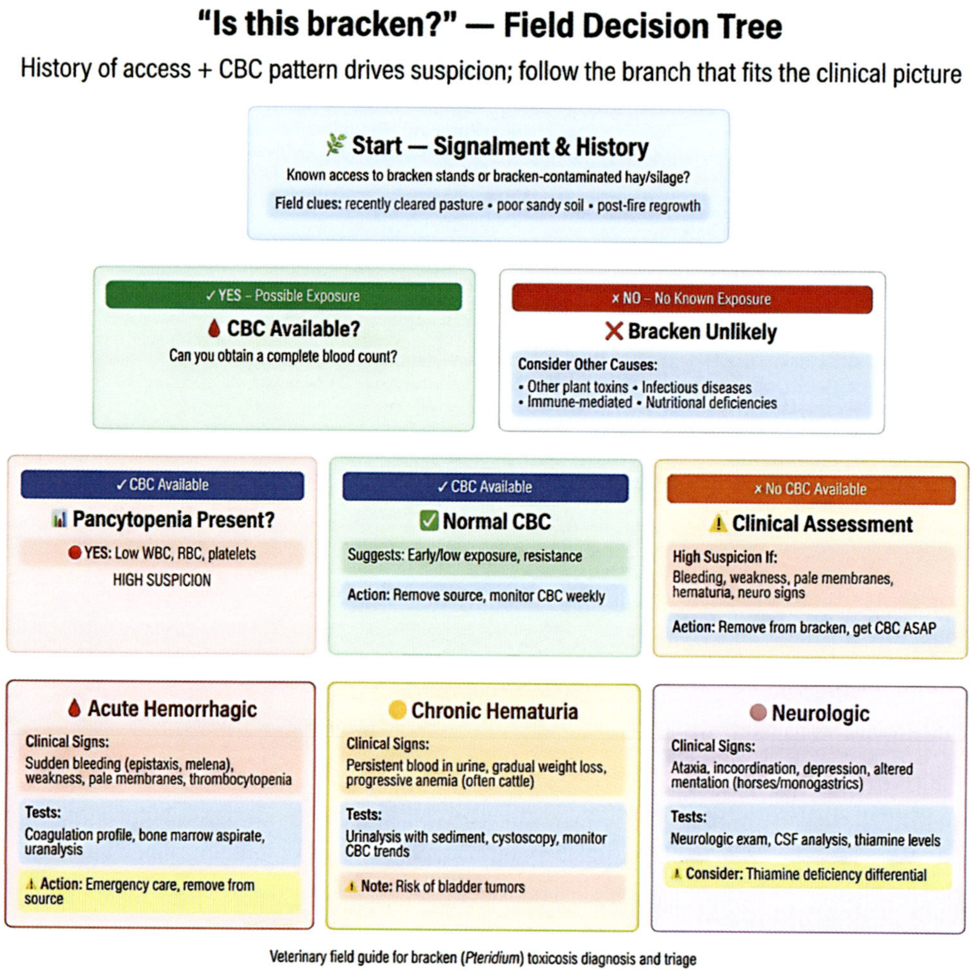

Figure 9.38 "Is this bracken?" – field decision tree. Rapid triage using access history, characteristic pasture ecology, and a basic work-up (CBC cytopenias, coag profile, urinalysis), with branches for acute hemorrhagic pattern, chronic hematuria, and thiamine-responsive neurologic disease. *Source:* Cope (2025b)/ Merck & Co.

In practice, a chronic intermittent hematuria and postmortem findings such as urinary bladder tumors and hemorrhages of the bladder help differentiate bracken fern poisoning from other hemorrhagic diseases and toxicoses (Cope, 2025b).

Treatment

Butyl alcohol and thiamine have been used as antidotes in bracken fern poisoning in cattle and horses, respectively. Fresh whole blood transfusions are also recommended. Fluid therapy should be instituted to counteract shock. In addition, antibiotic therapy may be required to prevent secondary bacterial infection. Figure 9.39 summarizes prevention/management on bracken-infested pastures to reduce future cases (Cope, 2025b).

Table 9.16 What to sample in suspected bracken cases (minimum panel + add-ons).

Test/sample	What it shows (expected findings)	How to collect/preserve (quick notes)	How to use/follow-up
CBC	Thrombocytopenia occurs first, followed by leukopenia; anemia develops later (Cope, 2025b).	EDTA whole blood; run promptly; make smears at field side if delay expected (Cope, 2025b).	If cytopenias present with compatible history → strong presumptive diagnosis; proceed to coag panel and (if PM) marrow exam (Cope, 2025b).
Coagulation profile	PT/aPTT are often normal; use coag panel mainly to rule out anticoagulant rodenticide/DIC and interpret alongside platelet count (Cope, 2025b).	Citrated plasma; minimize delay/keep cool; follow lab panel (PT/aPTT ± fibrinogen (Cope, 2025b).	Marked prolongation with normal platelets suggests rodenticide or DIC; in bracken, thrombocytopenia is typically prominent (Cope, 2025b).
Urinalysis	Hematuria (RBCs) in chronic exposures (enzootic hematuria); ± urothelial atypia/ neoplastic cells **may be seen** on cytology in chronic cases (Xu 1992, Cope, 2025b).	Fresh urine (cystocentesis or clean midstream); cytology slide if possible (Cope, 2025b).	Persistent/intermittent hematuria in older cattle → image/examine bladder and consider biopsy if feasible (Cope, 2025b).
Postmortem: bone marrow (rib/sternum or femur)	Hypocellular/aplastic marrow; "gelatinous transformation/ serous atrophy" in severe cases (Cope, 2025b) National Toxicology Program, 2024).	Imprints/smears from cut surface; formalin-fix a core; photograph gelatinous change; avoid blood contamination (Cope, 2025b; National Toxicology Program, 2024).	Marrow aplasia with field history + CBC cytopenias supports acute bracken toxicosis (Cope, 2025b).
Postmortem: spleen and liver (± GI)	Context for hemorrhages, secondary lesions; rule-outs (sepsis, viral disease) (Cope, 2025b).	Representative sections in 10% NBF for histology; fresh pieces if ancillary tests planned (Cope, 2025b).	Use with marrow findings to confirm pattern and exclude differentials (Cope, 2025b).
Histology targets (chronic cattle)	Urinary bladder: hyperplasia/ dysplasia to neoplasia; vascular ectasia; lesions consistent with enzootic hematuria (Xu 1992, Cope, 2025b).	Multiple bladder mucosal biopsies/sections; include gross lesions and normal-appearing areas (Cope, 2025b).	If neoplasia present, consider BPV context (see optional PCR) and herd/ pasture investigation (Cope, 2025b)
Optional: BPV PCR (research/ cluster)	Papillomavirus infection is a possible cofactor in enzootic hematuria/cancer syndrome; BPV (especially BPV-2) is commonly detected in bladder tumors in bracken-associated enzootic hematuria contexts (Xu 1992, Cope, 2025b).	Target bladder lesions or urine cell pellets; follow lab primer/panel guidance (Cope, 2025b).	Positive BPV does not exclude bracken exposure; interpret alongside histology and farm history (Cope, 2025b).
Rule-outs to note	Anticoagulant rodenticide toxicosis; septicemias/ vasculitis; BVDV/BNP context for marrow changes; urolithiasis or Leptospira for hematuria; other causes of PEM/thiamine deficiency in equids/monogastrics.	Match samples to differential (e.g., rodenticide assay, culture/PCR, viral testing, imaging.	A compatible history of access to bracken plus CBC cytopenias remains the strongest field pattern for bracken.

CBC (pancytopenia), coag profile, urinalysis (chronic hematuria), postmortem marrow/spleen/liver, bladder histology (chronic), optional BPV PCR; with collection notes and rule-outs (Cope, 2025; National Toxicology Program, 2024).

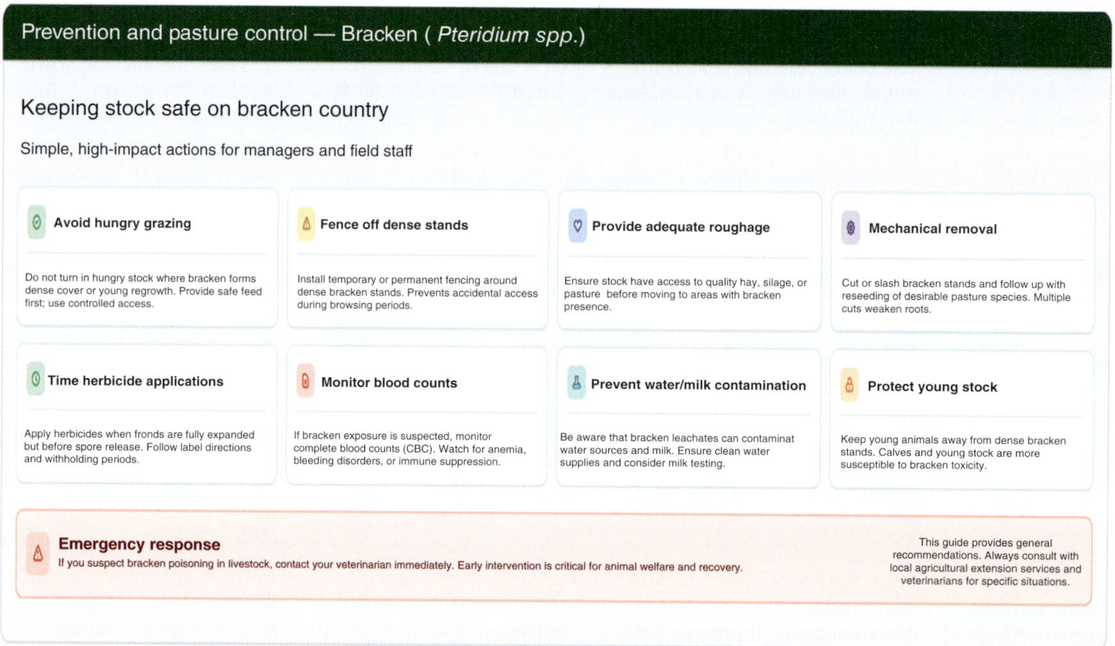

Figure 9.39 Prevention and pasture control on bracken country. Practical management: avoid hungry grazing on dense stands; fence/remove bracken, re-grass, and monitor at-risk cattle (older animals) for intermittent hematuria. *Source:* Cope (2025b)/ Merck & Co.

Nitrate and Nitrite Poisoning

Nitrates and nitrites are water-soluble compounds. Nitrates (NO_3^-) are added to the soil to be used by plants to form their protein either through the use of fertilizers (e.g., ammonium and potassium nitrate) or the conversion of atmospheric nitrogen (N) by nitrogen-fixing bacteria. The plant protein is either utilized by the animals for their growth and development or is returned to the soil through decay. Nitrogen is again returned to the atmosphere and enters the cycle through the conversion of animal metabolic waste such as urea and ammonia to nitrites and/or ammonia. Thus, nitrate plays an important role in this animal–plant inter-relationship. For orientation to where livestock exposures emerge in this cycle, see Figure 9.40 (farm nitrogen cycle – exposure nodes: forage and water).

Sources

Nitrate and nitrite poisoning in domestic animals are due to the ingestion of water or plants high in nitrate content. Nitrates added to the soil through decaying organic matter, nitrogen fertilizers, or animal wastes leach into the groundwater and contaminate the well or reservoir. Water collected in a pond can also contain toxic levels of nitrates due to fertilizer runoff and may be an important source of nitrate

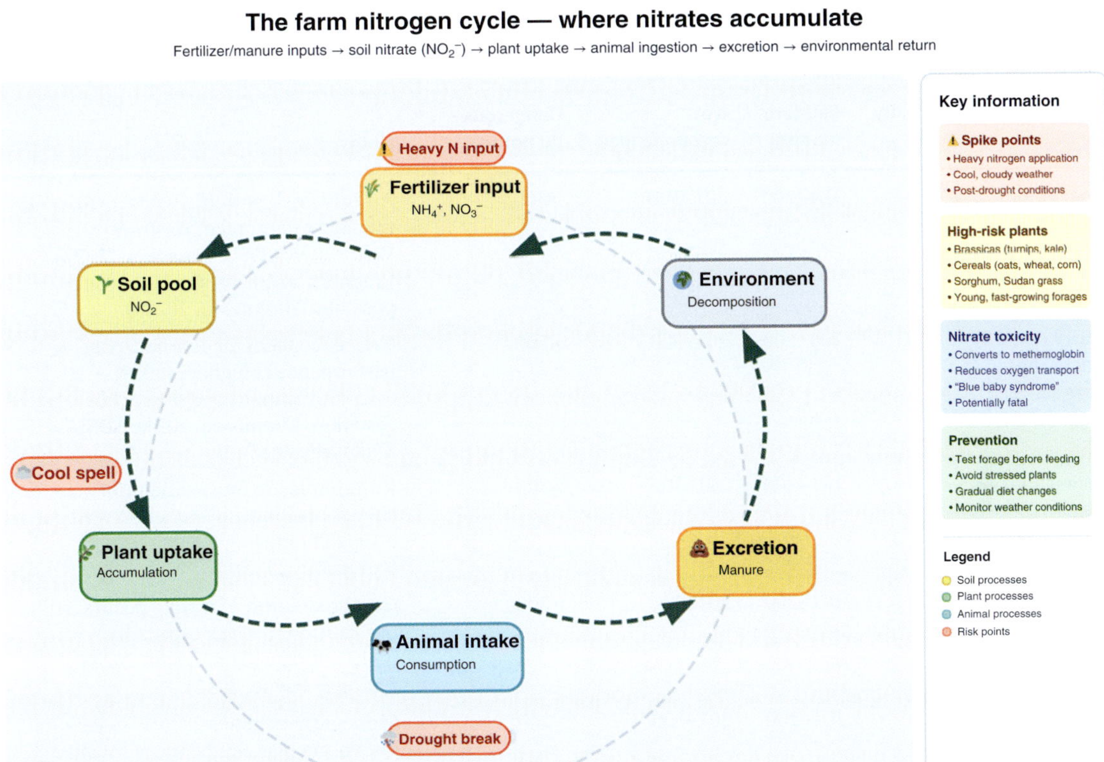

Figure 9.40 Farm nitrogen cycle – where toxic nitrate exposures arise. Illustrates fertilizer/manure inputs → soil nitrate pool → plant uptake, with two main livestock exposure nodes: (i) forage nitrate accumulation and (ii) groundwater/surface-water contamination via leaching/run-off. Also shows the return of N to the cycle (urea/ammonia) and how drought–rain whiplash or heavy N applications can transiently raise forage and water risk. Use this figure to orient field investigations before you dive into plant and water testing (introductory text; Gupta 2018; Thompson 2024b).

poisoning in farm animals (the leaching and runoff pathways are also highlighted in Figure 9.40). For drinking-water action bands by class of livestock, see Table 9.17.

Factors Influencing Nitrate Accumulation in Plants

Accumulation of nitrates by plants depends on several factors and has been reviewed in detail by Gupta, 2018; Thomson 2024b. A quick "risk windows" map that aligns with the points below is given in Figure 9.41.

Plant-Associated Factors

Taxonomical difference: Nitrate accumulation differs among species of plants and, in some cases, even among varieties of similar species (Gupta, 2018; Thompson 2024b). This difference is attributed to vartion in uptake and assimilation of nitrate.

Table 9.17 Water nitrate (NO_3–N) action bands by class of livestock – safe, caution, not recommended, dangerous – with notes on additive risk from high-nitrate forages.

Class of livestock	Generally safe	Caution/ monitor	Not recommended	Dangerous – do not use	Notes
Beef cattle	0–100	101–200	201–300	>300	Additive risk with high-nitrate forages; manage total intake (Rasby & Walz, 2025; SDSU Extension, 2022). Pregnant cows: avoid >100 where possible (Thompson, 2024a).
Dairy cattle (lactating/ pregnant)	0–100	101–200	201–300	>300	Greater concern for abortion/poor performance at higher intakes; err to the cautious end during late gestation (Thompson, 2024a; SDSU Extension, 2022).
Sheep and goats	0–100	101–200	201–300	>300	Ruminants are most susceptible; keep forage nitrate low when water >100 (Thompson, 2024a; SDSU Extension, 2022).
Horses	0–100	101–200	201–300	>300	Cecal reduction of nitrate occurs; still use caution if >100, especially with high-N forage (Thompson, 2024a; Zhang & Payne, 2017).
Swine	0–100	101–200	201–300	>300	Monogastrics generally less susceptible, but young pigs can be more sensitive; prefer ≤100 (Thompson, 2024a; Zhang & Payne, 2017).
Poultry	0–100	101–200	201–300	>300	Keep ≤100 where possible; avoid >100 if any additional stressors or poor water quality (Zhang & Payne, 2017).

Units are NO_3-N mg/L. To convert to nitrate ion (NO_3) mg/L, multiply by 4.4 (Merck Veterinary Manual – fish water quality tables).

Risk is additive across water + feed; when forage nitrate is elevated, treat the next stricter band as your action level (OSU Extension, 2017; SDSU Extension, 2022).

Pregnant stock/neonates: use stricter cutoffs; abortions have been reported after excessive nitrate exposure in cattle (Thompson, 2024a).

Source: Adapted from widely used U.S. extension guidance; units are mg/L NO_3–N; to convert to NO_3^- multiply by 4.43. References summarized in the footnotes of the uploaded table. Action bands were synthesized from widely used US extension guidance: safe ≤100, caution 100–300, and potentially toxic >300 mg/L NO_3-N (SDSU Extension, 2022; Minnesota Board of Animal Health, 2023). We split the "caution" band to flag 101–200 mg/L (monitor, balance with low-nitrate feed) vs. 201–300 mg/L (generally not recommended) and kept >300 mg/L as dangerous (Zhang & Payne, 2017; Rasby & Walz, 2025).

Part of plant: Nitrate concentration in plant tissues varies with the morphological parts (Most reports show the highest concentration in the stem. Normally, the lower portion of a plant tends to be higher in nitrate than the upper portion (Gupta, 2018; Thompson 2024b). The variation in nitrate content with plant parts appears to be associated with the site of nitrate reduction. Low nitrate reduction, which occurs in non-chlorophyllous tissue, accounts for the higher stem content compared to leaves.

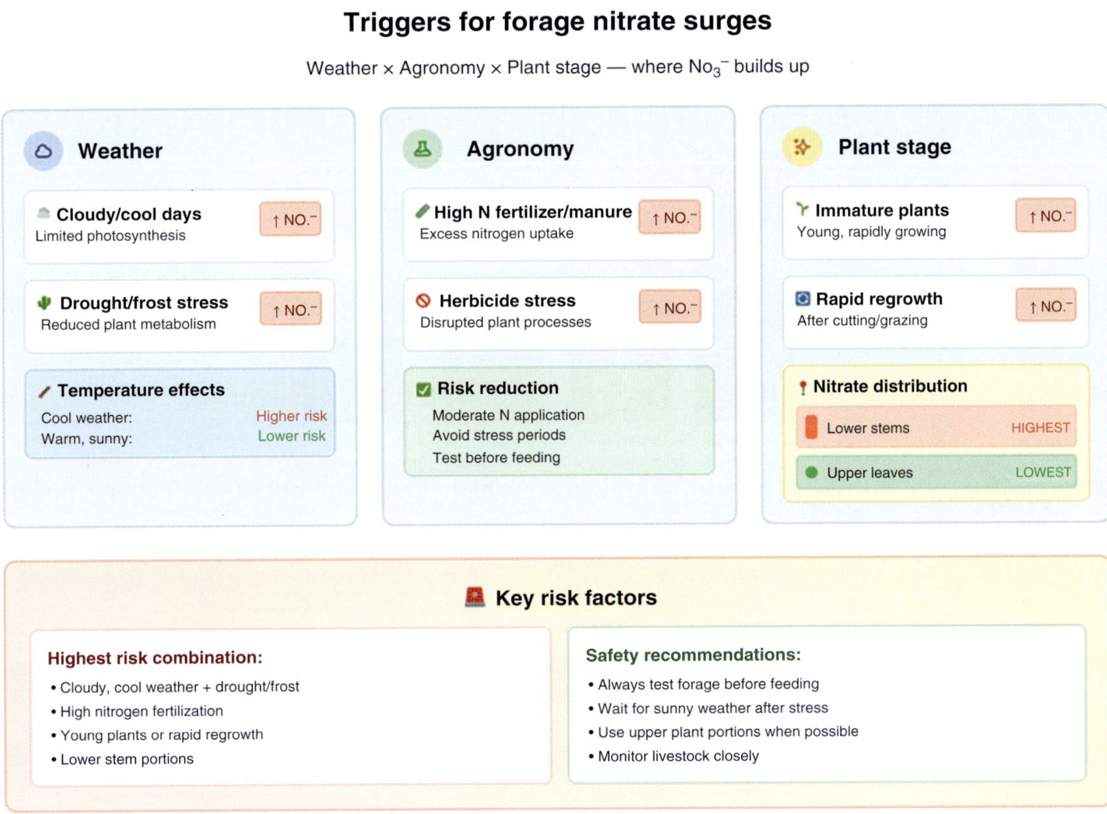

Figure 9.41 Why forage nitrate spikes – practical triggers. A quick "risk windows" map: heavy N fertilizer or slurry → rapid vegetative growth; cloudy/cool weather → reduced nitrate reduction in leaves; herbicide or drought stress → uptake without assimilation; and early-stage regrowth (pre-flowering) when plant demand and nitrate levels peak. These conditions often stack (e.g., drought followed by rain + high N), explaining sudden case clusters (Tucker 1971).

State of maturity: Nitrate content initially rises and then, after reaching its peak at about the flowering stage, declines as the plant matures. Nitrate content initially rises and then, after reaching its peak at about the pre-bloom (near-flowering) stage, declines as the plant matures (Tucker, 1971). The decline with maturity is due to greater dry-matter accumulation, high N demand for fruit/seed development, and waning soil N supply as the plant matures.

To help clinicians visualize which species, plant parts, and stages tend to run highest, refer to Figure 9.42; a concise list of nitrate-accumulating species with reported ranges is provided in Table 9.18.

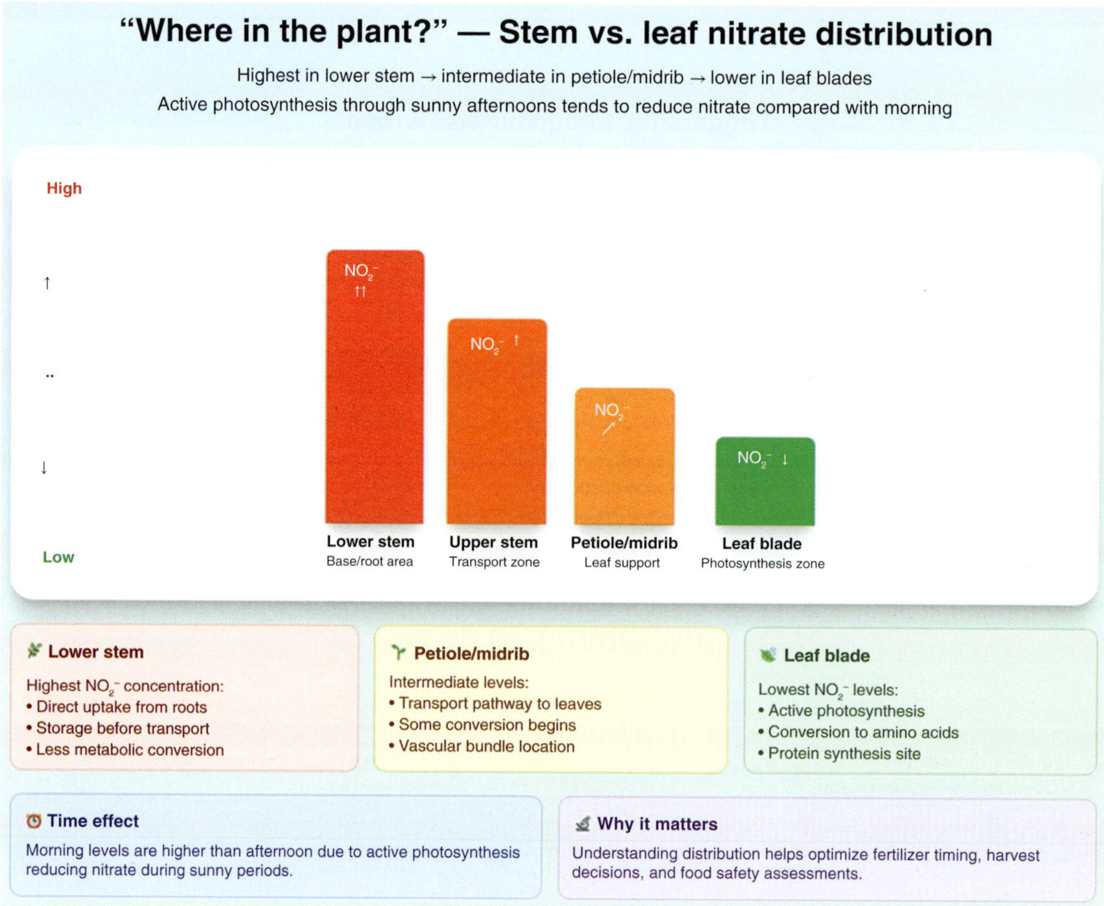

Figure 9.42 Where nitrate hides in the plant – stems and lower portions. Emphasizes that stems and lower plant parts typically carry higher nitrate than leaves/upper portions because non-chlorophyllous tissues have less nitrate-reductase activity. When sampling, cut low and include stems to avoid underestimating risk; this also explains why immature, fast-growing stands test "hotter" (Gupta 2018; Thompson 2024b). Emphasizes higher nitrate in stems/lower plant parts vs. leaves/upper parts.

Table 9.18 Nitrate-accumulating plants (NO_3–N, ppm): field-implicated species with reported ranges. Useful when triaging pasture risk by species composition (e.g., amaranths, foxtails, Napier grass).

Species	NO_3–N (ppm)	References
Spiny amaranth (*Amaranthus spinosus*)	4150–11000	Gupta (2018); Thompson (2024b)
Bristly foxtail (*Setaria verticillata*)	2900–6000	Gupta (2018); Thompson (2024b)
Guinea grass (*Panicum maximum*)	1500–2600	Gupta (2018); Thompson (2024b)
Para grass (*Brachiaria mutica*)	2700–400	Gupta (2018); Thompson (2024b)
Wire grass (*Eleusine indica*)	740–4100	Gupta (2018); Thompson (2024b)
	3500–33400	Gupta (2018); Thompson (2024b)
Bermuda grass (*Cynodon dactylon*)	460–1100	Gupta (2018); Thompson (2024b)
Ageratum (*Ageratum conyzoides*)	450–3900	Gupta (2018); Thompson (2024b)
Napier grass (*Pennisetum purpureum*)	2800–44000	Gupta (2018); Thompson (2024b)

Environmental Factors

Nitrogen supply: The content and form of soil nitrogen influence nitrate accumulation in plants. Plant nitrate is positively correlated with soil N supply (Gupta, 2018; Thompson 2024b) plant nitrate above ~0.15% is considered risky. Although most plants can use nitrate, nitrite, ammonium, and organic N, substantially higher plant nitrate levels are associated with nitrate fertilizers than with ammonium fertilizers at equivalent N amounts (Gupta, 2018).

Soil conditions: Acid soils, adequate moisture, low molybdenum, sulfur and phosphorus deficiency, and limited soil aeration favor nitrate uptake. Serious nitrate poisoning has been reported from drought-affected areas.

Other factors: Light, temperature, and herbicides can all increase accumulation; mechanisms vary and may stack (e.g., drought → rain + high N + cloudy days), explaining sudden case clusters. These stackable triggers are the ones highlighted in Figure 9.41.

Mechanism of Action

Nitrate ion per se is relatively nontoxic to mammals. The nitrate ion is readily absorbed and excreted by the kidney of the dog without ill-effects. Thus, the so-called "nitrate poisoning" is actually nitrite poisoning. Nitrate ions are readily reduced to nitrite ion in ruminants and herbivores, are rapidly absorbed, and cause toxicosis in these species. The nitrite ion oxidizes the ferrous (divalent) iron in hemoglobin to ferric (trivalent) forms, converting hemoglobin to methemoglobin. Since methemoglobin cannot carry oxygen, the affected animals develop hypoxia or anoxia and sudden death. Figure 9.43 shows this pathway at a glance, as well as the therapeutic target (reduction of MetHb).

Clinical Signs

Nitrate poisoning is usually acute and occurs within a few hours after ingestion of food or water containing high nitrate. Clinical signs appear when methemoglobin levels are about 40%, and affected animals normally die when levels reach 80–90%. Weakness, muscle tremors, staggering gait, severe dyspnea, and cyanotic mucous membranes were observed in nitrate-poisoned cattle (Gupta, 2018; Thompson 2024b). The affected cattle died in recumbency with a rapid weak pulse, severe respiratory distress, anoxia, and convulsions. Death is greatly influenced by stress and exertion. The blood becomes typically dark brown or "chocolate" colored (Gupta, 2018; Thompson 2024b). The affected animals also exhibit signs of abdominal pain, salivation, diarrhea, and frequent micturition – direct irritant effects of nitrate, especially those of non-plant origin. Figure 9.44 pairs the per acute time course with the classic "chocolate blood" look.

Pathophysiology

Nitrate- or nitrite-poisoned animals show characteristic signs related to anoxia and necropsy lesions related to severe methemoglobinemia. Cyanotic mucous membranes and dark brown, muddy, or chocolate-colored blood covering carcasses, gloves, and necropsy equipment are consistent findings. Variable petechial and ecchymotic hemorrhages of serosal surfaces (Gupta, 2018; Thompson 2024b) and congestion of the rumen or abomasum are also seen (Gupta, 2018). Nitrite and methemoglobin

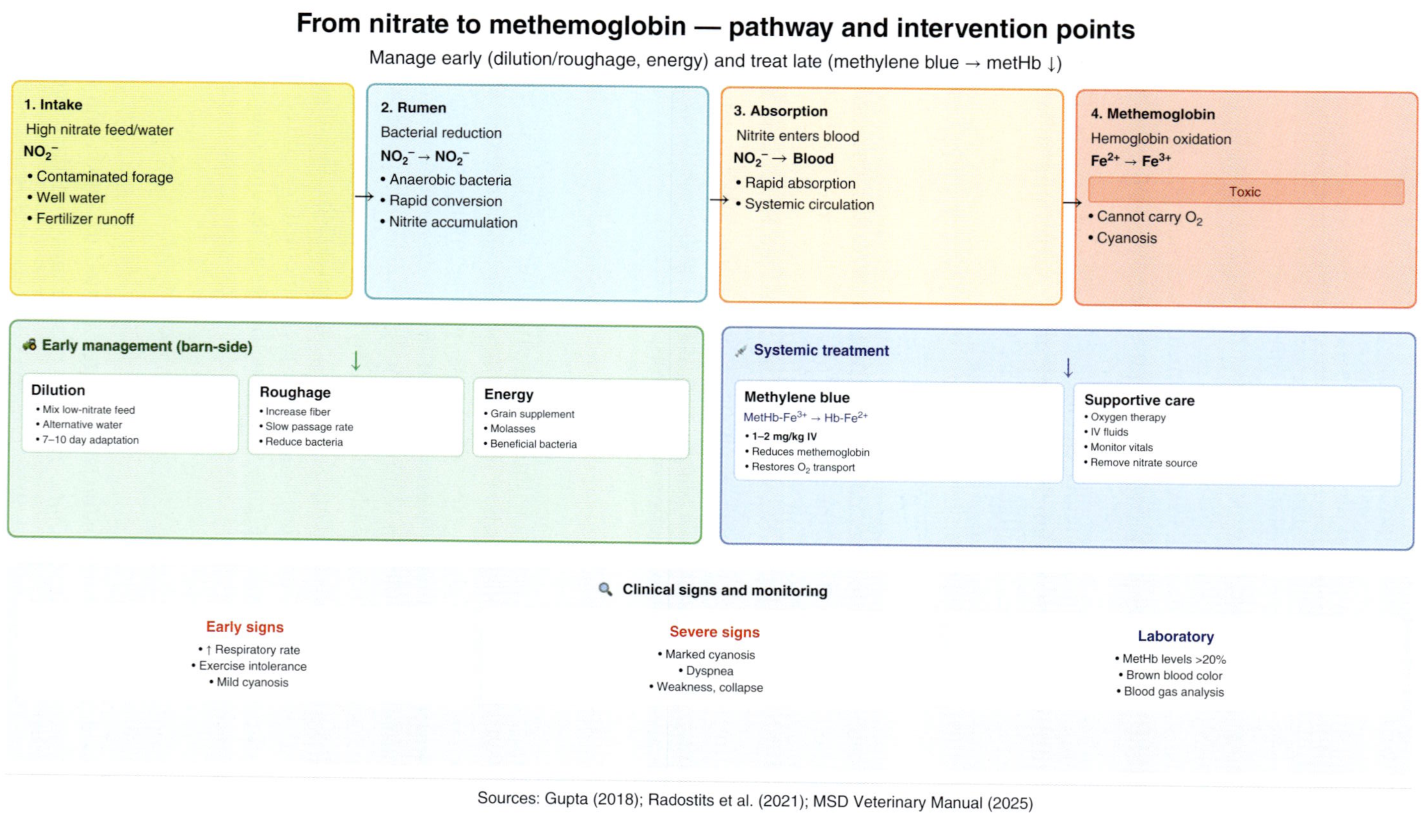

Figure 9.43 Nitrate → nitrite → methemoglobin: pathway and where treatment works. In ruminants, nitrate (NO_3^-) is reduced by rumen microbes to nitrite (NO_2^-), which oxidizes Hb(Fe^{2+}) to metHb(Fe^{3+}), impairing O_2 carriage and producing hypoxia; clinical signs appear around ~40% metHb, and death at ~80–90%. The diagram shows intervention points: remove the source, give methylene blue to reduce metHb back to functional Hb, and support oxygen delivery (Gupta 2018; Thompson 2024b).

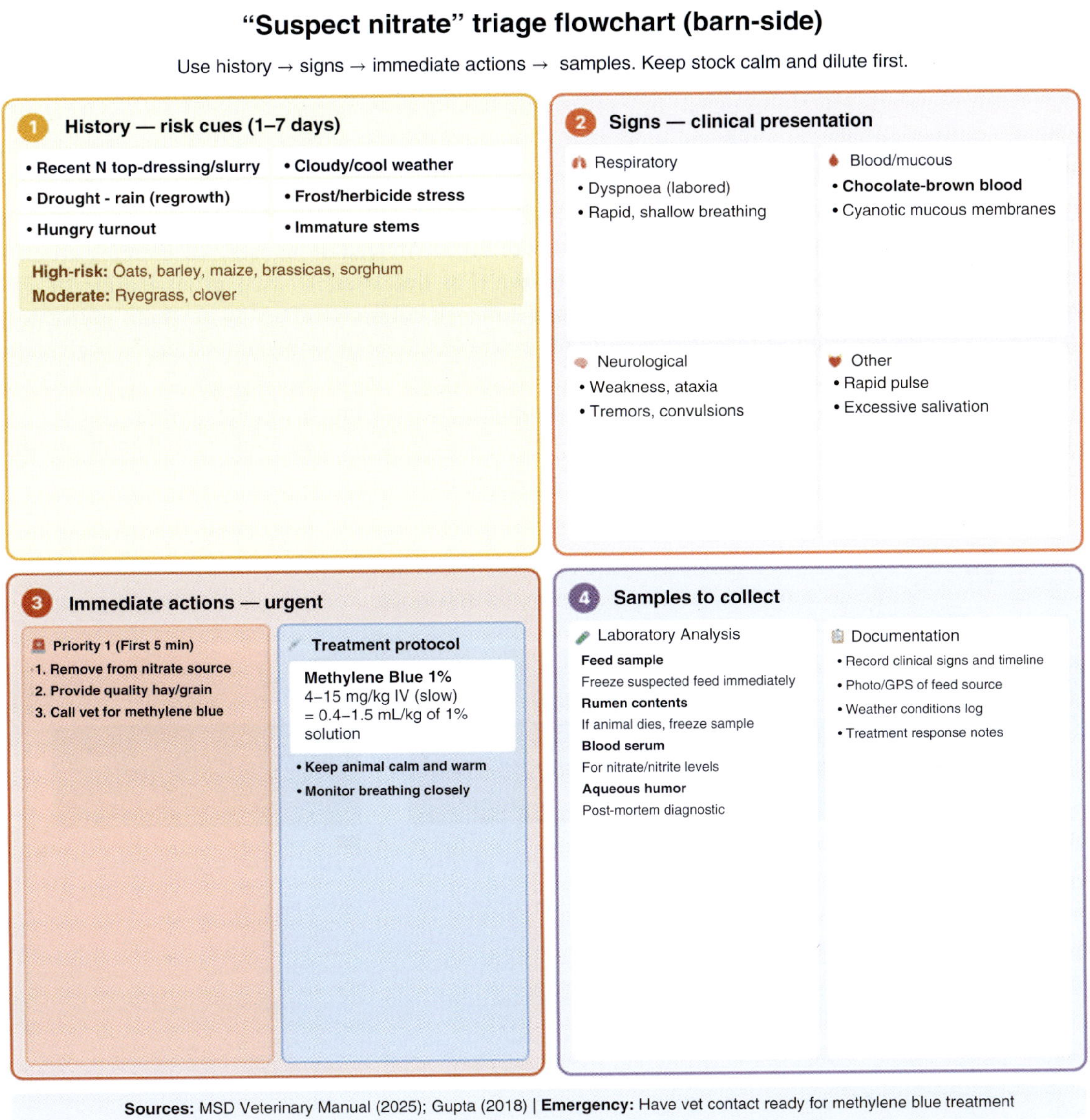

Figure 9.44 What to test, how to handle: barn-side screens and reference samples. Shows the field sequence – rapid plant screen (diphenylamine or commercial nitrate dipsticks), prioritized specimens (suspect forage, drinking water, ocular fluid, serum/EDTA), and preservation. Key handling messages: freeze feed/ingesta promptly; keep serum/ocular fluid cold; and remember nitrite/metHb kinetics (nitrite and metHb fall quickly in blood, while nitrate in urine and nitrite in chilled urine can remain detectable longer). *Source:* Gupta (2018) / with permission of Elsevier.

disappear rapidly from the circulation. Methemoglobin levels depend on serum nitrite. Nitrate is normally excreted in the urine when sublethal amounts are consumed; nitrite remains stable for up to 48 hours in stored urine samples.

Diagnosis

Confirmatory diagnosis of nitrate poisoning is based on the characteristic clinical signs, elevation of serum nitrite, methemoglobinemia, and high levels of nitrate in feed or ingesta. All samples submitted for nitrate/nitrite determinations must be frozen. For quick color-based prioritization of differentials at the crush-side, use Figure 9.45 (blood/mucosa color swatches – what each points to). A simple qualitative field test for the detection of nitrate or nitrite in suspected materials is given in Table 9.19.

When interpreting lab reports and preparing submissions, two practical aides follow: Table 9.20 provides unit conversions (NO_3^- ↔ NO_3-N; % ↔ ppm; water mg/L), and Table 9.21 lists diagnostic specimen handling (what to collect, how to preserve and ship).

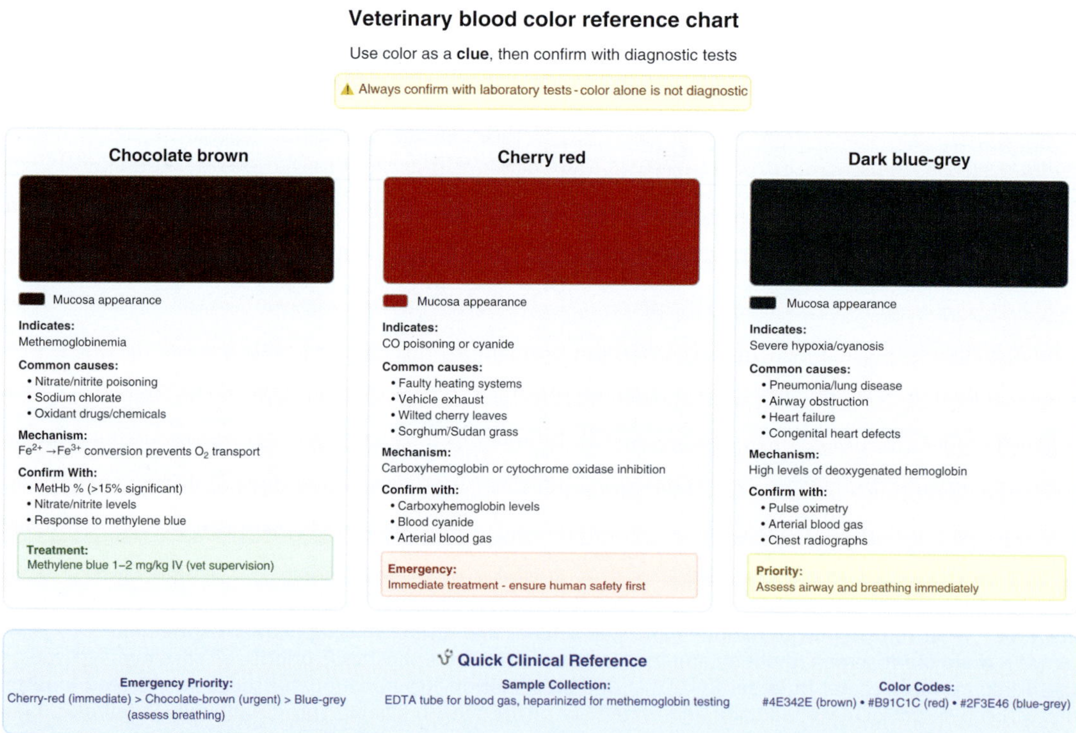

Figure 9.45 Differential blood/mucosa color swatches – rapid triage cues. Side-by-side reference for clinicians: chocolate-brown = methemoglobinemia (typical of nitrate/nitrite or sodium chlorate toxicosis); cherry-red = cyanide toxicity or carboxyhemoglobinemia; dark blue/gray = severe hypoxia/poor oxygenation. Use as a quick visual clue only – confirm with appropriate tests (e.g., metHb %, co-oximetry, cyanide assays) (Gupta 2018; Thompson 2024b).

Table 9.19 Qualitative barn-side tests for nitrate and nitrite (screening only).

Analyte	Field screening test (reagents and procedure)
Nitrate	1. Add 0.5 g diphenylamine in 20 mL of water. 2. Add sulfuric acid, q.s. to 100 mL. Cool the resulting solution store in a brown bottle. 3. Mix equal parts of the stock solution and 80% sulfuric acid. 4. Test suspected material by dropping one drop of reagent on the cut surface of the plant. 5. A color change from green to blue is positive reaction indicating more than 2% nitrate.
Nitrite	1. Reagents needed are: (i) sulfanilic acid (0.5 g in 150 mL of 20% glacial acetic acid) and (ii) α-naphythylamine hydrochloride prepared by dissolving (with heat) 0.2 g of the salt in 20% glacial acetic acid. 2. Add 2 mL of unknown sample to a test tube. Then add 2 mL of sulfanilic acid, followed by 2 mL α-naphytylamine. A pink to red color is positive for nitrites. The solutions applied to cut surfaces of plants in the same order will give a pink to red reaction if positive.

Step-by-step reagents and procedure for (i) the diphenylamine–sulfuric acid stem test for nitrate (one drop on a freshly cut plant surface; blue-green color change indicates a strongly positive reaction, historically used as a high-level screen) and (ii) a Griess-type reaction using sulfanilic acid and α-naphthylamine for nitrite (pink to red color in liquid samples or plant cuts signifies nitrite presence). Use as rapid presumptive screens only; confirm with quantitative laboratory analysis and handle suspect samples cold or frozen to limit ongoing microbial reduction/oxidation (see submission guidance in the chapter).

Table 9.20 Unit conversions at a glance (NO_3^- %, NO_3–N %, ppm; KNO_3^- NO_3^-). %↔ppm; NO_3–N↔NO_3^- (×/÷4.43); KNO_3 to NO_3^- and NO_3–N factors; worked examples; as-fed vs. DM notes (Gupta, 2018).

Conversion	Factor/ formula	Use it like...	Worked example
NO_3–N → NO_3^-	× 4.43	multiply NO_3–N by 4.43 to express as nitrate	1,000 ppm NO_3–N → 4,430 ppm NO_3^-
NO_3^- → NO_3–N	÷ 4.43	divide nitrate by 4.43 to express as NO_3–N	0.50% NO_3^- → 0.50 × 10,000 ÷ 4.43 ≈ 1,129 ppm NO_3–N
% → ppm	× 10,000	percent to parts per million	0.25% → 2,500 ppm
ppm → %	÷ 10,000	parts per million to percent	4,000 ppm → 0.40%
KNO_3 → NO_3^-	× 0.613	potassium nitrate to nitrate ion	1.0 g KNO_3 → 0.613 g NO_3^-
KNO_3 → NO_3–N	× 0.138	potassium nitrate to nitrate-nitrogen	1,000 mg KNO_3 → 138 mg NO_3–N
NO_3^- → KNO_3	÷ 0.613	nitrate ion to equivalent KNO_3 mass	620 mg NO_3^- → ~1,012 mg KNO_3
NO_3–N → KNO_3	÷ 0.138	nitrate-N to equivalent KNO_3 mass	100 mg NO_3–N → ~725 mg KNO_3
mg/L NO_3–N → mg/L NO_3^-	× 4.43	water reports	50 mg/L NO_3–N → 222 mg/L NO_3^-
mg/L NO_3^- → mg/L NO_3–N	÷ 4.43	water reports	300 mg/L NO_3^- → ~68 mg/L NO_3–N

Quick notes (for field use).

- Keep the **basis consistent** (as-fed vs. **dry matter**) when comparing forage results.
- In solids, **ppm ≈ mg/kg**; in water, **ppm ≈ mg/L** (at typical densities).
- The **4.43** factor comes from molecular weights: NO_3^- (62.0) / N (14.0) ≈ **4.43**.
- The **0.613** and **0.138** factors come from KNO_3 molecular weight ≈101.1: NO_3^-/KNO_3 = 62.0/101.1 ≈ **0.613**; N/KNO_3 = 14.0/101.1 ≈ **0.138**.
- Many labs report **NO_3–N** (especially in water). Always check the reporting form before applying thresholds (Gupta, 2018).

Standard analytical conversion factors summarized above (Gupta, 2018)/with permission of Elsevier.

Table 9.21 Diagnostic specimen handling for nitrate/nitrite: matrix, container/preservation, minimum volumes, and holding/transport recommendations from field to lab. Prioritizes freezing/rapid chilling to preserve nitrite, with ocular fluid and rumen contents highlighted for postmortem cases.

Matrix	Container and amount	Preservative	Temperature and storage	Hold time (maximum before analysis)	Notes (field tips)
Feed/forage (include stems and midribs)	Heavy-duty plastic bag for moist/green forage; paper bag for dry hay; aim ≥0.5–1 kg composite from multiple spots/bales	None	Moist/green: chill or freeze immediately; ship cold. Dry hay: room temperature in paper bag.	Same day or overnight; avoid warm transit for moist samples	Lower stems often have higher nitrate – take a representative composite and avoid storing moist forage warm in sealed plastic (University of Kentucky Veterinary Diagnostic Laboratory, 2022).
Water (the actual drinking source)	Clean plastic bottle (or lab kit bottle); fill and cap tightly; minimize headspace	Use lab-supplied preserved bottle if provided; otherwise none	Keep cold; ship with ice packs	Deliver to lab within ~24–30 h of collection (per lab/kit)	Flush lines; sample mid-flow; follow kit instructions (Penn State Agricultural Analytical Services Lab, 2023; Texas A&M Veterinary Medical Diagnostic Laboratory, 2024).
Rumen contents/ ingesta (PM or high-risk animal)	Leak-proof plastic jar/tube; double-bag	No additives (do not use formalin)	Freeze as soon as possible (refrigeration acceptable only for very rapid submission)	Submit as soon as possible; frozen samples maintain stability better	Supportive sample only – interpret alongside ocular fluid/plasma and suspect feed/water; rumen nitrate is not a reliable stand-in for dietary concentration (Missouri University Veterinary Medical Diagnostic Laboratory, n.d.-b; Thompson, 2024b).
Whole blood/ plasma; ± serum	Blood tubes; plasma (heparin) preferred antemortem; serum acceptable if required by lab	Standard anticoagulant for plasma; none for serum	Chill promptly; freeze if any delay (fresh whole blood is required if measuring methemoglobin)	Lab-dependent; contact the lab for specific limits	Plasma/serum nitrate is commonly used; check each lab's submission notes and panels (North Dakota State University Veterinary Diagnostic Laboratory, n.d.; Thompson, 2024b).

Table 9.21 (Continued)

Matrix	Container and amount	Preservative	Temperature and storage	Hold time (maximum before analysis)	Notes (field tips)
Ocular fluid (aqueous/ vitreous; PM)	Sterile syringe into plastic tube (≥1–5 mL; many labs accept 0.2–1 mL minimum) or submit whole eye	None	Refrigerate/ cold-pack; freeze if delay	Diagnostic window up to ~60 h postmortem (lab guidance); then keep cold or frozen	Preferred postmortem specimen for nitrate; collect ASAP and label side (Kansas State Veterinary Diagnostic Laboratory, 2015; Missouri University Veterinary Medical Diagnostic Laboratory, n.d.-a; Texas A&M Veterinary Medical Diagnostic Laboratory, n.d.; Guay, 2024

General footnotes (APA in-text):

- Plasma is preferred antemortem; ocular fluid is preferred postmortem; freeze specimens if analysis will be delayed (Thompson, 2024b).
- For water submissions, many programs ask for delivery within roughly 24–30 hours on ice (Penn State Agricultural Analytical Services Lab, 2023; Texas A&M Veterinary Medical Diagnostic Laboratory, n.d.; Guay, 2024).
- Forage: chill/freeze moist samples immediately; use paper bags for dry hay; ship overnight (University of Kentucky Veterinary Diagnostic Laboratory, 2022).
- Ocular fluid can remain diagnostically useful for ~60 hours after death; follow the receiving lab's collection/packaging instructions (Kansas State Veterinary Diagnostic Laboratory, 2015; Missouri University Veterinary Medical Diagnostic Laboratory, n.d.-a).

For one-look toxicant differentials by color/mechanism/first-aid, see Table 9.22; for a longer comparative list for teaching or QA checks, see Table 9.23.

A field outbreak example remains instructive: In one case of nitrate poisoning in cattle fed Napier grass, the average level of nitrate (NO_3^-) in the grass involved ranged between 28.3 and 44 mg/g, whereas the level from the "nontoxic" areas was 3.9 mg/g (Gupta, 2018; Thompson 2024b). Thus, that report agrees with Gupta (2018) that any pasture containing more than 10–15 mg/g of nitrate is potentially lethal to animals.

Treatment

The treatment of nitrate poisoning is directed toward converting methemoglobin back to hemoglobin – i.e., restoring the iron in hemoglobin to the divalent (Fe^{2+}) form. This is achieved by the intravenous administration of methylene blue 4 mg/kg in a 2–4% solution. Methylene blue is rapidly reduced to leukomethylene blue, which reduces methemoglobin ($Fe^{3+} \rightarrow Fe^{2+}$). The administration of methylene blue

Table 9.22 One-look blood/mucosa color differential in acute toxicoses, with mechanism and first-line treatment.

Toxicants	Blood color	Mechanism	Treatment
Nitrate/nitrite	Brown	Methemoglobinemia	Methylene blue
Sodium chlorate	Brown	Methemoglobinemia	Methylene blue
Cyanide	Cherry red	Cytochrome oxidases	Nitrite/thiosulfate inhibition
Carbon monoxide	Bright red	Carbon monoxide hemoglobin	Fresh air; oxygen + 5% CO_2
Carbon dioxide	Dark	Displacement	Oxygen; fresh air

Compact comparison of classic barn-side color cues and what they usually indicate:

- Chocolate-brown blood with cyanotic mucosae → methemoglobinemia from nitrate/nitrite or sodium chlorate; first-line therapy methylene blue (dose per text).
- "Cherry-red" blood → impaired oxygen delivery from cyanide (tissue hypoxia via cytochrome oxidase inhibition) or COHb from carbon monoxide; initial veterinary field antidotes for cyanide are nitrite/thiosulfate kits where indicated; for CO, oxygen (±5% CO_2 as per older guidance).
- Dark blood with asphyxial pattern → carbon dioxide displacement; oxygen/fresh air.

Use this table alongside the clinical course and source history; confirm with appropriate laboratory testing.

Table 9.23 Nitrate/nitrite (NO_3^-/NO_2^-) poisoning – extended quick-reference (teaching/QA).

Block	What to remember
Typical context/ triggers	Heavy N fertilizer/slurry, cloudy/cool spells limiting photosynthesis, drought → rain (lush regrowth), frost/herbicide damage, hungry turnout on immature stems; water from high-nitrate wells (Gupta, 2018; Thompson, 2024b).
Color cue	Chocolate-brown blood/mucosa → methemoglobinemia (Thompson, 2024b).
Mechanism (one-line)	Rumen microbes reduce $NO_3^- \rightarrow NO_2^-$; nitrite oxidizes Fe^{2+} (Hb) → Fe^{3+} (metHb), impairing O_2 carriage (Gupta, 2018; Thompson, 2024b).
Rapid clinical pattern	Dyspnea/tachypnea, weakness/ataxia, cyanosis, brown blood, sudden deaths; groups at pasture; pregnant stock at greater risk (Thompson, 2024b).
Immediate barn-side actions	Remove from source; feed hay/roughage first (dilute); keep calm/shaded; oxygen if available; start sampling (Gupta, 2018; Thompson, 2024b).
Specific therapy pointer	Methylene blue (MB) IV under veterinary supervision; many protocols start at ~4 mg/kg (1–4% solution) with one cautious repeat if needed (Thompson, 2024b; Gupta, 2018).
Priority samples (first hold)	Forage (include stems/midribs) and water – chill/freeze moist forage; whole blood/plasma antemortem; ocular (aqueous) fluid postmortem; label and ship cold (Thompson, 2024b; University of Kentucky Veterinary Diagnostic Laboratory, 2022).
Quick tests (field/ lab)	On-farm: stem-heavy composite + quick nitrate test (or picrate paper as a screen); lab: nitrate/nitrite in plasma/serum/ocular fluid, forage/water quantitation (Thompson, 2024b; University of Kentucky Veterinary Diagnostic Laboratory, 2022).
Key differentials to rule out	Cyanide (often cherry-red blood, peracute), urea/NPN (rumen alkalosis, ammonia odor), sodium chlorate/other oxidants (metHb + hemolysis) (Gupta, 2018; Thompson, 2024b).
Management to prevent relapse	Delay grazing after big N or rain/frost until several sunny days have passed, then test; prefer afternoon grazing; dilute high-NO_3 forage; consider ensiling but retest finished silage – reduction is variable (Gupta, 2018; Thompson, 2024b).
Residues/ regulatory note	MB use in food animals is extra-label in many jurisdictions – set milk/meat withholding per local policy (consult residue resources) (Thompson, 2024b).

One-page nitrate/nitrite quick-reference aligning context, color cue, mechanism, clinical pattern, first moves, therapy anchor, samples, tests, differentials, and prevention; color is supportive, not diagnostic – **confirm with tests** (Thompson, 2024b; Gupta, 2018).

Table 9.24 Methylene blue quick card (dose, repeat, caveats) for nitrate/nitrite methemoglobinemia.

Class/species	Dose and solution	Route and rate	Repeat	Key caveats and notes
Cattle (beef/dairy)	4 mg/kg IV as a 2–4% solution (start at 4 mg/kg) (Gupta, 2018; Thompson, 2024b).	Slow IV in sterile water or 0.9% NaCl; keep animals calm to limit O_2 demand (Thompson, 2024b).	If response is incomplete, repeat once after ~20–30 min; reassess exposure (Thompson, 2024b).	Remove source and dilute with hay; very high cumulative doses can worsen methemoglobinemia/hemolysis (Gupta, 2018; United States Pharmacopeial Convention/AAVPT, 2008).
Sheep and goats	4 mg/kg IV (2–4% solution); field recovery reported at 4 mg/kg (Simões et al., 2018; Thompson, 2024b).	Slow IV as above (Thompson, 2024b).	May repeat once after 20–30 min if needed (Thompson, 2024b).	Start low and monitor; provide fermentable carbohydrate to drive rumen nitrite → ammonia (Gupta, 2018).
Camelids (llama, alpaca)	Begin at the low end (~4 mg/kg IV) as a 2–4% solution; titrate cautiously (Thompson, 2024b).	Slow IV; minimize stress/exertion (Thompson, 2024b).	If required, one conservative repeat after 20–30 min with clinical reassessment (Thompson, 2024b).	Limited species-specific data – consider toxicologist input; control the source first (Gupta, 2018).

Start 4 mg/kg IV (2–4% solution), slow rate; may repeat once if needed; remove source; monitor for excessive cumulative dosing; residue/withholding cautions (Gupta, 2018; Simões et al., 2018; Thompson, 2024b; USP/AAVPT, 2008; FARAD, 2025).
Quick prep math. 1% = 10 mg/mL; 2% = 20 mg/mL; 4% = 40 mg/mL. Example: 4 mg/kg at 2% → 0.2 mL/kg (i.e., 20 mL/100 kg).
Residues and regulations (food animals). Use under a valid veterinarian-client-patient relationship (VCPR) and extra-label directions; set milk/meat withholding using local policy or FARAD (Food Animal Residue Avoidance Databank [FARAD], 2025).
Some references list wider ranges (e.g., up to 10–15 mg/kg in severe cases); many field protocols begin with 4 mg/kg and reassess (Gupta, 2018; Thompson, 2024b).

may be repeated because absorption of nitrate may continue from a full rumen. A quick-card for dose, preparation math, and cautions is provided in Table 9.24.

In addition to this, mineral oils should also be given orally to the affected animals to counteract the caustic effects of nitrate and accelerate its elimination through the feces. Ice-cold water may also be given to reduce rumen bacterial fermentation and release of nitrate from the plant materials.

Practical Prevention/Management Add-ons

Because many outbreaks follow management/weather events, two visual aids are included for day-to-day decisions: Figure 9.46 shows safe return-to-grazing timelines (after fertilizer, drought break, frost), and Figure 9.47 summarizes ensiling and nitrate – what fermentation fixes, and what it doesn't.

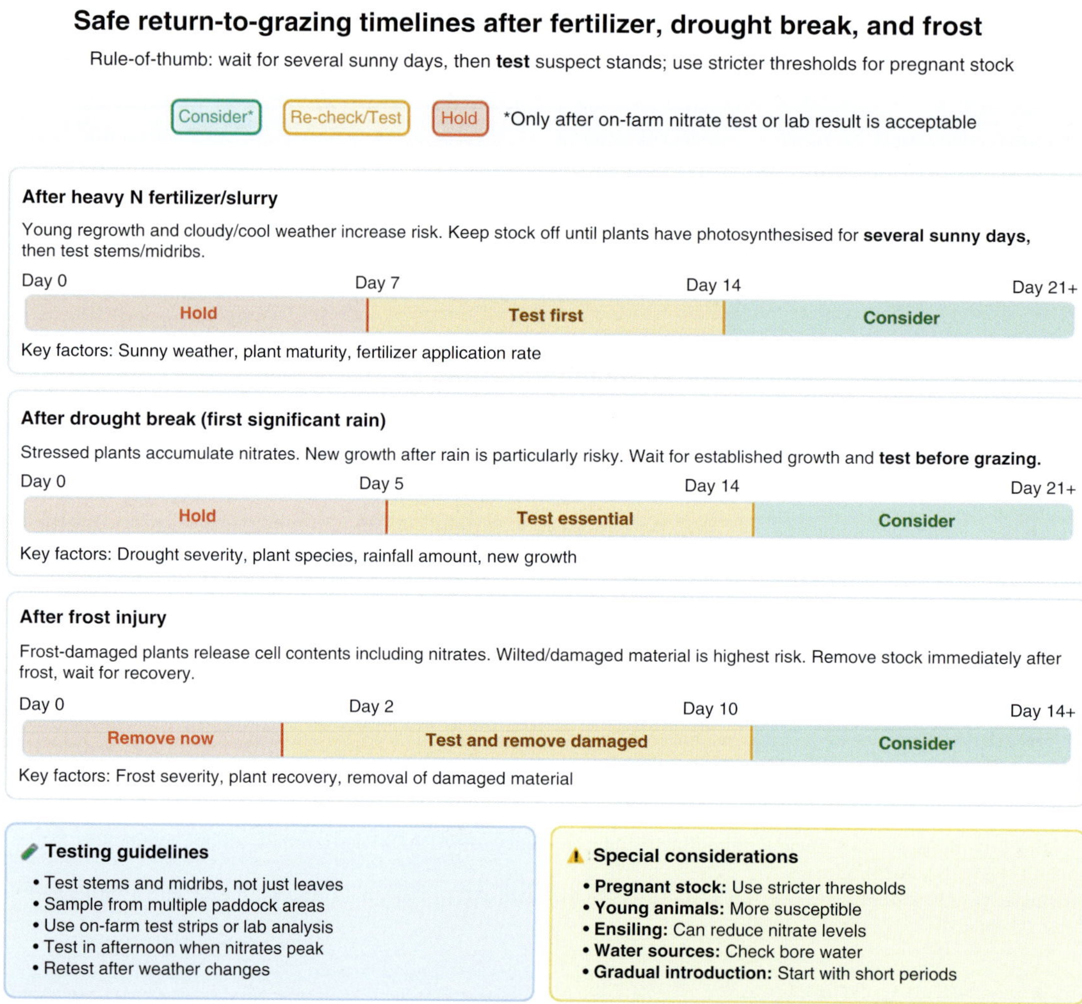

Figure 9.46 Safe return-to-grazing timelines after fertilizer use, drought break, and frost. Decision matrix showing conservative stand-down periods and when to test forage NO_3-N under three common spike scenarios: (i) recent nitrogen application (especially >50–100 kg N/ha), (ii) first green flush after drought, and (iii) post-frost regrowth. Notes added risks with cloudy weather and high-moisture forages; advises dilution, ensiling to completion (fermentation can reduce but not fully remove nitrate), and re-testing after weather changes. Adapted from synthesis on nitrate accumulation and plant stress responses (Gupta 2018; Thompson 2024b).

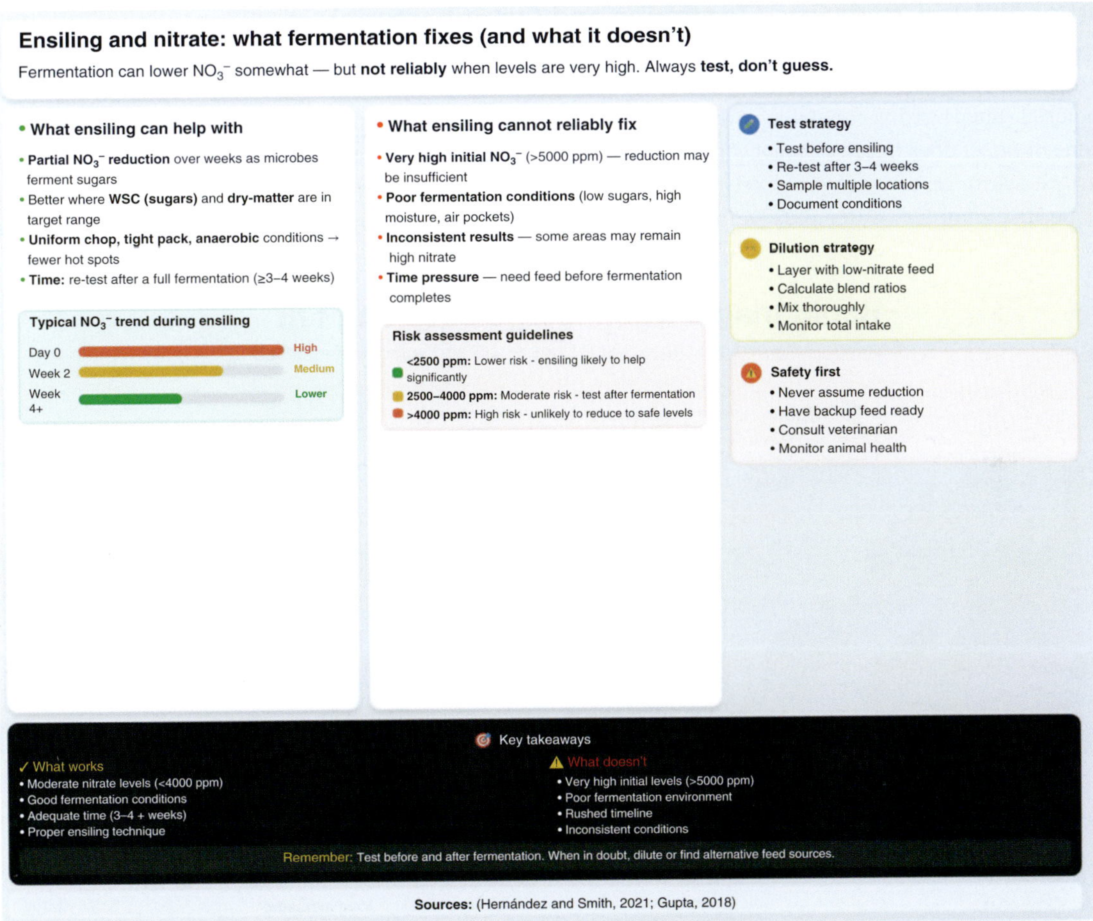

Figure 9.47 Ensiling and nitrate – what fermentation fixes (and what it doesn't). Conceptual pathway showing how proper ensiling can lower plant nitrate via microbial reduction ($NO_3^- \rightarrow NO_2^- \rightarrow NH_3$) during an anaerobic, well-packed, sealed fermentation, with typical but variable decreases after a full cure. Emphasizes limits: (i) early fermentation may transiently raise nitrite; (ii) poorly fermented/wet silage often retains hazardous nitrate; (iii) very high pre-ensiling nitrate remains unsafe after ensiling and requires dilution/reformulation; and (iv) finished silage must be tested before feeding. Notes good-practice levers (target DM, chop length, pack density, airtight seal, ≥3–6 weeks cure) and clarifies that nitrate risk is distinct from cyanide (prussic acid may dissipate with wilting/ensiling, but cyanide management follows separate guidance). Adapted from agronomic/toxicology syntheses on nitrate accumulation and forage conservation (Gupta 2018; Thompson 2024b).

Other Natural Toxicants (Zootoxins and Cyanobacteria)

While plant and fungal toxicoses dominate tropical practice, animal-origin toxins (zootoxins) and cyanobacterial (algal) toxins can drive per-acute losses and must stay in the differential – especially when the scene or onset does not fit a forage story (see Figure 9.48). Hot, still weather with nutrient-rich water and surface scum, or a witnessed/likely bite/handling event, are high-yield triage cues that immediately shape first samples (water plus scum; rumen/gastric contents; fresh/fixed liver) and on-farm controls

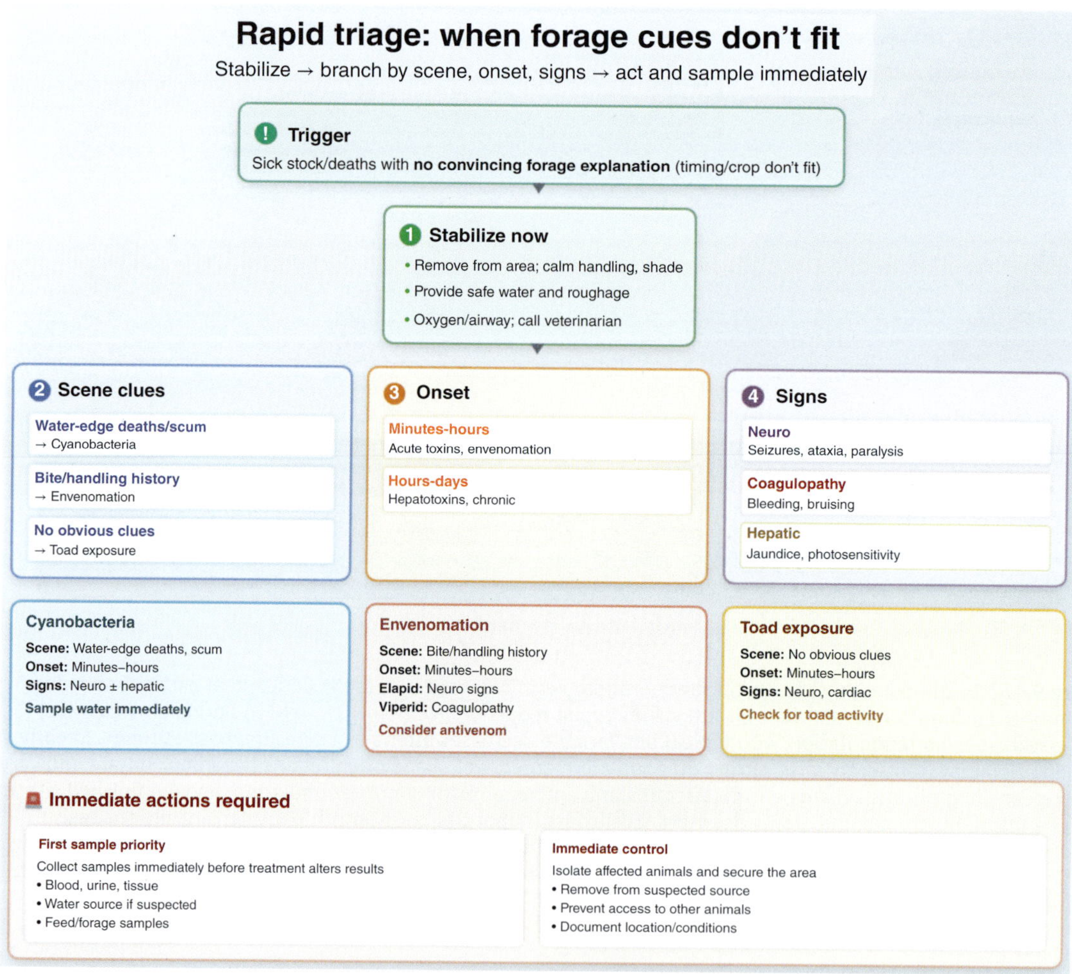

Figure 9.48 Rapid triage when forage cues don't fit. Flowchart for peracute toxicoses when typical forage patterns are absent. Branches on scene clues (e.g., water-edge deaths/scum; bite/handling history), onset (minutes–hours vs. hours–days), and dominant signs (neuro, coagulopathy, hepatic/photosensitization). Endpoints flag likely causes (cyanobacterial neurotoxins/hepatotoxins; elapid/viperid envenomation; toad exposure) with first samples and immediate controls. Adapted from standard veterinary guidance on algal poisoning, snakebite, and toad intoxication, and public health guidance on cyanotoxin sampling and risk control (Association of Public Health Laboratories, 2021; Gutiérrez et al. 2017; WHO, 2020).

(deny access; supply clean water; safe immobilization/antivenom pathways as indicated) (Association of Public Health Laboratories [Association of Public Health Laboratories], 2021; Bischoff, 2024; World Health Organization [WHO], 2020).

Zootoxins (Examples and Patterns)

Snakes (elapids/viperids): Expect rapid neuroparalysis/respiratory compromise (elapids) or coagulopathy/hemorrhage with painful edema (viperids). Typical scenes include paddock/yard encounters; look for fang marks, local swelling, or recumbency near the encounter site. Early priorities: scene safety, syndromic stabilization, coagulation monitoring, pain control, and antivenom when criteria are met (Gutiérrez et al., 2017; Gwaltney-Brant, 2024a).

Toads (bufotoxins): Profuse salivation, head shaking, vomiting, ataxia/seizures, arrhythmias; dogs are usual victims, but curious stock around troughs can be exposed. Immediate care: copious mouth/ocular rinsing (when safe), early decontamination, control of arrhythmias/seizures, thermoregulation, and strict removal of access to toads (Gwaltney-Brant, 2024b).

Field Sampling and Immediate Controls (Zootoxins)

Collect whole blood (complete blood count [CBC]/chemistry; PT/aPTT where viperid exposure suspected), urine (myoglobin/hematuria), and – if available – swabs from bite site before cleansing. Stabilize airway/breathing/circulation, use analgesia/sedation judiciously, and avoid aggressive wound manipulation (risk of further venom dispersion). Antivenom decisions are sign- and trend-based; document baseline coagulation parameters and reassess (Gwaltney-Brant, 2024a).

Cyanobacterial Toxins (Fresh/Brackish Water)

Warm, calm, eutrophic waters favor blooms; wind concentrates scum along margins where animals drink. Neurotoxins (anatoxin-a/-a(s), saxitoxins) cause tremors, fasciculations, dyspnea, and peracute collapse within minutes–hours; hepatotoxins (microcystins, nodularins) cause acute hepatic injury with potential photosensitization and high case fatality. First samples: bulk water (opaque/amber bottle, chilled), surface scum, rumen/gastric contents, fresh and fixed liver; chill/freeze promptly (some toxins are labile). Immediate controls: fence off suspect water; supply clean water; consider aeration/nutrient reduction; use algaecides cautiously (cell lysis → toxin release) (Association of Public Health Laboratories, 2021; Bischoff, 2024; WHO, 2020).

When to Suspect These Over Forage Toxicoses

Per-acute onset (minutes–few hours), multiple animals down near water, or dramatic neuro/respiratory signs → consider cyanobacterial neurotoxins (Association of Public Health Laboratories, 2021).

Acute hepatic crisis after scum exposure/weather shift → consider microcystins/nodularins (WHO, 2020).

Coagulopathy/local swelling (± fang marks) or rapid neuromuscular paralysis without a forage trigger → snake envenomation; hypersalivation + arrhythmias/seizures around troughs → toads (Gutiérrez et al., 2017; Gwaltney-Brant, 2024a; Gwaltney-Brant, 2024b) (Table 9.25).

Table 9.25 Zootoxins vs. cyanobacterial toxins – at-a-glance differential.

Group	Trigger/scene	Onset	Key signs (one-look)	Primary lesion/target	First samples to grab	Immediate controls (barn-side)
Elapids (cobras, kraits, mambas)	Snake encounter; little swelling at bite (kraits); night-time bites in sleeping animals/handlers	30 min–6 h (can be faster with high dose)	Cranial nerve palsies (ptosis, dysphagia), progressive flaccid paralysis, ± mild local pain (spitting cobras may cause ocular injury)	Neurotoxic α/β-toxins at NMJ (post-/pre-synaptic), ± PLA_2	Photo/ID of snake (if safe), serum, EDTA blood; wound swab for venom immunoassay where available; baseline CK	Airway/oxygen, pressure-immobilization bandage for slender-fang elapids (if trained), antivenom early when indicated; minimize movement; avoid cutting/sucking/tourniquets
Viperids (pit vipers, adders)	Snake seen; painful swelling and bruising at bite; pasture edges, rock piles	Minutes–hours	Severe local edema, hemorrhage, coagulopathy (oozing wounds), tachycardia, shock; possible neuro signs with some species	Vasculotoxic/hemotoxic; endothelial injury, DIC, myonecrosis	CBC, PT/aPTT, fibrinogen, type and crossmatch; site photos; serum CK; retained feed/water for QA	Antivenom if criteria met; IV fluids, analgesia (avoid NSAIDs if coagulopathy), limb support; do not use tight tourniquets or incision/suction
Toads (bufonids; cane toad)	Dog or stock mouthing toad near water/troughs; foamy salivation	Minutes (0–60 min)	Profuse salivation, head shaking, vomiting (pets), arrhythmias, ataxia/seizures; in livestock: drooling, collapse	Bufadienolide cardiac glycosides (Na^+/K^+-ATPase inhibition), catecholamine effects	Oral swabs/foam, gastric contents (early), ECG, serum K^+; identify toad if safe	Copious mouth rinse (water), activated charcoal if early and safe; control arrhythmias (e.g., lidocaine for V-tach, vet-directed), benzodiazepines for seizures; remove access to toads
Cyanobacterial neurotoxins (anatoxin-a, anatoxin-a(s), saxitoxins)	Warm, eutrophic ponds; scums/pea-soup water; calm sunny run → animals drink at margins	Minutes–hours	Tremors, fasciculations, hypersalivation, dyspnea; rapid respiratory paralysis/death in heavy exposures	NMJ/ion channel targets: nicotinic agonist (anatoxin-a), AChE inhibitor (anatoxin-a(s)), Na^+ channel block (saxitoxins)	Water (dark bottle, cold), scum mat, rumen/gastric contents; vomitus; whole blood for gases	Fence off water, provide alternate supply; oxygen/ventilation as available; atropine may help muscarinic signs with anatoxin-a(s); otherwise supportive; notify lab/public health
Cyanobacterial hepatotoxins (microcystins, nodularins)	Same ponds/lagoons; bloom die-off or wind-blown scums	Hours–1–2 d	Depression, anorexia, vomiting/diarrhea, shock, later photosensitization; high case fatality	Acute hepatic necrosis (centrilobular→massive), hemorrhagic liver; inhibits PP1/PP2A	Serum chem (ALT/AST, bilirubin, PT/aPTT); liver (fresh and fixed), water/scum; rumen contents	Remove water access, aggressive IV fluids, hepatoprotective/supportive care; activated carbon/cholestyramine if early; shade; report bloom and warn neighbors

AChE, acetylcholinesterase; CK, creatine kinase; NMJ, neuromuscular junction; PLA_2, phospholipase A_2; PT/aPTT, prothrombin time/activated partial thromboplastin time.
Fast field differential using scene + onset + one-look signs to sort snake/toad envenoming from cyanobacterial neurotoxins vs. hepatotoxins, with primary target, first samples, and immediate barn-side controls summarized (Association of Public Health Laboratories, 2021; WHO 2020).

References

Abdullah, A. S. (1994). Natural toxicants affecting animal health and production (Inaugural lecture, Universiti Pertanian Malaysia). Available at: http://psasir.upm.edu.my/id/eprint/1116/1/LG_396_P4_S981_no.11.pdf

Adams, L. G., Dollahite, J. W., Romane, W. M., Bullard, T. L., & Bridges, C. H. (1969). Cystitis and ataxia associated with sorghum ingestion by horses. *Journal of the American Veterinary Medical Association, 155*(3), 518–524. PMID: 5816060.5816060

Adaska, J. M., Rimoldi, G., Blanchard, P. C., Champagne, J., Poppenga, R. H., & Mostrom, M. (2018). Multiple episodes of 1080 (sodium monofluoroacetate) intoxication in a California calf-raising operation. *Journal of Veterinary Diagnostic Investigation, 30*(5), 747–751. https://doi.org/10.1177/1040638718781435

Allison, M. J., Mayberry, W. R., Mcsweeney, C. S., & Stahl, D. A. (1992). Synergistes jonesii, gen. nov., sp.nov. : A Rumen Bacterium That Degrades Toxic Pyridinediols. *Systematic and Applied Microbiology, 15*(4), 522-529. https://doi.org/10.1016/s0723-2020(11)80111-6

Alshannaq, A., & Yu, J.-H. (2017). Occurrence, Toxicity, and Analysis of Major Mycotoxins in Food. *International Journal of Environmental Research and Public Health, b*(6), 632. https://doi.org/10.3390/ijerph14060632

Arnold, M. 2021, 'FAQs about cyanide or "prussic acid" poisoning in ruminants', Ohio *BEEF* Cattle Letter, Ohio State University Extension Beef Team, 3 Nov 2021, viewed 22 Jan 2026, https://u.osu.edu/beef/2021/11/03/faqs-about-cyanide-or-prussic-acid-poisoning-in-ruminants/

Association of Public Health Laboratories (APHL) 2021, *Cyanotoxins: A Guidance Document for Public Health Laboratories: Laboratory User Guide*, November 2021, APHL, Silver Spring, MD, viewed 22 Jan 2026, https://www.aphl.org/aboutAPHL/publications/Documents/EH_2021_Cyanotoxin_Guide.pdf

Avellaneda-Cáceres, A., Lee, S. T., Ruiz, Á., Sandoval, G. V., Colque-Caro, L. A., Cook, D., Aguirre, L. S., Uzal, F. A., & Micheloud, J. F. (2025a). Oxalate nephropathy in cattle associated with the consumption of *Megathyrsus maximus* in Argentina. *Journal of Veterinary Diagnostic Investigation, 37*(5), 813–816. https://doi.org/10.1177/10406387251336265

Bailey, E. A., Iyer, R. S., Stone, M. P., Harris, T. M., & Essigmann, J. M. (1996). *Mutational properties of the primary aflatoxin B1–DNA adduct. Proceedings of the National Academy of Sciences of the USA, 93*(4), 1535–1539. https://doi.org/10.1073/pnas.93.4.1535

Bajracharya, G. B., & Bajracharya, B.(2022). A comprehensive review on Nepalese wild vegetable food ferns. *Heliyon, 8*(11), e11687. https://doi.org/10.1016/j.heliyon.2022.e11687

Barth, A. T., et al. (1994). *Coffee Senna (Senna occidentalis) poisoning in cattle in Brazil. Vet Hum Toxicol., 36*(6), 541–545.

Bennett, J. W., & Klich, M. (2003). Mycotoxins. *Clinical Microbiology Reviews, 16*(3), 497–516. https://doi.org/10.1128/CMR.16.3.497-516.2003. PMID: 12857779

Bildfell, R., 2024. Pyrrolizidine Alkaloidosis in Animals (Seneciosis, Senecio Poisoning, Ragwort Toxicity). MSD Veterinary Manual (Professional Version). Reviewed/Revised Apr 2022; Modified Sept 2024. Accessed 22 Jan 2026.

Bischoff, K., 2024. Algal poisoning of animals. Merck Veterinary Manual (Professional Version). Reviewed/Revised Jul 2021; Modified Sept 2024. Available at: https://www.merckvetmanual.com/toxicology/algal-poisoning/algal-poisoning-of-animals (accessed 22 Jan 2026).

Bookbinder, L. 2024, 'Overview of photosensitization in animals', MSD Veterinary Manual (Professional Version), reviewed/revised/modified Mar 2024, viewed 21 Jan 2026, <https://www.msdvetmanual.com/integumentary-system/photosensitization/overview-of-photosensitization-in-animals>.

Buonvino, S., Arciero, I., & Melino, S. (2022). Thiosulfate-cyanide sulfurtransferase a mitochondrial essential enzyme: from cell metabolism to the biotechnological applications. *International Journal of Molecular Sciences*, *23*(15), 8452. https://doi.org/10.3390/ijms23158452

Burrows, G. E. (1981). Cyanide intoxication in sheep; therapeutics. *Veterinary and Human Toxicology*, *23*(1), 22–28. (PMID: 6789546)

Burrows, G. E., & Way, J. L. (1979). Cyanide intoxication in sheep: Enhancement of efficacy of sodium nitrite, sodium thiosulfate, and cobaltous chloride. *American Journal of Veterinary Research*, *40*(5), 613–617.

Carvalho, T., Pinto, C., & Peleteiro, M. C. (2006). Urinary bladder lesions in bovine enzootic haematuria. *Journal of Comparative Pathology*, *134*(4), 336–346. https://doi.org/10.1016/j.jcpa.2006.01.001

Centers for Disease Control and Prevention. (2024, September 6). *Ricin – Chemical fact sheet.*

Cope, R. B. 2024. Important poisonous plants of Australia. MSD Veterinary Manual (Professional Version). Reviewed/Revised Nov 2023; Modified Sept 2024. Available at: https://www.msdvetmanual.com/toxicology/poisonous-plants/important-poisonous-plants-of-australia (accessed Day Month Year).

Cope, R. B. (2025a). *'Cyanide poisoning in animals', Merck Veterinary Manual (Professional Version).* Merck & Co., Inc. reviewed/revised Apr 2021, modified Jul 2025, viewed 21 Jan 2026, https://www.merckvetmanual.com/toxicology/cyanide-poisoning/cyanide-poisoning-in-animals

Cope, R. B. (2025b). Bracken fern and other fern poisoning in animals. In *MSD Veterinary Manual (Professional Version).* Merck & Co., Inc. reviewed/revised modified Aug 2025, viewed 21 Jan 2026, https://www.msdvetmanual.com/toxicology/bracken-fern-and-other-fern-poisoning/bracken-fern-and-other-fern-poisoning-in-animals

Cornell University College of Veterinary Medicine. n.d.-a. *NST image database – image ID 11422.*

Cornell University College of Veterinary Medicine. n.d.-b. *NST image database – image ID 12385.*

CSIROpedia (CSIRO). 2015. Leucaena toxicity solution publications. Last updated 9 November 2015. Available at: https://csiropedia.csiro.au/leucaena-toxicity-solution-publications/ (accessed 22 January 2026).

Dalzell, S. A., Shelton, H. M., Mullen, B. F., Larsen, P. H., & McLaughlin, K. G. (2006). *Leucaena: A guide to establishment and management.* Meat & Livestock Australia Limited. ISBN 978-1-74191-013-1

Dalzell, S. A., Burnett, D. J., Dowsett, J. E., Forbes, V. E., & Shelton, H. M. (2012). Prevalence of mimosine and DHP toxicity in cattle grazing Leucaena leucocephala pastures in Queensland, Australia. *Animal Production Science*, *52*(5), 365–372. https://doi.org/10.1071/AN11236

De Angelis, A., Gasco, L., Parisi, G., & Danieli, P. P. (2021). A multipurpose leguminous plant for the Mediterranean countries: *Leucaena leucocephala* as an alternative protein source: a review. *Animals (Basel)*, *11*(8), 2230. https://doi.org/10.3390/ani11082230. PMID: 34438688

Diab, A. M., Salem, R. M., El-Keredy, M. S. A., Ali, G. I. E., & El-Habashi, N. (2018). Experimental ochratoxicosis A in Nile tilapia and its amelioration by some feed additives. *International Journal of Veterinary Science and Medicine*, *6*(2), 149–158. https://doi.org/10.1016/j.ijvsm.2018.09.004

Dzombak, D. A., Ghosh, R. S., & Wong-Chong, G. M. (Eds.). (2006). *Cyanide in Water and Soil: Chemistry, Risk, and Management.* CRC Press. https://doi.org/10.1201/9781420032079

EFSA Panel on Contaminants in the Food Chain (CONTAM). (2004). Opinion of the Scientific Panel on Contaminants in the Food Chain related to aflatoxin B_1 as undesirable substance in animal feed. *EFSA Journal*, *2*(39), 1–27. https://doi.org/10.2903/j.efsa.2004.39

EFSA Panel on Contaminants in the Food Chain (CONTAM). (2011). Scientific Opinion on the risks for animal and public health related to the presence of T-2 and HT-2 toxin in food and feed. *EFSA Journal*, *9*(12), 2481. https://doi.org/10.2903/j.efsa.2011.2481

EFSA Panel on Contaminants in the Food Chain (CONTAM). (2012b). Scientific Opinion on ergot alkaloids in food and feed. *EFSA Journal*, *10*(7), 2798. https://doi.org/10.2903/j.efsa.2012.2798

EFSA Panel on Contaminants in the Food Chain (CONTAM). (2017a). Risks to human and animal health related to the presence of deoxynivalenol and its acetylated and modified forms in food and feed. *EFSA Journal*, *15*(9), 4718. https://doi.org/10.2903/j.efsa.2017.4718

EFSA Panel on Contaminants in the Food Chain (CONTAM). (2017b). Risks for animal health related to zearalenone and its modified forms in feed. *EFSA Journal*, *15*(7), 4851. https://doi.org/10.2903/j.efsa.2017.4851

EFSA Panel on Contaminants in the Food Chain (CONTAM). (2018). Risks for animal health related to the presence of fumonisins, their modified forms and hidden forms in feed. *EFSA Journal*, *16*(5), e05242. https://doi.org/10.2903/j.efsa.2018.5242. PMID: 32625894

EFSA Panel on Contaminants in the Food Chain (CONTAM). (2023). Risks for animal health related to the presence of ochratoxin A (OTA) in feed. *EFSA Journal*, *21*(11), 8375. https://doi.org/10.2903/j.efsa.2023.8375

EFSA Panel on Contaminants in the Food Chain (CONTAM). (2024). Risks for animal health related to the presence of ergot alkaloids in feed. *EFSA Journal*, *22*(1), e8496. https://doi.org/10.2903/j.efsa.2024.8496

Fernández, M., Pérez, V., Fuertes, M., Benavides, J., Espinosa, J., Menéndez, J., García-Pérez, A. L., & Ferreras, M. C. (2021). Pathological study of facial eczema (Pithomycotoxicosis) in Sheep. *Animals*, *11*(4), 1070. https://doi.org/10.3390/ani11041070

Flora of Pennsylvania. (n.d.). Pteridium aquilinum (bracken fern). *Flora of Pennsylvania*. viewed 22 Jan 2026, https://www.paenflowered.org/apgii/polypodiales/dennstaedtiaceae/pteridium/pteridium-aquilinum

Food Animal Residue Avoidance Databank (FARAD). 2025. *Food Animal Residue Avoidance Databank (FARAD)*. Updated 30 June 2025. (accessed 21 January 2026).

Food Standards Australia New Zealand (FSANZ) 2005, Cyanogenic glycosides in cassava and bamboo shoots: a human health risk assessment (Technical Report Series No. 28), FSANZ, Canberra, viewed 21 Jan 2026, https://www.foodstandards.gov.au/sites/default/files/publications/Documents/28_Cyanogenic_glycosides.pdf.

FutureBeef. (2017, July 19; reviewed 2025, July 15). Leucaena rumen inoculum – composition and activity. FutureBeef. Available at: https://futurebeef.com.au/resources/leucaena-rumen-inoculum-composition-activity/ (accessed 15 January 2026).

FutureBeef. (2022, November 18). Leucaena inoculum for cattle. FutureBeef. Available at: https://futurebeef.com.au/resources/leucaena-inoculum/ (accessed 21 January 2026).

Garland, T. 2024, 'Gossypol poisoning in animals', MSD Veterinary Manual (Professional Version), Merck & Co., Inc., Rahway, NJ, USA, reviewed/revised Oct 2020, modified Sept 2024, viewed 21 Jan 2026, https://www.msdvetmanual.com/toxicology/poisonous-plants/gossypol-poisoning-in-animals

Gleadow, R. M., & Møller, B. L. (2014). Cyanogenic glycosides: synthesis, physiology, and phenotypic plasticity. *Annual Review of Plant Biology*, *65*, 155–185. https://doi.org/10.1146/annurev-arplant-050213-040027. PMID:24579992

Graham, S. R., Dalzell, S. A., Nguyen, T. N., Davis, C. K., Greenway, D., McSweeney, C. S., & Shelton, H. M. (2013). Efficacy, persistence and presence of *Synergistes jonesii* in cattle grazing leucaena in Queensland: on-farm observations pre- and post-inoculation. *Animal Production Science*, *53*(10), 1065–1074. https://doi.org/10.1071/AN12301

Gruss, S.M., Johnson, K.D. , Johnson, S.K., Holman, J.D., Obour, A., Aiken, R.A. & Tuinstra, M.R. 2022, Managing the Prussic Acid Hazard in Sorghum (MF3607), Kansas State University Agricultural Experiment Station and Cooperative Extension Service, *Kansas State University, published June 2022, viewed*22Jan 2026, https://bookstore.ksre.ksu.edu/pubs/managing-the-prussic-acid-hazard-in-sorghum_MF3607.pdf

Guay, M. (2024). *Avoid nitrate toxicity with routine testing*. Texas A&M Veterinary Medical Diagnostic Laboratory (TVMDL), 11 October. Available at: https://tvmdl.tamu.edu/avoid-nitrate-toxicity-with-routine-testing/. (accessed 22 January 2026)

Gupta, R. C. (Ed.). (2018). *Veterinary toxicology: Basic and clinical principles* (3rd ed.). Academic Press.

Gutiérrez, J. M., Calvete, J. J., Habib, A. G., Harrison, R. A., Williams, D. J., & Warrell, D. A. (2017). Snakebite envenoming. *Nature Reviews Disease Primers*, *3*, 17063. https://doi.org/10.1038/nrdp.2017.63. PMID: 28905944

Gwaltney-Brant, S. M. (2024a). *'Snakebites in animals', Merck Veterinary Manual (Professional Version).* Merck & Co., Inc. reviewed/revised Jan 2022, modified Sept 2024, viewed 21 Jan 2026, https://www.merckvetmanual.com/toxicology/snakebite/snakebites-in-animals

Gwaltney-Brant, S. M. (2024b). *'Toad poisoning in dogs and cats', Merck Veterinary Manual (Professional Version).* Merck & Co., Inc. reviewed/revised Jan 2022, modified Sept 2024, viewed 21 Jan 2026, https://www.merckvetmanual.com/toxicology/toad-poisoning/toad-poisoning-in-dogs-and-cats

Hammond, A. C. (1995). Leucaena toxicosis and its control in ruminants. *Journal of Animal Science*, *73*(5), 1487–1492. https://doi.org/10.2527/1995.7351487x. PMID: 7665380

Haque, M. R., & Bradbury, J. H. (2002). Total cyanide determination of plants and foods using the picrate and acid hydrolysis methods. *Food Chemistry*, *77*(1), 107–114. https://doi.org/10.1016/S0308-8146(01)00313-2

Hatzade, R. I., Salve, P. D., Waghmare, S. P., & Bhikane, A. U. (2020). Management of clinical case of subabul (*Leucaena leucocephala*) poisoning in a goat kid. *The Pharma Innovation Journal*, *2020*(9), 11S, 98–100S.

Hirono, I., Ito, M., Yagyu, S., Haga, M., Wakamatsu, K., Kishikawa, T., Nishikawa, O., Yamada, K., Ojika, M., & Kigoshi, H. (1993). Reproduction of Progressive Retinal Degeneration(Bright Blindness) in Sheep by Administration of Ptaquiloside Contained in Bracken. *Journal of Veterinary Medical Science*, *55*(6), 979-983. https://doi.org/10.1292/jvms.55.979

Hirono, I., Kono, Y., Takahashi, K., Yamada, K., Niwa, H., Ojika, M., Kigoshi, H., Niiyama, K., & Uosaki, Y. (1984. *Veterinary Record*, *115*(15), 375–378.

Holman, J., Roozeboom, K.L., Mengel, D.B. & Blasi, D.A. 2012, Prussic Acid Poisoning (MF3040), *Kansas State University Agricultural Experiment Station and Cooperative Extension Service, published Mar 2012, viewed*22Jan 2026, https://bookstore.ksre.ksu.edu/pubs/prussic-acid-poisoning_MF3040.pdf

Jerry, C. 2024, *Poisonings in Poultry*, Merck Veterinary Manual (Professional Version). Reviewed/Revised Jan 2024; Modified Sept 2024.

Jindal, N., Mahipal, S. K., & Mahajan, N. K. (1993). Occurrence of aflatoxin in compound poultry feeds in Haryana and effect of different storage conditions on its production. *Indian Journal of Animal Sciences*, *63*, 71–73.

Joint FAO/WHO Food Standards Programme, Codex Committee on Contaminants in Foods (CCCF). 2019. Discussion paper on the establishment of MLs for HCN in cassava and cassava-based products and occurrence of mycotoxins in these products. CX/CF 19/13/14. 13th Session, Yogyakarta, Indonesia, 29 April–3 May 2019.

Jones, R. J., & Megarrity, R. G. (1986). Successful transfer of DHP-degrading bacteria from Hawaiian goats to Australian ruminants to overcome the toxicity of leucaena. *Australian Veterinary Journal*, *63*(8), 259–262. https://doi.org/10.1111/j.1751-0813.1986.tb02990.x. PMID: 3790013

Kansas State University Research and Extension 2022. Managing the prussic acid hazard in sorghum (MF3607).

Kansas State Veterinary Diagnostic Laboratory (KSVDL) 2015, 'Bovine nitrate sampling', Diagnostic Insights (March 2015 issue), Kansas State University, viewed 21 Jan 2026, <https://www.ksvdl.org/resources/news/diagnostic_insights/march2015/Bovine_Nitrate_Sampling.html>.

K-State Agronomy eUpdate. (2022, July 14). *Managing the prussic acid hazard in sorghum.*

Lajis, N. H., Abdullah, A. S., Salim, S. J., Bremner, J. B., & Khan, M. N. (1993). Epi-sarsasapogenin and epi-smilagenin: two sapogenins isolated from the rumen content of sheep intoxicated by *Brachiaria decumbens*. *Steroids*, *58*(8), 387–389. https://doi.org/10.1016/0039-128X(93)90043-M

Leong, L. E. X., Spittal, M. J., Hefford, M. A., & Pernthaner, A. (2017). Fluoroacetate in plants: distribution, toxicity to livestock, and microbial detoxification – a review. *Journal of Animal Science and Biotechnology*, *8*, 55. https://doi.org/10.1186/s40104-017-0180-6. PMID:28674607

Low, S. G. (2015). Signal grass (Brachiaria decumbens) toxicity in grazing ruminants. *Agriculture*, *5*(4), 971–990. https://doi.org/10.3390/agriculture5040971

Lozano, M. C., Martinez, N. M., & Diaz, G. J. (2017). Content of the Saponin Protodioscin in Brachiaria spp. from the Eastern Plains of Colombia. *Toxins*, *9*(7), 220. https://doi.org/10.3390/toxins9070220. PMID: 28703748

Malir, F., Ostry, V., Pfohl-Leszkowicz, A., & Novotna, E. (2013). Ochratoxin A: developmental and reproductive toxicity—an overview. *Birth Defects Research Part B: Developmental and Reproductive Toxicology*, *98*(6), 493–502. https://doi.org/10.1002/bdrb.21091

Mannaa, M., & Kim, K. D. (2017). Influence of Temperature and Water Activity on Deleterious Fungi and Mycotoxin Production during Grain Storage. *Mycobiology*, *45*(4), 240–254. https://doi.org/10.5941/MYCO.2017.45.4.240. PMID: 29371792

McGlone, M. S., Wilmshurst, J. M., & Leach, H. M. (2005). An ecological and historical review of bracken (*Pteridium esculentum*) in New Zealand. *New Zealand Journal of Ecology*, *29*(2), 165–184, viewed 22 Jan 2026. https://newzealandecology.org/nzje/2269.pdf

Merck KGaA (Sigma-Aldrich). (2018). *70185 Czapek Dox Agar (data sheet).* Merck KGaA.

Minnesota Board of Animal Health n.d., Guidance on nitrates in livestock water supply, Minnesota Board of Animal Health, Saint Paul, MN.

Missouri University Veterinary Medical Diagnostic Laboratory n.d.-a, 'Nitrate in ocular fluid', MU VMDL (Analytical Chemistry and Toxicology), viewed 21 Jan 2026, https://vmdl.missouri.edu/toxicology/nitrate-in-ocular-fluid/.

Missouri University Veterinary Medical Diagnostic Laboratory n.d.-b, 'Sample collection – Toxicology', MU VMDL, viewed 21 Jan 2026, https://vmdl.missouri.edu/sample-collection-toxicology/.

Mostrom, M.S. 2024, 'Mycotoxin-associated estrogenism and vulvovaginitis in animals', MSD Veterinary Manual (Professional Version), Merck & Co., Inc., reviewed/revised Nov 2021, modified Sept 2024, viewed 21 Jan 2026, https://www.msdvetmanual.com/toxicology/mycotoxicoses/mycotoxin-associated-estrogenism-and-vulvovaginitis-in-animals

National Toxicology Program 2024, 'Bone marrow – Gelatinous transformation', NTP Nonneoplastic Lesion Atlas, National Institute of Environmental Health Sciences, last updated 24 May 2024, viewed 21 Jan 2026, <https://ntp.niehs.nih.gov/atlas/nnl/hematopoietic-system/bone-marrow/GelatinousTransformation>.

Ng, P. C., Hendry-Hofer, T. B., Brenner, M., Mahon, S. B., Boss, G. R., Maddry, J. K., & Bebarta, V. S. (2021). *Efficacy of oral administration of sodium thiosulfate in a large, swine model of oral cyanide toxicity. Journal of Medical Toxicology*, *17*(3), 257–264. https://doi.org/10.1007/s13181-021-00836-5

North Dakota State University Veterinary Diagnostic Laboratory n.d., 'Nitrate (Serum or ocular fluid)', NDSU VDL Tests, viewed 21 Jan 2026, https://www.vdl.ndsu.edu/tests/nitrate/.

Oklahoma State University Extension. (2017). *Prussic Acid Poisoning (PSS-2904).* Oklahoma State University Extension Fact Sheet. (accessed 21 January 2026)

Penn State Agricultural Analytical Services Laboratory, 2023. Livestock drinking water sample submission form (Rev. 06/23). The Pennsylvania State University. Available at: https://agsci.psu.edu/aasl/water-testing (accessed 22 January 2026).

Peterson, M. E., & Talcott, P. A. (Eds.). (2013). *Small Animal Toxicology* (3rd ed.). Elsevier/Saunders.

Petrikovics, I., Budai, M., Kovacs, K., & Thompson, D. E. (2015). Past, present and future of cyanide antagonism research: From the early remedies to the current therapies. *World Journal of Methodology*, *5*(2), 88–100. https://doi.org/10.5662/wjm.v5.i2.88

Pitt, J. I., & Hocking, A. D. (2022). *Fungi and Food Spoilage* (4th ed.). Springer. https://doi.org/10.1007/978-3-030-85640-3

Rasby, R. & Walz, T. 2025, Water Requirements for Beef Cattle (G2060), Nebraska Extension Publications (NebGuide), University of Nebraska–Lincoln, last revised 26 Feb 2025, viewed 21 Jan 2026, https://extensionpubs.unl.edu/publication/g2060/water-requirements-for-beef-cattle.

Richards, C., Zhang, H., Step, D.L. & Strickland, G. 2017, Prussic Acid Poisoning (PSS-2904), Oklahoma State University Extension Fact Sheet, *Oklahoma State University, viewed*22Jan 2026, https://extension.okstate.edu/fact-sheets/prussic-acid-poisoning

Riet-Correa, B., Castro, M. B., Lemos, R. A., Riet-Correa, G., Mustafa, V., & Riet-Correa, F. (2011). Brachiaria spp. poisoning of ruminants in Brazil. *Pesquisa Veterinária Brasileira*, *31*(3), 183–192. https://doi.org/10.1590/S0100-736X2011000300001

Ringot, D., Chango, A., Schneider, Y.-J., & Larondelle, Y. (2006). Toxicokinetics and toxicodynamics of ochratoxin A, an update. *Chemico-Biological Interactions*, *159*(1), 18–46. https://doi.org/10.1016/j.cbi.2005.10.106

Salam Abdullah, A., & Rajion, M. A. (1990). Signal grass (*Brachiaria decumbens*) toxicity in sheep: changes in rumen microbial populations and volatile fatty acid concentrations. *Veterinary and Human Toxicology*, *32*(5), 444–445. *(No DOI.)*

Salim, J. M., Lee, G. E., Salam, M. R., Shahimi, S., Pesiu, E., Jani, J. M., Horsali, N. A. I., Shahrudin, R., Nor, S. M. M., Chong, J. L., Mohamad, F., Raffi, A., & Nikong, D.(2020). A checklist of vascular plants and uses of some species for livelihood-making in Setiu Wetlands, Terengganu, *Malaysia. PhytoKeys*, *160*, 7–43. https://doi.org/10.3897/phytokeys.160.52946

Sandu, D., 2024. Aflatoxicosis in poultry. MSD Veterinary Manual (Professional Version). Reviewed/Revised Dec 2023; Modified Sept 2024. Available at: https://www.msdvetmanual.com/poultry/mycotoxicoses-in-poultry/aflatoxicosis-in-poultry (accessed 22 January 2026).

SDSU Extension. (2022, September 9). *Nitrates and livestock water quality*. South Dakota State University Extension. (Written collaboratively by Adele Harty and Ken Olson). https://extension.sdstate.edu/nitrates-and-livestock-water-quality

Sharma, O. P., Sharma, S., Pattabhi, V., Mahato, S. B., & Sharma, P. D. (2007). *A review of the hepatotoxic plant Lantana camara. Critical Reviews in Toxicology*, *37*(4), 313–352. https://doi.org/10.1080/10408440601177863

Shelton, H. M., Kerven, G. L., & Dalzell, S. A. (2019). An update on leucaena toxicity: Is inoculation with *Synergistes jonesii* necessary? *Tropical Grasslands–Forrajes Tropicales*, *7*(2), 146–153. https://doi.org/10.17138/tgft(7)146-153

Shelton, H.M., Dalzell, S., Tomkins, N. & Buck, S. 2021, Leucaena: The productive and sustainable forage legume, 2nd edn, Meat & Livestock Australia Limited, published Nov 2021, viewed 22 Jan 2026, <https://www.mla.com.au/globalassets/mla-corporate/research-and-development/program-areas/grazing-and-pasture-management/leucaena/leucaena-productive-sustainable-forage-legume.pdf>.

Silva, F., Garcês, A., Magalhães, C., & Pires, I. (2023). Diseases in Ruminants Associated with *Pteridium aquilinum* Ingestion. *Biology and Life Sciences Forum.*, *24*(1), 8. https://doi.org/10.3390/IECT2023-14800

Simões, J. G., Medeiros, R. M. T., Medeiros, M. A., Olinda, R. G., Dantas, A. F. M., & Riet-Correa, F. (2018). Nitrate and nitrite poisoning in sheep and goats caused by ingestion of *Portulaca oleracea*. *Pesquisa Veterinária Brasileira*, *38*(8), 1549–1553. https://doi.org/10.1590/1678-5150-PVB-5550

Sykes, C. A., Filigenzi, M., Uzal, F. A., & Poppenga, R. H. (2023). Yellow oleander (Thevetia peruviana) toxicosis in 4 goats. *Journal of Veterinary Diagnostic Investigation*, *35*(5), 563–567. https://doi.org/10.1177/10406387231186190

Texas A&M Veterinary Medical Diagnostic Laboratory (TVMDL) (n.d.) Nitrates – Fluids (Colorimetric) (Test Code 1049). TVMDL. Available at: https://tvmdl.tamu.edu/tests/nitrates-fluids-colorimetric/ (accessed 22 January 2026).

Thompson, L. J. (2024a). *'Nonprotein nitrogen poisoning in animals (Ammonia toxicosis, urea poisoning)', Merck Veterinary Manual (Professional Version).* Merck & Co., Inc. Reviewed/Revised Apr 2021; Modified Sept 2024, viewed 21 Jan 2026

Thompson, L. J. (2024b). *'Nitrate and nitrite poisoning in animals', Merck Veterinary Manual (Professional Version).* Merck & Co., Inc. Reviewed/Revised Apr 2021; Modified Sept 2024, viewed 21 Jan 2026

Tucker, B. B. (1971). *Nitrate Nitrogen Accumulation in Summer Forages.* In Report of the Twenty-Eighth Southern Pasture and Forage Crop Improvement Conference, Oklahoma State University, Stillwater, Oklahoma, July 6–8, 1971 (USDA-ARS Plant Science Research Division, PSR-47-71), pp. 67–80.

United States Pharmacopeial Convention (USP) & American Academy of Veterinary Pharmacology and Therapeutics (AAVPT) 2008, 'Methylene Blue (Veterinary—Systemic)', USP Veterinary Pharmaceutical Information Monographs, viewed 22 Jan 2026.

University of Adelaide, Mycology Online. (2025). *Aspergillus (morphology on Czapek–Dox agar).* The University of Adelaide. Available at: https://mycology.adelaide.edu.au/fungal-descriptions-and-antifungal-susceptibility/hyphomycetes-conidial-moulds/aspergillus. (accessed 22 January 2026)

University of Kentucky Veterinary Diagnostic Laboratory 2022, Forage-related disorders in cattle: Nitrate poisoning—2022 update (sampling and shipping guidance),University of Kentucky, updated 25 Jul 2022.

Vetter, J. (2009). A biological hazard of our age : Bracken fern [Pteridium aquilinum (L.) Kuhn] — A Review. *Acta Veterinaria Hungarica*, *57*(1), 183-196. https://doi.org/10.1556/avet.57.2009.1.18

Walter, S. L. (2002). Acute penitrem A and roquefortine poisoning in a dog. *Canadian Veterinary Journal*, *43*(5), 372–374. PMID: 12001505. PMCID: PMC339273

Weaver, C. M., & Trucksess, M. W. (2010). Determination of Aflatoxins in Botanical Roots by a Modification of AOAC Official MethodSM 991.31 : Single-Laboratory Validation. *Journal of AOAC INTERNATIONAL*, *93*(1), 184–189. https://doi.org/10.1093/jaoac/93.1.184

Wilk-Zasadna, I., & Minta, M. (2009). Developmental toxicity of ochratoxin A in rat embryo midbrain micromass cultures. *International Journal of Molecular Sciences*, *10*(1), 37–49. https://doi.org/10.3390/ijms10010037. PMID: 19333434

Wilk-Zasadna, I., & Minta, M. (2009). Developmental toxicity of ochratoxin A in rat embryo midbrain micromass cultures. *International Journal of Molecular Sciences*, *10*(1), 37–49. https://doi.org/10.3390/ijms10010037. PMID: 19333434

Wilson, B. J., & Harbison, R. D. (1973). *Rubratoxins. Journal of the American Veterinary Medical Association*, *163*(11), 1274–1276. (Review). PMID: 4593856

Worbs, S., Köhler, K., Pauly, D., Avondet, M.-A., Schaer, M., Dorner, M. B., & Dorner, B. G. (2011). Ricinus communis intoxications in human and veterinary medicine—A summary of real cases. *Toxins*, *3*(10), 1332–1372. https://doi.org/10.3390/toxins3101332

World Health Organization (WHO) 2020, Cyanobacterial toxins: microcystins, Background document for development of WHO Guidelines for drinking-water quality and Guidelines for safe recreational water environments, WHO, Geneva, WHO/HEP/ECH/WSH/2020.6, viewed 22 Jan 2026, https://cdn.who.int/media/docs/default-source/wash-documents/wash-chemicals/microcystins-background-201223.pdf.

Xu, L. R. (1992). Bracken poisoning and enzootic haematuria in cattle in China. *Research in Veterinary Science*, *53*(1), 116–121. https://doi.org/10.1016/0034-5288(92)90095-J. PMID: 1410808

Zhang, H., & Payne, J. (2017). Livestock and poultry drinking water quality: Understanding your water test report (L-256). *Oklahoma State University Extension.* Available at: https://extension.okstate.edu/fact-sheets/print-publications/l/understanding-your-water-test-report-l-256.pdf (accessed 22 January 2026)

10

Therapeutic Agents and Toxicity

Drugs are among our most powerful tools in tropical veterinary practice and, paradoxically, among our most frequent sources of preventable harm. Unlike environmental or natural toxins, therapeutic agents enter animals because we (or owners) intend to help. In the tropics, however, the margin between dose and danger narrows: heat and dehydration amplify exposure, parasite pressure drives repeat or stacked dosing, over-the-counter access and informal supply chains enable misuse, and counterfeit or substandard products complicate both efficacy and safety. This chapter brings those realities into focus and translates them into field-ready recognition, response, and prevention.

We frame drug toxicities through a few recurring lenses. First is the toxidrome approach: cholinergic crises from organophosphates/carbamates; neuroexcitation from pyrethroids and select antimicrobials; α_2-agonist sedation from amitraz; and hepato-/nephrotoxic patterns from nonsteroidal anti-inflammatory drugs (NSAIDs), paracetamol (especially cats), and aminoglycosides. Recognizing the dominant pattern in minutes dictates the first hour of care – sample before you wash, decontaminate smartly, give the right antidote early, control tremors or seizures, stabilize temperature and perfusion, and set a monitoring plan (renal, electrocardiogram [ECG]/creatine kinase [CK], ocular, as indicated).

Second is species and genetic susceptibility. Cats' limited glucuronidation makes permethrin and paracetamol uniquely dangerous; MDR1 variants in collie-type dogs lower the threshold for macrocyclic-lactone neurotoxicity; equids are exquisitely sensitive to ionophores; rabbits should not receive fipronil. These red flags recur across casework and deserve explicit "do-not-use/handle-with-care" cues.

Third is regional use and stewardship. Levamisole with an organophosphate "on the same day," closantel overdosing in small ruminants for *Haemonchus*, prolonged oxytetracycline in resistant pneumonias, or off-label human NSAIDs in dogs are not isolated mishaps – they are patterns. We treat them as such, pairing practical algorithms with owner/handler scripts and withdrawal/residue reminders. One Health externalities – such as vulture mortality from veterinary diclofenac, fish kills with pyrethroid runoff, and dung fauna impacts of macrocyclic lactones – are included where management choices ripple beyond the patient.

This chapter bridges earlier foundations (absorption, distribution, metabolism, and excretion [ADME] modifiers; diagnostics and sampling; pesticide syndromes; metals and natural toxins) and applies them to therapeutic classes most relevant in tropical systems: antimicrobials (sulfonamides, nitrofurans, aminoglycosides, fluoroquinolones, tetracyclines), anthelmintics/antiprotozoals (macrocyclic lactones, levamisole, benzimidazoles, closantel, ionophores, diminazene), ectoparasiticides (OPs/carbamates, pyrethroids, amitraz, fipronil/isoxazolines), anti-inflammatories/analgesics (NSAIDs, paracetamol), and sedatives/anesthetics. Each brief centers on use in the tropics, hallmark signs, red-flag species, first-hour actions (including antidotes), monitoring, and prevention – supported by quick-reference tables and flowcharts.

Our aim is pragmatic: help you act decisively when a treatment turns toxic and help you design protocols that keep it from happening again.

Practical Framework for Drug Toxicity in the Tropics

In tropical practice, heat load, dehydration, pregnancy, juvenile growth plates, and preexisting hepatic/renal disease can turn otherwise routine exposures into clinically significant toxicoses. This section offers a fast, field-usable lens you can apply before you even know the exact agent; an at-a-glance toxidrome triage is provided to operationalize first-hour decisions (see Figure 10.1).

Host factors: Species and genetics matter. Cats' limited glucuronidation explains their heightened risk with certain xenobiotics and drugs (e.g., permethrin spot-ons, paracetamol) and the need to avoid canine-only products on felines (Kahn & Line, 2020). Collie-type dogs with the ABCB1/MDR1 deletion are far more susceptible to macrocyclic-lactone–associated neurotoxicity at doses tolerated by other breeds; dose discipline and, where available, genotyping/phenotype awareness reduce risk (Kahn & Line, 2020). Equids are exquisitely sensitive to ionophores (e.g., monensin), with myocardial necrosis at exposures safe for ruminants (Gupta, 2018). Field experience and extension reports also note breed/species variability in organophosphate tolerance, warranting conservative use where baseline sensitivity is uncertain (Kahn & Line, 2020). Lagomorphs should not receive fipronil because of reported seizures and fatalities (Kahn & Line, 2020). A compact "Do-Not-Use/Use-With-Caution" matrix summarizes these red-flag pairings for rapid recall (Figure 10.2).

Environmental amplifiers: High ambient temperatures accelerate dermal absorption from pour-on ectoparasiticides and increase metabolic demand; combine that with dehydration and the kidney becomes the first collateral victim (notably with aminoglycosides and NSAIDs) (Gupta, 2018). Intense UV exposure in the tropics also brings out photosensitizing liabilities of some antimicrobials (e.g., tetracyclines), especially on lightly pigmented skin (Gupta, 2018). These host- and environment-level multipliers are mapped against exemplar drug classes in a single schematic (Figure 10.3).

Use patterns that tilt risk: Three recurrent patterns drive cases in the tropics. (i) human medicines in animals (e.g., ibuprofen/diclofenac in dogs; off-label human ciprofloxacin substituted for enrofloxacin), (ii) depot/long-acting formulations that outlast changing physiology or co-morbidities, and (iii) dose-stacking to "overcome resistance" (e.g., levamisole plus an organophosphate within 24 hours; escalated macrocyclic-lactone doses), which narrows safety margins and multiplies toxidromes (Gupta, 2018; Kahn & Line, 2020). The triad –Host × Drug × Environment – provides a simple mental model to anticipate these pitfalls (Figure 10.3).

Universal first 60 minutes (mini-checklist). Act by toxidrome while you're still confirming the agent:

- Airway–breathing–circulation, oxygen, IV access.
- **Sample first (before washing or emesis)**: serum/whole blood (chemistry, ± cholinesterase if OP/carbamate suspected), urine, and any suspect product/feed/vomitus; baseline glucose/electrolytes; ECG/CK if myopathy (ionophores) is in play (Cornell AHDC, 2023; MSU VDL, 2023).
- **Decontaminate**: dermal wash with mild detergent; gastrointestinal (GI) decon only if safe (no seizures/caustics/aspiration risk); single-dose activated charcoal where indicated (Kahn & Line, 2020).

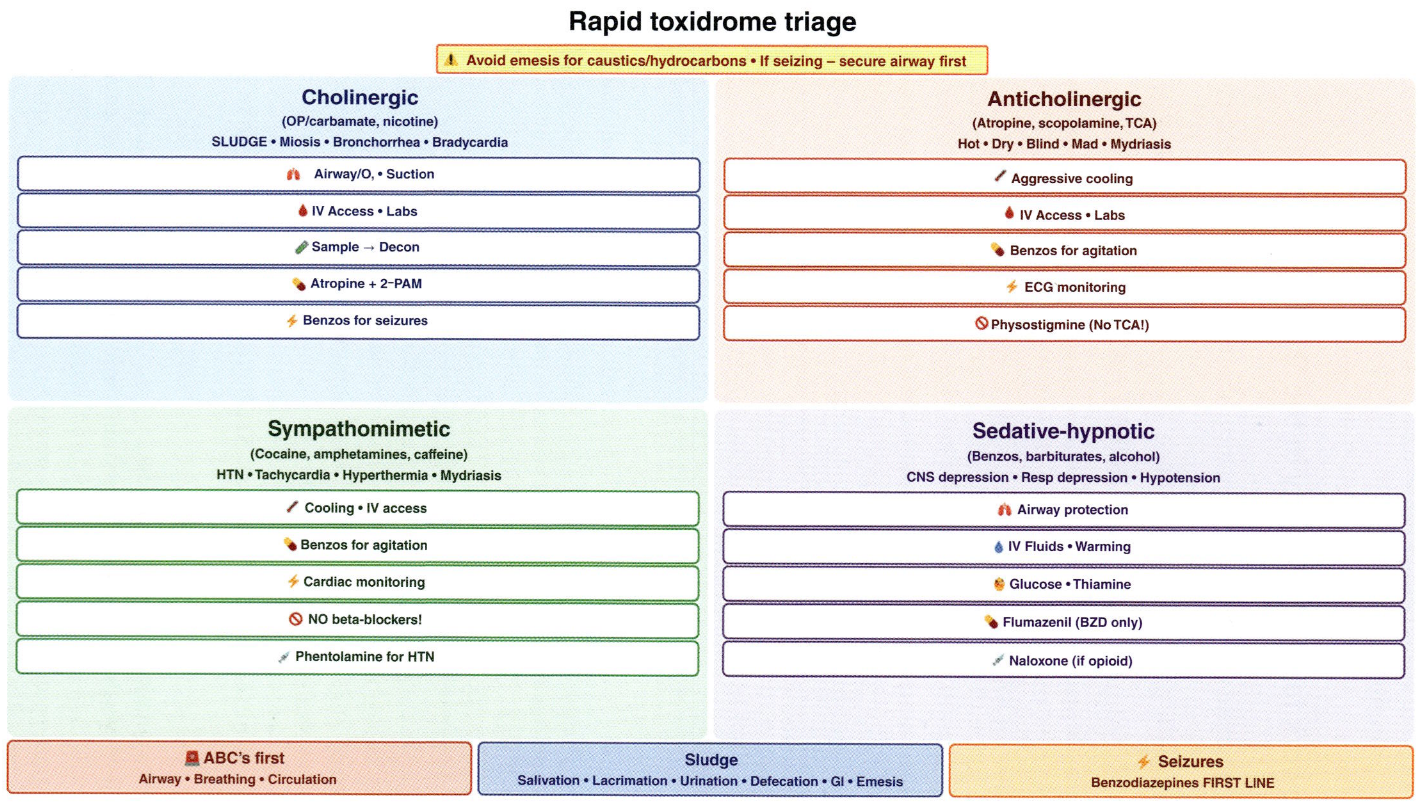

Figure 10.1 Rapid toxidrome triage: predominant signs guide classification into cholinergic (OP/carbamate), neuroexcitation (e.g., pyrethroids, methylxanthines), α_2-agonist sedation (amitraz), or hepato/nephrotoxic patterns, with first-hour actions/antidotes appended to each branch (adapted for tropical veterinary settings). *Sources:* Merck Veterinary Manual (online edition, 2023–2024 updates); Gupta (2018).

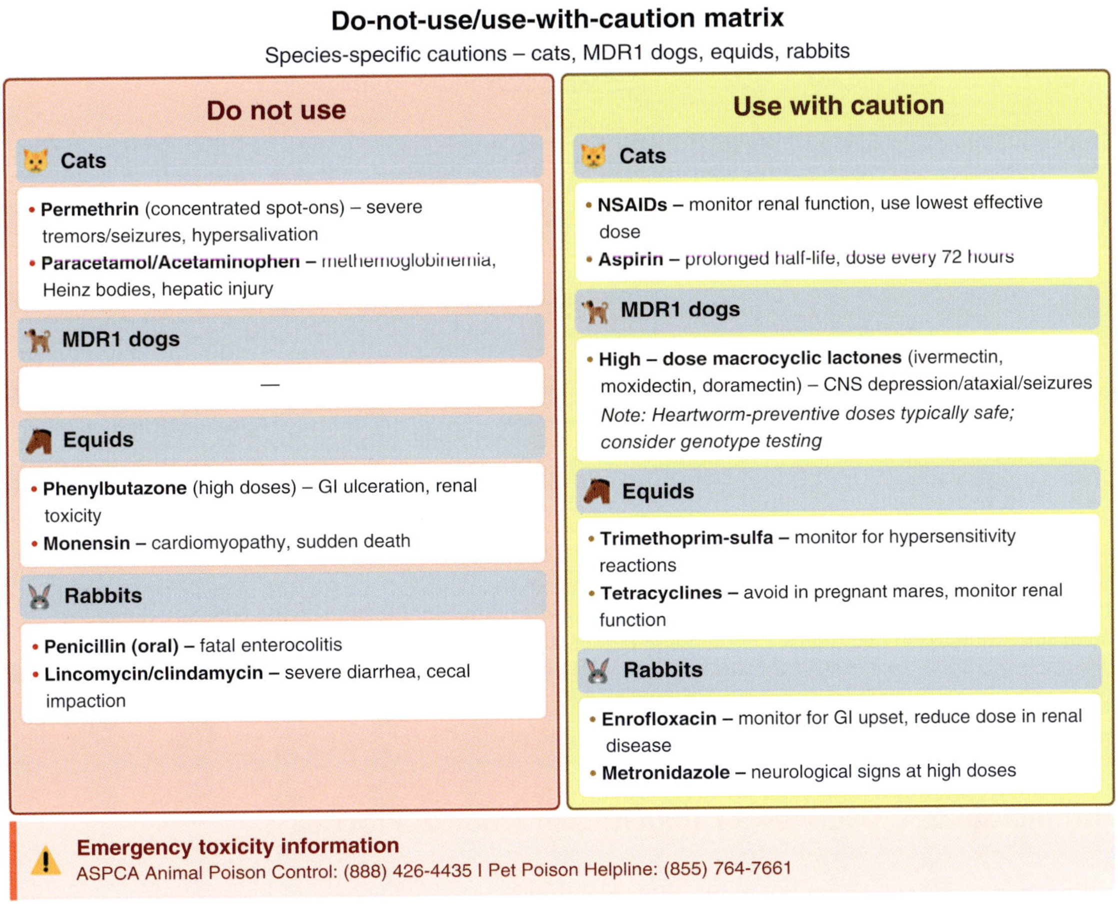

Figure 10.2 Do-Not-Use/Use-with-Caution matrix: high-risk pairings (cats–permethrin/paracetamol; MDR1 dogs–high-dose macrocyclic lactones; equids–ionophores; rabbits–fipronil) with brief rationales and safer alternatives. *Source:* Kahn and Line (2020); Gupta (2018).

- **Antidote early when appropriate**: atropine ± oxime for OPs; atipamezole/yohimbine for amitraz; N-acetylcysteine (NAC) for feline paracetamol (Kahn & Line, 2020).
- **Control tremors/seizures**: (methocarbamol for pyrethroid tremors; benzodiazepines/propofol as needed), correct temperature, start isotonic fluids, and set a monitoring plan (e.g., daily renal panel for aminoglycosides/NSAIDs; ECG/CK for ionophores; ocular checks for closantel/enrofloxacin cats) (Gupta, 2018; Kahn & Line, 2020).

A first-hour playbook condenses these actions by toxidrome for quick bedside use (Table 10.1).

Why this framework. You may not know the bottle, but you will recognize the pattern: cholinergic (OP/carbamate), neuroexcitation (pyrethroids, metronidazole), α_2-sedative (amitraz), or hepato/nephrotoxic (paracetamol, NSAIDs, aminoglycosides). This lets you stabilize the patient, protect diagnostic yield, and avoid the common missteps – washing away the evidence, delaying antidotes, or compounding toxicity with the wrong adjuncts – while you confirm the agent and plan definitive care

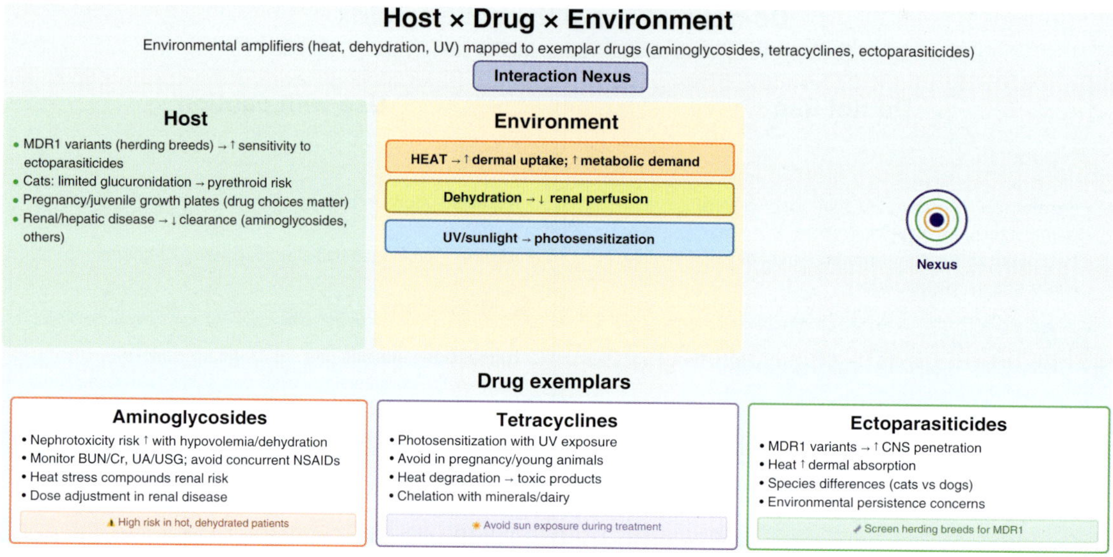

Figure 10.3 Host × Drug × Environment schematic: heat, dehydration, and UV exposure mapped to exemplar classes (aminoglycosides, tetracyclines, ectoparasiticides), illustrating how environmental stressors shrink therapeutic windows in the tropics. *Source:* Gupta (2018); Kahn and Line (2020).

(Kahn & Line, 2020; MSU VDL, 2023). For rapid orientation to the four dominant patterns, use the decision-tree in Figure 10.1 alongside the checklists in Table 10.1.

Antimicrobials – Overview of Toxicities in Tropical Practice

Antimicrobials are indispensable in the tropics, but heat stress, dehydration, high pathogen pressure, and variable supply chains (OTC access, counterfeit/substandard risks) narrow safety margins and shape the pattern of adverse events (Gupta, 2018; Kahn & Line, 2020). To orient the reader at a glance, Figure 10.4 maps each major antimicrobial class to its signature toxicity, early marker, and first-hour priority, with tropical amplifiers annotated (see Figure 10.4).

Class-characteristic toxicities recur predictably: nephrotoxicity with aminoglycosides, idiosyncratic immune-mediated reactions with sulfonamides, cartilage injury in juveniles with fluoroquinolones, retinal degeneration in cats with enrofloxacin, esophageal injury/photosensitivity with tetracyclines, and neurotoxicity with metronidazole at higher or prolonged dosing (Gupta, 2018; Kahn & Line, 2020). Field amplifiers include dehydration (raising aminoglycoside/NSAID renal risk), UV exposure (unmasking tetracycline photosensitivity), and prolonged or stacked courses adopted to "overcome resistance," which increase the likelihood of cumulative toxicity (Gupta, 2018). Practical stewardship therefore centers on weight-based dosing, the shortest effective duration, early monitoring of the target organ (e.g., a renal panel with aminoglycosides), and species-specific cautions (e.g., feline glucuronidation limits; MDR1 herding breeds) (Kahn & Line, 2020). Table 10.2 converts these principles into a one-page "Stewardship-at-a-Glance" guide keyed by class, hallmark toxicity, early labs/signs, first-hour actions, monitoring cadence, and "avoid in ... " red flags (see Table 10.2). This overview sets up the class briefs that follow, beginning with sulfonamides.

Table 10.1 First-hour playbook by toxidrome (dogs/cats; adapt to species): likely culprits (scene clues), do-now 0–15 minutes, Next 15–60 minutes, labs/monitoring, and "avoid" list.

Toxidrome	Likely culprits (scene clues)	Do-now 0–15 min	Next 15–60 min	Labs/monitoring	"Avoid" list
Cholinergic	Organophosphates and carbamates (agri/pet insecticides, recent dips), nicotine; SLUDGE/DUMBELS, miosis, bronchorrhea (Merck Veterinary Manual, 2024a, 2024b).	Airway and oxygen; suction secretions; atropine to effect for muscarinic signs; control seizures with diazepam; start dermal wash or single-dose AC only after airway protected (Merck Veterinary Manual, 2024a).	If OP suspected: add pralidoxime (2-PAM) early; do not use 2-PAM for pure carbamate exposures. Continue decon, temperature control, IV fluids (Merck Veterinary Manual, 2024a, 2024b).	Baseline PCV/TP, glucose, electrolytes, BUN/Cr; consider blood/RBC cholinesterase where available; ECG for brady/tachyarrhythmias (Merck Veterinary Manual, 2024a).	No emesis with neurological/respiratory compromise; avoid phenothiazines and morphine; avoid 2-PAM in pure carbamate poisoning (Merck Veterinary Manual, 2024a, 2024b).
Neuroex-citation	Tremorgenic mycotoxins ("moldy rubbish"), pyrethrins/pyrethroids (esp. cats, recent spot-on), strychnine baits, methylxanthines (chocolate); tremors/seizures, hyperthermia, mydriasis (Merck Veterinary Manual, 2023a, 2023b, 2024c, 2024d).	Stop seizures/tremors: diazepam ± methocarbamol; begin active cooling if hyperthermic; start IV fluids. Decon only once controlled (Merck Veterinary Manual, 2023a, 2023b).	If refractory: phenobarbital/propofol per status protocols; multi-dose AC for methylx-anthines; bathe cats with topical pyrethroid exposure; continue fluids and temperature control (Merck Veterinary Manual, 2023b, 2024c).	ECG/HR, temperature, electrolytes (K^+/Mg^{2+}), CK; chemistry as indicated (Merck Veterinary Manual, 2024e).	Do not attempt emesis during uncontrolled tremors/seizures; avoid unsupervised at-home decon (Merck Veterinary Manual, 2023a, 2023b).
α_2-sedation (amitraz)	Ingested tick-collar pieces, dip exposure; sedation, bradycardia, hypotension, hypothermia, hyperglycemia (Merck Veterinary Manual, 2024f).	Supportive care, warm patient, IV fluids; remove collar/dermal wash (Merck Veterinary Manual, 2024f).	Reverse with atipamezole (or yohimbine) when moderate–severe; monitor glucose and temperature; single-dose AC if ingestion and protected airway (Hugnet et al., 1996; Merck Veterinary Manual, 2024f).	Glucose, electrolytes, ECG/HR, temperature; chemistry if prolonged depression (Merck Veterinary Manual, 2024f).	Avoid routine atropine as sole therapy for bradycardia (treat the α_2-agonism instead); no emesis in depressed patients (Merck Veterinary Manual, 2024f).
Hepato/nephrotoxic	Nephro: ethylene glycol (sweet puddle/garage), lilies (cats). Hepato: acetaminophen (cats), NSAIDs, aflatoxin-contaminated feed; GI upset, icterus, PU/PD, abdominal pain (Merck Veterinary Manual, 2024g, 2023c, 2024h, 2023d).	Start IV crystalloids; antiemetic; single-dose AC where appropriate. EG: begin fomepizole (dogs) or ethanol protocol asap. APAP (cats): start N-acetylcysteine early. Remove remaining plant/product; aggressive fluids for lily exposures (Merck Veterinary Manual, 2024g, 2023c, 2024h).	Add hepatic/GI support (e.g., SAMe/silybin); consider cholestyramine for enterohepatic toxins (e.g., aflatoxins, select drugs). Ongoing diuresis and urine-output tracking (Merck Veterinary Manual, 2023d, 2024e).	Chem panel (ALT/AST, ALP, bilirubin), PT/INR; BUN/Cr, electrolytes, UA/USG; for lilies, recheck renal values q24 h × 72 h; ECG if hyperkalemia risk (Merck Veterinary Manual, 2023c, 2024e).	Avoid additional nephro/hepatotoxins (NSAIDs, high-dose acetaminophen, contrast agents); do not delay antidotes while awaiting labs/imaging (Merck Veterinary Manual, 2024g, 2024h).

AC, activated charcoal; APAP, acetaminophen; EG, ethylene glycol; PT/INR, prothrombin time/international normalized ratio.
Sources: Merck Veterinary Manual (online edition, 2023–2024 updates); Hugnet et al. (1996) for α_2-agonist reversal guidance.

Renal | Hepatic | Neurologic/Ototoxic | Retinal/Ocular | Hematologic/Immune | GI/Esophageal | Musculoskeletal

Antimicrobial class	Signature toxicity	Early markers	Primary prevention
Renal			
Aminoglycosides (gentamicin, tobramycin)	Acute tubular necrosis, nephrotoxicity	Rising creatinine, ↓GFR, proteinuria	Monitor levels, dose adjustment, hydration
Vancomycin	Acute kidney injury	Serum creatinine elevation, oliguria	TDM, avoid concurrent nephrotoxins
Hepatic			
Isoniazid	Hepatotoxicity, DILI	Elevated ALT/AST, bilirubin	Baseline LFTs, regular monitoring
Rifampin	Cholestatic hepatitis	↑Alkaline phosphatase, jaundice	Monitor liver enzymes
Neurologic/ototoxic			
Aminoglycosides	Ototoxicity (vestibular/cochlear)	Hearing loss, tinnitus, vertigo	Audiometry monitoring
Metronidazole	Peripheral neuropathy, CNS toxicity	Numbness, tingling, ataxia	Limit duration, neuro monitoring
Retinal/ocular			
Ehambutol	Optic neuritis	Visual field defects, color vision changes	Regular ophthalmologic exams
Chloroquine/HCQ	Retinal toxicity, maculopathy	Visual field changes, pigmentation	Annual retinal screening
Hematologic/immune			
Chloramphenicol	Bone marrow suppression	Pancytopenia, ↓blood counts	Regular CBC monitoring
TMP-SMX	Bone marrow suppression, hemolysis	Thrombocytopenia, anemia	Monitor blood counts, folate
GI/esophageal			
Clindamycin	C. difficile-associated diarrhea	Diarrhea, abdominal pain, colitis	Judicious use, monitor symptoms
Broad-spectrum ABx	AAD, dysbiosis	Loose stools, GI upset	Narrow spectrum when possible
Musculoskeletal			
Fluoroquinolones	Tendinopathy, tendon rupture	Tendon pain, swelling, ↓mobility	Avoid in high-risk patients
Corticosteroids	Muscle weakness, osteoporosis	Proximal weakness, bone loss	Minimize duration, Ca/VitD

TDM = Therapeutic Drug Monitoring; DILI = Drug-Induced Liver Injury; AAD = Antibiotic-Associated Diarrhea; HCQ = Hydroxychloroquine

Figure 10.4 Antimicrobial map and toxicity overview (tropical context). Schematic linking antimicrobial classes to signature toxicities (e.g., aminoglycosides → nephrotoxicity; sulfonamides → idiosyncratic immune-mediated events; fluoroquinolones → juvenile cartilage injury; enrofloxacin in cats → retinal degeneration; tetracyclines → oesophagitis/photosensitivity; metronidazole → neurotoxicity), with early markers and "first-hour" actions highlighted; environmental amplifiers (heat, dehydration, UV) annotated. *Source:* Gupta (2018), Kahn and Line (2020).

Table 10.2 Antimicrobials – Stewardship-at-a-Glance.

Class	Common tropical use	Hallmark toxicity	Early labs/signs	First-hour actions	Monitor	Avoid in ...
Aminoglycosides (gentamicin, amikacin)	Severe G – sepsis; ICU; topical otic	Nephrotoxicity (acute tubular necrosis); ± ototoxicity (Giguère et al., 2013; Merck Veterinary Manual, 2024; Papich, 2020)	Rising BUN/Cr in 24–72 h; ↓ USG; casts; ↓ urine output	Stop/hold drug; IV crystalloids; eliminate co-nephrotoxins (NSAIDs, contrast, loops); consider once-daily dosing if therapy must continue (Papich, 2020; Giguère et al., 2013)	Daily hydration/ urine output; BUN/Cr q24–48 h	Preexisting renal disease; dehydrated patients
Fluoroquinolones (enrofloxacin, marbofloxacin)	UTI, mixed G–/ resp infections; rickettsial adjunct	Cats: acute retinal degeneration (dose-related enrofloxacin); juveniles: cartilage injury (Gelatt, 2014; Papich, 2020)	Cats: mydriasis, sudden vision loss; juveniles: lameness	Stop drug at first vision change; switch class; light protection pending evaluation (Gelatt, 2014)	Vision checks first 48–72 h with higher feline doses; growth-age restrictions	High-dose enrofloxacin in cats; growing large-breed dogs
Tetracyclines (doxycycline, oxytetracycline)	*Ehrlichia*/ *Anaplasma*, leptospirosis, hemoplasmas	Esophagitis/stricture in cats with dry-pilling (Papich, 2020; Plumb, 2018)	Dysphagia, ptyalism, regurgitation within hours–days	Stop tablets; give water/ food; start GI protectants (e.g., sucralfate); image if severe (Plumb, 2018)	Swallowing comfort; intake; weight	Cats: avoid dry pilling; late pregnancy/ young (tooth/ bone effects)
Macrolides (erythromycin, azithromycin, clarithromycin)	Foal *Rhodococcus equi* (with rifampin)	Severe/fatal colitis in adult horses; rare hyperthermia in foals (Giguère et al., 2013)	Horses: diarrhea/ colic; foals: panting, very high temp	Do not use in adult horses; isolate diarrheic cases; fluids/anti-endotoxin; protect mares from exposure when foals treated (Giguère et al., 2013)	Temp, fecal output; liver enzymes with rifampin	Adult horses; mares exposed to treated foals
Lincosamides (clindamycin, lincomycin)	Anaerobes, protozoa; oral wounds	Fatal dysbiosis in hindgut fermenters (rabbits, guinea pigs); severe colitis in horses/ruminants (Carpenter & Marion, 2018; Giguère et al., 2013)	Acute watery diarrhea, rapid decline	Contraindicated in rabbits/ GP/horses; stop drug; aggressive fluids; consider cholestyramine ± metronidazole per protocol (Carpenter & Marion, 2018)	Hydration, fecal output	Rabbits, guinea pigs, hamsters, chinchillas, ruminants, adult horses

(*Continued*)

Table 10.2 (Continued)

Class	Common tropical use	Hallmark toxicity	Early labs/signs	First-hour actions	Monitor	Avoid in ...
Sulfonamides ± trimethoprim	UTIs, skin, coccidiosis	Idiosyncratic KCS ("dry eye"), polyarthritis, hepatopathy (Merck Veterinary Manual, 2024; Plumb, 2018)	↓ Schirmer tear test; mucoid ocular discharge; fever, arthralgia	Stop drug; ocular lube ± cyclosporine; baseline CBC/chem (Plumb, 2018)	CBC; ALT/ALP; Schirmer tear tests during prolonged therapy	Breeds with ocular surface disease; long courses
Chloramphenicol (phenicols)	Deep sepsis/anaerobes when resistance limits options	Bone-marrow suppression (idiosyncratic); human exposure hazard (Giguère et al., 2013; Plumb, 2018)	Neutropenia/thrombocytopenia; lethargy, pallor	Stop drug; PPE for handlers; supportive care; avoid in food animals (Plumb, 2018)	CBC q7–10 d during courses	Food-producing animals; caution in households with pregnant people
Rifampin (often with macrolide in foals)	*R. equi* pneumonia (foals)	Hepatotoxicity, orange body fluids; CYP induction (Giguère et al., 2013; Plumb, 2018)	↑ ALT/AST ± bilirubin; anorexia/lethargy	Reduce/stop; hepatoprotectants; review drug interactions (Giguère et al., 2013)	Weekly chem panel during therapy	Preexisting hepatic disease
Nitroimidazoles (metronidazole)	Anaerobic enteritis, protozoa	Neurotoxicity at higher/ELDU doses (Peterson & Talcott, 2013; Plumb, 2018)	Ataxia, nystagmus, tremors; seizures in severe cases	Stop drug; supportive care; diazepam for severe signs per local protocols (Peterson & Talcott, 2013)	Neuro exam until resolved	Very young/neurological patients; high-dose or prolonged courses
Polymyxins (polymyxin B/colistin)	Horses: anti-endotoxin adjunct	Nephrotoxicity (dose-related); neuro signs at higher doses; risk ↑ with aminoglycosides (Giguère et al., 2013)	Rising creatinine; ataxia with cumulative dosing	Aggressive IV fluids; avoid co-nephrotoxins; lowest effective dose/short courses (Giguère et al., 2013)	BUN/Cr daily while on therapy	Azotemic/dehydrated patients; concurrent aminoglycosides
β-lactams (penicillins/cephalosporins)	Broad use – skin/soft tissue, mastitis, UTIs	Oral use in rabbits/GP: lethal enterocolitis; otherwise hypersensitivity (Carpenter & Marion, 2018; Giguère et al., 2013)	Rabbits: abrupt watery diarrhea, rapid deterioration	Never give orally to rabbits/GP; if exposed → withdraw drug, fluids, anti-endotoxin protocols (Carpenter & Marion, 2018)	Fecal output/hydration in hindgut fermenters; watch for anaphylaxis	Rabbits/GP (oral route); known β-lactam allergy

ELDU, extralabel drug use; GP, guinea pigs; KCS, keratoconjunctivitis sicca; USG, urine specific gravity.
Class-by-class summary of common tropical use, hallmark toxicity, early labs/signs, first-hour actions, monitoring, and avoid-in species/situations. Evidence anchors include Merck Veterinary Manual (online), Papich (2020), Giguère et al. (2013), Plumb (2018), Gelatt (2014), Carpenter & Marion, (2018), and Peterson and Talcott (2013).

Sulfonamides

Source

Sulfonamides are synthetic antibacterial compounds widely used in veterinary practice to treat bacterial infections. They are white, amphoteric powders – sparingly soluble in water but readily soluble in alkaline or strong acid solutions. The basic sulfonamide scaffold and its relationship to p-aminobenzoic acid (PABA) are shown in Figure 10.5 (Giguère et al., 2013; Papich, 2020).

Although clinical utility has been tempered by resistance and the availability of newer antibiotics, sulfonamides remain common in veterinary medicine – these medicines are often effective, inexpensive, and widely available (Giguère et al., 2013). Common veterinary agents include sulfathiazole, sulfapyridine, sulfamethoxazole, and sulfadiazine (Giguère et al., 2013). Trimethoprim–sulfonamide combinations (typically 1:5) provide pharmacologic synergy and extend spectrum (Giguère et al., 2013).

Toxicity

Sulfonamide toxicity is reported in calves, poultry, cats, and dogs after individual dosing or inclusion in feed/water. Three patterns occur: acute (drug shock), chronic/renal, and hypersensitivity (Giguère et al., 2013; Papich, 2020). The acute form is classically associated with rapid IV administration. The chronic/renal form, more common, reflects renal tubular irritation and crystalluria with potential

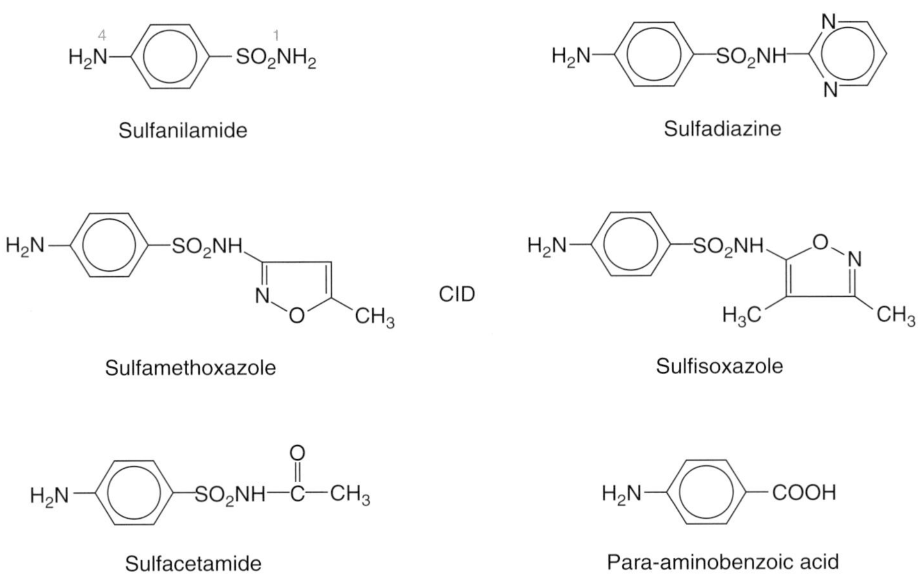

Figure 10.5 Chemical structures of p-aminobenzoic acid (PABA) and representative sulfonamides (sulfanilamide, sulfadiazine, sulfamethoxazole, sulfisoxazole, sulfacetamide). *Source:* Adapted from Giguère et al. (2013) and Papich (2020).

urethral obstruction (Giguère et al., 2013; Papich, 2020). Hypersensitivity reactions can follow prolonged/repeated dosing and include respiratory difficulty and urticaria.

Intrinsic solubility and acetylated metabolites influence risk; high renal excretion favors crystal formation, especially in carnivores with acidic urine (Papich, 2020). Dehydration or poor water access increases risk for chronic toxicosis (Papich, 2020).

Mechanism of Action (Toxicity)

The mechanism for the acute "drug shock" syndrome is uncertain. The renal form is due to intraluminal crystal formation → mucosal irritation, hematuria, and obstruction. Sulfonamides and metabolites are relatively insoluble in acidic urine (Papich, 2020). Hypersensitivity is presumed immune-mediated (Giguère et al., 2013).

Clinical Signs

High IV doses (e.g., sulfabromomethazine in cattle) have produced visual disturbance, muscular weakness, ataxia, and collapse (Gelatt, 2014). The chronic uremic form presents with anorexia, depression, collapse, hematuria, albuminuria, and oliguria; sulfonamide crystals may be visible at the external urinary meatus (Gupta, 2018). Hypersensitivity may manifest with fever, bronchospasm/asthma-like signs, and urticaria (Kahn & Line, 2020).

Pathophysiology

Postmortem findings in chronic/uremic cases include crystals throughout the urinary tract and hemorrhagic changes consistent with obstruction and tubular damage (Gupta, 2018).

Diagnosis

Diagnosis of chronic or hypersensitivity syndromes relies on exposure history and compatible signs. Chronic (uremic) cases can be difficult to confirm if treatment was owner-initiated. Urinalysis (pH, crystals), CBC/chemistry, and (in dogs on longer courses) Schirmer tear testing help detect complications early (Kahn & Line, 2020). The crystalluria pathway and key decision points are summarized in Figure 10.6.

Treatment

For acute drug shock, halt or slow the infusion, provide supportive care, and treat signs. For chronic/renal cases, stop therapy, rehydrate, and alkalinize urine (IV alkalinizing fluids ± oral alkalinizing electrolytes) (Papich, 2020). For hypersensitivity, withdraw the drug and manage signs (e.g., antihistamines; adrenaline/epinephrine for severe urticaria/bronchospasm) (Kahn & Line, 2020). A one-page quick reference comparing the three syndromes is provided in Table 10.3.

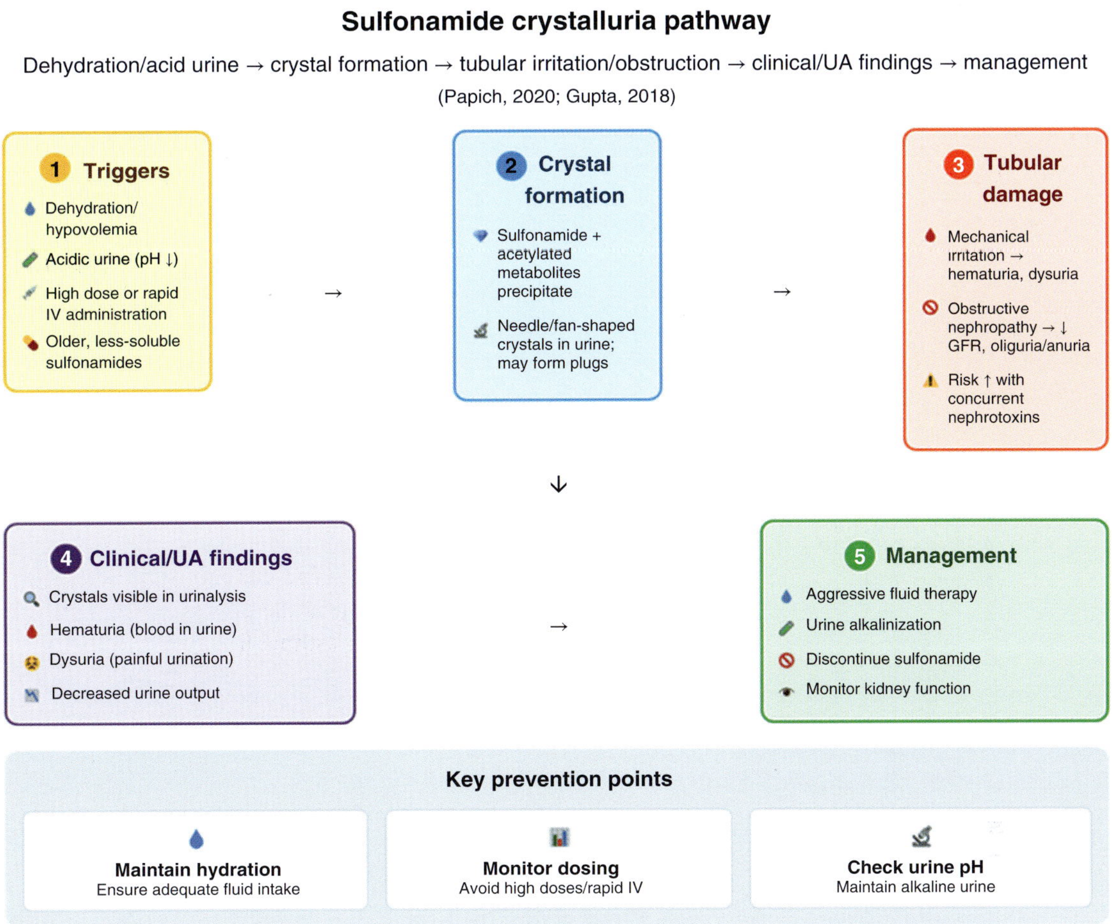

Figure 10.6 Sulfonamide crystalluria pathway – dehydration/acid urine → crystal formation → tubular irritation/obstruction → clinical/urinalysis findings → management steps. *Source:* Papich (2020) and Gupta (2018).

Nitrofurans

Source

Nitrofurans are yellow, crystalline, sparingly water-soluble synthetic agents with antibacterial and anticoccidial activity. Their antimicrobial effect depends on the 5-nitro moiety (Figure 10.7). Historical/legacy use includes nitrofurazone, nitrofurantoin, nifuratel, nifuroxazide/nifuroquine, and furazolidone; utility is limited by poor solubility and toxicity, and activity diminishes in alkaline media (Constable et al., 2016; Papich, 2020).

Table 10.3 Sulfonamides: acute vs. chronic vs. hypersensitivity toxic syndromes (quick reference).

Syndrome	Typical context	Key signs	First actions	Monitoring	Prevention cues
Acute (dose/solubility related)	High dose or rapid IV; dehydrated patient; acidic urine; older, less-soluble sulfas; concurrent nephrotoxins.	Vomiting/diarrhea; hematuria, crystalluria, dysuria; lumbar/renal pain; oliguria/anuria; azotemia.	Stop sulfonamide. IV crystalloids (aim diuresis); consider urinary alkalinization (e.g., sodium bicarbonate) if crystalluria; antiemetic/analgesia; remove co-nephrotoxins.	UA (USG, sediment for crystals), BUN/Cr q24–48 h; urine output; electrolytes/acid–base.	Ensure hydration before and during therapy; avoid high/rapid doses; prefer modern, more soluble sulfas; adjust dose in renal compromise.
Chronic cumulative (tear film/hepatic/endocrine)	Courses ≥1–2 weeks (esp. trimethoprim–sulfa) in dogs.	KCS ("dry eye") – mucoid discharge, blepharospasm, photophobia; hepatopathy (↑ALT/ALP, anorexia/lethargy); transient hypothyroxinemia.	Stop drug. Ocular lube ± topical cyclosporine; consider hepatoprotectants (e.g., SAMe/silybin); client warning for delayed resolution of TT4.	Schirmer tear test baseline and during therapy; ALT/ALP weekly while on; TT4 if long courses or clinical signs.	Avoid dry-eye–prone breeds or long courses; use minimum effective duration; baseline/periodic tear test and chemistry; counsel owners on early ocular signs.
Hypersensitivity/idiosyncratic (multisystem)	7–21 d after start (or sooner on re-exposure); breed predisposition reported (e.g., Doberman Pinschers).	Fever, polyarthritis, skin eruptions/mucosal ulceration; hepatitis; ± IMHA/ITP; lymphadenopathy; rarely aseptic meningitis.	Immediately discontinue drug; anti-inflammatory to immunosuppressive corticosteroids if systemic immune-mediated disease; supportive care (fluids, analgesia); manage organ-specific issues (e.g., ocular therapy, hepatopathy).	CBC/platelets daily then q48–72 h; ALT/ALP, bilirubin; UA/proteinuria; ± coagulation if hepatitis severe.	Absolute avoidance of sulfonamides lifelong after a reaction; flag medical record; avoid concurrent hepatotoxins; use alternatives when feasible.

Source: Giguère et al. (2013), Papich (2020), Kahn and Line (2020), and Gupta (2018).

Figure 10.7 Chemical structure of nitrofurans used in veterinary medicine (e.g., nitrofurazone, nitrofurantoin, furazolidone). Author's illustration; structures redrawn from standard chemical data. See Constable et al. (2016) and Papich (2020).

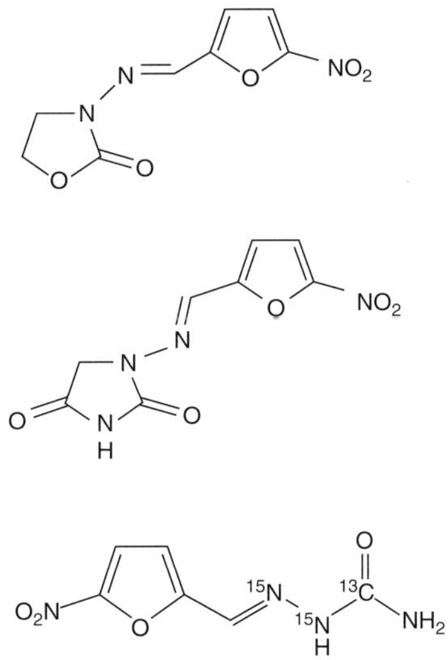

Furazolidone

Nitrofurantoin

Nitrofurazone

Toxicity

Toxicity relates to GI absorption rate and water solubility. In calves, continuous nitrofurazone dosing at ≈30 mg/kg/day may cause death within ~5 days; 15 mg/kg/day can cause hyperexcitability/convulsions by ~19 days and death by ~27 days; 10 mg/kg/day yields variable toxicity and reduced weight gain; 5 mg/kg/day is generally tolerated (Papich, 2020). Furazolidone tends to be less acutely toxic than nitrofurazone, likely due to lower GI absorption (Constable et al., 2016).

Mechanism of Action (Toxicity)

Nitrofurans undergo reduction to reactive intermediates that inhibit multiple enzymes of aerobic carbohydrate oxidation (e.g., pyruvate and succinate dehydrogenases), demonstrated in mammalian tissues and bacterial cultures (Constable et al., 2016). In susceptible animals, impaired cerebral glucose oxidation explains neurological manifestations (Gupta, 2018). See Figure 10.8 for a schematic of pathway targets and clinical correlations.

Clinical Signs

Field and experimental reports describe furazolidone toxicosis in calves and pigs (Constable et al., 2016; Gupta, 2018). In calves, prolonged oral administration (e.g., 5–10 mg/kg/day for weeks) has been associated with hemorrhagic diathesis, profuse fetid diarrhea, pale mucous membranes, tachycardia, pyrexia (40–42°C), rapid progression to recumbency, epistaxis, prolonged clotting times, and neurological signs (circling, muscle rigidity); thrombocytopenia may occur (Constable et al., 2016; Papich, 2020). Ducks are more sensitive than chicks to nitrofurazone in feed (Papich, 2020).

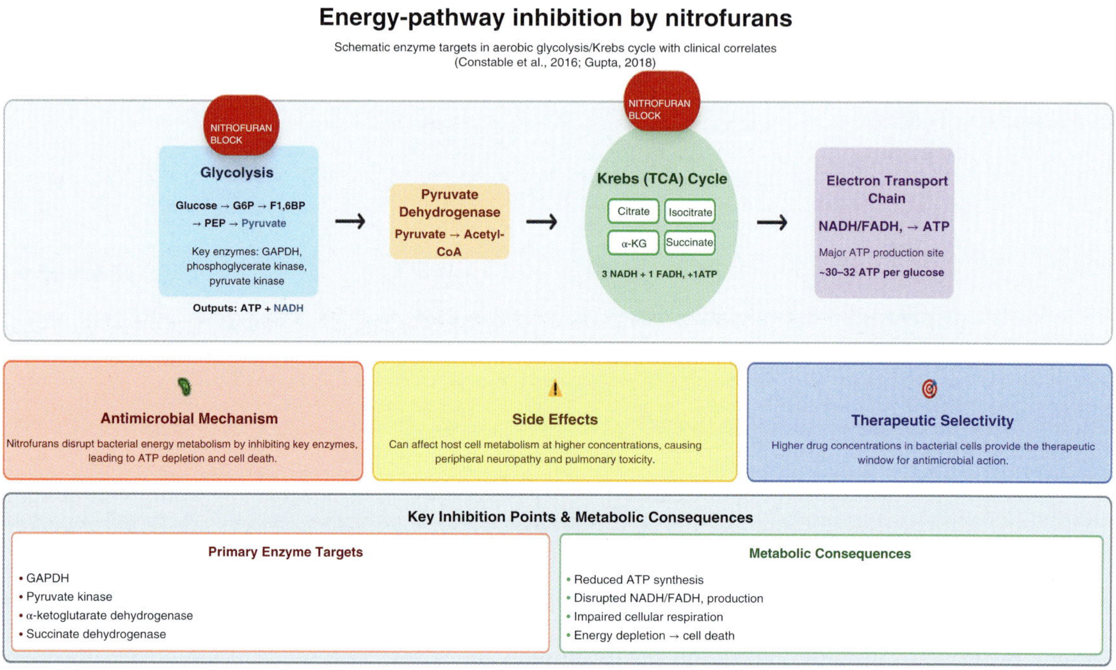

Figure 10.8 Energy-pathway inhibition by nitrofurans – enzyme targets in aerobic glycolysis/Krebs cycle with clinical correlates (neurological signs, diarrhea). *Source:* Constable et al. (2016) and Gupta (2018).

Pathophysiology

Neurological signs reflect cerebral energy failure from inhibited aerobic oxidation. Thrombocytopenia with furazolidone exposure is consistent with bone marrow suppression, and dehydration from severe diarrhea contributes to weakness and recumbency (Constable et al., 2016; Gupta, 2018).

Treatment

Immediate withdrawal of the nitrofuran or medicated feed is essential; many cases improve once medication stops (Constable et al., 2016). Provide supportive care: correct dehydration and electrolyte/acid–base derangements, manage uremia if present, and monitor coagulation parameters (Papich, 2020). A bedside summary of agents, dose/exposure patterns, timelines, and key signs/labs is provided in Table 10.4.

Aminoglycosides

Source

Aminoglycosides are concentration-dependent, bactericidal antibiotics used widely in tropical practice for Gram-negative sepsis, pneumonia, uterine, and musculoskeletal infections across species. Frequent field use is driven by availability, rapid kill, and cost – often in dehydrated or critically ill animals where

Table 10.4 Nitrofurans: dose, time-to-toxicity, and key clinical/lab features.

Agent	Typical dose/exposure	Time course	Dominant signs	Lab abnormalities (e.g., platelets, coagulation)	First actions	Outcome
Nitrofurantoin	Dogs/cats: commonly used as urinary antiseptic at ~**3–5 mg/kg PO q8–12 h** (formulation dependent); overdose or prolonged courses ↑ risk (Papich, 2020).	**Hours–days** for GI intolerance/hypersensitivity; **>1–2 weeks** for hepatic or neurological effects (Papich, 2020).	Nausea/vomiting, anorexia; lethargy; pruritic rash/fever (hypersensitivity); rare peripheral neuropathy with long courses (Papich, 2020).	Mild–moderate **↑ALT/AST**; ± **eosinophilia** with hypersensitivity; UA may show sterile pyuria; cytopenias uncommon (Papich, 2020).	**Stop drug**; antiemetic/GI support; treat hypersensitivity as indicated; switch class guided by culture and susceptibility (Papich, 2020).	**Good** if recognized early – typically resolves within days after withdrawal (Papich, 2020).
Furazolidone *(historical; prohibited in food animals in many jurisdictions)*	Past exposure via **medicated feed/bolus** or dosing errors; ELDU discouraged/illegal in food species (Constable et al., 2016).	**Days–weeks** of therapy, sooner if overdosed (Constable et al., 2016).	Depression, reduced appetite; **neurological signs** (tremor, ataxia); diarrhea; possible cardiopulmonary intolerance in young stock (Constable et al., 2016).	**Leukopenia or thrombocytopenia** possible; ↑ **liver enzymes**; acid–base/electrolyte derangements with diarrhea; coagulation changes uncommon (Constable et al., 2016).	**Immediate withdrawal**; fluids/electrolytes; nutritional support; control tremors/seizures if present; verify legal status and residues (Constable et al., 2016).	**Variable** – favorable if discontinued promptly; prolonged/high exposure can be **poor** in young or debilitated animals (Constable et al., 2016).
Nitrofurazone *(topical; systemic use discouraged)*	**Topical** wound preparations; **systemic absorption** ↑ with large open surfaces/occlusion; accidental **ingestion** possible (Constable et al., 2016; Papich, 2020).	**Days–weeks** with repeated/large-area use; **hours–days** after ingestion (Constable et al., 2016; Papich, 2020).	Local dermatitis/irritation; vomiting if ingested; with sustained exposure: **weakness, pallor** from marrow effects (Constable et al., 2016).	**Cytopenias** (neutropenia, **thrombocytopenia**; rarely pancytopenia); mild **↑ALT/AST**; prolonged bleeding if platelets low (Constable et al., 2016).	**Discontinue** product; CBC/chem and wound-care revision; supportive care (transfusion if severe thrombocytopenia); select alternatives (Constable et al., 2016; Papich, 2020).	**Good** after cessation for mild cases; guarded if **aplastic-type marrow suppression** occurs (Constable et al., 2016).

Many nitrofurans are banned or tightly restricted in food animals; confirm local regulations.
Source: Papich (2020) and Constable et al. (2016).

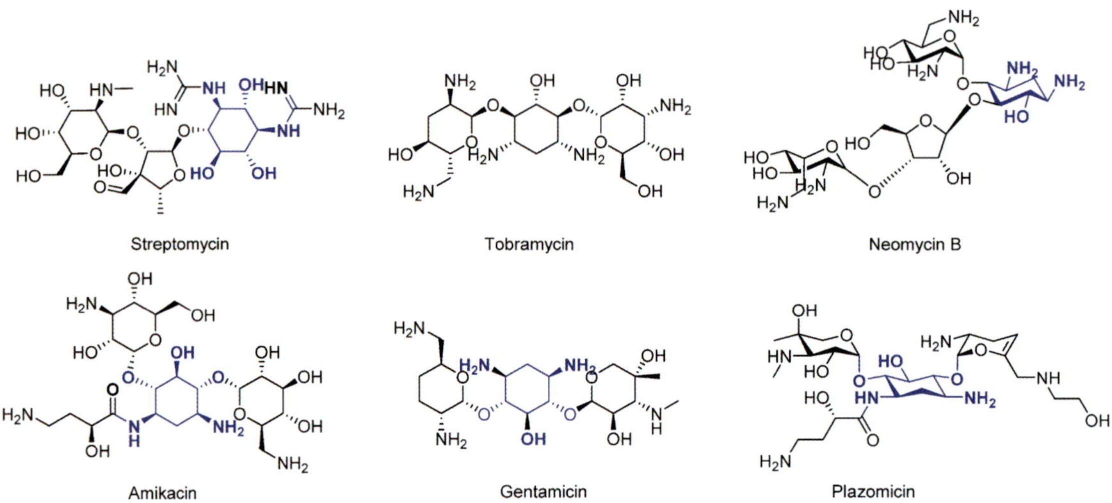

Figure 10.9 Representative aminoglycoside structures and aminocyclitol cores. Examples (gentamicin C complex, amikacin, neomycin, streptomycin) with conserved ring system and typical side-chain substitutions highlighted. *Source:* Adapted from Serio et al. (2018).

renal safety margins are narrowed (Giguère et al., 2013; Kahn & Line, 2020; Papich, 2020). Representative chemical scaffolds and side-chain differences are shown in Figure 10.9 (adapted from Serio et al., 2018).

Toxicity

The hallmark adverse effect is non-oliguric acute kidney injury (AKI) from proximal tubular cell damage, typically emerging after several days of therapy; early markers include rising urea/creatinine and granular casts on urinalysis (Gupta, 2018; Kahn & Line, 2020). Ototoxicity (cochlear and/or vestibular) occurs across species – with cats relatively more susceptible – and neuromuscular blockade is uncommon but reported with rapid IV boluses or concurrent neuromuscular blockers (Kahn & Line, 2020; Papich, 2020). Risk rises with dehydration, advanced age, preexisting renal disease, and concurrent nephrotoxins (e.g., NSAIDs, loop diuretics) (Gupta, 2018).

Mechanism of Action (Toxicity)

Aminoglycosides are filtered and taken up by proximal tubular epithelial cells via megalin-mediated endocytosis, accumulating in lysosomes/mitochondria and causing acute tubular necrosis. In the inner ear, they injure hair cells, producing cochlear/vestibular dysfunction (Gupta, 2018; Peterson & Talcott, 2013).

Clinical Signs

AKI: Polyuria/polydipsia or normal urine output with azotemia after 3–5 days, lethargy, inappetence (Gupta, 2018). Ototoxicity: hearing loss, head tilt, ataxia (cats > dogs) (Kahn & Line, 2020). Neuromuscular blockade: peri-anesthetic weakness or apnea (rare) (Papich, 2020).

Pathophysiology

Histopathology shows proximal tubular necrosis with isosthenuria; auditory pathology shows loss of hair cells and spiral ganglion degeneration (Gupta, 2018).

Diagnosis

History of exposure and timing; serum chemistry (blood urea nitrogen [BUN]/creatinine), urinalysis (casts), hearing/vestibular exam; consider therapeutic drug monitoring (trough just before the third dose) if therapy must continue (Giguère et al., 2013; Kahn & Line, 2020). A concise first-hour algorithm is provided in Figure 10.10 to guide stabilization and sampling.

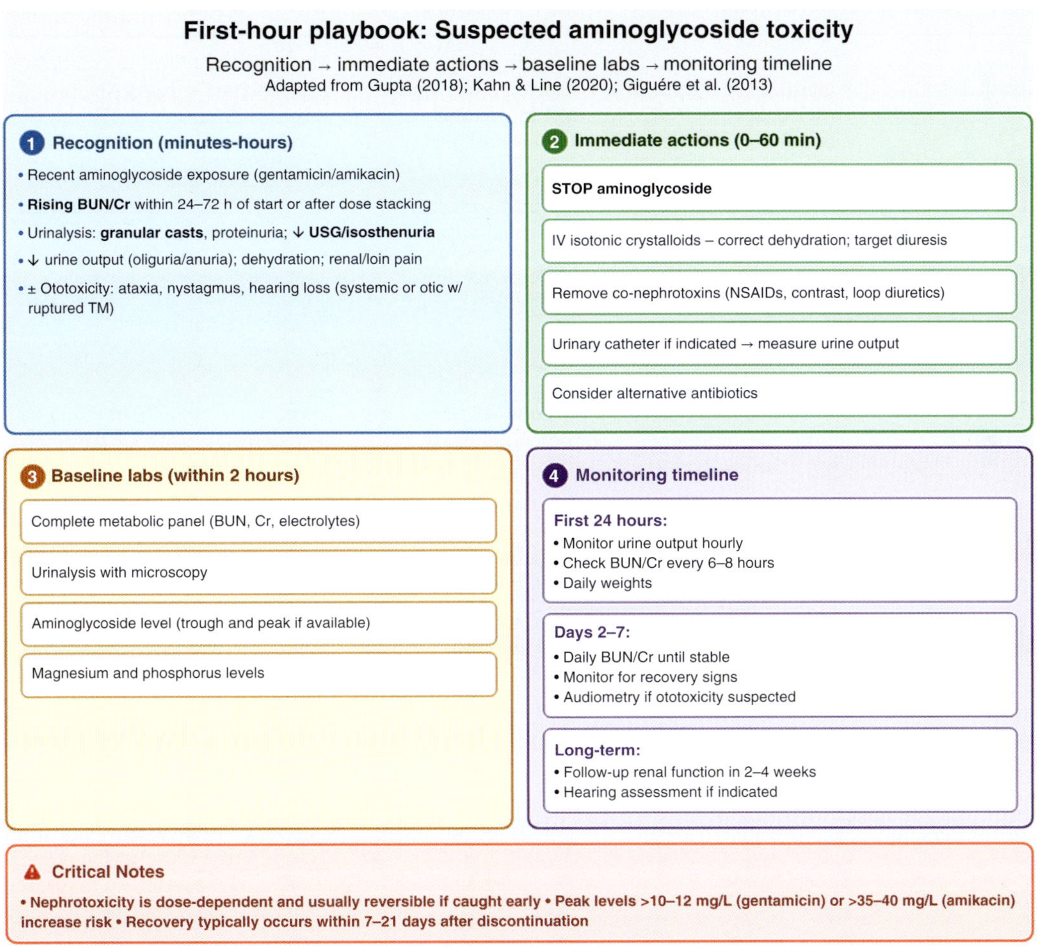

Figure 10.10 First-hour playbook for suspected aminoglycoside toxicity – recognition (rising BUN/Cr, casts), immediate actions (stop drug, fluids), initial labs (baseline and q24–48 h renal panel), and monitoring timeline. *Source:* Gupta (2018); Kahn and Line (2020); Giguère et al. (2013).

Treatment

Stop the drug; start isotonic crystalloids to correct dehydration, discontinue other nephrotoxins, and monitor renal indices q24–48 h; manage vestibular signs supportively. Preventive strategies include once-daily/extended-interval dosing where appropriate and routine therapeutic drug monitoring (TDM) on prolonged courses (Giguère et al., 2013; Papich, 2020). A bedside risk/monitoring checklist appears in Table 10.5.

Table 10.5 Aminoglycosides – risk factors, early markers, and monitoring cadence.

Risk factor	What to check	When to recheck	Action threshold
Dehydration/ hypovolemia	Hydration status, weight, urine output, UA (USG, **casts**), BUN/Cr, electrolytes (K^+/Mg^{2+})	After fluid resuscitation; then **q24 h** inpatient (or sooner if oliguria)	Any **upward trend** in creatinine or **new casts → hold AG**, optimize fluids, treat AKI protocol
Pre-existing renal disease/age extremes (geriatric, neonate)	Baseline renal panel + UA; consider GFR estimate if available	**q24–48 h** while on therapy; sooner if clinical change	Any deterioration from baseline (Cr/BUN, USG) → **pause/adjust AG** or switch class
Concurrent nephrotoxins (NSAIDs, radiocontrast, amphotericin B, loop diuretics)	Full med list; renal panel; **K^+/Mg^{2+}** (ototoxic synergy with loops)	Daily labs while co-exposed	If co-nephrotoxin cannot be stopped or labs drift → **stop AG**/ choose alternative
Cumulative exposure/ prolonged course	Day count; cumulative mg/kg; UA sediment; daily dose interval	UA **q24–48 h**; reassess indication **daily**	Appearance of **casts** or rising Cr despite fluids → **discontinue** or de-escalate therapy
High trough concentration (TDM)	**Trough** just before 3rd dose; peak if using target-peak strategy	After any dose/ interval change; then per protocol (e.g., weekly if prolonged)	**Detectable/above target trough → extend interval or reduce dose**; aim near-zero trough
Sepsis, hypotension, low perfusion	MAP/BP, lactate, perfusion parameters; urine output	Continuous hemodynamic checks; renal labs **q24 h**	Persistent hypotension/oliguria or rising Cr → **hold AG** until perfusion normalized
Topical otic AG with suspected TM rupture	Otoscopy; vestibular/ hearing signs (ataxia, nystagmus); caregiver reports	**Daily** while on otic meds	TM not intact or neurologic/ ototoxic signs → **stop ototopical AG**; use non-ototoxic alternative
Multiple daily dosing/ dose stacking	Regimen review (favor once-daily/extended-interval when appropriate)	TDM after regimen change	If interval too short or accumulation evident (rising trough/Cr) → **switch to extended interval** or alternate drug
Electrolyte disorders (hypo-Mg^{2+}/K^+)	Serum **Mg^{2+}/K^+**	**q24–48 h** or with diuretic use	Correct abnormalities; if persistent with AG on board → **pause AG** due to ↑ oto/ nephrotox risk

Table 10.5 (Continued)

Risk factor	What to check	When to recheck	Action threshold
Outpatient therapy	Owner diary: appetite, water intake/urination; arrange labs	**24–48 h** after start, then per risk (q48–72 h)	Missed checks or symptom report + any lab drift → **stop AG** and reassess plan

Columns: Risk factor | What to check | When to recheck | Action threshold.
Source: Giguère et al. (2013), Papich (2020), and Gupta (2018).

Fluoroquinolones

Source

Used for serious Gram-negative and mixed infections in small animals and horses; regulation in food animals varies by jurisdiction. In tropical practice, off-label human ciprofloxacin is sometimes substituted for veterinary products, producing variable exposure and risk (Giguère et al., 2013; Kahn & Line, 2020; Papich, 2020). Representative chemical structures for commonly used agents are shown in Figure 10.11 to anchor class identity before toxicity details.

Toxicity

Class concerns include articular cartilage injury in juveniles, central nervous system (CNS) excitation/ lowered seizure threshold, and idiosyncratic feline retinal degeneration with enrofloxacin (Kahn &

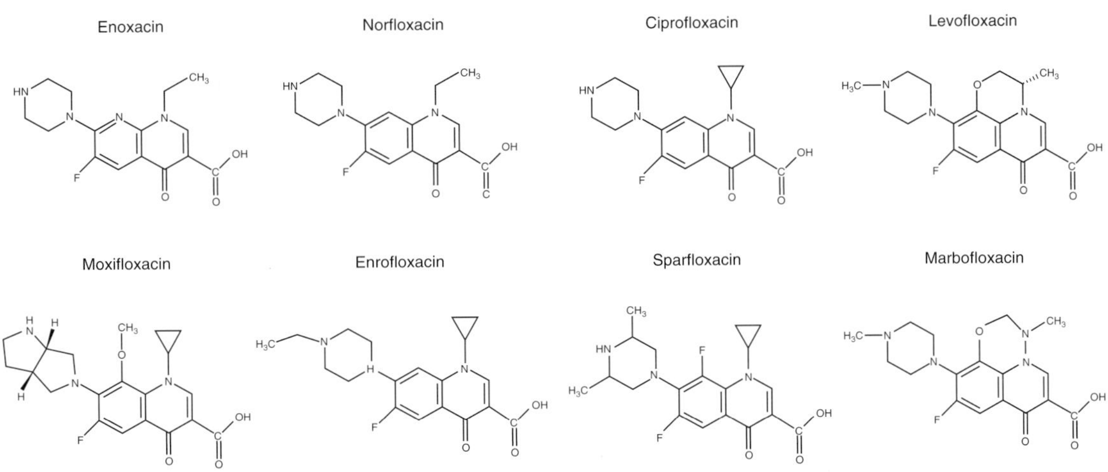

Figure 10.11 Chemical structures of common veterinary fluoroquinolones. Core quinolone scaffold with representative substitutions for enrofloxacin, ciprofloxacin, and marbofloxacin. *Source:* Adapted from Giguère et al. (2013) and Papich (2020).

Line, 2020; Papich, 2020). Retinopathy has followed higher-than-recommended dosing or IV administration and, rarely, label dosing in susceptible cats – presenting as acute blindness with fixed, dilated pupils (Gelatt, 2014; Papich, 2020). A one-page risk map summarizing who is most vulnerable (juveniles, cats on enrofloxacin, seizure-prone patients, dehydration/renal impairment, high-dose or rapid IV use, polypharmacy) appears in Figure 10.12.

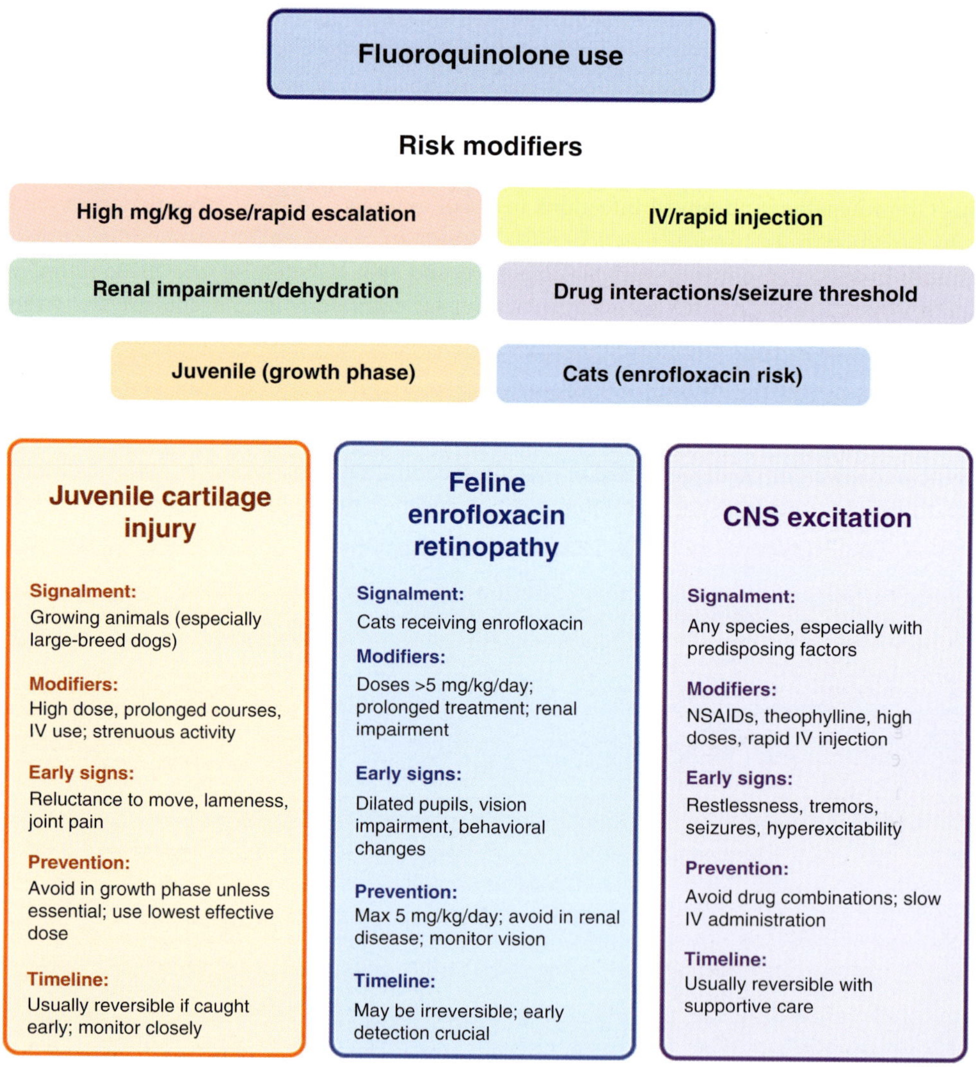

Figure 10.12 Fluoroquinolone risk map (tropical practice). Visual summary of major toxicities – juvenile cartilage injury, feline enrofloxacin retinopathy, and CNS excitation – with key modifiers (dose, IV use, renal disease, polypharmacy). *Source:* Giguère et al. (2013), Gelatt (2014), Kahn and Line (2020), and Papich (2020).

Mechanism of Action (Toxicity)

In growing animals, fluoroquinolones chelate Mg^{2+} in cartilage and disrupt chondrocyte matrix synthesis, leading to erosions of weight-bearing cartilage (Giguère et al., 2013). In cats, enrofloxacin has been associated with photoreceptor/retinal pigment epithelial damage – phototoxic/oxidative mechanisms are proposed (Gelatt, 2014). At high CNS concentrations, the class can antagonize γ-aminobutyric acid (GABA), lowering the seizure threshold (Kahn & Line, 2020).

Clinical Signs

Juveniles: Lameness and reluctance to move after several doses or prolonged courses (Giguère et al., 2013). Cats: sudden vision loss, mydriasis unresponsive to light; fundus – tapetal hyperreflectivity and vessel attenuation (Gelatt, 2014). CNS: agitation, tremor, or seizures at excessive doses or in predisposed patients (Kahn & Line, 2020).

Pathophysiology

Articular chondrocyte injury and fissuring of cartilage plates; retinal photoreceptor degeneration in cats; and usually reversible CNS signs in dogs when the drug is withdrawn (Gelatt, 2014; Giguère et al., 2013).

Diagnosis

Age/exposure history; orthopedic exam for juveniles; feline ophthalmic exam (menace/PLR, fundus ± ERG if available) for suspected retinopathy; review dose, route, and renal status (which alters exposure) (Gelatt, 2014; Papich, 2020).

Treatment

Discontinue the drug; protect affected cats from bright light; manage seizures with benzodiazepines if needed; switch to alternatives (e.g., marbofloxacin, orbifloxacin, pradofloxacin) as indicated; avoid class use in growing animals unless benefits outweigh risks (Kahn & Line, 2020; Papich, 2020). A bedside safe-use guardrail table (by patient group) is provided in Table 10.6.

Tetracyclines

Source

Broad-spectrum, inexpensive, and common in tropical practice for respiratory, tick-borne, and mixed infections. Oral and parenteral forms are used across species (Giguère et al., 2013; Papich, 2020). Representative chemical scaffolds for three members of the class are shown in Figure 10.13, which anchors class identity before toxicity details (Giguère et al., 2013; Papich, 2020).

Table 10.6 Fluoroquinolones – signature toxicities and safe-use guardrails. Patient-group rows (e.g., cats on enrofloxacin, growing animals, seizure-prone, renal impairment/dehydration, high-dose/rapid IV, polypharmacy) with columns for Hallmark risk, Early sign/test, First actions, Avoid/prefer.

Patient group	Hallmark risk	Early sign/test	First actions	Avoid/prefer
Cats (on enrofloxacin)	Dose-related retinal degeneration → acute blindness (Gelatt, 2014; Papich, 2020)	Mydriasis, reduced PLR; sudden vision change; ERG abnormalities if available (Gelatt, 2014)	Stop enrofloxacin immediately, protect from bright light, switch class; urgent ophthalmoscopic evaluation (Gelatt, 2014; Papich, 2020)	Avoid high-dose/IV enrofloxacin and use caution in renal disease; prefer feline-approved alternatives (e.g., pradofloxacin, marbofloxacin) when appropriate (Papich, 2020)
Growing animals (juvenile dogs/foals)	Articular cartilage injury → lameness (Giguère et al., 2013; Papich, 2020)	Reluctance to move, joint pain/ lameness during therapy	Defer/avoid FQ during growth if alternatives exist; rest; discontinue if orthopedic signs emerge (Giguère et al., 2013)	Avoid routine FQ in growth phase; prefer alternatives or shortest, lowest-effective dosing if essential (Papich, 2020)
Seizure-prone patients/low seizure threshold	CNS excitation (agitation, tremor, seizures) (Kahn & Line, 2020; Papich, 2020)	Disorientation, tremor; caregiver reports of new neurological signs	Stop FQ; manage seizures per protocol; correct electrolytes; review interacting drugs (Kahn & Line, 2020)	Avoid rapid IV administration and pro-convulsant co-meds (e.g., theophylline, certain NSAIDs); prefer non-FQ alternatives when feasible (Papich, 2020)
Renal impairment/ dehydration	Drug accumulation → ↑ risk of CNS/GI adverse effects (Kahn & Line, 2020; Papich, 2020)	Rising creatinine; reduced urine output; clinical dehydration	Rehydrate first; reduce dose/extend interval based on renal function; monitor closely (Papich, 2020)	Avoid high mg/kg and fixed q12 h in azotemia; prefer individualized dosing with interval extension + monitoring (Kahn & Line, 2020)
High-dose or rapid IV use (any species)	Exaggerated toxicity: CNS signs; in cats, retinal risk escalates (Gelatt, 2014; Papich, 2020)	Post-dose agitation, tremor; in cats, early mydriasis/PLR change	Slow/avoid IV push; switch to PO/IM where appropriate; reduce dose (Papich, 2020)	Avoid IV bolus and aggressive up-titration; prefer slow infusion (if IV necessary) and conservative dosing
Cats with pre-existing ocular disease or bright-light exposure	Photosensitized retinopathy risk heightened (Gelatt, 2014)	Light sensitivity, dilated pupils, visual deficits	Stop FQ; dark/ low-light precautions; ophthalmology consult (Gelatt, 2014)	Avoid enrofloxacin; prefer feline-safer FQs/non-FQ options and lowest effective dose (Papich, 2020)
Polypharmacy (drug interactions)	Lowered seizure threshold/altered exposure (Giguère et al., 2013; Papich, 2020)	New neuro signs after starting interacting meds; review med list	Deprescribe/replace interacting agents (e.g., theophylline); adjust FQ dose; monitor (Papich, 2020)	Avoid pro-convulsants and unnecessary CNS-active co-meds; prefer spaced administration away from cation-containing foods/ antacids to ensure predictable exposure (Kahn & Line, 2020)

FQ, fluoroquinolone; GI, gastrointestinal; IM, intramuscular; IV, intravenous; PLR, pupillary light reflex; PO, oral.
Source: Gelatt (2014), Giguère et al. (2013), Kahn and Line (2020), and Papich (2020).

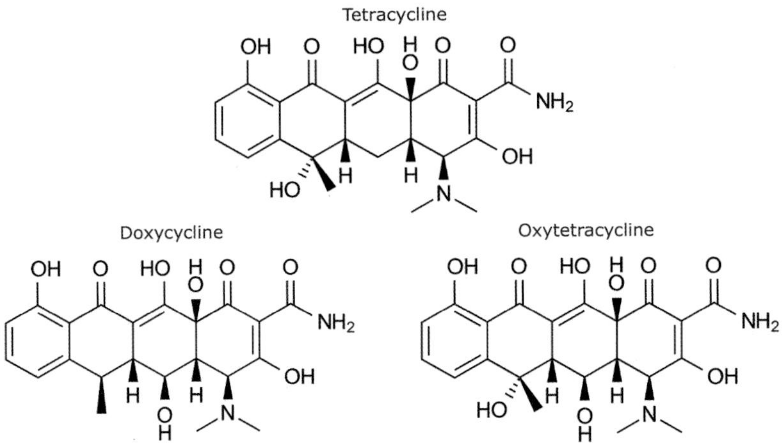

Figure 10.13 The chemical structure of three tetracycline antibiotics. Representative structures commonly used in veterinary medicine (e.g., oxytetracycline, doxycycline, minocycline). *Source:* Adapted from Giguère et al. (2013) and Papich (2020).

Toxicity

Typical issues include GI upset/dysbiosis, esophagitis, and esophageal stricture in cats with dry-pilled doxycycline, photosensitivity, tooth discoloration, and enamel hypoplasia in young animals, and hepatic injury at high doses or in susceptible patients (Gupta, 2018; Kahn & Line, 2020; Papich, 2020). Horses and other hindgut fermenters are at risk of antibiotic-associated colitis with some oral tetracyclines (Kahn & Line, 2020). A concise visual of these toxicity hotspots appears in Figure 10.14, highlighting where and why problems arise in clinical practice (Gupta, 2018; Kahn & Line, 2020; Papich, 2020).

Mechanism of Action (Toxicity)

Chelation of Ca^{2+} in developing teeth/bone explains discoloration and growth effects; photoactivated reactive species contribute to photosensitivity; pill esophagitis in cats results from local mucosal injury when tablets/capsules lodge in the esophagus (Gupta, 2018; Papich, 2020).

Clinical Signs

Cats (doxycycline): Dysphagia, hypersalivation, regurgitation days after dosing; later esophageal stricture (Kahn & Line, 2020; Papich, 2020).
Photosensitivity: Erythema/dermatitis on nonpigmented skin in strong sun exposure (Gupta, 2018).
Young animals: Permanent yellow-brown tooth discoloration (Kahn & Line, 2020).

Pathophysiology

Endoscopic evidence of esophageal ulceration/stricture in cats; phototoxic dermatitis on exposed skin; dental enamel incorporation of drug complexes during development (Gupta, 2018; Kahn & Line, 2020).

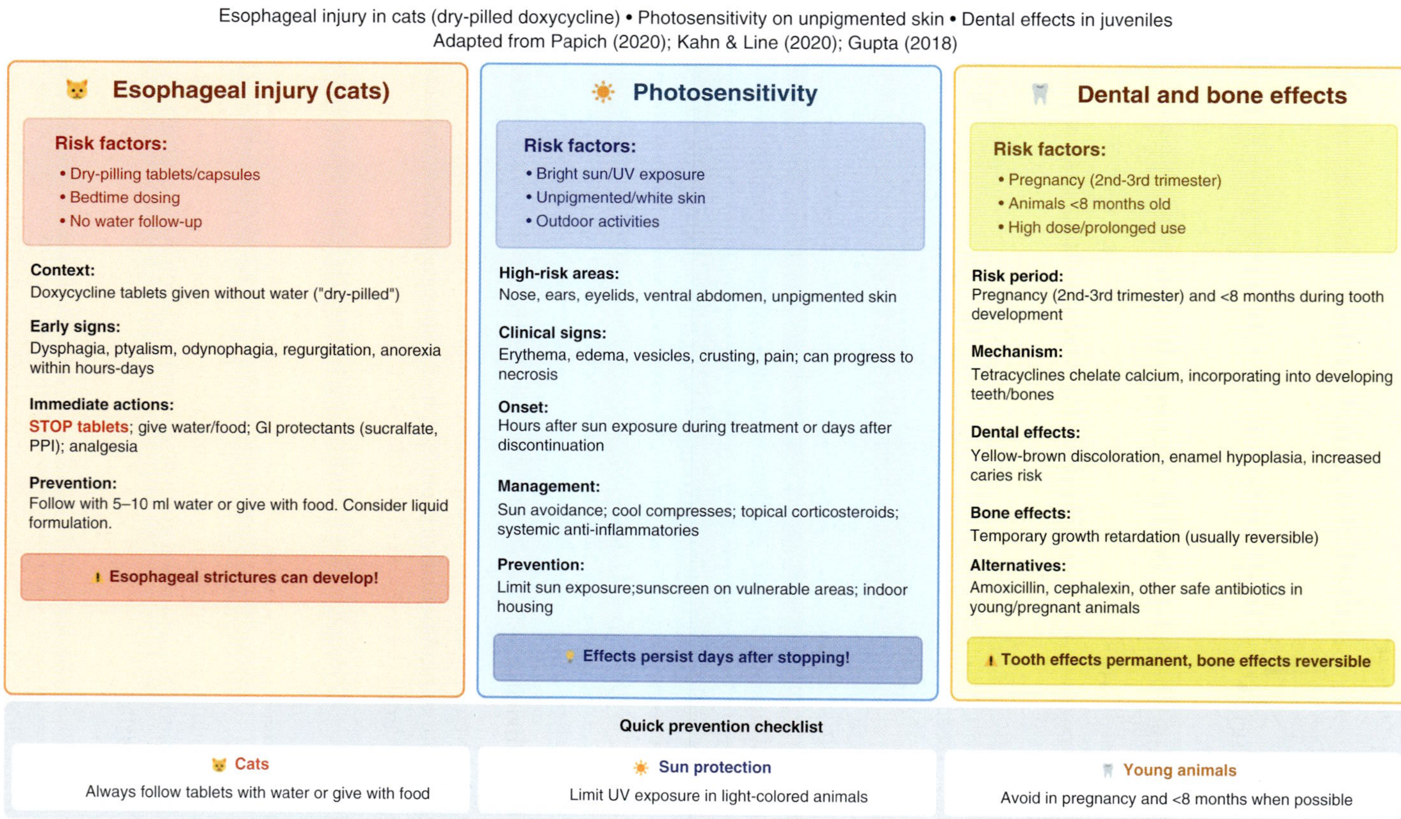

Figure 10.14 Tetracycline toxicity hotspots. Esophageal injury in cats (dry-pilled doxycycline), photosensitivity on unpigmented skin, and dental effects in juveniles with clinical cues and prevention notes. *Source:* Papich (2020); Kahn and Line (2020); and Gupta (2018).

Diagnosis

Exposure history; in cats, ask specifically about dry pilling. Thoracic radiographs or esophagoscopy for suspected stricture; complete blood count (CBC)/chemistry if hepatic injury suspected; consider species-specific risk factors (Kahn & Line, 2020; Papich, 2020).

Treatment

For pill esophagitis/stricture risk: Discontinue doxycycline, initiate sucralfate and a proton pump inhibitor (PPI) (e.g., omeprazole), and arrange endoscopic management if stricture forms. Prevention rule: never dry-pill cats – administer liquid formulations or follow tablets/capsules with ≥5–6 mL water or a small meal (Kahn & Line, 2020; Papich, 2020). For photosensitivity, limit UV exposure; for dental risks, avoid class use in late gestation/young animals where alternatives exist (Gupta, 2018). A scenario-based safety checklist is provided in Table 10.7 for bedside use (Gupta, 2018; Kahn & Line, 2020; Papich, 2020).

Table 10.7 Tetracyclines – administration safeguards and monitoring.

Scenario	Risk	Prevention (what to do)	Early sign	First actions
Cats given doxycycline as a “dry pill”	Esophagitis → stricture	Give with ≥5–6 mL water and/or small meal; avoid bedtime dosing; prefer liquid/paste formulations in cats	Dysphagia, ptyalism, painful swallow, regurgitation (hours–days)	Stop tablets/capsules; start GI protection (e.g., sucralfate, consider PPI), analgesia; switch to liquid; image if severe/persistent
Any species on tetracyclines with intense UV exposure	Photosensitivity dermatitis on unpigmented/sparse hair skin	Daytime UV avoidance; shade/clothing; lowest effective dose; owner education in sunny climates	Erythema, pruritus on white/薄-haired skin; ocular squinting	Reduce/stop drug; strict sun avoidance; topical wound/skin care; choose alternative class if needed
Pregnancy/juveniles in tooth–bone mineralization phase	Dental discoloration/hypoplasia; delayed bone growth	Avoid tetracyclines in late pregnancy/lactation and in growing animals when alternatives exist	Visible tooth discoloration; slowed growth	Discontinue; document findings; change class; counsel caregivers on prognosis/cosmesis
Swallowing dysfunction (megaesophagus, xerostomia)	Pill lodging → esophagitis	Use liquid formulation; feed “chaser” food/water; avoid recumbent dosing	Cough, regurgitation soon after dosing	Stop oral solid forms; switch to liquid; esophageal care as above

(Continued)

Table 10.7 (Continued)

Scenario	Risk	Prevention (what to do)	Early sign	First actions
High-dose/ prolonged courses	GI upset, hepatopathy (idiosyncratic/rare)	Baseline ALT/ALP/ bilirubin; give with food (if label allows); minimize duration	Anorexia, vomiting; rising ALT/ALP	Hold drug; supportive care; recheck serum biochemistry panel; select alternative agent
Co-administration with cations (iron, Ca^{2+}/Mg^{2+} antacids, dairy)	Treatment failure (chelation ↓ absorption)	Separate tetracycline dose by ≥2–3 h from cation products; avoid dairy with dose	Lack of clinical response	Educate owner; reschedule dosing; consider serum levels/ agent switch if needed
Parenteral oxytetracycline (large animals; horses/cattle)	Infusion reactions, phlebitis; injection-site pain/necrosis; nephrotoxicity (dehydration)	Dilute and give slowly IV (horses); limit IM volume/site; strict asepsis; ensure hydration; avoid extra-label routes	Local swelling/ pain; restlessness during infusion; rising creatinine	Stop/slow infusion; treat infiltration; analgesia/anti-inflammatories; fluids; adjust route/dose
Cats/dogs on minocycline	Vestibular signs (idiosyncratic)	Start at conservative dose; warn owners; avoid if prior intolerance	Disequilibrium, ataxia, nausea	Discontinue or reduce dose; antiemetics/ vestibular support; switch class
Concurrent hepatotoxins (e.g., azoles, high-dose acetaminophen in dogs)	Additive liver injury risk	Avoid combinations where possible; baseline and periodic chem panel	Early ALT rise; lethargy/ anorexia	Stop one/both agents; hepatoprotectants per protocol; monitor labs to trend recovery

ALT/ALP, alanine/aspartate aminotransferases; IM, intramuscular; IV, intravenous; PPI, proton-pump inhibitor.
Scenario-based checklist (risk → prevention → early sign → first actions), including never dry-pill cats, separate from cation products, sun avoidance advice, and avoidance in late pregnancy/juveniles.
Source: Papich (2020); Kahn and Line (2020); and Gupta (2018).

Brief Call-Outs – Chloramphenicol and Metronidazole

Chloramphenicol

Prolonged therapy can produce dose-dependent, reversible bone-marrow suppression (anemia, leukopenia, thrombocytopenia) in veterinary patients; moreover, the risk of idiosyncratic aplastic anemia in humans has led to its prohibition in food-producing animals in many jurisdictions because of residue concerns (Giguère et al., 2013; Kahn & Line, 2020; Plumb, 2018). When similar spectrum is needed in food animals, florfenicol is generally preferred where permitted (Kahn & Line, 2020; Plumb, 2018).

Metronidazole

Neurotoxicity is dose- and duration-related, most often presenting as vestibulo-cerebellar signs (ataxia, nystagmus, head tilt), tremors, or seizures; management is to stop the drug immediately and provide supportive care. Multiple veterinary references note that diazepam may hasten neurological recovery in affected dogs and cats (Kahn & Line, 2020; Papich, 2020; Peterson & Talcott, 2013).

To close the antimicrobials section, Table 10.8 consolidates the "what next?" pivot after recognition and stabilization – linking each signature toxicity to the immediate first steps and giving practical, culture-guided safer alternatives, with species/breed traps and regulatory constraints flagged (Gelatt, 2014; Giguère et al., 2013; Gupta, 2018; Kahn & Line, 2020; Papich, 2020; Peterson & Talcott, 2013; Plumb, 2018).

Anthelmintics and Antiprotozoals – Overview of Toxicities in Tropical Practice

Heavy parasite pressure, OTC access, depot/long-acting formulations, and off-label dose stacking in tropical systems narrow safety margins across these drug classes. Use the toxidrome cues below plus the first-hour actions, then lock in prevention and stewardship tailored to species, genetics, and environment (Gupta, 2018; Kahn & Line, 2020; Peterson & Talcott, 2013).

Macrocyclic Lactones (Ivermectin, Doramectin, Moxidectin)

Source

Endectocides used for nematodes and ectoparasites (pour-on, oral, injectable). Reliance is high in tropical livestock and working dogs; long-acting/depot products are common (Kahn & Line, 2020). ABCB1/MDR1 variants in collie-type dogs reduce blood–brain barrier P-glycoprotein (P-gp); chelonians are highly susceptible and should not receive this class (Gupta, 2018; Kahn & Line, 2020). Representative avermectin vs. milbemycin scaffolds are shown in Figure 10.15 to anchor class identity before toxicity details (Giguère et al., 2013; Papich, 2020).

Toxicity

Toxidrome: Progressive CNS depression → ataxia, tremors, cortical blindness, coma; mydriasis, hypersalivation; onset may be delayed with depot formulations. Amplifiers: extra-label/high doses; MDR1 genotype; dehydration or hepatic compromise; co-administration of P-gp/CYP inhibitors (e.g., azoles, macrolides, cyclosporine) or sedatives (Kahn & Line, 2020; Peterson & Talcott, 2013). A quick risk map appears in Figure 10.16.

Mechanism of Action (Toxicity)

At toxic CNS levels, macrocyclic lactones potentiate GABA_A and glutamate-gated chloride channels; P-gp deficiency (ABCB1) permits CNS accumulation (Gupta, 2018; Peterson & Talcott, 2013).

Table 10.8 Antimicrobials – signature toxicities and safer alternatives (tropical practice).

Drug/class	Typical tropical use	Hallmark toxicity	Species/breed traps	Antidote/first steps	Safer alternative (when)
Sulfonamides ± trimethoprim	Broad empirical coverage; coccidiosis support	Idiosyncratic hypersensitivity (fever, polyarthropathy, KCS, hepatopathy); crystalluria/obstruction	Dogs (e.g., Doberman lines), dehydrated patients, acidic urine	Stop drug; IV fluids/urinalysis; Schirmer tear test; manage immune-mediated signs	Amoxicillin–clavulanate or 1st/2nd-gen cephalosporin when culture allows; toltrazuril/ponazuril for coccidiosis (per label/regulation) (Giguère et al., 2013; Kahn & Line, 2020; Papich, 2020)
Nitrofurans (legacy)	Historic GI/UTI/coccidiosis; legacy stocks	Neurotoxicity; hemorrhagic diathesis; marrow suppression	Calves; ducklings > chicks; food animal residue bans	Withdraw immediately; fluids/electrolytes; monitor coagulation	Use labeled, permitted agents per culture: e.g., amoxicillin–clavulanate for UTIs; ceftiofur in cattle (jurisdiction dependent) (Constable et al., 2016; Kahn & Line, 2020; Papich, 2020)
Aminoglycosides (gentamicin/amikacin/neomycin/streptomycin)	Sepsis, pneumonia, uterine infections	Non-oliguric AKI; ototoxicity (± neuromuscular blockade)	Cats (oto risk), dehydrated ruminants, geriatrics, renal disease	Stop drug; crystalloids; stop nephrotoxins; monitor BUN/Cr q24–48 h	Ceftiofur (ruminants); amoxicillin–clavulanate (small animals) when susceptible; consider FQ only if juvenile/cat risks addressed (Giguère et al., 2013; Gupta, 2018; Kahn & Line, 2020; Papich, 2020)
Fluoroquinolones – juveniles (class)	Serious Gram-negatives	Articular cartilage injury	Growing dogs/foals	Discontinue; rest; switch class	Culture-directed β-lactam (e.g., amox-clav, cephalosporin) or doxycycline for tick-borne targets as indicated (Giguère et al., 2013; Kahn & Line, 2020; Papich, 2020)
Enrofloxacin – cats	Serious Gram-negatives in cats	Idiosyncratic retinal degeneration → acute blindness	Cats (higher doses/rapid IV ↑ risk)	Discontinue; reduce light exposure; ophthalmic monitoring	Pradofloxacin or marbofloxacin in cats when a FQ is essential; otherwise culture-guided β-lactam (Gelatt, 2014; Kahn & Line, 2020; Papich, 2020)

Tetracyclines – doxycycline (cats)	Tick-borne, respiratory	Esophagitis/stricture (dry-pilling)	Cats; poor pill-follow with water/food	Stop; sucralfate + PPI; endoscopic care if stricture	Liquid doxycycline or tablets strictly with ≥5–6 mL water/meal; for selected indications, azithromycin (disease-dependent) (Kahn & Line, 2020; Papich, 2020)
Tetracyclines (class)	Broad, vector-borne	Photosensitivity; dental discoloration in juveniles; hepatopathy at high dose	Light-skinned animals in high UV; late gestation/young	Sun avoidance; stop if severe; avoid in late gestation/juveniles	Consider non-photosensitizing alternatives guided by culture (e.g., amox-clav, macrolide for specific respiratory pathogens) (Gupta, 2018; Kahn & Line, 2020; Papich, 2020)
Chloramphenicol	Anaerobes, respiratory (small animals)	Dose-related marrow suppression; human aplastic-anemia risk	Food animals (residue prohibition)	Stop; monitor CBC	Florfenicol in food animals where legal; small-animal alternatives: amox-clav, clindamycin per culture (Giguère et al., 2013; Kahn & Line, 2020; Plumb, 2018
Metronidazole	Anaerobes; protozoa (Giardia)	Dose-related neurotoxicity (vestibulo-cerebellar)	Hepatic disease; high dose/long duration	Stop; supportive care; diazepam may hasten recovery	Clindamycin for anaerobes (site-specific); fenbendazole for Giardia (Kahn & Line, 2020; Papich, 2020; Peterson & Talcott, 2013)

Quick-reference crosswalk mapping drug/class → typical tropical use → hallmark toxicity → species/breed traps → antidote/first steps → safer alternative (when).

1) Select alternatives based on culture/susceptibility, site of infection, and patient comorbidities; verify label status and observe residue/withdrawal requirements for food animals.
2) Regulatory restrictions vary by jurisdiction (e.g., chloramphenicol and nitrofurans prohibited in food-producing animals; additional limits may apply to fluoroquinolones or nitroimidazoles); confirm locally before prescribing (Kahn & Line, 2020; Papich, 2020).
3) Doses are intentionally omitted here – consult your formulary/texts cited for current dosing and monitoring guidance (Giguère et al., 2013; Peterson & Talcott, 2013; Plumb, 2018).

Source: Giguère et al. (2013); Gupta (2018); Kahn and Line (2020); Papich (2020); Gelatt (2014); Plumb (2018); and Peterson and Talcott (2013).

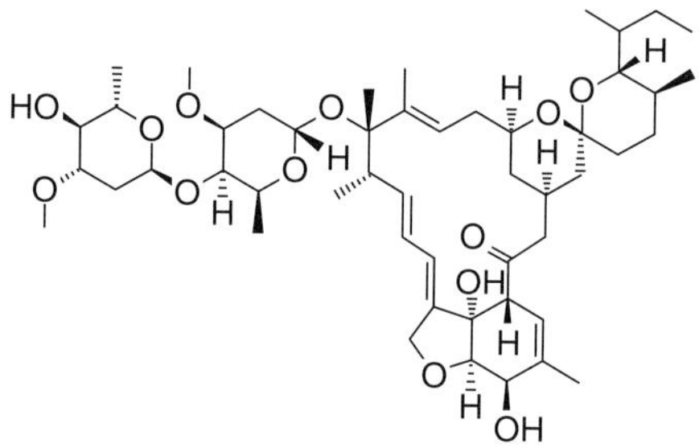

Ivermectin B1a 36.11.1a

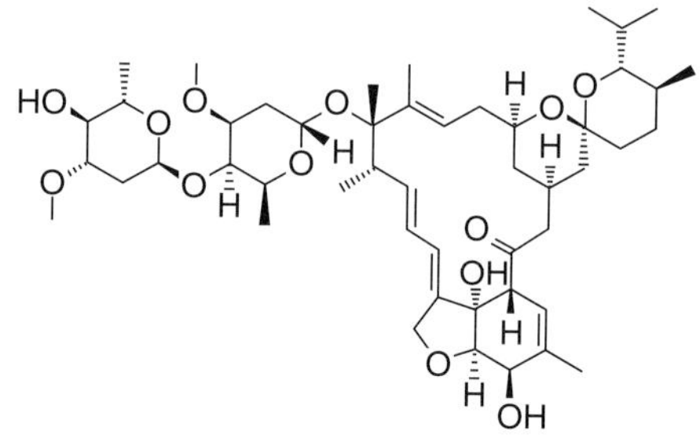

Ivermectin B1b 36.11.1b

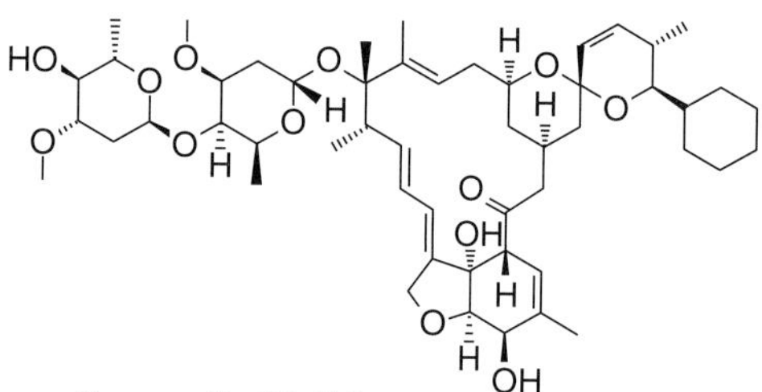

Doramectin 36.11.2

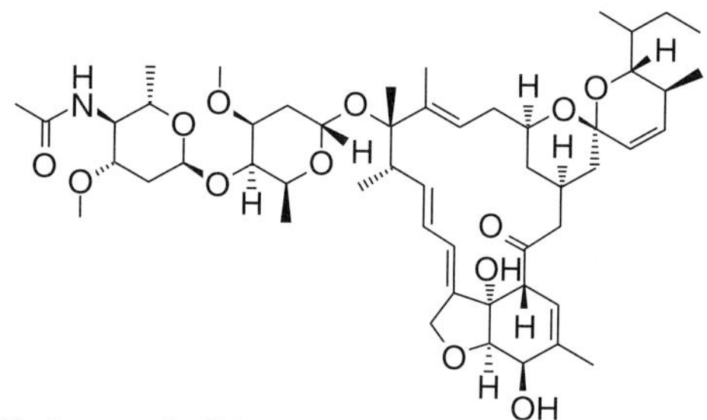

Eprinomectin B1a 36.11.3

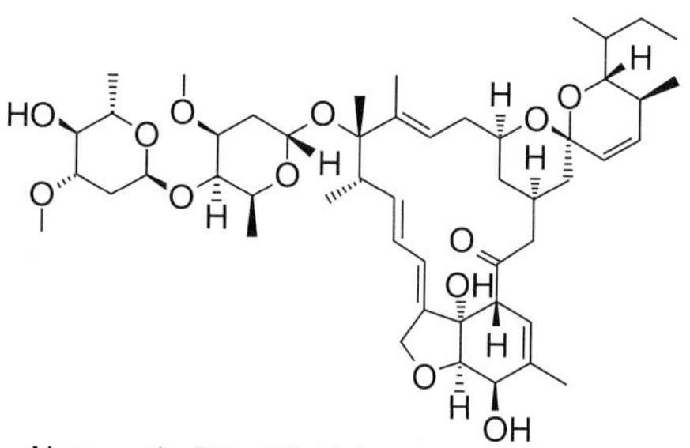

Abamectin B1a 36.11.4a

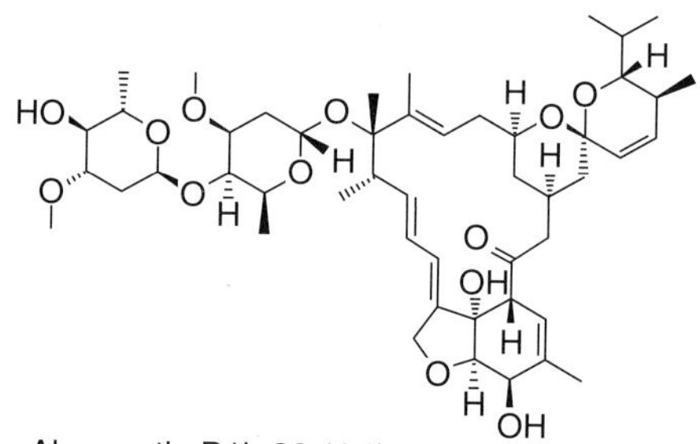

Abamectin B1b 36.11.4b

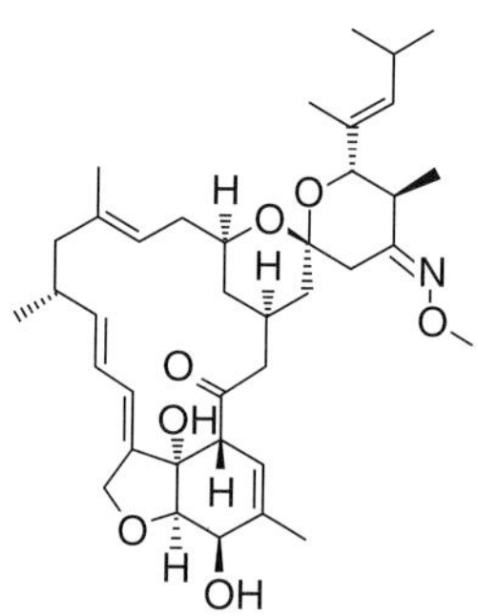

Moxidectin 36.11.5

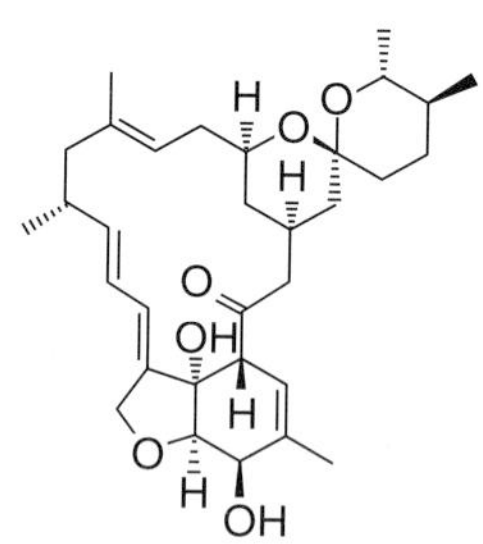

Milbemycin A1 36.11.6

Figure 10.15 Structure of macrocyclic lactone anthelmintics. Representative avermectins (e.g., ivermectin, doramectin) and milbemycins (moxidectin) highlighting shared macrocyclic lactone cores and key side-chain differences. *Source:* Adapted from Giguère et al. (2013) and Papich (2020).

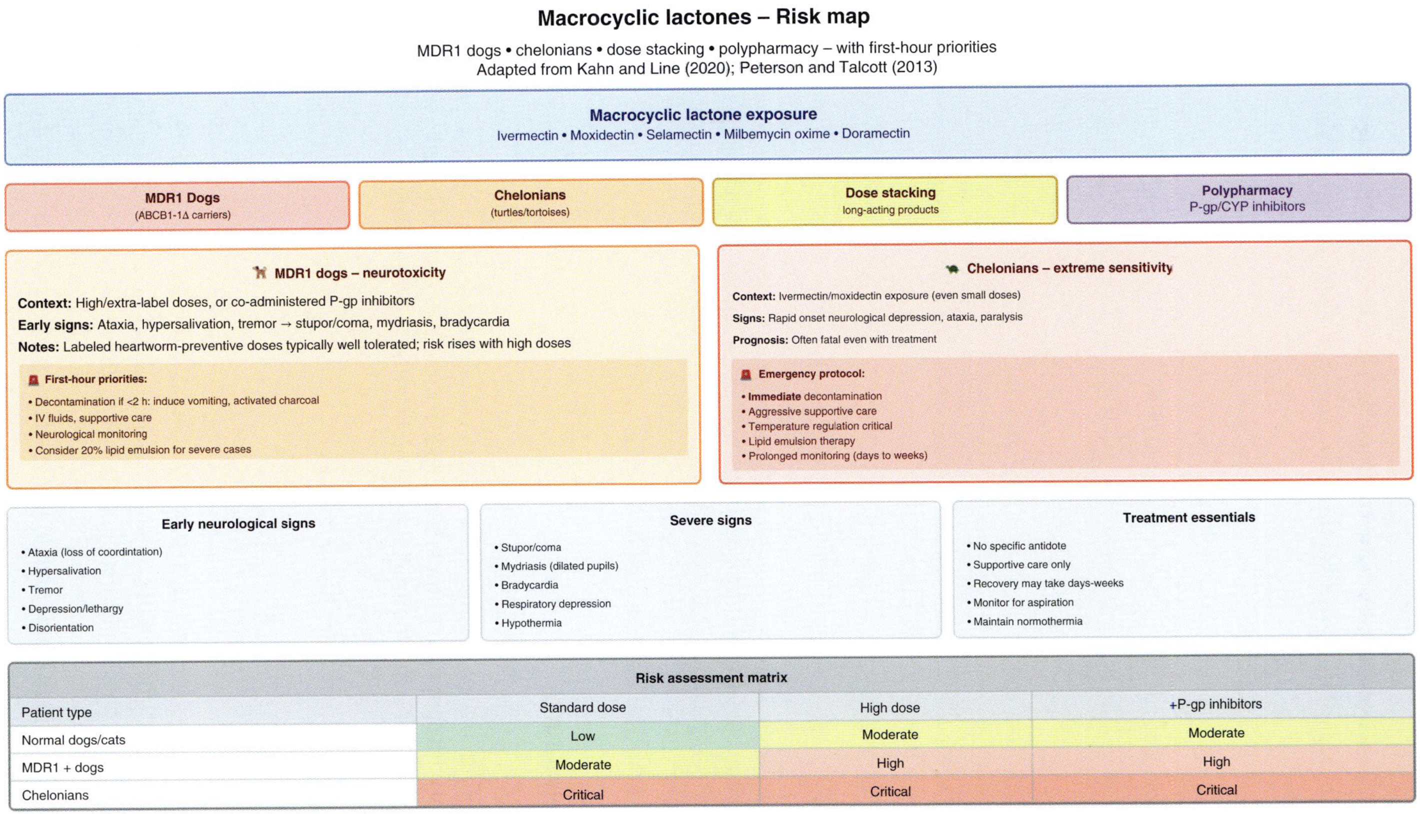

Figure 10.16 Macrocyclic lactones – risk map (tropical practice). MDR1/ABCB1 dogs, chelonians, dose stacking/long-acting products, and polypharmacy (P-gp/CYP inhibitors) with first-hour priorities (stabilize ABCs, avoid extra sedatives, consider lipid therapy in severe cases). *Source:* Kahn and Line (2020) and Peterson and Talcott (2013).

Clinical Signs

Quiet to obtunded mentation, ataxia, tremors, hypersalivation; absent menace with variable PLR; bradycardia/hypoventilation in severe cases (Kahn & Line, 2020). Signs may wax and wane or recur with long-acting products.

Pathophysiology

White-matter vacuolation/edema in brain; reversible retinal dysfunction described in some dogs (Gupta, 2018).

Diagnosis

Confirm product, route, dose, and stacking (pour-on + oral + long-acting). Consider ABCB1 testing (where available). Screen for OP/carbamate co-exposures. Drug quantitation in serum/fat may be available in specialized labs (Kahn & Line, 2020; Peterson & Talcott, 2013).

Treatment

Stabilize airway/ventilation and temperature; avoid additional GABAergic sedatives unless controlling seizures. Activated charcoal (if recent oral exposure and airway protected; repeat dosing may help with large/depot exposures). Intravenous lipid emulsion (ILE) is a reasonable adjunct in life-threatening neurotoxicity (case-series support). IV crystalloids, careful nursing, and low-stimulus care; vision may recover over days–weeks (Kahn & Line, 2020; Peterson & Talcott, 2013).

Prevention and Stewardship

Genotype ABCB1 dogs when feasible; dose discipline (no "extra for sarcoptic mange" beyond label); avoid P-gp/CYP inhibitors when possible; never use in chelonians; separate species during handling and prevent cross-licking with spot-ons (Kahn & Line, 2020). Table 10.9 provides a bedside checklist of exposure contexts → early signs → first-hour actions → monitoring → prevention (e.g., MDR1 dogs, depot products, polypharmacy, large-animal concentrates, chelonian exposure).

Levamisole

Source

Nicotinic anthelmintic for GI nematodes in small ruminants and cattle; widely used in tropical systems for *Haemonchus* control where rapid hematocrit decline drives urgent deworming. The therapeutic index is narrow, so weight estimation errors, stacked products, and same-day pesticide use can quickly tip into toxicosis (Gupta, 2018; Kahn & Line, 2020). A simple scaffold reference for the molecule is shown in Figure 10.17.

Table 10.9 Macrocyclic lactones – exposure contexts, early signs, first actions, monitoring, and prevention.

Exposure context	Early signs	First actions (0–60 min)	Monitoring	Prevention (genotype, dose discipline)
MDR1/ABCB1-1Δ dogs (Collie-type, Sheltie, Aussie; status unknown or high dose)	Ataxia, hypersalivation, tremor → stupor/coma; mydriasis; bradycardia	Stop drug; stabilize ABCs; control tremor/seizure per protocol; if oral and recent/asymptomatic: emesis per protocol → activated charcoal (consider repeat doses for large exposures); consider lipid emulsion in severe neurotoxicity	Neuro checks q2–4 h; HR/RR, SpO_2, temperature; glucose/electrolytes; observe ≥24–72 h (longer if depot/large dose)	Genotype before high-risk use; avoid extra-label high doses; use labeled HW-preventive doses only; document status in chart
Polypharmacy – P-gp/CYP inhibitors (e.g., azoles, macrolides, cyclosporine) or pro-convulsants	Faster onset/worse CNS depression; agitation/seizures	Hold macrocyclic lactone and interacting drug(s); manage seizures; charcoal if ingestion recent; admit	As above; add drug–drug review; consider longer observation for delayed recurrence	Audit med list; avoid unnecessary inhibitors/pro-convulsants; space or replace interacting agents
Dose stacking/multiple products/long-acting depot	Prolonged or biphasic CNS signs; relapse after partial recovery	Stop all products; confirm brands/strengths/routes; charcoal (repeat dosing may help with enterohepatic/depot exposure); supportive care	Extended observation (48–96 h); daily neuro exam; repeat electrolytes if fluids given	One product at a time; implement a cool-off interval when switching; weigh the patient and calculate mg/kg every time
Accidental topical ingestion (selamectin/moxidectin spot-on) or licking treated housemate	Hypersalivation, vomiting; ataxia/depression	Decontaminate skin (mild dish soap bath), prevent further licking; if ingestion <1–2 h and asymptomatic → emesis; charcoal as indicated; supportive care	Neuro/GI checks for 24–48 h; temperature	Separate treated animals until dry; apply correct dose to intact skin only; e-collar if needed
Concentrated large-animal products ingested by dogs/cats (pour-on/drench/injectable)	Rapid, severe CNS depression; tremors/seizures; apnea	As above plus early charcoal (repeat) and strong supportive care; consider lipid emulsion; ventilatory support if needed	ICU-level monitoring; blood gases as available	Do not store or use LA concentrates around pets; secure storage; species-correct products only
Chelonians (turtles/tortoises) exposure	Profound depression, paresis/paralysis, apnea; high fatality	Absolute avoidance is best; if exposed: immediate decontamination, oxygen/ventilation support, consult exotics/poison center	Continuous respiratory/neuro monitoring; prolonged care often required	Never use macrocyclic lactones in chelonians; flag hospital formulary; staff education
High-dose extra-label ivermectin/moxidectin (e.g., demodicosis protocols)	Dose-related CNS depression; vomiting; ataxia	Hold therapy, convert to safer regimen; treat as per MDR1 row if signs present	Daily neuro checks; revisit indication and alternatives	Prefer labeled options or safer alternatives; ABCB1 testing before high-dose protocols; start low/go slow with close rechecks

(*Continued*)

Table 10.9 (Continued)

Exposure context	Early signs	First actions (0–60 min)	Monitoring	Prevention (genotype, dose discipline)
Neonates/underweight/ill or dehydrated patients	Enhanced sedation/ataxia; hypothermia	Stabilize hydration/temperature first; hold drug; treat symptomatically	Temperature, glucose, electrolytes; neuro checks	Dose by current weight; avoid in unstable or dehydrated animals; ensure euvolemia before dosing
Outpatient adherence errors (missed then "double-dosed", wrong strength)	Variable; GI upset → CNS signs	Triage when/how much; do not "catch up"; consider charcoal if recent and asymptomatic	24–48 h observation if moderate overdose	Provide written calendars/alerts; use weight-appropriate single-dose products; dispense lowest effective strength
Topical exposure to abraded skin or open wounds	Faster onset of systemic signs at smaller amounts	Wash thoroughly; wound care; monitor; supportive care as needed	24–48 h neuro/temp checks	Apply only to intact skin; avoid peri-wound areas; owner handling instructions

ABCs, airway/breathing/circulation; CYP, cytochrome P450; HW, heartworm; P-gp, P-glycoprotein.
Rows include MDR1 dogs, polypharmacy, dose stacking/depot, accidental topical ingestion/licking, large-animal product ingestion by pets, chelonian exposure, high-dose extra-label protocols, neonates/ill/dehydrated, adherence errors, abraded-skin exposure; columns: Exposure context | Early signs | First actions (0–60 minutes) | Monitoring | Prevention.
Source: Kahn and Line (2020); Gupta (2018); Peterson and Talcott (2013).

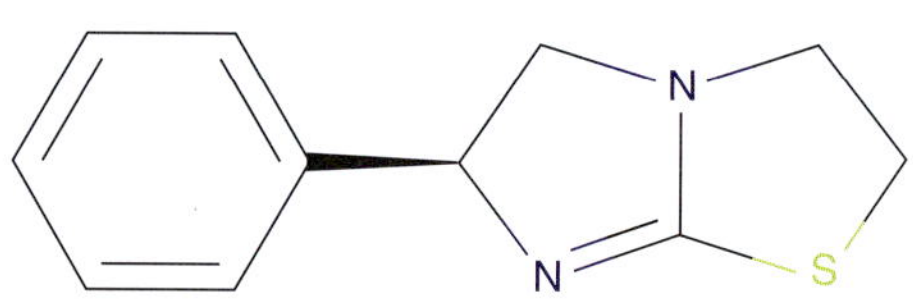

Figure 10.17 Chemical structure of levamisole. Author's schematic to aid class recognition; structure redrawn from standard pharmacology data. See Kahn and Line (2020) and Gupta (2018) for clinical use and safety context.

Toxicity

Toxidrome: Nicotinic cholinergic overstimulation – SLUD (salivation, lacrimation, urination, defecation), tachypnea/dyspnea, colic, muscle fasciculations → tremor, weakness, collapse; seizures may occur. High-risk interaction: same-day levamisole with organophosphates/carbamates (dips, sprays, feed additives) markedly increases severity (Gupta, 2018; Kahn & Line, 2020). A first-hour triage schematic appears in Figure 10.18.

Mechanism of Action (Toxicity)

Direct agonism at nicotinic acetylcholine receptors at the neuromuscular junction; additive/synergistic effects with acetylcholinesterase (AChE)-inhibiting OP/carbamate exposures amplify cholinergic tone (Gupta, 2018).

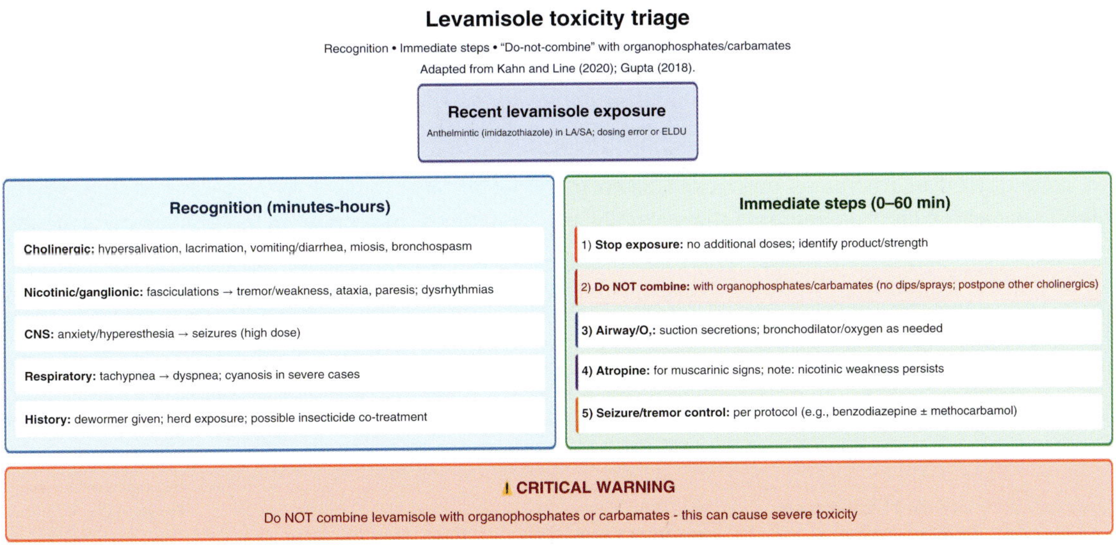

Figure 10.18 Levamisole toxicity triage. Recognition (SLUD, fasciculations, collapse), immediate steps (airway/O_2, atropine for muscarinic signs, diazepam for seizures), and explicit "do-not-combine" warning with organophosphates/carbamates. *Source:* Kahn and Line (2020) and Gupta (2018).

Clinical Signs

Onset within hours of dosing: profuse salivation and diarrhea, abdominal pain/colic, muscle fasciculation, ataxia/recumbency; hypoxemia may follow from airway secretions and respiratory muscle weakness; seizures in severe cases (Kahn & Line, 2020).

Pathophysiology

Overstimulation at the neuromuscular junction (NMJ) with secondary respiratory/metabolic compromise; severe cases may show acid–base derangements from hypoventilation and agitation (Gupta, 2018).

Diagnosis

Confirm dose (mg/kg) and species-specific plan (goats typically require different dosimetry than sheep); weigh animals (avoid eyeballing). Elicit OP/carbamate use in the last 24–48 hours. Differentiate from OP poisoning: blood cholinesterase activity is usually normal in levamisole toxicosis (Kahn & Line, 2020).

Treatment

Atropine for prominent muscarinic signs (salivation, bronchorrhea); diazepam for seizures; oxygen and suction as needed; IV crystalloids and temperature support. GI decontamination only if very recent and the airway is protected. Remove OP/carbamate co-exposures and avoid further cholinergic drugs (Gupta, 2018; Kahn & Line, 2020).

Prevention and Stewardship

No same-day OPs/carbamates or stacked dewormers; weigh accurately (use a scale or weight tape), follow species-specific dosimetry (goats vs. sheep), and defer treatment in debilitated or severely parasitized animals until stabilized (Kahn & Line, 2020).

Table 10.10 summarizes species/context-specific safeguards, early red flags, first steps, and a practical do-not-combine list for field teams.

Table 10.10 Levamisole – narrow therapeutic-index safeguards by species, red flags, and first steps.

Species/ context	Narrow TI safeguards (before dosing)	Red flags (early signs)	First steps (0–60 min)	Do-not-combine (high-risk co-exposures*)
Cattle (beef/ dairy)	Weigh accurately; label-dose only; avoid dehydrated, stressed, or severely parasitized animals until stabilized; do not stack dewormers the same day.	Hypersalivation, diarrhea, bradycardia; muscle fasciculations/ataxia; tachypnea → dyspnea.	Stop levamisole; airway/ O_2; atropine for muscarinic signs; control tremor/seizure per protocol; consider emesis/charcoal only if very recent ingestion and appropriate.	OP insecticides (e.g., dichlorvos, coumaphos, malathion), carbamates (carbaryl, carbofuran, propoxur); other cholinergics.
Sheep/ goats	Dose to current weight; avoid sick, late-gestation, or debilitated animals; separate from other cholinergics by label washout.	Hypersalivation, abdominal pain, diarrhea; weakness, ataxia.	As above; fluids/ temperature support; admit if respiratory effort increases.	OPs; carbamates; stacked deworming (same-day).
Swine	Calibrate dosing equipment; avoid extra-label mg/kg; withhold if febrile or dehydrated.	Vomiting/diarrhea; tremor; cyanosis if severe.	As above; antiemetics/ supportive care as needed.	OPs/carbamates; other cholinergic parasiticides.
Camelids	Use conservative label-equivalent dosing; avoid if anorectic or dehydrated; monitor closely first 2–4 h.	Salivation, weakness, ataxia; tachypnea.	Stop drug; oxygen and supportive care; consider referral if worsening.	OPs/carbamates; stacked products.
Horses (ELDU not preferred)	Prefer labeled equine anthelmintics; if used, strict weight-based dosing; avoid stressed/ ill horses.	Sweating, colic-like discomfort; salivation; ataxia.	Discontinue; symptomatic care; avoid further cholinergics.	OPs/carbamates; cholinergic GI prokinetics.

Table 10.10 (Continued)

Species/ context	Narrow TI safeguards (before dosing)	Red flags (early signs)	First steps (0–60 min)	Do-not-combine (high-risk co-exposures*)
Dogs/cats (generally avoid routine use)	Avoid unless compelling indication; verify product/strength; caution in small or compromised patients.	Hypersalivation, vomiting/diarrhea; tremor/seizure; bradycardia.	Stop exposure; airway/O_2; atropine for muscarinic signs; benzodiazepine for seizures; consider charcoal if appropriate and protected airway.	OP/carbamate flea/tick dips, sprays, collars; other cholinergics.

* Do-not-combine list (class examples): Organophosphates – dichlorvos, coumaphos, malathion; carbamates – carbaryl, carbofuran, propoxur. Avoid same-day or close-interval co-treatment; follow label washout intervals; never "stack" cholinergic parasiticides.
ELDU, extra-label drug use; O_2, oxygen; OP, organophosphate; TI, therapeutic index.
Rows by species/context (cattle; sheep/goats; swine; camelids; horses [ELDU]; dogs/cats) with columns for Narrow TI safeguards (before dosing), Red flags (early signs), First steps (0–60 minutes), and Do-not-combine (high-risk co-exposures).
Source: Kahn and Line (2020) and Gupta (2018).

Benzimidazoles (Albendazole, Fenbendazole)

Source

Broad-spectrum agents for GI nematodiasis (some cestodes/trematodes) across ruminants, equids, swine, and small animals; overall wide safety margin when label directions and timing are respected (Kahn & Line, 2020). A side-by-side of albendazole vs. fenbendazole chemical scaffolds is shown in Figure 10.19 to anchor class identity before safety nuances (Gupta, 2018; Kahn & Line, 2020).

Toxicity

Key cautions include albendazole teratogenicity – avoid during early pregnancy (organogenesis) – and rare bone-marrow suppression and hepatotoxicity with prolonged/high-dose regimens; malnutrition, heavy parasite burdens, and concurrent illness can amplify risk (Gupta, 2018; Kahn & Line, 2020). A species-specific "do-not-use" window graphic appears in Figure 10.20 (e.g., cattle and small ruminants – first ~30–45 days of gestation; equids – avoid T1; dogs/cats – prefer fenbendazole, avoid albendazole in pregnancy).

Mechanism of Action (Toxicity)

Benzimidazoles bind β-tubulin, disrupting microtubules; at sufficiently high mammalian exposures this impairs embryogenesis and other rapidly dividing host cells, explaining teratogenicity and occasional myelosuppression (Gupta, 2018).

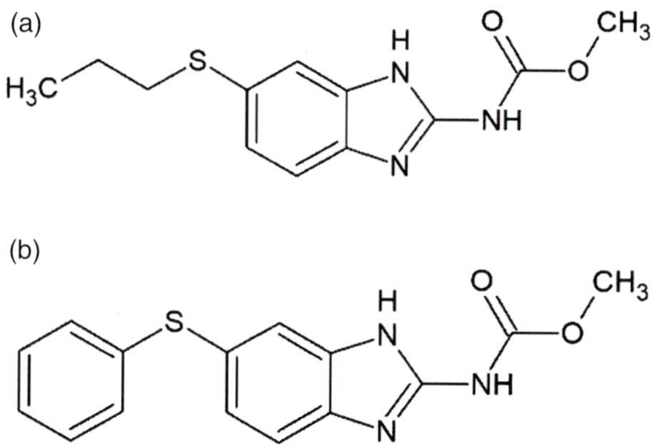

Figure 10.19 Chemical structures of (a) albendazole and (b) fenbendazole. Side-by-side structures highlighting the benzimidazole core and thio/oxy substituents used in veterinary practice. Adapted from standard pharmacology sources referenced in text (Gupta, 2018; Kahn & Line, 2020).

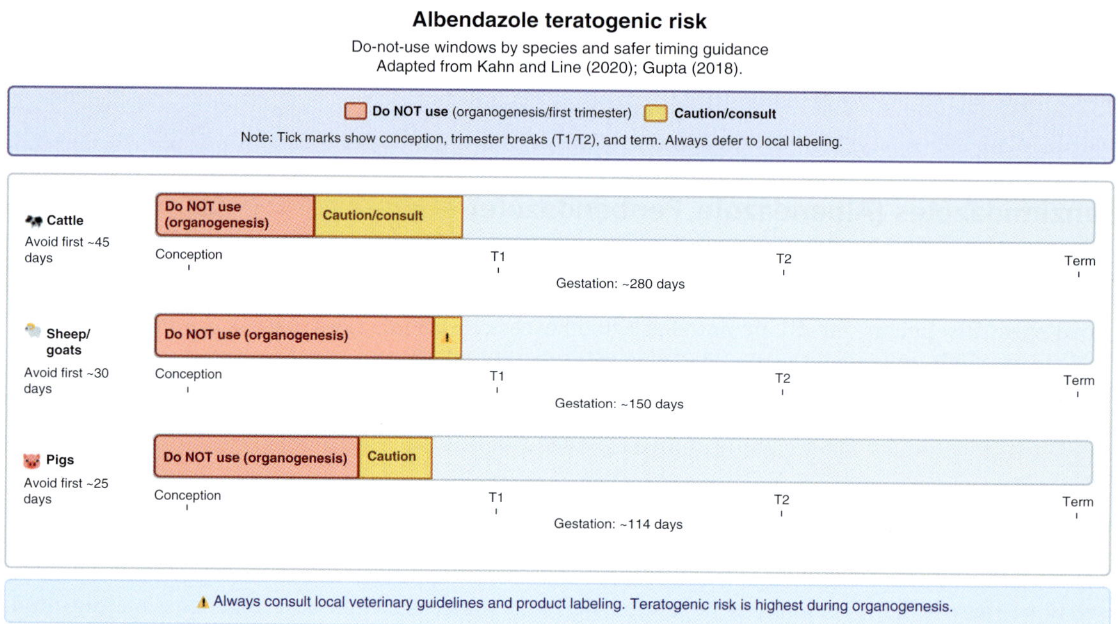

Figure 10.20 Albendazole teratogenic risk – do-not-use windows by species and safer timing guidance. Schematic showing first-trimester avoidance periods in cattle, sheep/goats, and equids, and small-animal cautions (prefer fenbendazole; avoid albendazole in pregnancy). *Source:* Kahn and Line (2020) and Gupta (2018).

Clinical Signs

Typically mild and nonspecific with overdoses (inappetence, lethargy). When given in vulnerable gestational windows: early embryonic loss or congenital anomalies. With idiosyncratic or prolonged/high-dose courses: pallor, petechiation (cytopenias), occasional alanine aminotransferase/alkaline phosphatase ALT/ALP elevations (Kahn & Line, 2020).

Pathophysiology

Disruption of organogenesis in early gestation; hypocellular bone marrow in rare idiosyncratic cases; hepatocellular stress with sustained high exposure (Gupta, 2018).

Diagnosis

Confirm pregnancy stage and exact dose/duration; for extended/high-dose courses obtain baseline CBC/chemistry and recheck periodically (Kahn & Line, 2020). Incorporate faecal egg count/faecal egg count reduction test (FEC/FECRT) to avoid unnecessary redosing that increases toxicity risk and selects for resistance (Gupta, 2018; Kahn & Line, 2020).

Treatment

Withdraw the drug and provide supportive care. For suspected marrow suppression: stop therapy and monitor CBC until recovery; for hepatic enzyme elevations: rest the liver (diet/fluids), recheck chemistries, and reassess the deworming plan/timing (Gupta, 2018; Kahn & Line, 2020).

Prevention and Stewardship

Stage pregnancy before albendazole; prefer fenbendazole where pregnancy safety is needed (follow regional labels). Avoid chronic high-dose regimens; schedule pre-breeding or postpartum deworming when feasible; base redosing on FEC/FECRT; do not "stack" anthelmintics the same day; rotate classes sensibly to preserve efficacy (Gupta, 2018; Kahn & Line, 2020). Table 10.11 converts these principles into a species-by-species checklist of risk windows, monitoring for prolonged courses, and stop rules (including small-animal cautions to avoid albendazole and prefer fenbendazole; do not use febantel in pregnant bitches/queens).

Table 10.11 Benzimidazoles – pregnancy and prolonged-course safeguards (species, risk window, monitoring, stop rules).

Species (examples)	Pregnancy risk window (do-not-use/use-with-caution)	Monitoring for prolonged or repeated courses	Stop rules (anytime during therapy)
Cattle (albendazole, fenbendazole, oxfendazole)	Avoid early gestation (organogenesis; label commonly cautions first ~45 d). Use caution through remainder of 1st trimester; follow country-specific labels/withdrawals.	Clinical: appetite, rumen fill, milk yield; fecal egg counts (FEC) to avoid unnecessary repeats. If high-dose/ELDU courses, consider chem panel (AST/ALT, bilirubin).	Pregnancy discovered in the avoid window; anorexia/lethargy after dosing; >2× rise in liver enzymes from baseline; abortions or malformations in herd – halt program and review timing/agent.
Sheep/goats (albendazole, fenbendazole)	Avoid first ~30–45 d of gestation; caution for remainder of T1.	Clinical condition, FEC; in intensive/repeat protocols consider periodic chem panel.	Any early embryonic loss spike; >2× ALT/AST from baseline; persistent inappetence – stop and switch timing/agent.

(Continued)

Table 10.11 (Continued)

Species (examples)	**Pregnancy risk window (do-not-use/ use-with-caution)**	**Monitoring for prolonged or repeated courses**	**Stop rules (anytime during therapy)**
Camelids (fenbendazole; limited data for albendazole)	Avoid early gestation; prefer fenbendazole if treatment unavoidable (consult regional guidance).	Weight/BCS, appetite; FEC; for extended courses consider chem panel.	Worsening anorexia/ depression; abnormal chemistry trends; pregnancy confirmed in avoid window – discontinue and reassess.
Equids (horses) (fenbendazole, oxibendazole; albendazole use varies)	Avoid T1; use equine-labeled options and timing per label; reserve off-label benzimidazoles only with risk–benefit rationale.	Clinical: appetite, manure quality; FEC reduction tests (FECRT) to avoid overuse. In multi-day high-dose regimens, consider baseline/ endpoint chem panel.	Colic/anorexia temporally linked to dosing; abnormal liver enzymes; mare confirmed early pregnant when product not labeled – pause and consult.
Swine (fenbendazole, albendazole in some regions)	Avoid early gestation per label; caution later in T1.	Production metrics (gain, feed intake); FEC as indicated.	Maternal illness after dosing; reproductive losses temporally associated – stop and review label timing.
Dogs (fenbendazole; avoid albendazole; febantel combos not for pregnant bitches)	Prefer fenbendazole where pregnancy safety data support use; avoid albendazole/febantel in pregnancy unless a label specifically allows.	Baseline CBC/biochemistry panel if course >10–14 d or high dose; recheck q1–2 week (ALT/ALP, ± bilirubin), watch GI tolerance.	CBC cytopenia, ALT/ALP >2–3× baseline, intractable vomiting/anorexia, neurological signs; pregnancy identified when product is contraindicated – stop and change plan.
Cats (fenbendazole ELDU in many locales; do not use febantel in cats)	Avoid albendazole (myelotoxic/hepatotoxic risk); if deworming pregnant queens, use feline-appropriate alternatives per label.	Baseline and q1–2 week CBC/chem for extended courses; monitor appetite/ behavior.	Any cytopenia, ALT/ALP rise >2× baseline, persistent GI intolerance; discontinue immediately if pregnancy and product is not feline-pregnancy approved.
Mixed-species herds	Plan pre-breeding deworming to avoid early gestation across groups; never "stack" multiple anthelmintics on the same day in bred animals.	Lot-level outcomes (abortions, weak neonates) after treatment; sample chem panels if high-dose/ herd-wide courses are used.	Clustered repro events post-treat – stop program, investigate timing/agent/ resistance, and consult label/ regulator.

BCS, body condition score; CBC, complete blood count; chem, serum biochemistry; ELDU, extra-label drug use; FEC, fecal egg count; FECRT, fecal egg count reduction test; T1, first trimester.

Rows: Cattle; Sheep/Goats; Camelids; Equids; Swine; Dogs; Cats; Mixed-species herds. Columns: Pregnancy risk window (do-not-use/use-with-caution) | Monitoring for prolonged/repeated courses | Stop rules. Includes general safeguards (pre-breeding/postpartum deworming, baseline/recheck CBC/chem for >10–14 d courses, FEC/FECRT use, follow current labels/withdrawals).

General safeguards

Prefer pre-breeding or postpartum deworming when feasible; document risk–benefit if treating during pregnancy.

For courses lasting >10–14 days or involving high doses/repeats, get baseline CBC/chem and recheck q1–2 weeks until 1–2 weeks after completion.

Use FEC/FECRT to avoid unnecessary redosing and resistance selection.

Always follow current product labeling and regional pregnancy/withdrawal guidance.

Source: Kahn and Line (2020) and Gupta (2018).

Salicylanilides (Closantel, Rafoxanide)

Source

Flukicides and key *Haemonchus* tools in small ruminants/cattle, where liver fluke and wireworm co-exist (Kahn & Line, 2020). To anchor class identity before safety details, Figure 10.21 shows representative salicylanilide structures used in veterinary practice (closantel, rafoxanide, oxyclozanide).

Toxicity

The signature problem is delayed optic neuropathy/retinal degeneration → partial to complete blindness (sheep/goats), often with weakness and ataxia. Risk is amplified by dosing errors, malnutrition/hyperproteinemia (↑ free drug), intercurrent illness, and stacking with other salicylanilides (Gupta, 2018; Kahn & Line, 2020). A practical timeline + what to document schematic appears in Figure 10.22 to guide field teams during the first days after exposure.

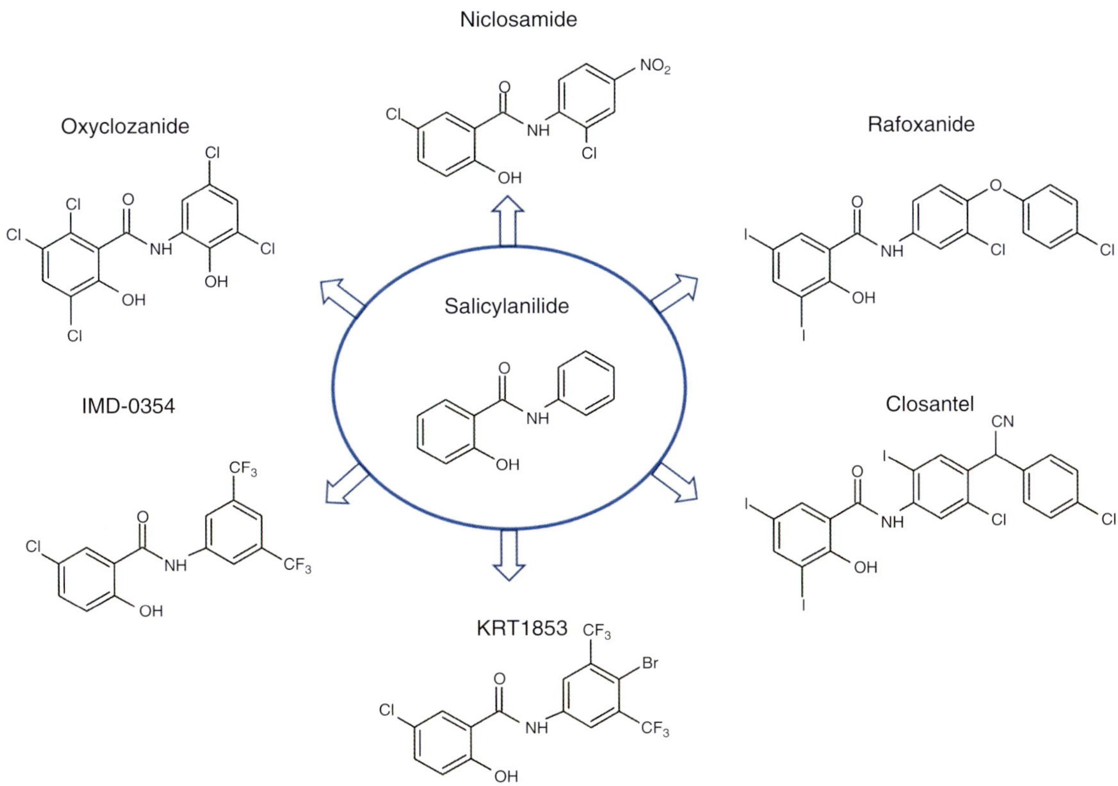

Figure 10.21 Structures of salicylanilides. Representative structures (closantel, rafoxanide, oxyclozanide) highlighting the salicylanilide core used in veterinary flukicides. *Source:* Adapted from standard pharmacology references cited in text.

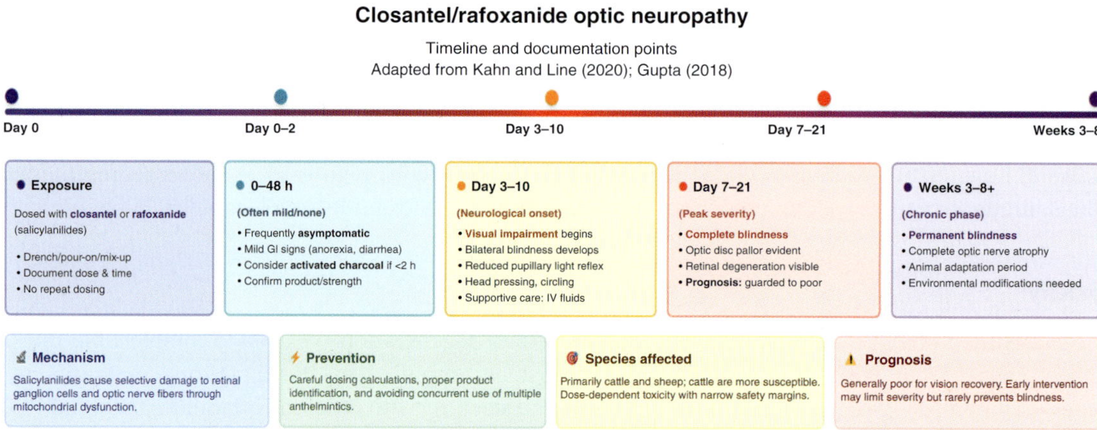

Figure 10.22 Closantel/rafoxanide optic neuropathy – timeline and documentation points. Day-by-day cues from exposure to visual loss with "what to record" (dose, mg/kg; product/lot; PLR/menace, fundus photos; ERG if available) to support monitoring and case investigation. *Source:* Kahn and Line (2020) and Gupta (2018).

Mechanism of Action (Toxicity)

At host-toxic exposures, evidence points to mitochondrial dysfunction and optic nerve/myelin injury; closantel's primary antiparasitic action (uncoupling helminth oxidative phosphorylation) can affect host tissues when overdosed (Gupta, 2018).

Clinical Signs

Progressive visual loss over days, absent menace; pupils may be dilated with reduced or inconsistent pupillary light reflex (PLR); ataxia/weakness variably present (Kahn & Line, 2020).

Pathophysiology

Optic disc swelling that progresses to pallor/atrophy; retinal degeneration on fundus exam; characteristic electroretinogram (ERG) abnormalities when available (Gupta, 2018; Kahn & Line, 2020).

Diagnosis

Get an accurate dose history (mg/kg), product concentration, route, and device calibration; record body condition/albumin. Perform ophthalmic documentation (menace/PLR, fundus photographs; ERG if available). Rule out differentials (polioencephalomalacia, OP toxicity, infectious ocular disease) (Kahn & Line, 2020).

Treatment

Immediate withdrawal of the drug. There is no specific antidote; institute supportive nursing, safe penning for visually impaired stock, hydration/nutrition support, and serial ocular/neuro checks. Prognosis for vision is guarded, especially once ERG/fundus changes are established (Kahn & Line, 2020).

Prevention and Stewardship

Do not exceed label dose; weigh accurately (no eyeballing); verify product concentration/units; avoid use in malnourished/ill animals; do not stack salicylanilides the same day; spot-audit drench gun/syringe output during mass-treat days (Gupta, 2018; Kahn & Line, 2020). A bedside, species- and context-specific safeguard grid is provided in Table 10.12.

Table 10.12 Salicylanilides – dose guardrails, red flags (malnutrition/illness), and actions after overdose.

Agent/species context	Dose guardrails (before you treat)	Red flags (malnutrition/ illness and co-factors)	Actions after overdose (0–60 min, then ongoing)
Closantel – cattle (drench/ injectable)	Weigh each animal; label mg/kg only; calibrate drench-gun/ syringe; one flukicide at a time (no same-day "stacking"); verify product strength and species labeling.	Low BCS/albumin, dehydration, heavy parasitism, hepatic compromise; concurrent salicylanilide use; dosing by visual guess; equipment mis-calibration.	Stop further doses; confirm product/ lot and exact mg/kg. If oral and <2 h and animal safe: consider activated charcoal; dermal exposure: wash with mild detergent. Admit; pen safely (vision may decline days later). Begin daily ocular/neuro checks (PLR/menace, pupil photos). Supportive care; there is no antidote.
Rafoxanide – sheep/goats	Dose to current weight; avoid extra-label high mg/kg; respect milk/ meat withdrawals; do not combine with other salicylanilides the same day.	Thin, ill, late-gestation, hypoproteinemic animals; concurrent hepatotoxins; recent stressful handling/ transport.	As above. Early course often mild GI only; still document exposure and schedule rechecks days 3–10 for emerging vision change. Support hydration and nutrition; low-stress handling.
Oxyclozanide – cattle/sheep	Follow label; avoid repeat dosing sooner than recommended; check drench delivery (air locks, worn seals).	Debilitated animals; diarrhea/dehydration; polypharmacy.	Withhold additional doses; manage GI upset; monitor chemistry (± bilirubin/enzymes) and hydration. If ingestion was recent and safe: charcoal. Observe at least 24–48 h, longer if signs evolve.
Closantel/ rafoxanide combo days (mass-treat, herd)	One product per day; weigh groups or use scales at chute; log each batch/lot; spot-audit gun output each pen.	Multiple operators, rushed processing, mixed concentrations on hand, language/label confusion.	Halt the line if errors suspected; reconcile inventory used vs. headcount; trace animals dosed. Early warning to staff: watch for mydriasis/PLR loss in coming week(s). Escalate to ophthalmology/ diagnostics if deficits appear.
Off-label species (dogs/cats/ chelonia)	Avoid use; choose labeled alternatives.	Any exposure is a red flag; very narrow margin in some non-ruminants.	Treat as toxic exposure: decontaminate promptly (emesis if appropriate and airway-protected; charcoal), admit for neuro/ocular monitoring; consider toxicological consultation.

(Continued)

Table 10.12 (Continued)

Agent/species context	Dose guardrails (before you treat)	Red flags (malnutrition/ illness and co-factors)	Actions after overdose (0–60 min, then ongoing)
Malnourished/ cachectic any species	Delay until nutritional status improved; correct dehydration; consider albumin/ chem panel where feasible.	Low albumin (↑ free drug), concurrent illness, fever.	If already dosed: heightened monitoring; lower threshold for inpatient care; support calories/ fluids; schedule serial ocular exams through day 21.
Hepatic compromise	Consider alternative anthelmintic or defer; adhere strictly to label; avoid repeats.	Prior liver disease, concurrent hepatotoxins.	Baseline and follow-up chemistry; supportive care; consult before any redose.

BCS, body condition score; PLR, pupillary light reflex.
Contexts (e.g., closantel – cattle, rafoxanide – small ruminants, oxyclozanide, mass-treat herd days, off-label species, malnourished/hepatic compromise) with columns for Dose guardrails (before you treat), Red flags, Actions after overdose (0–60 minutes, then ongoing), plus a bottom box on "what to document" in every suspected overdose.
What to document for every overdose/suspected overdose

Product and **lot/expiry**, exact **mg/kg**, route, device calibration check, who administered; animal IDs/weights; co-exposures; timeline (dose → first sign → peak); **ocular/neuro findings;** lab trends; pharmacovigilance report if indicated.
Source: Kahn and Line (2020) and Gupta (2018).

Diminazene Aceturate

Source

Trypanocide (IM only) for cattle, small ruminants, and camels in tsetse/trypanosome belts (Constable et al., 2016; Kahn & Line, 2020). To anchor the drug identity before safety nuances, the chemical structure is shown in Figure 10.23.

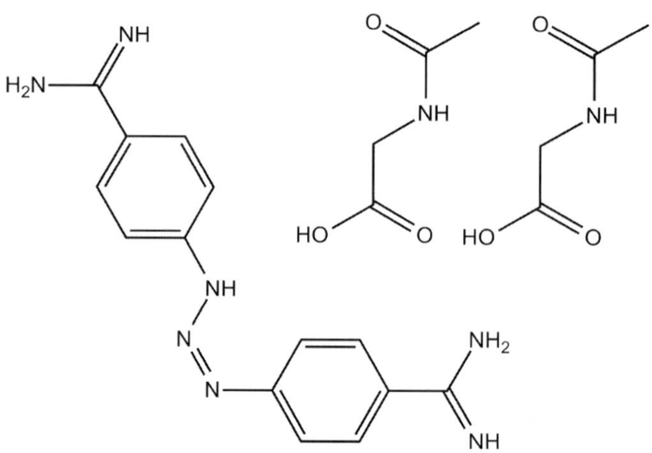

Figure 10.23 Chemical structure of diminazene aceturate. Author's schematic for class recognition in tropical practice. See Constable et al. (2016) and Kahn and Line (2020) for clinical use and safety context.

Toxicity

Delayed neurotoxicity (24–72 hours postinjection): Agitation → ataxia → seizures, vocalization, hyperesthesia; risk rises with overdose, repeat/high cumulative dosing, and hepatic/renal compromise (Constable et al., 2016; Kahn & Line, 2020). A practical onset–severity ladder with first-hour actions appears in Figure 10.24.

Mechanism of Action (Toxicity)

Not fully defined; reports implicate brainstem/cortical neuronal injury and cerebral edema at toxic exposures (Gupta, 2018; Kahn & Line, 2020).

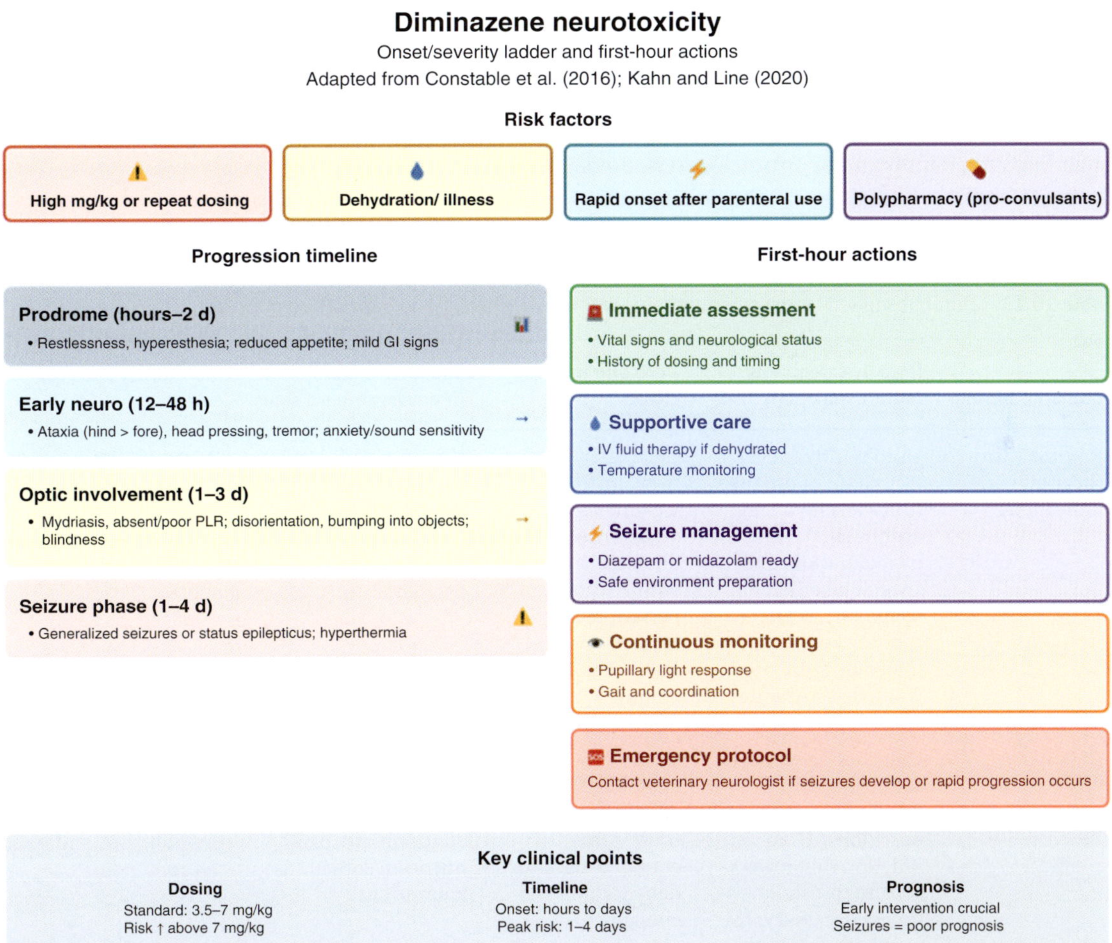

Figure 10.24 Diminazene neurotoxicity – onset/severity ladder and first-hour actions. Timeline from injection (0 h) to 24–72 h for emergence/worsening of neuro signs, with a prioritized first-hour bundle (airway/O_2, seizure control, fluids, temperature and electrolyte/glucose checks). *Source:* Constable et al. (2016) and Kahn and Line (2020).

Clinical Signs

Restlessness, pacing or circling, staggering/ataxia, recumbency, seizures; temperature may be normal or febrile (Constable et al., 2016).

Pathophysiology

Cerebral edema and neuronal degeneration in severe cases; prolonged seizures may lead to secondary rhabdomyolysis (Gupta, 2018).

Diagnosis

Audit dose (mg/kg) and interval carefully; confirm IM route (never IV); check renal/hepatic status. Reserve CSF sampling for select differentials once stabilized (Constable et al., 2016; Kahn & Line, 2020).

Treatment

Seizure control (benzodiazepines → add phenobarbital if needed), anti-edema measures where indicated, quiet housing, temperature control, IV crystalloids, and correction of glucose/electrolytes. Avoid further dosing (Constable et al., 2016; Kahn & Line, 2020). A bedside, scenario-based safeguard and supportive bundle is provided in Table 10.13.

Table 10.13 Diminazene – IM-only safeguards, dose/interval checks, and supportive bundle.

Scenario/setting	IM-only safeguards (before injection)	Dose and interval checks	Supportive bundle (if adverse/neuro signs)	Monitoring and stop rules
Routine case (healthy, correct indication)	Use IM only (never IV); confirm product (diminazene aceturate), concentration, and species labeling; weigh on a scale; aspirate before injection; split large volumes across sites.	Calculate mg/kg from current weight; verify syringe/needle; double-check math with a second person; respect label re-dose interval and any cumulative mg/kg limits.	If mild post-injection malaise only: rest, hydration, NSAID per label/clinic policy for injection-site soreness.	Recheck within 24–48 h; if any neuro or visual change emerges at any time → escalate to neuro pathway below.
Debilitated/ dehydrated/ febrile	Consider deferring or stabilizing first (fluids, fever control, nutrition); avoid sedation that lowers seizure threshold unless necessary; IM only with smallest practical per-site volume.	Use lowest effective labeled dose; avoid repeats until stable; correct weight for dehydration changes.	Begin fluids, temperature control; low-stress environment; early nutrition support as appropriate.	If mentation worsens, ataxia or tremor appears → stop further doses, admit, and start neuro bundle.

Table 10.13 (Continued)

Scenario/setting	IM-only safeguards (before injection)	Dose and interval checks	Supportive bundle (if adverse/neuro signs)	Monitoring and stop rules
High exposure risk (repeat dosing, recent prior dose, or uncertain history)	Verify last administration (date, mg/kg, lot); do not "top up" because of missed doses; IM only.	Confirm minimum interval has elapsed; cap total cumulative mg/kg; if uncertain, withhold and monitor/retreat plan.	Not applicable unless signs occur – keep patient under observation longer post-dose (clinic or supervised).	If any signs within 24–72 h (ataxia, mydriasis, seizures) → treat as toxicity and document exposure timeline.
Polypharmacy/ pro-convulsant co-meds	Review meds for agents that lower seizure threshold (e.g., certain fluoroquinolones, theophylline); avoid same-day triggers where possible.	Do not exceed label dose; extend interval or choose alternatives if interactions can't be avoided.	If tremor/anxiety appears: quiet room, benzodiazepine per protocol; consider phenobarbital if seizures recur.	Observe closely for 24–72 h; if seizures occur, permanently discontinue diminazene for that patient and update chart.
Small animal use (where permitted)	IM only; accurate weight; avoid in unstable, hypoglycemic, or actively seizuring patients; have IV access and oxygen ready.	Conservative, label-compliant dosing; avoid repeats unless clinically essential and interval met.	First-hour package: stop drug; oxygen/ airway, IV fluids, benzodiazepine for seizures ± methocarbamol for tremors; manage hyperthermia; check glucose and electrolytes and correct.	Neuro checks q2–4 h (mentation, gait, pupils/PLR, menace), vitals (HR/RR/SpO_2/ temperature); escalate to ICU if refractory seizures.
After suspected overdose/ calculation error	Do not give any additional doses; secure vial/syringe for lot and volume reconciliation; notify team lead.	Re-calculate true mg/kg; record exact time, route, lot/expiry; identify any co-exposures.	Start toxicity bundle (see below); consider early activated charcoal only if an oral exposure occurred and airway is protected (not applicable to IM).	Admit. Monitor at least 24–72 h (severity often escalates over this window). Report per pharmacovigilance policy.

ICU, intensive care unit; IM, intramuscular; PLR, pupillary light reflex; O_2, oxygen.
Scenario-based grid (healthy routine case; debilitated/dehydrated/febrile; high-exposure risk; polypharmacy; small-animal use where permitted; suspected overdose) with columns for IM-only safeguards, dose and interval checks, supportive bundle, and monitoring/stop rules; includes a standardized toxicity bundle and owner/herd alerts.
Airway/O_2, quiet environment; control hyperthermia.
Seizure control: benzodiazepine per protocol → add phenobarbital if needed; methocarbamol for tremor/rigidity.
Fluids (isotonic) and glucose/electrolyte correction.
Documentation: exact dose (mg/kg), time, product/lot, concurrent drugs; serial neuro chart (mentation, ataxia score, pupil size/PLR, menace).
Owner/herd alerts: warn that signs can emerge or worsen up to 72 h post-injection; arrange rechecks.
Source: Constable et al. (2016) and Kahn and Line (2020). Toxicity "supportive bundle" (when neurotoxicity is suspected or confirmed).

Strict dose/interval adherence; do not "top up" missed doses; IM only; avoid repeat high doses; screen for renal/hepatic compromise when feasible; review polypharmacy for agents that lower the seizure threshold (Kahn & Line, 2020).

Ionophores (Monensin, Lasalocid, Salinomycin)

Source

Anticoccidials and feed-efficiency modifiers in ruminants/poultry. Horses are exquisitely sensitive, and feed-mill cross-contamination is a classic cause of equine fatalities in tropical production systems (Gupta, 2018; Kahn & Line, 2020). To anchor class identity before toxicity details, representative ionophore structures are shown in Figure 10.25 (monensin, lasalocid, salinomycin).

Toxicity

Toxidrome (species-patterned):

Equids: rapid weakness, tachycardia/arrhythmia, colic, diaphoresis → collapse/sudden death.
Cattle: dose-dependent myopathy with weakness/recumbency; dark urine possible.
Dogs/cats: accidental feed exposure → skeletal ± cardiac myopathy.
Potentiators: formulation errors, cross-fed rations, and drug interactions (e.g., some macrolides/pleuromutilins in swine/poultry) increase risk/severity (Gupta, 2018; Kahn & Line, 2020). A succinct organ/biomarker map appears in Figure 10.26.

Mechanism of Action (Toxicity)

Transmembrane cation transport → mitochondrial dysfunction, ATP depletion, and myocyte necrosis, especially in high-metabolic tissues (Gupta, 2018).

Clinical Signs

Equids: acute weakness, tachyarrhythmias, colic, dyspnea; rapid deterioration possible.
Cattle/small ruminants: anorexia, weakness, ataxia, recumbency; myoglobinuria may occur.
Companions (dogs/cats): lethargy, muscle pain/weakness; arrhythmias if cardiac involvement (Kahn & Line, 2020).

Pathophysiology

Cardiac and skeletal muscle necrosis; elevations in CK/AST and cardiac troponin (cTnI); ECG may reveal conduction blocks or ventricular arrhythmias (Gupta, 2018; Kahn & Line, 2020).

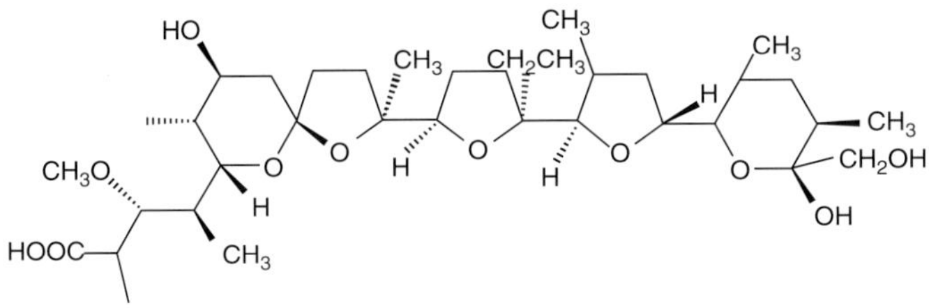

Monensin (MW 670)

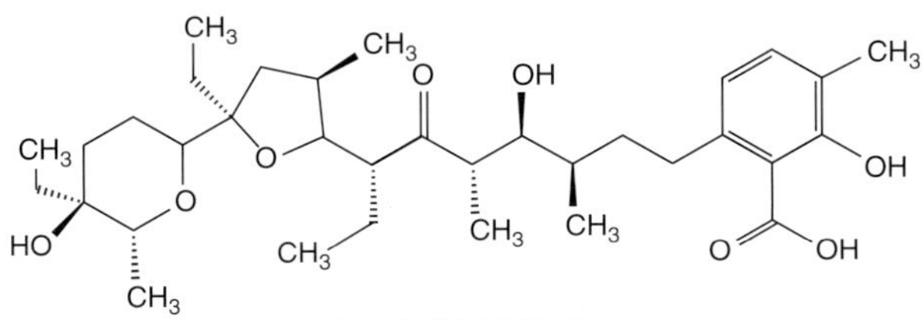

Lasalocid (MW 590)

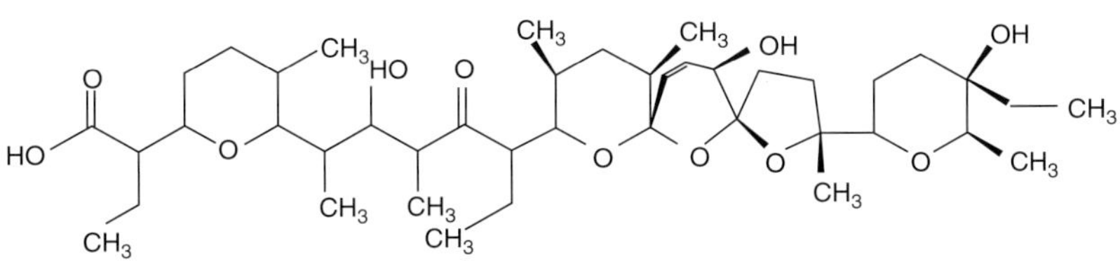

Salinomycin (MW 750)

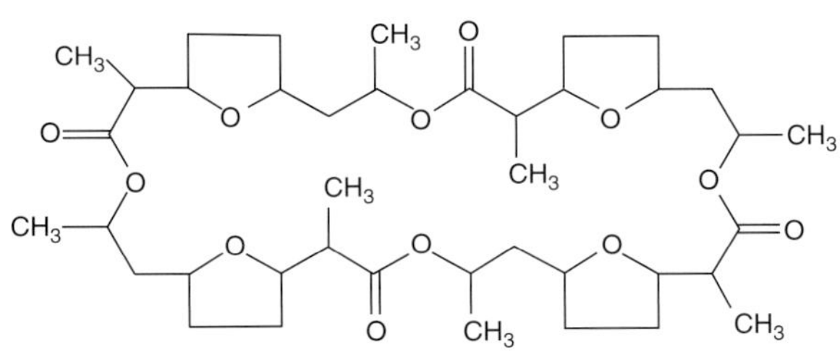

Nonactin (MW 736)

Figure 10.25 Structures of ionophores. Representative veterinary ionophores (e.g., monensin, lasalocid, salinomycin) highlighting shared scaffold features relevant to potency and species sensitivity. *Source:* Adapted from standard pharmacology references cited in text.

Diagnosis

Immediate source removal (hold suspect batch), run CK/cTnI, electrolytes/acid–base; ECG and serial biomarkers; necropsy of fatalities; submit feed samples for ionophore assay; look for mill cross-contamination or mis-sequenced mixing runs (Kahn & Line, 2020).

Ionophore toxicity

Target organs and biomarkers (heart vs skeletal muscle) with expected ECG/biomarker patterns
Adapted from Gupta (2018); Kahn and Line (2020).

Common ionophores: monensin, lasalocid, salinomycin, narasin. **Typical contexts:** feed-mill mix-up, wrong-species exposure, cumulative intake.
Species tendency: Equids/camelids → heart-predominant; cattle → heart ± skeletal; small animals/poultry → skeletal-predominant (dose-dependent).

Heart (cardiomyocyte injury)

Clinical picture:

- Weakness, collapse, dyspnea; exercise intolerance; sudden death.
- Congestive signs (tachycardia, jugular pulse, pulmonary edema).

Biomarkers (typical pattern)

- Cardiac troponin I (cTnI): ↑↑ early (6–24 h), may peak 24–48 h.
- CK (total/MB): ↑ mild–moderate; AST: ↑ mild; myoglobinuria uncommon.
- Lactate/acid–base derangements with shock.
- Echocardiography: hypokinesis/poor systolic function (if available).

ECG expectations

- Ventricular premature complexes (VPCs), bigeminy; ventricular tachycardia.
- Conduction blocks (1°–2° AV), ST–T abnormalities; sinus tachycardia.
- Atrial fibrillation (large animals); ventricular fibrillation (terminal).

Skeletal muscle (rhabdomyolysis)

Clinical picture:

- Muscle stiffness, reluctance to move; recumbency, "sawhorse" stance.
- Dark/red-brown urine (myoglobinuria); muscle pain/tenderness.

Biomarkers (typical pattern)

- CK (creatine kinase): ↑↑↑ massive (>10,000–100,000+ U/L)
- AST: ↑↑ marked; LDH: ↑↑; aldolase: ↑↑ (if measured).
- Myoglobin (serum/urine): ↑↑↑ early, then clears rapidly.
- Cardiac troponin I: normal–mild ↑ (unless concurrent cardiac injury).

Secondary complications

- Acute kidney injury (AKI) from myoglobinuria/tubular necrosis.
- Hyperkalemia, hyperphosphatemia, hypocalcemia (cell lysis).
- Compartment syndrome (swelling); DIC in severe cases.

Key diagnostic differences

Parameter	Heart-predominant	Muscle-predominant
Primary biomarker	Cardiac troponin I ↑↑	CK ↑↑↑ (massive)
Clinical signs	Weakness, dyspnea, collapse	Stiffness, dark urine, recumbency
ECG changes	VPCs, arrhythmias, blocks	Usually normal (unless severe)
Complications	Congestive heart failure	Acute kidney injury

Clinical pearls

Timing matters:
Cardiac troponin peaks early (6–24 h), CK can stay elevated for days

Species differences:
Horses/llamas more cardiac-sensitive; poultry more muscle-sensitive

Figure 10.26 Ionophore toxicity – target organs and biomarkers. Heart vs. skeletal muscle targets with expected biomarkers (CK/AST, cTnI) and typical ECG patterns, to guide early testing and triage. *Source:* Gupta (2018) and Kahn and Line (2020).

Treatment

Aggressive supportive care: IV fluids, correct electrolytes/acid–base; control arrhythmias and avoid excessive catecholamines; analgesia and strict rest. Prognosis in horses is guarded–poor even with early intervention (Gupta, 2018; Kahn & Line, 2020). A species-specific monitoring grid is provided in Table 10.14 (baseline → 6–12 h → 24–48 h → ~72 h with disposition triggers).

Prevention and Stewardship

Feed-mill QA: Validated formulas/ppm, micro-ingredient scale calibration, documented sequencing and line flushing, clear bin/auger labeling ("NO HORSES"), medicated-feed tags, transport clean-outs, retain samples, and deviation/CAPA logs. On farms with equids and ruminants, never interchange rations and institute driver sign-offs (Gupta, 2018; Kahn & Line, 2020). The QA checklist is appended within Table 10.14.

To wrap, Table 10.15 "sweeps the floor" by condensing each drug class into its therapeutic window, red-flag species/contexts, classic field pitfalls, pregnancy "do/don't," and what to monitor next. Use it side-by-side with the class briefs and action grids (Tables 10.9–10.14): e.g., neuro checks after macrocyclic lactones; SLUD/neuromuscular watch after levamisole; pregnancy timing and CBC/chem for prolonged benzimidazoles; ocular/PLR + ERG vigilance with salicylanilides; dose/interval audit for diminazene; and CK/cTnI/ECG for ionophores (Gupta, 2018; Kahn & Line, 2020; Peterson & Talcott, 2013). The table also reinforces simple, high-yield housekeeping in tropical programs: weigh – don't guess; calibrate drench guns/syringes; one dewormer per day (no stacking); pre-breeding or postpartum timing when feasible; and FEC/FECRT-guided redosing to curb toxicity and slow resistance.

Ectoparasiticides – Toxicities in Tropical Practice

High heat/humidity, frequent dermal/topical use (pour-ons, dips, spot-ons), and over-the-counter (OTC) access make ectoparasiticide toxicoses a recurring problem in the tropics. Heat and occlusion increase dermal flux and depot effect; dehydration, anemia, and concurrent cholinergic or α_2-acting drugs further narrow safety margins (Gupta, 2018; Kahn & Line, 2020; Peterson & Talcott, 2013). To orient triage, Figure 10.27 maps the major classes to their signature toxidromes and first-hour priorities: cholinergic crisis for organophosphates/carbamates (decon → oxygen/ventilation → atropine; oxime early for OPs), neuroexcitation for pyrethroids (bath → methocarbamol/benzodiazepine; temperature control; consider ILE for refractory cases), α_2-agonist syndrome for amitraz (remove/wash → yohimbine/atipamezole → fluids/warmth), and species-specific cautions (see individual agent sections; e.g., rabbit contraindication under fipronil/isoxazolines). Use this map to stabilize by toxidrome, sample early (blood/serum ± cholinesterase where relevant), then decontaminate and treat while confirming the agent and exposure route (Gupta, 2018; Kahn & Line, 2020; Peterson & Talcott, 2013). See Figure 10.27.

Table 10.14 Ionophores – monitoring grid (CK/troponin/ECG by species) and feed-mill QA checklist.

Species/ setting	Dominant target	Baseline (time 0)	6–12 h	24–48 h	~72 h	Disposition triggers (anytime)	Notes
Equids (horses, donkeys)	Heart ≫ skeletal	cTnI, CK, AST; ECG; lactate; electrolytes; ± echo if dyspneic	Trend cTnI, ECG	Peak risk for cTnI/ arrhythmia – repeat cTnI, ECG; CK/AST	cTnI and ECG; CK/AST to confirm down-trend	cTnI rising or >ULN ×2, ventricular arrhythmias, syncope, worsening CHF signs → ICU/echo	Exercise restriction; avoid catecholaminergics; IV fluids, O_2 as indicated
Cattle (beef/ dairy)	Heart ± skeletal	cTnI, CK, AST; ECG if available; electrolytes	CK (early), cTnI	Repeat cTnI + CK/AST	CK should fall; AST may still rise	cTnI ↑ from baseline, VPCs/ VT, recumbency, dark urine → admit	Watch for feed cohort "clusters"; monitor pen-mates
Small ruminants (sheep/goats)	Mixed; dose-dependent	CK, AST; consider cTnI; ECG if feasible	CK	CK/AST; ± cTnI if cardiac signs	CK down, AST plateau	Persistent CK ↑, myoglobinuria, arrhythmia → admit	Hydration, shade; check feed source immediately
Camelids	Heart-predominant	cTnI, CK/AST; ECG	cTnI	cTnI + ECG; CK/AST	cTnI/ECG	cTnI ↑ or rhythm change → hospitalize/echo	Often low reserve – monitor closely for 72 h
Swine	Skeletal ≥ heart	CK, AST; ± cTnI; ECG if available	CK	CK/AST; ± cTnI	CK ↓, AST peak	Recumbency, CK extreme ↑, acidosis → aggressive fluids	Check group feed bin and sequencing records
Poultry	Skeletal	CK; AST (lab dependent)	CK	CK/AST (sentinel birds)	Trend in flock	Sudden deaths, weakness clusters → pull feed	Flock-level sampling; necropsy for confirmation

Dogs/cats (accidental feed exposure)	Skeletal ± heart	CK, AST; cTnI if any cardiac sign; ECG; electrolytes	CK; cTnI if suspect cardiac	CK/AST (and cTnI if indicated)	CK ↓, AST slower	Seizures, arrhythmia, rising cTnI, renal compromise → ICU	Treat pain, fluids; strict rest

AST, aspartate aminotransferase; CHF, congestive heart failure; CK, creatine kinase; cTnI, cardiac troponin I; ECG, electrocardiogram; ULN, upper limit of normal; VPCs, ventricular premature complexes; VT, ventricular tachycardia.

Species rows (equids, cattle, small ruminants, camelids, swine, poultry, dogs/cats) with columns for Baseline (time 0), 6–12 h, 24–48 h, ~72 h, and Disposition triggers, followed by a feed-mill/on-farm QA checklist (formulation/batching, sequencing/flushing, labeling/segregation, transport cleanout, inventory/traceability, and actions when exposure is suspected).

Feed-mill/on-farm QA checklist for ionophore prevention

Formulation and batching

- Signed formula with ionophore name, target ppm, species (no equid use) and version control.
- Micro-ingredient scale calibration log; verify premix potency and lot numbers.
- Batch ticket reconciliation: theoretical vs. actual weigh-backs (±1–2% tolerance).

Sequencing and flushing

- Segregated bins for ionophore premix; color-coded lines.
- Documented mixer sequencing: non-medicated → ionophore batches → flush (appropriate carrier) → non-target species last.
- Flush records (amount, material, destination) retained.

Labeling and segregation

- Clear bin/auger labels; "NO HORSES" signage where equids are present.
- Medicated-feed tags on every delivery; species and ppm prominently printed.
- Transport and auger cleanout between species; driver sign-off.

Inventory and traceability

- Lot-to-lot trace (premix → batch → truck → farm/bin); retain samples (e.g., 60–90 days).
- Deviations/CAPA log (near-misses included); staff training records up-to-date.

When exposure suspected

- Immediate hold on suspect feed; isolate bins/augers; sample feed for ionophore assay.
- Create an animal timeline (start of new feed → first signs), identify cohort mates, and start the monitoring grid above for sentinels.
- Notify veterinarian/producer network and, if applicable, regulator/insurer.

Source: Kahn and Line (2020) and Gupta (2018).

Table 10.15 Anthelmintics and antiprotozoals – safety margins and red flags (tropical practice).

Class (examples)	Therapeutic window	Red-flag species/ contexts	Typical field pitfalls	"Do/Don't" in pregnancy	Monitoring
Benzimidazoles (albendazole, fenbendazole, oxfendazole, triclabendazole)	Moderate (agent-dependent). Albendazole narrower (myelotoxic/ hepatotoxic at high/ prolonged doses).	Small animals on albendazole; camelids (limited data); debilitated/ hypoproteinemic stock.	Dosing by eye; repeat high-dose courses; poor feed mixing; stacking with other dewormers "same day."	Do: use fenbendazole where label allows; schedule pre-breeding. Don't: use albendazole in T1 (organogenesis).	If >10–14 d or high dose: CBC/chem q1–2 week; watch appetite/behavior. Use FEC/FECRT to avoid unnecessary repeat.
Macrocyclic lactones (ivermectin, doramectin, moxidectin, eprinomectin)	Wide at label in target species; narrow in MDR1-mutant dogs; high-dose ELDU narrows.	MDR1 dogs (Collie-type), chelonians, some birds; debilitated neonates; heavy co-exposures (sedatives).	"Dose stacking" (topical + injectable + oral); guessing weights; accidental ingestion of pour-ons; dog on spinosad + high ivermectin.	Generally OK at label in food animals/equids; avoid high-dose ELDU in pregnant dogs; follow species labels.	Neuro checks if at-risk: mentation/ ataxia, PLR; in dogs, observe 24–48 h after high exposure.
Imidazothiazoles (levamisole)	Narrow TI (2× error can be severe).	Heat-stressed, dehydrated, parasitized or thin animals; camelids; small ruminants at high dose.	Mis-calibrated drench-gun; combining with OP/ carbamates; repeated doses too close.	Avoid in early gestation; otherwise use label-compliant single doses only. Don't combine with cholinergics/OPs.	Observe 4–12 h for nicotinic signs (tremor, salivation, bradycardia); temp/ HR; provide quiet pen; stop program if neuro signs.
Tetrahydropyrimidines (pyrantel, morantel)	Wide (low systemic absorption).	Severe debility; concurrent cholinergic agents (additive effects).	Underdosing (resistance selection); confusing pamoate vs. tartrate strength.	Generally safe at label across species; still follow local labels.	Minimal: GI tolerance, FEC/ FECRT post-treatment to confirm effect.
Isoquinolines (praziquantel, epsiprantel)	Wide at label.	Very young neonates (age/weight limits); severe hepatic disease.	Tablet splitting/dose miscalc; off-label high repeats.	Generally compatible with pregnancy at label (check product).	Monitor GI tolerance; no routine labs needed for single courses.
Salicylanilides/ flukicides (closantel, rafoxanide, oxyclozanide)	Moderate–narrow; long half-life; optic neuropathy risk if overdosed.	Non-ruminants (dogs/cats, equids); malnourished/ hypoproteinemic ruminants.	Visual weight estimates; stacking flukicides; wrong concentration; mass-treat line errors.	Don't use in small animals. In ruminants: avoid early gestation; use label only.	Ocular/neuro checks days 3–21 (PLR/ menace, pupil photos); hydration; chem (albumin/ enzymes) if ill.

Depsipeptides (emodepside – cats/dogs)	Generally wide at label.	Kittens/puppies below label age; fragile, low-weight patients; MDR1 dogs (caution, limited data).	Off-label dosing; combining with other neuro-active meds.	Avoid if label says "not evaluated" in pregnancy/lactation.	Watch for ataxia, salivation first 24 h; otherwise minimal labs for single use.
Amino-acetonitrile derivatives (monepantel – sheep)	Wide at label.	Off-label species; very thin sheep; high parasite burdens with die-off risk.	Dose miscalc in mixed flocks; resistance assumption without FEC.	Labeled as safe in pregnant ewes (check local label).	FEC/FECRT at 7–14 d; clinical appetite/BCS.
Arsenicals (adulticide) (melarsomine – dogs)	Narrow; injection-site and thromboembolism risks.	Cats (not indicated); dogs with class III/IV HW disease; cachectic.	Wrong site depth; exercise post-dose; skipping anti-inflammatory/adjunct protocol.	Use only when indicated; defer breeding activity; risk–benefit in pregnancy.	Respiratory status, pain/lameness, D-dimer/hematology per protocol; strict exercise restriction.
Organophosphates/carbamates (trichlorfon, coumaphos; some regions)	Narrow; cholinergic toxicity.	Cats, Brahman-type cattle, stressed/heat-loaded animals.	Wrong dilution; mixing with levamisole; repeated close intervals.	Generally avoid in pregnancy unless label explicitly allows.	Cholinergic signs (SLUD), HR/RR/temp; have atropine/2-PAM protocols ready (per OP).

CBC, complete blood count; chem, serum biochemistry; FEC/FECRT, fecal egg count/fecal egg count reduction test; HW, heartworm; MDR1, ABCB1 gene variant; OP, organophosphate; PLR, pupillary light reflex; TI, therapeutic index; T1, first trimester.

Cross-walk of Class → Therapeutic window → Red-flag species/contexts → Typical field pitfalls → "Do/Don't" in pregnancy → Monitoring, aligned to the toxidromes and first-hour actions summarized in this section.

Columns: Class | Therapeutic window | Red-flag species | Typical field pitfalls | "Do/Don't" in pregnancy | Monitoring.

Quick reminders;

- Weigh – don't guess. Calibrate drench guns/syringes each session.
- One dewormer per day (no stacking), and verify product concentration and species labeling.
- Prefer pre-breeding or postpartum timing when feasible; document risk–benefit if treating during pregnancy.
- Use FEC/FECRT to direct therapy and slow resistance; avoid reflex redosing.

Source: Gupta (2018), Kahn and Line (2020), and Peterson and Talcott (2013).

Ectoparasiticides → Toxidromes → First-hour priorities

Class map of ectoparasiticides → hallmark toxidromes → first-hour priorities
Adapted from Kahn and Line (2020); Gupta (2018)

Class	Hallmark toxidrome	First-hour priorities
Pyrethrins/pyrethroids (permethrin) Cats sensitive; dermal exposures common.	**Neuroexcitation/tremor-seizure** Paresthesia, tremor → seizures; ± hyperthermia.	• Decontamination (dermal wash) • Seizure control (diazepam) • Temperature monitoring • Supportive care
Organophosphates/carbamates Feed dips, sprays; cholinergic risk.	**Cholinergic crisis** SLUD, miosis, bradycardia, dyspnea; fasciculations, weakness.	• Atropine administration • Pralidoxime (2-PAM) if available • Decontamination • Respiratory support
Amitraz Collars/dips for dogs/livestock.	**α, -agonist sedation / bradycardia** CNS depression, hypotension, hypothermia; hyperglycemia.	• Yohimbine (α, antagonist) • Warming support • IV fluids for hypotension • Monitor glucose levels
Fipronil Topical spot-ons; do not use in rabbits.	**GABA-block neuroexcitation** Ataxia → seizures; cats/dogs; rabbits: severe systemic tox.	• Seizure control (diazepam) • Decontamination • **Rabbits: intensive supportive care** • Monitor neurological status
Isoxazolines (fluralaner, afoxolaner, sarolaner) Oral/topical flea/tick preventatives.	**GABA/glutamate block** Tremor, ataxia → seizures; generally well-tolerated at therapeutic doses.	• Seizure control if needed • Decontamination (if recent) • Supportive care • Monitor for neurological signs

Quick reference notes

Species sensitivities:
- Cats: pyrethrin/pyrethroid sensitive
- Rabbits: Fipronil contraindicated
- Dogs: Generally more tolerant

Common exposures:
- Dermal: Spot-ons, dips, sprays
- Oral: Accidental ingestion
- Cross-species application

Figure 10.27 Class map of ectoparasiticides → hallmark toxidromes → first-hour priorities. Visual cross-walk linking organophosphates/carbamates (cholinergic crisis), pyrethroids (neuroexcitation), amitraz (α_2-agonist toxidrome), and fipronil/isoxazolines (species-specific cautions) to initial decontamination and treatment steps used in tropical practice. Author's schematic; *Source:* Gupta (2018), Kahn and Line (2020), and Peterson and Talcott (2013).

Organophosphates/Carbamates

Source

Agricultural dips/sprays (dogs, ruminants), crop insecticides repurposed onto animals, and legacy flea collars/sprays are common sources. In the tropics, human-handled "crop OPs" used on pets and backyard ruminants are a frequent exposure pattern (Kahn & Line, 2020; Peterson & Talcott, 2013). To anchor class identity before clinical content, Figure 10.28 shows the core carbamate and organophosphate functional groups alongside other pesticide scaffolds for contrast.

Toxicity

Cholinergic crisis with SLUDGE-M (salivation, lacrimation, urination, defecation, GI cramps, emesis, miosis), bronchorrhea/bronchospasm, muscle fasciculations → weakness and respiratory failure risk. OPs irreversibly inhibit AChE with time-dependent aging; carbamates inhibit AChE reversibly and generally for a shorter duration (Gupta, 2018; Peterson & Talcott, 2013). For a one-glance triage sequence (recognition → decon → atropine/oxime timing), see Figure 10.29.

Mechanism (Toxicity)

AChE inhibition → excess acetylcholine at muscarinic, nicotinic, and central sites. In OP poisoning, the phosphorylated AChE ages, limiting benefit from oximes after several hours; carbamate–AChE complexes spontaneously dissociate, explaining the typically shorter clinical course (Peterson & Talcott, 2013).

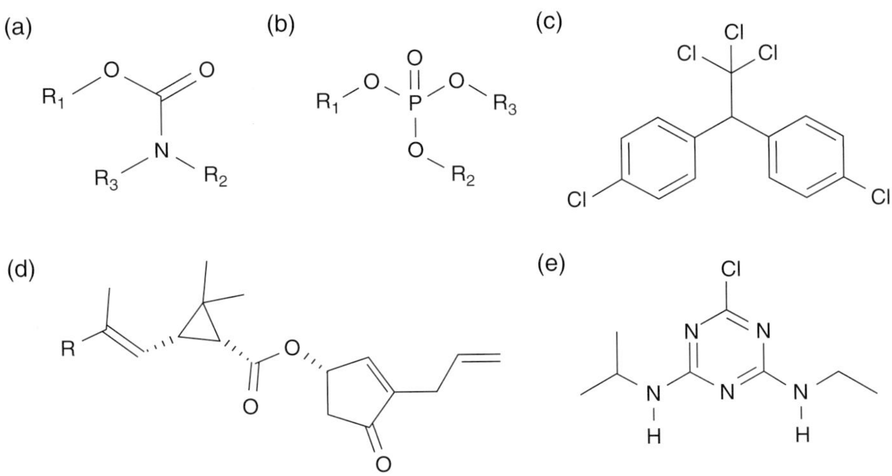

Figure 10.28 Primary pesticide functional groups (reference panel). (a) Carbamate, (b) organophosphate functional group, with additional panels (c) organochlorine (DDT), (d) the first pyrethroid (allethrin), and (e) a triazine herbicide (atrazine) for structural contrast. Author's figure; created with ChemDraw.

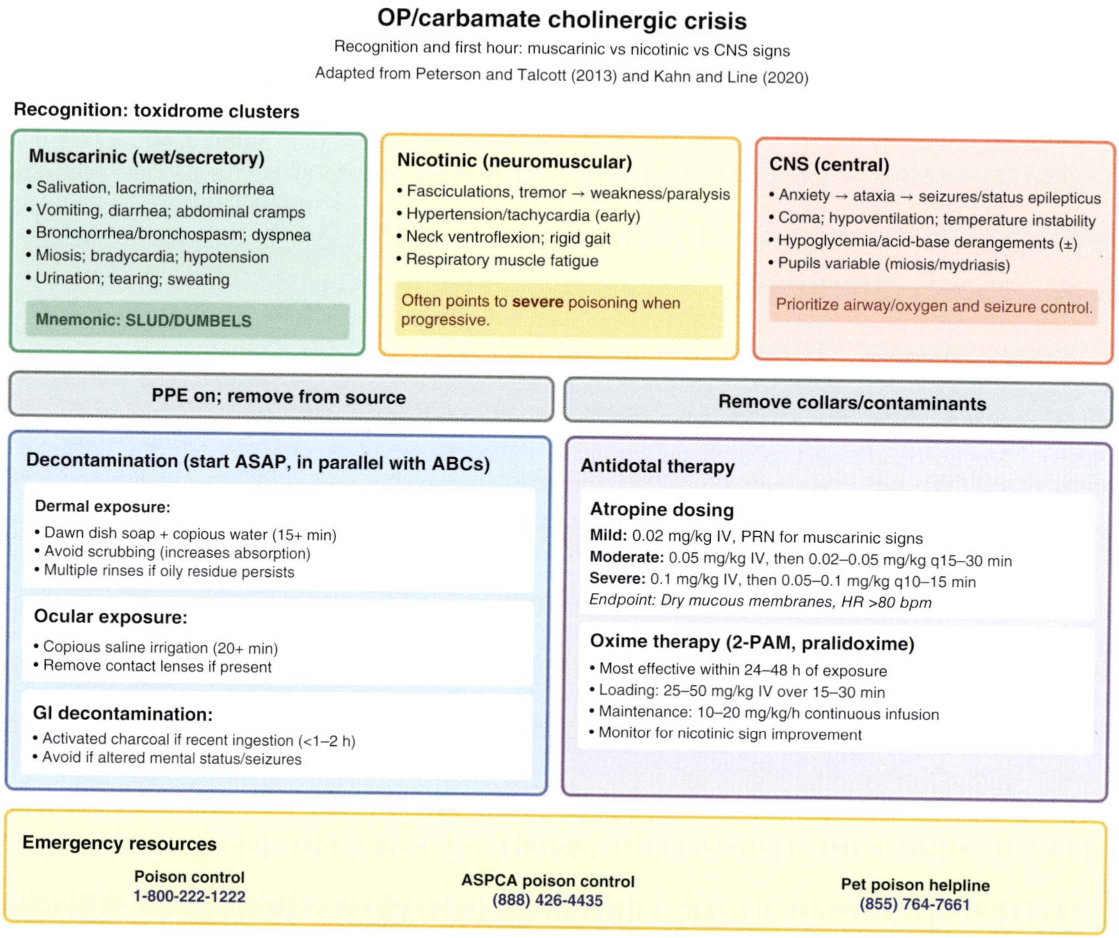

Figure 10.29 OP/carbamate cholinergic crisis – recognition and the first hour. Muscarinic vs. nicotinic vs. CNS signs and the decontamination → atropine → oxime (OP only, early) sequence, with sampling tips. *Source:* Peterson and Talcott (2013) and Kahn and Line (2020).

Clinical Signs

Cats/dogs/ruminants: Salivation, dyspnea/wheezes, bradycardia, miosis, fasciculations → weakness/paralysis, seizures in severe cases; hypoxemia and hyperthermia may be secondary to sustained tremor (Kahn & Line, 2020).

Diagnosis

Elicit exposure history (dip vat, crop insecticide, indoor foggers). Where available, obtain cholinesterase testing (RBC/whole-blood AChE preferred; plasma pseudocholinesterase [pseudo-ChE] as a trend). Rule out levamisole co-administration (adds nicotinic signs and complicates triage). Collect samples before bathing if feasible (Kahn & Line, 2020).

Treatment

Dermal decontamination (mild detergent; clip if matted), oxygen/ventilatory support, and atropine titrated to dry bronchial secretions/adequate heart rate (for muscarinic signs). Oxime (pralidoxime/obidoxime) early for OPs (ideally before aging); do not give oximes for pure carbamate exposures. Control seizures with benzodiazepines; give IV crystalloids and manage temperature/glucose/electrolytes (Kahn & Line, 2020; Peterson & Talcott, 2013). For a side-by-side "what to do now" grid (OPs vs. carbamates), see Table 10.16.

Prevention and Stewardship

No "crop OPs" on pets. Train and monitor dip-vat operations; never pair with levamisole the same day; label-rate only; warn about household contamination (bedding, car seats, child contact) (Kahn & Line, 2020).

Pyrethroids (Permethrin, Cypermethrin, Deltamethrin)

Source

Topical spot-ons, sprays, and dips remain the dominant exposure routes in tropical practice; canine permethrin products are the classic source of feline toxicosis in mixed-species homes (Kahn & Line, 2020; Peterson & Talcott, 2013). To anchor class identity before safety details, Figure 10.30 illustrates representative pyrethroid structures (permethrin, deltamethrin, α-cypermethrin) and isomer notes relevant to potency.

Toxicity

Cats: Rapid-onset neuroexcitation with generalized tremors, hypersalivation, seizures, and hyperthermia.
Dogs: Tremor/ataxia at very high doses or with concentrated pour-ons.
Aquatic species/invertebrates: Highly sensitive – flag run-off and pond exposures on farms (Gupta, 2018; Kahn & Line, 2020). A stepwise care pathway appears in Figure 10.31 for quick triage.

Mechanism (Toxicity)

Prolonged opening of voltage-gated Na^+ channels → repetitive neuronal firing; at very high tissue levels, GABA_A antagonism contributes to seizures (Peterson & Talcott, 2013).

Clinical Signs

Minutes–hours after exposure (accelerated by licking/occlusion): facial twitching → whole-body tremor → seizures; mydriasis common; hyperthermia from sustained muscle activity (Kahn & Line, 2020).

Table 10.16 OPs vs. carbamates – bedside differences and immediate actions.

Agent class	Exposure context	Key signs (recognition)	Do now (first hour)	Labs	Oxime?	Pitfalls (tropics)
Organo-phosphates (OPs)	Dips/sprays, foggers, crop sprays; concentrate spills; poor PPE; hot/humid conditions → ↑ dermal absorption; feed contamination.	Muscarinic: SLUD, bronchorrhea/bronchospasm, miosis, bradycardia. Nicotinic: fasciculations → weakness/paralysis, tachy→brady. CNS: agitation → seizures/coma. Often more prolonged course.	PPE on; remove from source/collars. Dermal decon with detergent ×2–3. ABCs: suction, O_2, IV access, temp control. Atropine titrated to drying of bronchial secretions/adequate HR. Pralidoxime (2-PAM) early (reactivates AChE before aging). Diazepam for seizures/tremor; isotonic fluids; correct glucose/electrolytes.	Whole-blood/RBC AChE (most specific) and/or plasma/pseudo-ChE (trend). Blood gas/ lactate, glucose, electrolytes; ± CK. Repeat at 24–48 h.	Yes. Start 2-PAM ASAP; repeat/infuse 24–48 h if weakness persists; stop when strength returns and cholinergic signs controlled with minimal atropine.	Decanted/relabeled pesticides; banned/obsolete OPs still in use; delaying atropine while bathing; inadequate 2-PAM supply; heat stress increasing absorption; stacking with levamisole or other cholinergics; poor ventilation during fogging.
Carbamates (carbaryl, propoxur, etc.)	Flea powders, garden sprays, premises dusts; ingestion of concentrates; dermal in cats.	Muscarinic-predominant SLUD/miosis; nicotinic weakness usually milder/shorter (reversible AChE inhibition); CNS signs possible but often less sustained than OPs.	Same PPE/source control and dermal/ocular decon. Atropine for muscarinic signs; diazepam if seizures; airway/O_2, IV fluids; correct glucose/electrolytes. Observe 24–48 h.	As above; RBC AChE may be depressed but rebounds faster; recheck at 24–48 h.	Generally no. Oximes are not routinely indicated for pure carbamate poisoning (reversible inhibition); prioritize atropine + support. If exposure uncertain/mixed, it's reasonable to treat as OP (give oxime) while clarifying.	Concentrate mis-dilution on farm; use of carbamate dips in cats; reliance on plasma ChE alone (false negatives); concurrent use with amitraz/other cholinergics; delaying care while attempting home bathing; counterfeit or highly concentrated products in informal markets.

AChE, acetylcholinesterase; ChE, cholinesterase; HR, heart rate; O_2, oxygen; SLUD, salivation, lacrimation, urination, diarrhea.
Columns: Agent class | Exposure context | Key signs | Do now (first hour) | Labs | Oxime? | Pitfalls (tropics). Rows detail OPs and carbamates with practical pearls (e.g., aging, RBC AChE, heat-amplified dermal absorption, levamisole stacking).

- **Atropine endpoint** is drying of bronchial secretions and improved ventilation – not mydriasis.
- Begin antidotes **in parallel** with decontamination when airway/ventilation is threatened.
- For severe respiratory muscle weakness, consider ventilatory support where available.

Source: Peterson and Talcott (2013); Gupta (2018); Kahn and Line (2020).

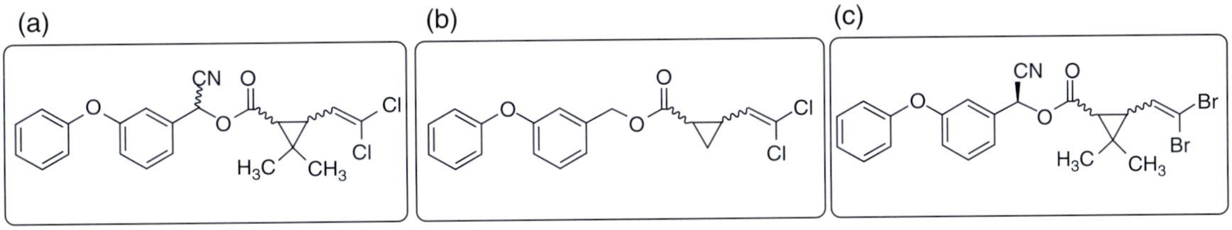

Figure 10.30 Structures of common pyrethroids used in veterinary practice. (a) Permethrin (cis/trans isomers); (b) deltamethrin; (c) α-cypermethrin (racemic). Structural features that influence potency and mammalian safety are highlighted.

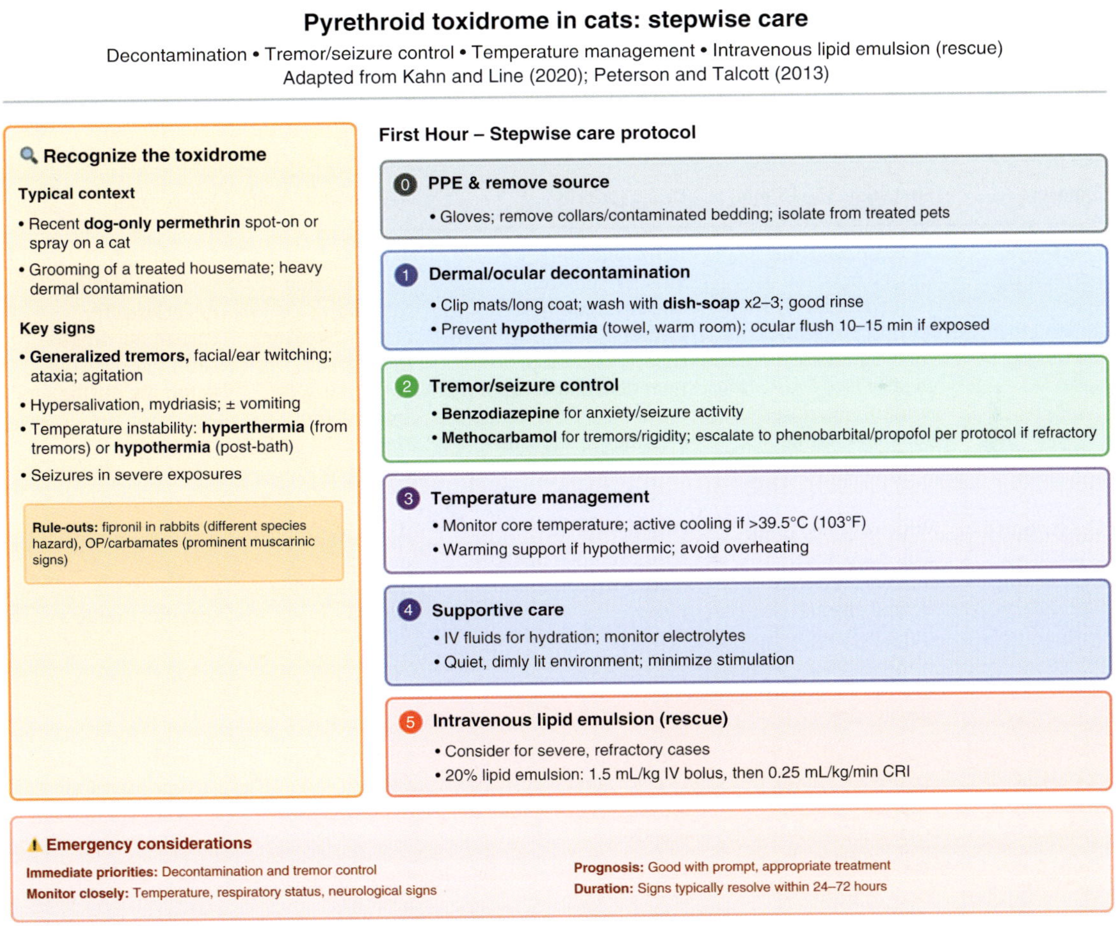

Figure 10.31 Pyrethroid toxidrome in cats – stepwise care. Decontamination (bath), tremor/seizure control (methocarbamol → benzodiazepine/propofol), temperature management, and ILE as rescue, with notes on relapse monitoring. *Source:* Kahn and Line (2020) and Peterson and Talcott (2013).

Diagnosis

History of dog-only product on a cat, heavy pour-on, aerosol exposure in a closed room, or grooming of a freshly treated animal. Diagnosis is clinical; no routine confirmatory lab is required (Peterson & Talcott, 2013).

Treatment

Dermal decon: Bathe with a mild detergent (repeat if oily film persists); protect the eyes and airways.
Control tremors/seizures: Methocarbamol (first-line for tremors/rigidity), benzodiazepines for anxiety/seizures; escalate to phenobarbital/propofol if refractory.
Temperature management: Active cooling/warming to normothermia; correct electrolytes/glucose if deranged.
Rescue: Intravenous lipid emulsion (ILE) may be considered for severe refractory neurotoxicity (case-series support) (Kahn & Line, 2020; Peterson & Talcott, 2013). For dosing intervals, relapse expectations, and environmental cautions, use Table 10.17 at bedside.

Table 10.17 Pyrethroid exposures – first-hour bundle and monitoring.

Exposure	First steps (0–15 min)	Drugs (priority)	Temperature plan	Watch-outs
Dog-only permethrin spot-on applied to a cat (classic case)	PPE; isolate from treated pets; clip if needed and dish-soap baths ×2–3 with thorough rinse; ocular flush if face contaminated; remove collars/bedding.	Benzodiazepine for anxiety/seizure; methocarbamol for tremors/ rigidity → escalate to phenobarbital/propofol if refractory; IV crystalloids; consider ILE rescue in severe cases.	Prevent hypothermia after baths (towels, warm air); treat hyperthermia from tremors (fans, cool IV fluids) until < 39.5°C.	Do not induce emesis when tremoring; never use OP/ carbamate dips as “antidotes”; avoid ketamine during active seizures; expect relapse of tremors – observe.
Cat groomed a recently treated dog (secondary dermal/oral)	Wipe residue; single dish-soap bath; remove access to treated animal; consider single-dose AC only if ingestion was recent, alert, and airway-safe.	Often lower requirements: benzo ± methocarbamol; fluids PRN.	As above; most need only normothermia checks.	Re-exposure risk if co-housed; educate owner on species-specific products.
Dog self-licked or punctured tube (oral + dermal)	Rinse mouth with small water/food slurry; no forced emesis if symptomatic; bathe dermal site.	Antiemetic; benzo if anxious; methocarbamol if tremoring; escalate if seizures.	Monitor; cool only if hyperthermic.	Aspiration risk from solvents; separate from cats in home.
Aerosol/fogger in closed room (inhalation ± dermal)	Move to fresh air; oxygen; bronchodilator if bronchospasm; wipe/ quick bath if residue; ocular irrigation if eyes irritated.	Benzo if agitation/ tremor; methocarbamol PRN.	Usually minimal – avoid chilling if wet.	Hydrocarbon carrier pneumonitis risk; ensure ventilation; avoid further exposure.

Table 10.17 (Continued)

Exposure	First steps (0–15 min)	Drugs (priority)	Temperature plan	Watch-outs
Ocular splash	Irrigate 10–15 min with isotonic fluid; remove residues from periocular hair.	Topical analgesia per clinic protocol; systemic sedation only if needed for irrigation.	N/A	Fluorescein stain and recheck – ulcer/ keratitis possible; avoid topical steroids unless directed.
Livestock dip/ spray overexposure (field)	Remove from spray line; shade/fresh air; rinse with water + mild detergent; remove contaminated tack.	Sedation rarely needed; if tremors → diazepam ± methocarbamol (availability dependent); IV/PO fluids.	Manage heat stress aggressively; avoid chilling.	Stacked products (e.g., OP + pyrethroid); wrong dilution; herd-level re-exposure from contaminated pens.
Large-volume concentrate ingestion (small animal)	Airway protection; no emesis if symptomatic; consider AC if early and safe; bathe if any dermal contamination.	Rapid benzo → methocarbamol; escalate to phenobarbital/ propofol; ILE rescue for severe neurotoxicity.	Active cooling if hyperthermic; warm if hypothermic post-bath.	Hydrocarbon solvent aspiration; electrolyte shifts (K, Ca, Mg) worsen tremors – correct.
Post-bath relapse/ hypothermia	Dry thoroughly; warm environment/forced warm air; reassess neuro status; continue quiet/dark setting.	Usually none beyond earlier protocol; repeat methocarbamol if tremors recur.	Rewarm to normothermia; then maintain.	Bradycardia from hypothermia; prolonged sedation can mask recurrence – observe 12–24 h.

AC, activated charcoal; ILE, intravenous lipid emulsion; OP, organophosphate.
Scenario rows (e.g., dog-only spot-on applied to a cat, grooming a treated dog, aerosol/fogger exposure, livestock dips, large-volume ingestion) with columns for Exposure | First steps | Drugs (priority) | Temperature plan | Watch-outs, plus a universal monitoring footer (neuro checks, vitals, electrolytes).
Monitoring (all scenarios)
Neuro checks q2–4 h, HR/RR/SpO_2/temp; electrolytes (K, Ca, Mg) and glucose if tremors are prolonged.
Observe 12–24 h (longer if severe ingestion). Document product name, concentration, amount, and time of exposure.
Source: Peterson and Talcott (2013) and Kahn and Line (2020).

Prevention and Stewardship

Never apply canine permethrin to cats; segregate wet/treated pets until fully dry; educate owners on label checks and species icons; post fish-safety warnings near ponds/aquaculture; avoid heat/occlusion that amplifies dermal absorption in the tropics (Kahn & Line, 2020).

Amitraz

Source

Tick collars and topical dips are the primary formulations; occasional ingestion of collars or dip concentrate occurs in dogs. Cats should not receive amitraz (Gupta, 2018; Kahn & Line, 2020). To anchor the drug identity before safety details, the chemical structure is shown in Figure 10.32.

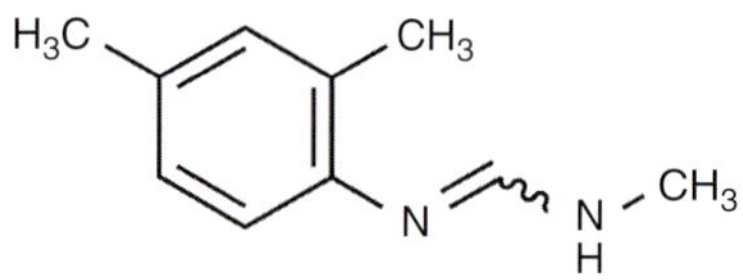

Figure 10.32 Chemical structure of amitraz. Author's schematic to anchor drug identity before toxicity discussion. See Kahn and Line (2020) and Gupta (2018) for clinical use and safety context.

Toxicity

α_2-agonist toxidrome: Sedation, bradycardia, hypotension, hypothermia, hyperglycemia, GI stasis/ileus; severe cases progress to CNS depression/coma (Kahn & Line, 2020). Collars left on during bathing or heat/occlusion can increase dermal uptake in tropical environments, deepening sedation and bradycardia. A first-hour triage ladder appears in Figure 10.33, aligning recognition with immediate reversal and monitoring.

Mechanism (Toxicity)

Central and peripheral α_2-adrenoceptor agonism → reduced sympathetic outflow; decreased GI motility; transient inhibition of insulin secretion yields stress hyperglycemia (Peterson & Talcott, 2013).

Clinical Signs

Depression/ataxia, bradycardia, hypothermia; pupils may be miotic or mydriatic; hyperglycemia on chemistry profile. Collar ingestion adds foreign-body/obstruction risk (Kahn & Line, 2020).

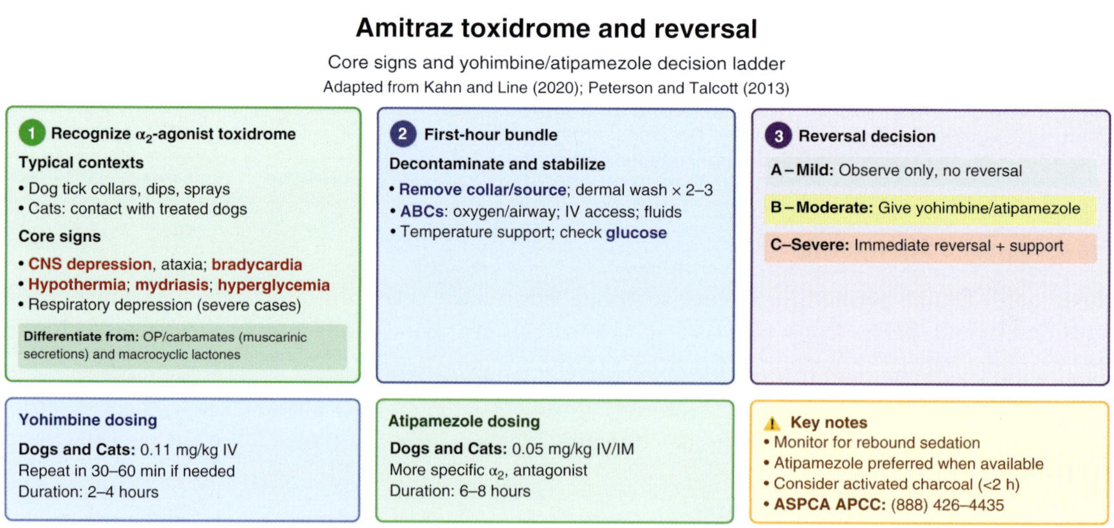

Figure 10.33 Amitraz toxidrome and reversal – first-hour priorities. Core signs (sedation, bradycardia, hypothermia, hyperglycemia, ileus) with a yohimbine/atipamezole decision ladder, temperature and glucose checkpoints, and relapse monitoring. *Source:* Kahn and Line (2020) and Peterson and Talcott (2013).

Diagnosis

Recent collar application or dip? The bradycardia + hypothermia + hyperglycemia triad is suggestive. Consider co-exposures to β-blockers or other α_2-acting sedatives that can magnify effects (Peterson & Talcott, 2013).

Treatment

Remove collar/wash thoroughly (mild detergent; dry to normothermia).

Reverse clinically significant sedation/bradycardia with atipamezole or yohimbine, titrated to effect.

IV crystalloids, oxygen as needed; avoid atropine unless clearly indicated (may worsen hypertension/arrhythmias).

Warm to normothermia; treat ileus if present. GI decontamination only for early, significant ingestion and never in a sedate patient without airway protection (Kahn & Line, 2020; Peterson & Talcott, 2013).

A scenario-based reversal/monitoring protocol (with doses and discharge criteria) is summarized in Table 10.18 for bedside use.

Table 10.18 Amitraz – first-hour reversal and monitoring protocol (by scenario).

Exposure	Reversal (drug/dose and timing)	Fluids/temperature	Glucose	Discharge criteria
Dog ingested amitraz collar (oral)	If moderate–severe sedation/bradycardia: atipamezole dogs 50 μg/kg IM (may repeat q1–3 h) or yohimbine dogs 0.1 mg/kg IV slow (or IM) → reassess 15–30 min.	Isotonic crystalloids if hypotensive; maintain airway/O_2 as needed; passive warming if hypothermic.	Check at presentation, then q2–4 h × 12–24 h; treat marked hyperglycemia per clinic protocol.	Awake/ambulatory, HR/BP stable without ongoing reversal, normothermic, eating, urinating; no relapse for ≥4–6 h after last antagonist dose.
Dog wearing collar/heavy dermal dip (dermal ± inhalation)	Remove collar/source; for persistent CNS depression/bradycardia: atipamezole 50 μg/kg IM or yohimbine 0.1 mg/kg IV/IM; repeat if relapse.	Bathe with mild detergent; dry thoroughly; active rewarming if post-bath hypothermia.	As above.	As above, plus skin clean/dry and owner instructed on product handling.
Cat secondary exposure (collar/dip on dog; grooming)	Decontamination first. If sedation/bradycardia: atipamezole cats 100 μg/kg IM (may repeat q1–3 h) or yohimbine 0.05–0.1 mg/kg IV/IM; monitor closely.	Warm, quiet environment; fluids if hypotensive; oxygen if needed.	Baseline, then q2–4 h for 12–24 h (cats often show transient hyperglycemia).	Bright, eating, normothermic, HR appropriate, no relapse ≥6 h after last antagonist; owners separate pets after treatment.

(Continued)

Table 10.18 (Continued)

Exposure	Reversal (drug/dose and timing)	Fluids/temperature	Glucose	Discharge criteria
Concentrate ingestion (small animal)	Early airway control. Prompt reversal as above (choose one antagonist); consider repeat dosing if relapse.	IV crystalloids; address hypoventilation; manage temperature (cool if hyperthermic from agitation).	Baseline and q2–4 h; manage significant derangements.	As above; extended observation (overnight) recommended.
Livestock dip/spray overexposure	Remove from spray line; shade. If clinically depressed/bradycardic: α_2-antagonist per large-animal protocol (e.g., atipamezole or regional LA antagonist); vet supervision.	Oral/IV fluids as needed; manage heat stress or chilling after rinsing.	Spot-check if feasible; trend clinical recovery.	Ambulatory, eating/ ruminating, HR/RR/ Temp acceptable; no relapse several hours post-reversal.
Mild dermal exposure (any species), stable vitals	No routine reversal – decon + observation; escalate to antagonist only if bradycardia/hypotension/ CNS depression develops.	Dry, warm, quiet stall/ward.	One check at baseline; repeat if mentation changes.	Normal mentation and vitals after observation window (typically 6–12 h).

BP, blood pressure; HR, heart rate; IM, intramuscular; IV, intravenous; O_2, oxygen; RR, respiratory rate.
Rows for collar ingestion (oral), dermal/dip exposure, secondary feline exposure, concentrate ingestion, livestock overexposure, and mild dermal contact; columns: Exposure | Reversal (drug/dose and timing) | Fluids/temperature | Glucose | Discharge criteria. Notes emphasize reversing only when clinically indicated, avoiding emesis in sedate patients, and observation windows to detect relapse.
Notes (first hour): reverse only if clinically indicated; treat bradycardia when hemodynamically significant (reversal often corrects it). Avoid inducing emesis in sedate patients or dermal-only exposures. Avoid agents that lower seizure threshold (e.g., ketamine during active depression).
Source: Peterson and Talcott (2013) and Kahn and Line (2020).

Prevention and Stewardship

No amitraz in cats; ensure child safety around collars; avoid co-administration with other sedatives; instruct owners to remove collars before bathing and to separate treated pets until fully dry (Kahn & Line, 2020).

Fipronil/Isoxazolines

Source

Topical fipronil (spot-ons, sprays) is widely used in dogs/cats but is contraindicated in rabbits. Isoxazolines (e.g., fluralaner, afoxolaner, sarolaner) are popular oral/topical ectoparasiticides in dogs/cats (Kahn &

Line, 2020; Papich, 2020). To anchor identity before safety details, Figure 10.34 shows the chemical structure of fipronil.

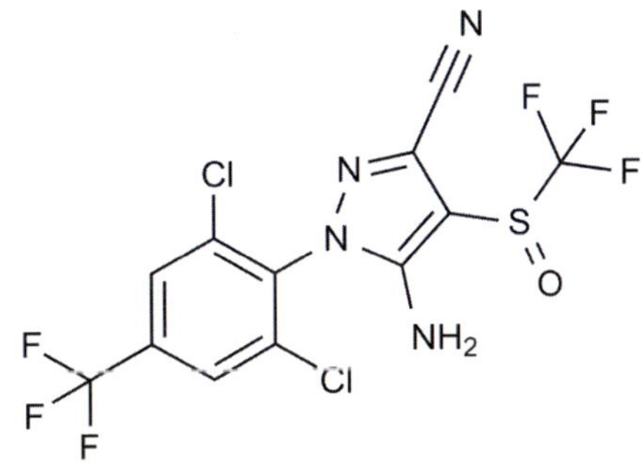

Figure 10.34 Chemical structure of fipronil. Schematic to anchor compound identity prior to toxicity discussion. See Kahn and Line (2020) and Papich (2020) for clinical use and safety context.

Toxicity

Fipronil: Generally a wide margin in dogs/cats, but rabbits – reports of seizures and fatalities; avoid use in lagomorphs.

Isoxazolines: Overall favorable safety profile; rare neurological events (tremor, ataxia, seizures) are reported – use caution in epileptic or seizure-prone pets and discuss risk–benefit with owners (Kahn & Line, 2020; Papich, 2020; Peterson & Talcott, 2013). A quick "who should not get what" risk map is provided in Figure 10.35.

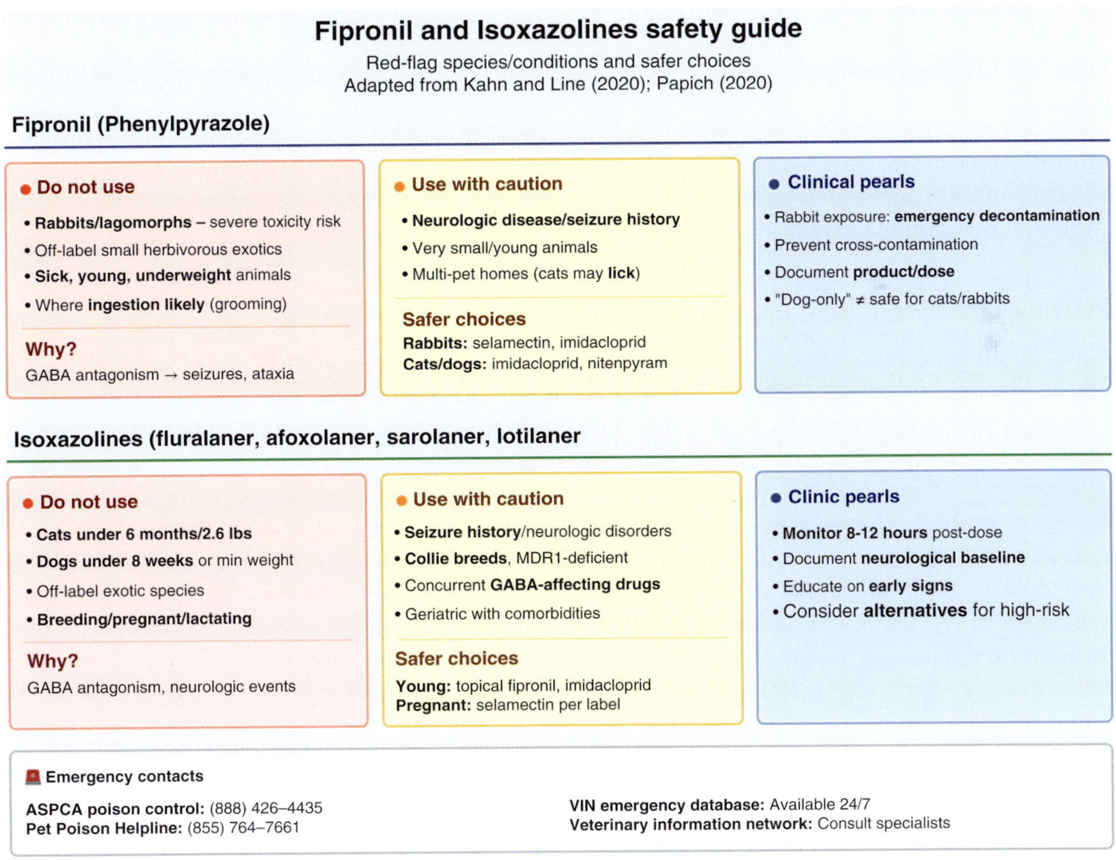

Figure 10.35 Fipronil and isoxazolines – who should not get what. Red-flag species/conditions (e.g., rabbits – avoid fipronil; epileptic pets – caution with isoxazolines) and safer choices. *Source:* Kahn and Line (2020) and Papich (2020).

Mechanism (Toxicity)

Fipronil: Antagonism at GABA_A-gated chloride channels (insects ≫ mammals).
Isoxazolines: Selective antagonism at GABA_A and glutamate-gated chloride channels in arthropods; rare CNS spillover is suspected in predisposed animals (Kahn & Line, 2020; Papich, 2020).

Clinical Signs

Fipronil (rabbits): Anorexia, neurological signs (tremor/seizure), death.
Dogs/cats: Occasional GI upset or mild neuro signs when misused/ingested.
Isoxazolines (dogs/cats): Infrequent tremor/ataxia/seizure soon after dosing in susceptible pets (Kahn & Line, 2020; Papich, 2020).

Diagnosis

Confirm species (strictly no rabbits for fipronil), formulation, dose, and timing. For isoxazolines, screen for seizure history and potential drug interactions; diagnosis is clinical (Kahn & Line, 2020).

Treatment

Fipronil: Wash dermal exposures with mild detergent; supportive care; control seizures if present.
Isoxazolines: Supportive management of rare neurological events (benzodiazepines if needed); most cases are self-limiting (Kahn & Line, 2020; Papich, 2020).

Prevention and Stewardship

Do not use fipronil in rabbits/lagomorphs; use species-specific products; separate pets until topicals are fully dry; counsel owners of seizure-prone pets about rare isoxazoline neuro events; avoid aquatic contamination (Kahn & Line, 2020; Papich, 2020). A practical counseling and safety checklist appears in Table 10.19.

To "sweep the floor" of this subsection, use Table 10.20 as your one-page, bedside checklist. It aligns each ectoparasiticide class with its hallmark toxidrome, antidote (if any), decontamination steps, tremor/seizure control, and species-specific cautions – including the rabbit and fish warnings that so often matter in tropical mixed-animal settings. It also reminds clinicians to start antidotes in parallel with decontamination when airway/ventilation is threatened, to keep wet animals away from aquaria/ponds and discard rinse water safely, and to separate housemates until topicals are fully dry to prevent oral exposure from grooming. Use it side-by-side with the class briefs above to drive the first hour, then pivot to monitoring and stewardship.

Anti-inflammatories and Analgesics – Overview of Toxicities in Tropical Practice

Analgesics and anti-inflammatories are used daily in tropical practice, where heat stress, dehydration, malnutrition, and easy OTC access to human products narrow safety margins and magnify familiar risks. Three patterns dominate casework. (i) owner-administered human drugs (ibuprofen, diclofenac,

Table 10.19 Fipronil/isoxazolines – species cautions and counseling checklist.

Patient type	OK/avoid	What to tell owners (counseling points)	Plan if signs occur
Rabbits/ lagomorphs	**Avoid fipronil** (contraindicated). Consider safer alternatives (e.g., selamectin, imidacloprid, lime–sulfur for mites) per vet guidance. Isoxazolines: generally **avoid off-label**.	Never use dog/cat fipronil on rabbits. Prevent cross-contact with recently treated pets; keep housing, bedding, and feeders free of residue.	If exposed: immediate dermal decontamination (mild detergent), keep warm, seek veterinary care urgently. Bring product/lot. Watch for ataxia, tremor, seizures.
Healthy adult cat	**Fipronil:** labeled feline products acceptable. **Isoxazolines:** acceptable when labeled.	Use species-specific product; keep cats separated until topical is dry. Prevent licking (e-collar, isolation). Give oral isoxazolines **with food** as labeled.	If hypersalivation, tremor, ataxia: wash off residue; **do not induce emesis**; seek care. Veterinary team: benzodiazepine for seizures; supportive care.
Cat with seizure history/ active neuro disease	**Fipronil:** use with caution; avoid ingestion. **Isoxazolines: use with caution** (post-marketing neurological events). Consider alternatives (selamectin/imidacloprid) if risk > benefit.	Discuss risk–benefit and obtain informed consent. Start when stable, monitor closely for 24–48 h. Avoid stacking other neuro-active drugs same day.	Stop exposure; contact clinic immediately if tremor/ataxia/seizure. Clinic: anticonvulsant protocol; supportive care. Document and report AE.
Kittens (< label age/weight)	Prefer **label-approved** products only; avoid off-label fipronil/isoxazoline use.	Dose strictly by weight; keep warm and dry after any bath. Store products away from children/pets.	If dosing error: call clinic/ poison line; bring box; monitor glucose/temp.
Healthy adult dog	**Fipronil:** labeled canine products acceptable. **Isoxazolines:** acceptable when labeled.	Give oral isoxazolines with food if indicated; keep dogs separated from cats/rabbits after topicals until dry. No bathing for label interval unless allowed.	Vomiting once after oral dose can be normal; persistent neuro signs (tremor, ataxia, seizure) → seek care. Bring product/lot.
Dog with seizure history/ active neuro disease	**Isoxazolines: use with caution**; consider alternatives if recent seizures. **Fipronil:** use carefully; prevent ingestion.	Explain small risk of neurological effects; avoid same-day use of other neurological actives; start when dog is stable; observe closely for 24–48 h.	If signs: stop exposure, seek care; clinic to treat seizures and provide supportive care; consider AE reporting.
Geriatric or hepatic/renal compromise (cat or dog)	Prefer products with wider safety margins; use **label doses** only.	Start low-stress; confirm no drug interactions; recheck if appetite/behavior changes.	If lethargy, inappetence, neurological signs: withhold further doses and contact clinic.
Multipet households (cat/dog/rabbit mix)	**Do not use fipronil on rabbits.** For cats/dogs, use species-specific labels.	Apply topical products in **separate rooms**; prevent grooming of wet product; launder bedding; record date/lot.	If a non-target pet licks product or shows signs: rinse mouth with small water amount, bathe exposed area, seek care.

(Continued)

Table 10.19 (Continued)

Patient type	OK/avoid	What to tell owners (counseling points)	Plan if signs occur
Pregnant/ lactating	Follow **label**; if not specifically approved, consider alternatives (selamectin/imidacloprid). Avoid off-label isoxazolines/ fipronil without clear justification.	Use only if benefit outweighs risk; discuss environmental control to reduce chemical load.	If adverse effects: stop product and contact clinic; supportive care as indicated.

AE, adverse event.
Rows by patient type (rabbits; healthy adult cat/dog; seizure-prone pets; kittens/puppies; geriatric or hepatic/renal compromise; multipet households; pregnant/lactating), with columns OK/avoid, owner counseling points, and plan if signs occur; includes concise owner handout one-liners. Owner handout one-liners.
Species-specific products only; keep pets separated until topical is dry.
Do not stack multiple ectoparasiticides the same day.
Keep the box/lot number; call if tremor, ataxia, seizures, or persistent vomiting occur.
Source: Papich (2020) and Kahn and Line (2020).

paracetamol) to pets; (ii) prolonged/depot courses in livestock and horses during drought, transport, or concurrent disease; and (iii) drug stacking (e.g., NSAID plus steroid) that multiplies GI and renal injury (Kahn & Line, 2020; Papich, 2021; Peterson & Talcott, 2013). Species biology is pivotal: Cats' limited glucuronidation makes paracetamol uniquely dangerous (methemoglobinemia, hepatic injury), while horses risk right dorsal colitis (RDC) on phenylbutazone. One Health considerations matter too – diclofenac residues in livestock carcasses contributed to vulture die-offs in South Asia, prompting restrictions and meloxicam adoption where available (Kahn & Line, 2020). Use the overview map in Figure 10.36 to triage by toxidrome and lock in the first-hour priorities (e.g., NAC for feline paracetamol; PPI + sucralfate ± misoprostol and fluids for NSAIDs; avoid NSAID–steroid combinations) while you confirm exposure and tailor ongoing care (Hall & Langston, 2020; Papich, 2021; Peterson & Talcott, 2013).

Nonnarcotic Analgesics (Paracetamol/Aspirin/Salicylates)

Source

The nonnarcotic analgesics commonly used as antipyretics/analgesics are aspirin (acetylsalicylic acid), sodium salicylate, and paracetamol (acetaminophen). The core scaffolds are shown in Figure 10.37, anchoring class identity before toxicity details (Papich, 2021).

Toxicity

Cats are highly susceptible to salicylates and paracetamol (Papich, 2021). Case reports document feline aspirin/paracetamol poisonings (Hall & Langston, 2020; Ko & Payton, 2022). In an experimental series, daily aspirin 33–63 mg/kg for ~35 days produced toxic hepatitis in ~50% of cats (Dowling, 2020). Dogs

Table 10.20 Ectoparasiticides – antidotes and first-hour actions.

Agent/class	Toxidrome (hallmark)	Antidote	Decon (start in parallel with ABCs)	Seizure/tremor control (priority)	Special notes (rabbits/fish)
Pyrethrins/pyrethroids (incl. permethrin)	Neuroexcitation → facial twitching, tremors → seizures, hyperthermia from muscle activity	None (supportive). ILE rescue if severe	Clip mats; dish-soap baths ×2–3 with thorough rinse; ocular irrigation 10–15 min if exposed; prevent post-bath hypothermia	Benzodiazepine for anxiety/seizures → methocarbamol for tremors; escalate phenobarbital/propofol if refractory	Rabbits: generally tolerate pyrethroids better than fipronil but avoid heavy exposures; use safer alternatives when possible. Fish: extremely toxic – keep run-off and wet animals away from aquaria/ponds
Organophosphates (OPs)	Cholinergic crisis (muscarinic SLUD, bronchorrhea/bronchospasm; nicotinic fasciculations/weakness; CNS seizures)	Atropine for muscarinic signs; pralidoxime (2-PAM) for OP (early); repeat per protocol	Dermal wash with mild detergent; ocular irrigation; consider activated charcoal if early, airway safe	Diazepam for seizures/tremor; control secretions/bronchospasm; fluids, O_2	Rabbits: avoid exposure; rapid decon if contaminated. Fish: highly sensitive – never allow OP run-off into tanks/ponds
Carbamates	Cholinergic, often shorter-lived vs. OP	Atropine; oximes generally not indicated for pure carbamate poisoning	As for OPs	Diazepam; supportive care	Same aquatic precautions as OPs; separate treated animals from aquaria until fully dry
Amitraz (α_2-agonist)	CNS depression, bradycardia, hypothermia, mydriasis; hyperglycemia	Yohimbine or atipamezole (choose one; repeat if relapse)	Remove collar/source; dermal wash ×2–3; dry and warm	Sedation usually improves after reversal; benzodiazepine only if needed (avoid ketamine during active depression)	Rabbits: avoid collars/dips; decon aggressively if exposed. Fish: toxic – keep collars/solutions away from water bodies
Fipronil (phenylpyrazole)	GABA-block neuroexcitation → ataxia → seizures; GI upset	None (supportive)	Dermal wash; ocular irrigation; limit oral exposure (prevent grooming)	Benzodiazepine ± methocarbamol; escalate per seizure protocol	Rabbits: contraindicated – do not use; emergency decon if exposure. Fish: very toxic – no run-off to aquaria

(Continued)

Table 10.20 (Continued)

Agent/class	Toxidrome (hallmark)	Antidote	Decon (start in parallel with ABCs)	Seizure/tremor control (priority)	Special notes (rabbits/fish)
Isoxazolines (fluralaner, afoxolaner, sarolaner, lotilaner)	Rare idiosyncratic tremor/ataxia/seizure reports	None	Oral products: no decon; if topical, wipe residue and bathe once if needed	Benzodiazepine first-line; standard seizure care	Rabbits: avoid off-label use unless specialist-directed. Fish: keep tablets/spot-ons and rinse water away from tanks
Macrocyclic lactones used as ectoparasiticides (selamectin, moxidectin, high-dose ivermectin)	CNS depression/ataxia (↑ risk in MDR1 dogs; dose stacking)	None; consider ILE rescue in severe cases	Dermal wash if topical; remove collars; observe	Benzodiazepine if agitation/seizure (uncommon); airway support for coma	Rabbits: selamectin often used under vet guidance; avoid large-animal pour-ons. Fish: ivermectin is highly toxic – strictly avoid contamination
Neonicotinoids (imidacloprid, etc.)	Usually GI-predominant (hypersalivation, vomiting); neurological signs uncommon	None	Rinse mouth; wipe/bathe dermal residues; ocular irrigation if irritated	Rarely needed; antiemetic/supportive care	Rabbits: imidacloprid often acceptable when prescribed; avoid ingestion of wet product. Fish: toxic – prevent run-off
Spinosyns (spinosad/spinetoram)	GI upset ± tremor; can potentiate ivermectin neurotoxicity	None	None usually; treat symptomatically	Benzodiazepine if tremor; antiemetic	Rabbits: limited data – prefer alternatives unless specialist-directed. Fish: toxic – avoid water contamination

ILE, intravenous lipid emulsion; MDR1, ABCB1 gene mutation (P-gp deficiency); OP, organophosphate; SLUD, salivation, lacrimation, urination, diarrhea. Crosswalk of Agent/class → Toxidrome → Antidote → Decontamination → Seizure/tremor control → Special notes (rabbits/fish), with footnoted reminders on initiating antidotes alongside ABCs and preventing aquatic exposure/runoff; includes guidance to keep topicals from housemates until fully dry.

- Start antidotes in parallel with decon when airway/ventilation is threatened.
- Keep wet animals away from aquaria/ponds; discard rinse water safely.
- For topicals, separate housemates until fully dry to prevent oral exposure (grooming).

Source: Gupta (2018), Kahn and Line (2020), and Peterson and Talcott (2013); table framework per author's worksheet.

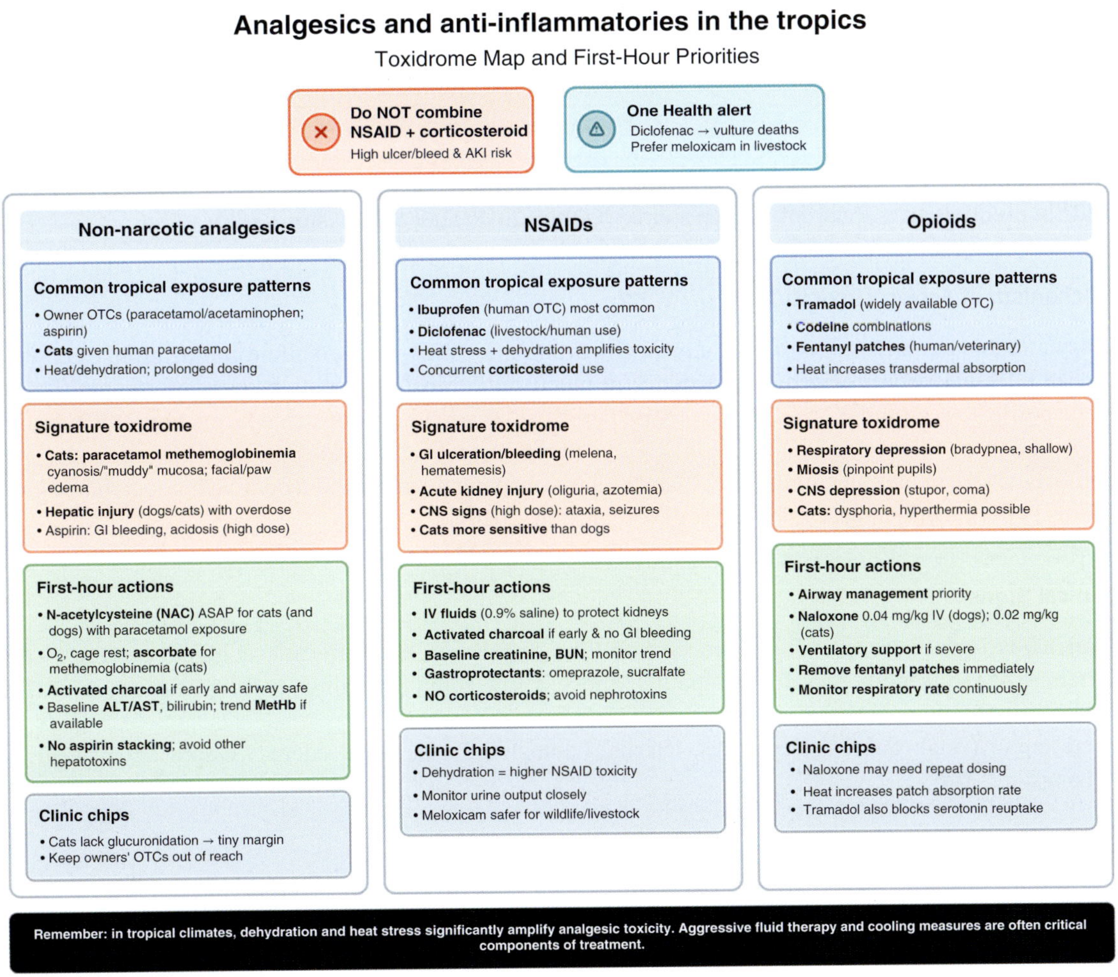

Figure 10.36 Overview of common exposure patterns, toxidromes, and first-hour priorities for non-narcotic analgesics, NSAIDs, and corticosteroids in tropical practice. Heat stress, dehydration, and human OTC use narrow safety margins; avoid NSAID–steroid combinations. One Health: diclofenac residues have been implicated in vulture mortality; meloxicam is preferred where available. *Source:* Hall and Langston (2020); Kahn and Line (2020); Papich (2020, 2021); Peterson and Talcott (2013). AKI, acute kidney injury; PPI, proton-pump inhibitor; OTC, over-the-counter.

Figure 10.37 Structural formulas of common non-narcotic analgesics. Aspirin (acetylsalicylic acid), sodium salicylate, and paracetamol (acetaminophen). Schematic to support class recognition prior to mechanistic and clinical content. *Source:* Adapted from Papich (2021).

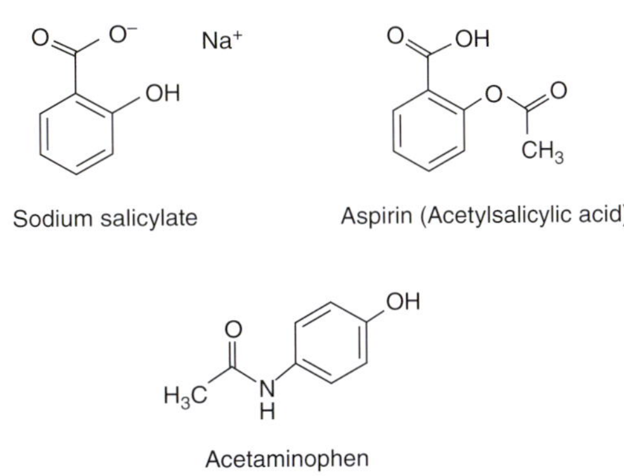

may progress from GI upset to CNS signs at high exposures (Phillips & Graham, 2019). Sheep can develop non-cardiogenic pulmonary edema even at therapeutic salicylate doses (Papich, 2021).

Feline paracetamol cues: Early facial edema, ptyalism, brown ("chocolate") mucous membranes, and low/erratic pulse-ox suggest methemoglobinemia with evolving hepatic injury; combination human cold/flu products are a frequent hidden source (Gupta, 2018; Hall & Langston, 2020).

Mechanism of Action (Toxicity)

Salicylates and paracetamol undergo hepatic glucuronidation and glycine/sulfate conjugation. Cats synthesize UDP-glucuronic acid but have deficient glucuronyl transferase activity, slowing clearance and predisposing to accumulation (Klaassen, 2019; Papich, 2021). Acidic feline urine favors nonionic tubular reabsorption of salicylates (Papich, 2021). Paracetamol bioactivation yields N-acetyl-p-benzoquinone imine (NAPQI), depleting glutathione → centrilobular hepatic necrosis and oxidative hemoglobin injury (Heinz bodies, methemoglobinemia) (Hall & Langston, 2020).

Clinical Signs

Aspirin/salicylates: Depression, anorexia, vomiting, hyperpnea, hyperthermia; at higher exposure – GI hemorrhage/ulcer, anemia, toxic hepatitis, and seizures/coma (Dowling, 2020; Jones & Park, 2021; Phillips & Graham, 2019).

Paracetamol (cats): anorexia, cyanosis, icterus, hemoglobinuria, facial edema (Gupta, 2018; Hall & Langston, 2020).

Pathophysiology

Aspirin: Gastric erosions/ulcers (topical irritation plus COX inhibition), anemia; hepatic injury; marrow hyperplasia sometimes noted at necropsy (Jones & Park, 2021).

Paracetamol (cats): Methemoglobinemia/Heinz-body hemolysis with centrilobular hepatic necrosis (Hall & Langston, 2020).

Diagnosis

Exposure history (including human combination products), species, and dose; CBC/chemistry; urinalysis. Co-oximetry (if available) confirms methemoglobinemia – note that conventional pulse oximetry is unreliable in this context (Hall & Langston, 2020).

Treatment

Early gastric decontamination (only with a protected airway) and activated charcoal for recent ingestions (Papich, 2021).

Enhance elimination/support: IV crystalloids; consider urine alkalinization (IV $NaHCO_3$) for significant salicylate toxicity (correct K^+ to enable alkalinization); diuresis as indicated (Papich, 2021). Peritoneal dialysis may be considered in severe cases when available (Ko & Payton, 2022).

Antidote (paracetamol): NAC – for example, 140 mg/kg loading, then q8 h × 2 additional doses (PO/IV) as per protocol (Fisher & Thompson, 2021; Wilson & Sutton, 2022). Avoid methylene blue in cats; consider ascorbate as an adjunct for methemoglobinemia (Hall & Langston, 2020). Include hepatic support (e.g., SAMe) during recovery where appropriate.

Nonsteroidal Anti-inflammatory (NSAID) Drugs

Source

In tropical systems, NSAID exposures cluster around three predictable contexts: (i) owner-administered human OTCs to pets (ibuprofen, diclofenac); (ii) prolonged or high-intensity equine phenylbutazone/flunixin use during transport, lameness, or competition; and (iii) ambient heat/dehydration/malnutrition, which narrows renal perfusion reserves and amplifies GI injury (Kahn & Line, 2020; Papich, 2020; Peterson & Talcott, 2013). Variable supply chains, depot/long-acting regimens, and concurrent disease (CKD, parasitism) further reduce safety margins.

Toxicity – Clinical Phenotypes

Dogs/cats (human NSAIDs, esp. ibuprofen/diclofenac). Early nausea, vomiting, hematemesis/melena, abdominal pain; with progression: perforating ulcer, anemia, shock. Renal involvement (often after large or repeated dosing, or in dehydration) presents with isosthenuria/azotemia, hyperkalemia, and oliguria/PU-PD patterns (Kahn & Line, 2020; Papich, 2020).

Horses (phenylbutazone > flunixin). RDC with protein-losing enteropathy after high or prolonged dosing – colic, soft feces/diarrhea, ventral edema, weight loss, and hypoalbuminemia; concurrent gastric squamous ulcer disease may coexist (Kahn & Line, 2020).

Population/One Health signals. Diclofenac residues in livestock carcasses were linked to vulture mortality in South Asia, spurring restrictions and meloxicam adoption as a raptor-safer alternative where available (Kahn & Line, 2020).

Mechanism (Why Tropical Contexts Hurt More)

Prostaglandin withdrawal. NSAIDs inhibit COX enzymes; reduced PGE_2/PGI_2 compromises mucosal blood flow, mucus/bicarbonate secretion, and epithelial restitution, predisposing to erosions/ulcers. In the kidney – especially under hypovolemia/heat stress – loss of vasodilatory prostaglandins limits afferent arteriolar dilation, precipitating prerenal → intrinsic AKI (Kahn & Line, 2020; Papich, 2020).

Topical/enterohepatic factors. Local mucosal irritation plus enterohepatic recirculation (e.g., ibuprofen, naproxen) prolongs exposure and recrudescent signs. Heat-driven dehydration, angiotensin-converting enzyme (ACE) inhibitors/diuretics, and concurrent steroids synergize GI/renal injury – the "triple-whammy" physiology (Papich, 2020; Peterson & Talcott, 2013).

Equine RDC special case. Prostaglandin depletion in the right dorsal colon impairs mucosal perfusion and barrier integrity in a high-load segment, explaining protein loss and mural thickening detectable on ultrasound (Kahn & Line, 2020).

Clinical Signs and Diagnosis

Small animals. Hematemesis/melena, abdominal pain, lethargy; BUN/creatinine rise, isosthenuria, electrolyte derangements if renal. Consider concurrent coagulopathy with severe GI bleeding. History often reveals human OTC or long-acting veterinary NSAID, sometimes stacked with a steroid (Kahn & Line, 2020).

Equine (RDC). Colic of variable intensity, soft feces/diarrhea, edema, weight loss; hypoalbuminemia out of proportion to other changes. Right dorsal colon ultrasound may show mural thickening; monitor TP/albumin trend (Kahn & Line, 2020).

Work-up. Minimum database: CBC/chemistry (BUN/Cr, electrolytes), UA, fecal occult blood (small animals); albumin q24–48 h and focused ultrasound in horses with RDC risk. Clarify exact drug, dose, duration, hydration status, and co-medications (Kahn & Line, 2020; Peterson & Talcott, 2013).

Management – First Hour to 72 Hours

Decontamination. Dogs: consider emesis within ~2 hours if safe, then activated charcoal (repeat for enterohepatic NSAIDs as per protocol). Cats: charcoal if protected airway. Do not induce emesis in compromised patients (Peterson & Talcott, 2013).

GI protection bundle. PPI (acid suppression) + sucralfate (mucosal bandage) ± misoprostol (especially for NSAID-induced ulcers) (Kahn & Line, 2020; Papich, 2020).

Renal support. Isotonic crystalloids 24–72 h targeting euvolemia and perfusion; monitor urine output, electrolytes, and azotemia trajectory (Kahn & Line, 2020).

Equine RDC care. Stop NSAID; IV fluids, stall rest; dietary rest (low-bulk, complete feeds), and serial albumin. Ultrasound-guided monitoring of right dorsal colon thickness to track response (Kahn & Line, 2020).

Escalation. Treat anemia/hyperproteinemia supportively; manage perforation/sepsis per standard critical care pathways. Never combine NSAID + corticosteroid; institute washout when switching NSAIDs (Kahn & Line, 2020; Peterson & Talcott, 2013).

Prevention and Stewardship (Field Rules)

No human NSAIDs for pets. Use veterinary-labeled products only; avoid multi-NSAID or NSAID–steroid combinations; respect washouts (Kahn & Line, 2020; Papich, 2020).

Hydration first. Delay elective NSAID dosing in heat stress, dehydration, or travel; rehydrate and reassess renal risk (Kahn & Line, 2020).

Risk triage. CKD/geriatrics: baseline chem/UA, conservative dosing, early recheck. Horses: avoid high/prolonged phenylbutazone, watch albumin, use targeted durations (Kahn & Line, 2020).

One Health. Where relevant, avoid diclofenac in food animals; meloxicam is the raptor-safer alternative (Kahn & Line, 2020).

Corticosteroids

Source

Glucocorticoids (e.g., dexamethasone, prednisolone) are widely used as anti-inflammatory and immunosuppressive agents across species. In tropical systems, high infectious-disease prevalence, heat/dehydration, malnutrition, and reliance on depot/long-acting formulations narrow safety margins and complicate monitoring (Kahn & Line, 2020; Papich, 2020). The core structures for two commonly used agents are shown to anchor class identity before safety details (Figure 10.38).

Toxicity (High-Yield)

Cross-species: Iatrogenic Cushingoid changes (polyuria-polydipsia (PU-PD), muscle catabolism), infection flares, GI ulcer/bleed – risk markedly increased with concurrent NSAIDs (Kahn & Line, 2020).
Cats: Insulin resistance → diabetes; UTIs may be subclinical (Papich, 2020).
Horses: Laminitis concern; delayed wound healing (Kahn & Line, 2020).
Ruminants/equids: Induction of parturition near term; neonatal viability concerns (Kahn & Line, 2020).

Mechanism of Action (Toxicity)

Glucocorticoids suppress leukocyte trafficking and cytokines and blunt fever, potentially unmasking or worsening infections; they reduce GI mucosal protection and delay restitution, synergizing with NSAIDs to cause ulcers/bleeding; they increase hepatic gluconeogenesis and peripheral insulin antagonism (hyperglycemia/diabetes risk in cats); they drive protein catabolism and alter hoof/laminar physiology (laminitis risk in horses). In late gestation (ruminants/equids), fetal maturation/parturition can be triggered (Kahn & Line, 2020; Papich, 2020).

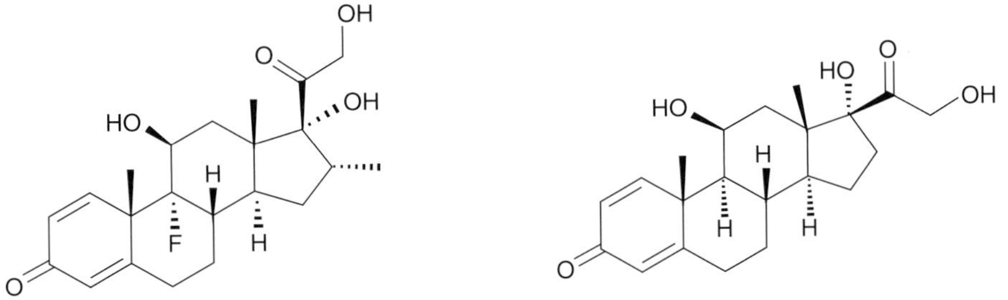

Figure 10.38 Chemical structures of dexamethasone and prednisolone. *Source:* Adapted from Kahn and Line (2020) and Papich (2020).

Clinical Signs

PU/PD/PP, panting, muscle wasting, thin skin; GI pain/melena/hematemesis with ulceration (especially if on an NSAID). Cats: hyperglycemia/ketonuria; recurrent/occult UTIs. Horses: foot soreness, stance change – laminitis watch (Kahn & Line, 2020; Papich, 2020).

Pathophysiology

GI: Prostaglandin loss + impaired restitution → erosions/ulcers; additive risk with NSAIDs.

Endocrine/metabolic: HPA-axis suppression with prolonged/high doses; hyperglycemia and lipid shifts (cats).

Musculoskeletal/hoof: Protein catabolism; altered perfusion/laminar metabolism (laminitis predisposition) (Kahn & Line, 2020; Papich, 2020).

Diagnosis

History (drug, dose, duration, depot use, NSAID co-exposure), hydration/nutritional status.

Dogs/cats: CBC/chem/UA (glucose); consider urine culture in cats.

Horses: Hoof exam/laminitis risk; ulcer history.

Ruminants/equids near term: Confirm gestational stage before dosing (Kahn & Line, 2020; Papich, 2020).

Treatment (Adverse Effects)

1) Stop NSAID co-therapy; institute PPI + sucralfate (± misoprostol) for suspected GI injury; manage anemia/transfuse as indicated.
2) **Infections**: culture-guided antimicrobials; taper or cease steroid if feasible.
3) **Hyperglycemia (cats)**: dietary plan, ± insulin; reassess steroid indication and dose.
4) **Equine laminitis**: stall rest, hoof support, analgesia; reconsider steroid plan.
5) **HPA suppression/tapering**: if ≥7–10 days or high-dose courses, taper rather than abrupt stop; typical approach is 10–25% dose reductions every 1–2 weeks, slowing/holding the taper for red flags (GI bleed, infection flare, hyperglycemia in cats, laminitis signs in horses) (Kahn & Line, 2020; Papich, 2020).

Prevention and Stewardship

Use the lowest effective dose for the shortest duration; avoid depot injections when close titration/monitoring is needed; never stack with NSAIDs; screen for infectious disease before high-dose therapy in febrile animals when feasible; plan a taper for courses >7–10 days; monitor glucose/UTIs (cats), albumin/GI bleed risk (dogs), and laminitis signs (horses). Use Table 10.23 at bedside to tailor mitigation by species and context (Kahn & Line, 2020; Papich, 2020).

Taken together, this subsection gives you a “see it–stabilize it–prevent it” pathway for three high-frequency drug groups in the tropics. Start with the toxidrome map (Figure 10.36) to triage fast; then

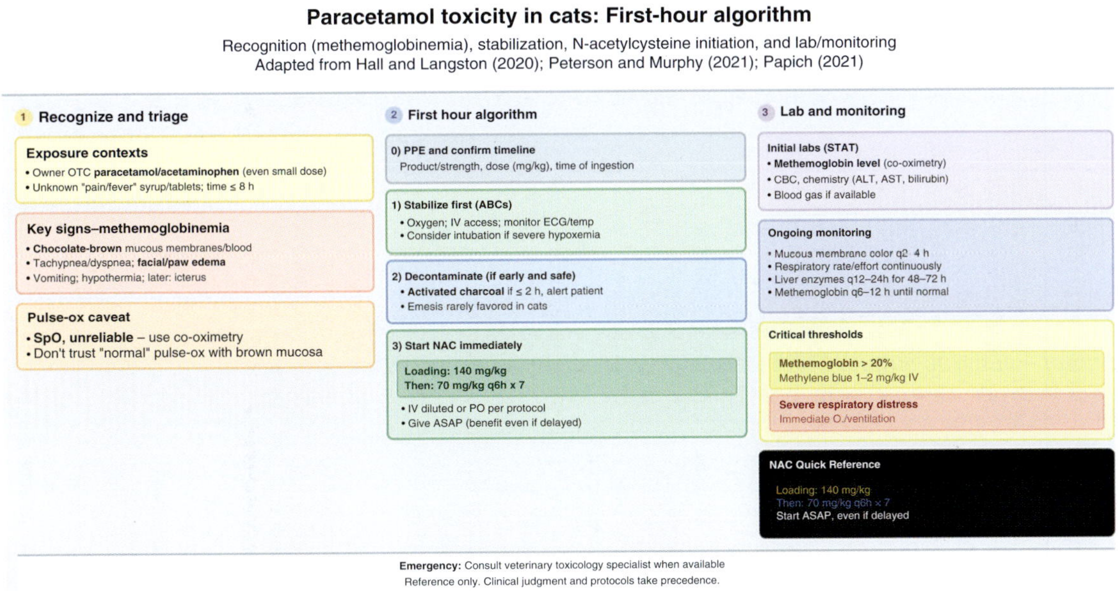

Figure 10.39 Paracetamol in cats – first-hour algorithm. Recognition of methemoglobinemia (chocolate mucosa; pulse-ox unreliability), immediate stabilization, N-acetylcysteine initiation, and early lab/monitoring checkpoints. *Source:* Hall and Langston (2020); Peterson and Murphy (2021); Papich (2021).

move class by class: use Figure 10.37 to anchor nonnarcotic analgesic chemistry and Figure 10.39 for the feline paracetamol first-hour algorithm (NAC early, pulse-ox caveats), with Table 10.21 as the bedside checklist. For NSAIDs, pair mechanism and field amplifiers with Figure 10.40, manage cases using the first-72-hour bundle and RDC cues in Figure 10.41, and keep dosing/monitoring guardrails handy in Table 10.22. For corticosteroids, confirm indication and risks up front, consult Table 10.23 for species-specific mitigation (no NSAID stacking, infection screens, diabetes/laminitis watch), and follow the taper/"slow-or-hold" prompts in Figure 10.42. As you finalize your case notes, document the exact product, dose, timing, hydration status, and any co-medications; these details determine both prognosis and stewardship decisions for the next patient (Kahn & Line, 2020; Papich, 2020, 2021; Peterson & Talcott, 2013).

Sedatives/Anesthetics (Briefs) – Tropical Context

High heat and humidity, dehydration, and malnutrition shrink safety margins for CNS-depressant drugs in the tropics. Add frequent field anesthesia/sedation (working dogs, equids, wildlife), depot formulations, and owner improvisation, and two toxidromes dominate casework: (i) barbiturate overdose/exposure with profound CNS and respiratory depression (including scavenging of euthanized carcasses by dogs and wild carnivores); (ii) α_2-agonist effects (xylazine/medetomidine/dexmedetomidine) with bradycardia, hypotension, hypoventilation, hypothermia, and hyperglycemia. Stabilize by toxidrome: for barbiturates, secure the airway early, ventilate, support perfusion and temperature, and consider intralipid only in

Table 10.21 Nonnarcotic analgesics – species sensitivities, toxic cues, and first-hour actions.

Species – drug	Exposure cues	Immediate actions	Antidote/alkalinization	Monitoring (0–48 h)	Do-not-use
Cat – paracetamol (acetaminophen)	Owner OTC (tablet/syrup) even "small" dose; combo cold meds. Brown/chocolate mucosa, dyspnea, facial/paw edema, vomiting, depression.	Oxygen, quiet/warm; IV access. Activated charcoal if ≤2 h and airway-safe (no emesis if compromised).	N-acetylcysteine: load 140 mg/kg, then 70 mg/kg q6 h × 7 (IV diluted or PO) per protocol. Ascorbate adjunct; SAMe hepatic support.	MetHb % (co-oximetry if available) q4–6 h until <10%; smear for Heinz bodies; ALT/AST, bilirubin; glucose, electrolytes/ acid–base; PCV/TP; UA.	Methylene blue (cats) – contraindicated. Avoid NSAIDs/steroids; no further paracetamol.
Cat – salicylate (aspirin/ pepto-bismol)	Single large or repeated dosing; dehydration/heat. Vomiting, melena, tachypnea (resp. alkalosis → metabolic acidosis), hyperthermia.	IV crystalloids; PPI + sucralfate; external cooling if hyperthermic. Activated charcoal if ≤2 h and safe.	No antidote. Urinary alkalinization (IV $NaHCO_3$) if severe tox/ acidemia; correct K^+ to facilitate alkalinization.	Acid–base/blood gas; electrolytes (K^+); renal panel; PCV/TP, fecal occult blood; ± coagulation.	Avoid NSAID or steroid stacking; avoid chronic aspirin without vet supervision (very slow clearance).
Dog – paracetamol	Overdose or chronic high dose; combo cold meds. Vomit, lethargy; ± methemoglobinemia at very high doses.	IV access; activated charcoal if ≤2 h (airway-safe); antiemetic; oxygen if dyspneic.	N-acetylcysteine as above (load/maintenance). SAMe liver support. (Avoid methylene blue unless specialist-directed.)	ALT/AST, bilirubin; PT/ INR if severe; glucose, electrolytes; ± MetHb % if cyanotic/brown blood.	Avoid NSAID co-administration; avoid repeat dosing in hepatic disease.
Dog – salicylate	Owner aspirin for pain or bismuth-subsalicylate; long-acting/stacked dosing; dehydration/heat. GI upset, melena, hyperventilation, fever.	Stop salicylate; IV crystalloids; PPI + sucralfate; external cooling if needed; activated charcoal if early.	No antidote. Urinary alkalinization with IV $NaHCO_3$ for moderate–severe cases; correct K^+; consider dialysis in life-threatening tox where available.	Acid–base; electrolytes (K^+); renal panel; PCV/TP, fecal occult blood; ± coagulation.	No NSAID–steroid overlap; avoid other NSAIDs.
Sheep – paracetamol	Accidental access to human OTCs; flock medicating errors. Depression, anorexia; ± brown mucosa (rare), vomiting uncommon.	Remove source; IV/PO fluids; activated charcoal (rumen) if early; shelter from heat.	N-acetylcysteine (extrapolated protocols) when significant ingestion; vitamin C adjunct considered.	Liver enzymes, bilirubin; hydration status; ± MetHb % if brown mucosa/ dyspnea; fecal output.	Avoid extra-label use for analgesia; do not stack with other hepatotoxins.
Sheep – salicylate	Off-label aspirin for pain/ fever; dehydration/heat; dosing errors. Anorexia, melena, depression; ± rumen hypomotility.	Stop drug; IV/PO fluids; shade/cooling; GI protection (PPI/sucralfate per clinic protocol); consider repeated charcoal if large ingestion.	No antidote. Urinary alkalinization (IV $NaHCO_3$) in moderate–severe tox/acidemia; correct K^+.	Acid–base; electrolytes, renal panel; fecal occult blood; hydration/rumen motility.	Avoid NSAID stacking; avoid late-gestation high doses; do not combine with steroids.

MetHb, methemoglobin; PPI, proton-pump inhibitor; SAMe, S-adenosyl-L-methionine; UA, urinalysis.
Rows by species (cat, dog, sheep) and drug (salicylate/paracetamol) with columns: Exposure cues, Immediate actions, Antidote/alkalinization, Monitoring (0–48 h), and Do-not-use (e.g., methylene blue in cats).
Source: Dowling (2020); Duarte and Harper (2020); Fisher and Thompson (2021); Hall and Langston (2020); Jones and Park (2021); Papich (2021); Peterson and Murphy (2021); Phillips and Graham (2019); Weiss and Berger (2019); Wilson and Sutton (2022).

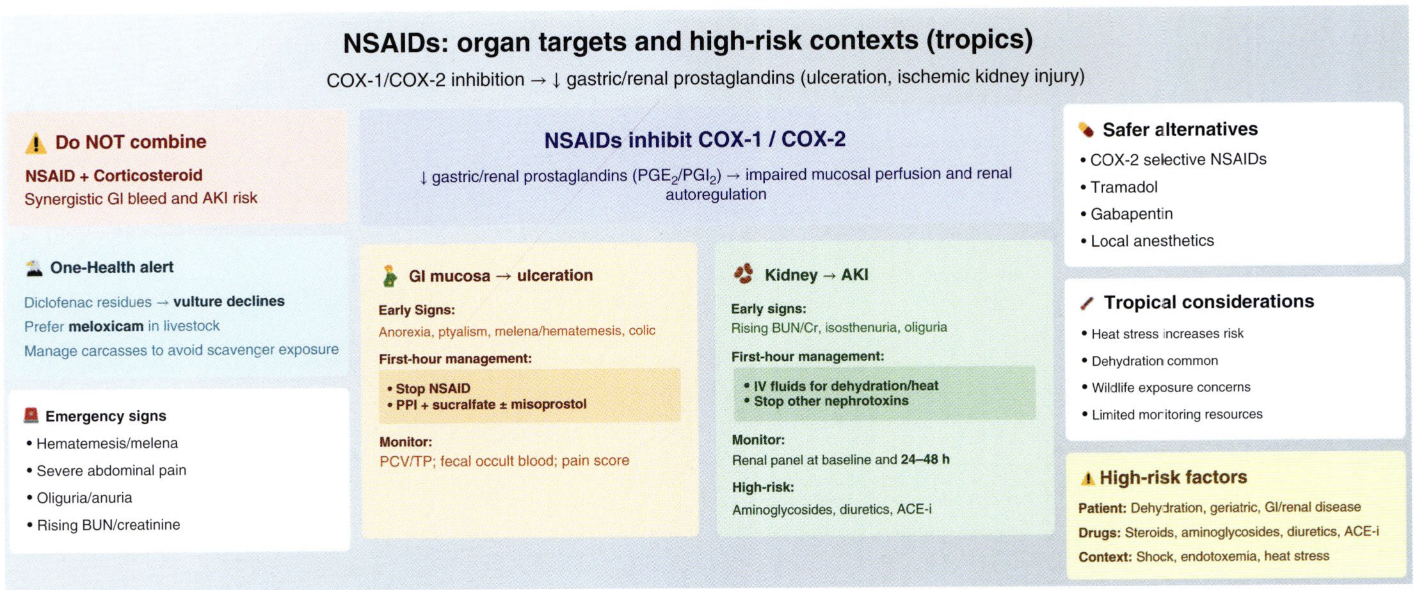

Figure 10.40 NSAIDs in the tropics – exposure patterns, target organs, and field amplifiers. Owner OTC use, prolonged courses, and heat/dehydration map to the principal targets: gastric/intestinal mucosa and kidney; in horses, the right dorsal colon is uniquely vulnerable. Insets flag dehydration, concurrent nephrotoxins (ACE-inhibitors, diuretics), and steroid co-administration as risk multipliers. *Source:* Kahn and Line (2020); Papich (2020); Peterson and Talcott (2013).

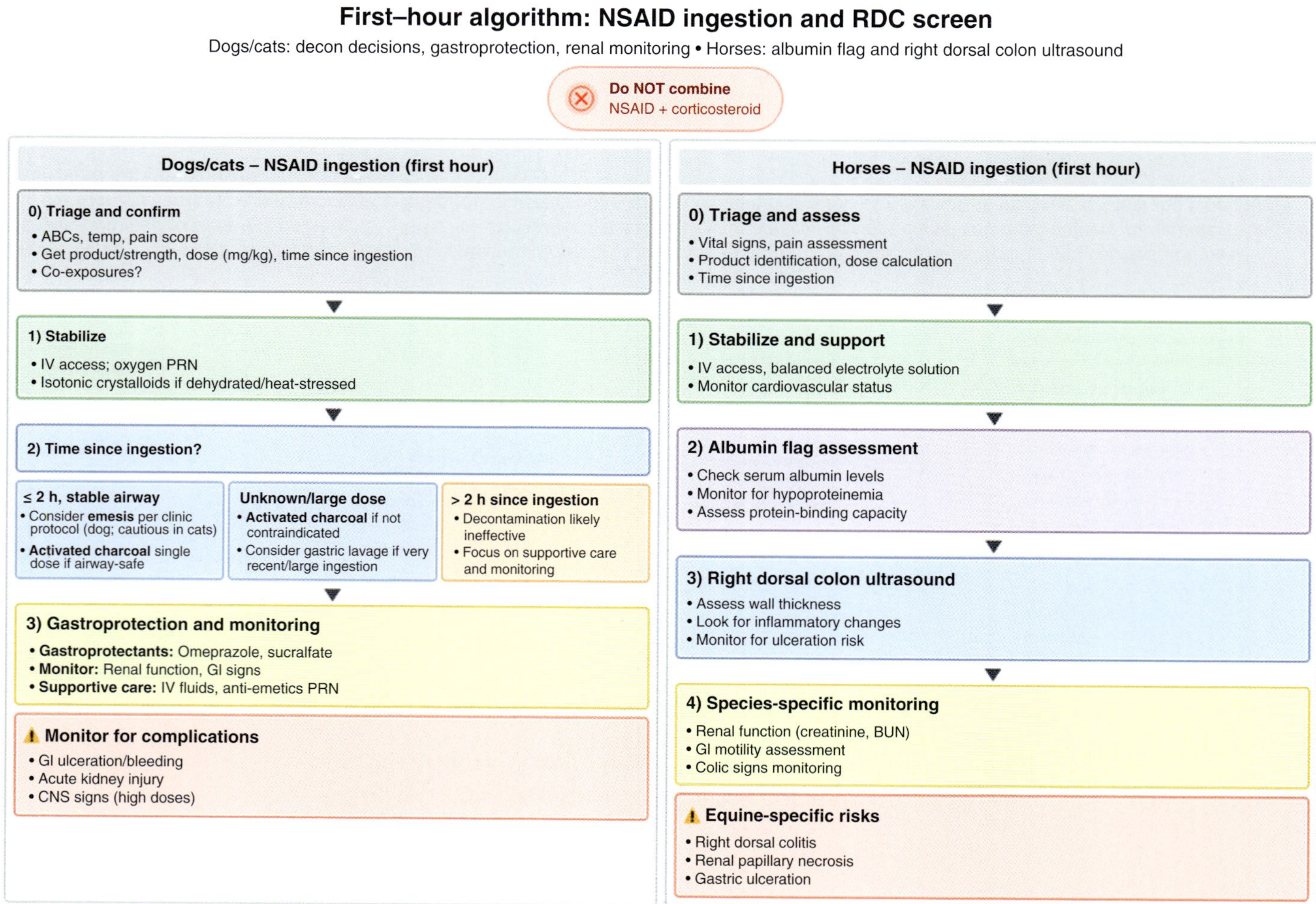

Figure 10.41 First-hour algorithm for NSAID exposures (dogs/cats) with equine RDC branch. Decision nodes for safe decontamination, gastroprotection bundle, renal monitoring/warning thresholds, and an equine pathway that flags albumin trending and right dorsal colon ultrasound checkpoints. *Source:* Peterson and Talcott (2013); Kahn and Line (2020).

Table 10.22 NSAIDs – species-specific toxic exposure cues and first-hour actions (bedside).

Drug/context	Species	Likely toxic exposure	Immediate actions	GI protection	Renal watch (0–48 h)	Do-not-combine	One Health note
Ibuprofen/naproxen (human OTC) ingestion	Dog	Single large dose or repeated access; vomiting, melena, abdominal pain	Stop NSAID; IV crystalloids if dehydrated; consider emesis ≤2 h (per protocol) and single-dose activated charcoal if airway-safe	PPI (omeprazole) + sucralfate ± misoprostol (ulcer risk)	Baseline & 24–48 h BUN/Cr, electrolytes; USG/UA, urine output; PCV/TP, fecal occult blood	Steroids, other NSAIDs, aminoglycosides/diuretics/ACE-i	—
Carprofen/meloxicam overdose or stacking	Dog	Double dosing, multi-product use; anorexia, vomiting	Stop drug; fluids; antiemetic; no further NSAIDs	PPI + sucralfate ± misoprostol	Renal panel now & 24–48 h; USG/UA; stool for melena	Steroids; nephrotoxins	—
Meloxicam repeats/human NSAID exposure	Cat	Off-label repeats or owner OTC; inappetence, vomiting	Stop drug; fluids (IV/SC); no emesis if unstable; charcoal if early & protected airway	PPI + sucralfate (± misoprostol with caution in pregnancy)	Renal panel, USG/UA at 0 and 24–48 h; weight/hydration trend	Steroids; other NSAIDs	—
Phenylbutazone/flunixin high dose or prolonged course	Horse (equid)	Colic/diarrhea, ventral edema, low albumin → suspect RDC	Stop NSAID; IV fluids; stall rest; high-fiber/low-bulk ration	Omeprazole + sucralfate ± misoprostol	Trend TP/albumin q24–48 h; US of right dorsal colon; renal panel if dehydrated	Steroids; long-stem hay early; product stacking	—
Flunixin field use in heat/dehydration	Cattle/Buffalo	Heat stress, diarrhea/endotoxemia; melena, weak	Stop NSAID; fluids/shade; treat primary disease	PPI/sucralfate per protocol	Renal panel if feasible; fecal blood; hydration	Steroids; nephrotoxins	Prefer meloxicam; avoid diclofenac (vulture risk)

(Continued)

Table 10.22 (Continued)

Drug/context	Species	Likely toxic exposure	Immediate actions	GI protection	Renal watch (0–48 h)	Do-not-combine	One Health note
NSAIDs off-label/stacked	Sheep/Goat	Dosing errors; dehydration; melena, anorexia	Stop NSAID; fluids (IV/PO); cooling; charcoal if early	PPI + sucralfate	Renal panel if available; fecal occult blood	Steroids; other NSAIDs	—
Flunixin/ketoprofen during heat/transport	Camelid	Dehydration; “colic-like” signs, anorexia	Stop NSAID; cool/quiet; IV fluids	PPI + sucralfate	Renal panel; USG/UA; monitor weight/hydration	Steroids; nephrotoxins	—
Any NSAID with CKD/geriatric	Dog/Cat	Therapeutic dose in renal compromise; inappetence, PU/PD	Stop NSAID; gentle IV/SC fluids; review all meds	PPI + sucralfate	BUN/Cr, electrolytes; USG/UA; output	Steroids; diuretics/ACE-i unless coordinated	—
Any NSAID + aminoglycoside/diuretic/ACE-i	Any SA/LA	Additive nephrotoxicity; rising creatinine, casts	Stop NSAID; stop/adjust co-nephrotoxins; correct dehydration	As above	Close renal panel and electrolytes at 0 and 24–48 h; USG/UA; output	This combination; steroids	—
Diclofenac in food animals	Cattle/Buffalo	Legal/illegal use; residue risk in carcasses	Prefer alternatives; document product/lot; carcass controls	Use meloxicam if NSAID needed	As feasible per field setting	Steroids; stacking	Diclofenac → vulture mortality; meloxicam preferred

ACE-i, angiotensin-converting enzyme inhibitor; AKI, acute kidney injury; LA, large animals; PCV/TP, packed cell volume/total protein; RDC, right dorsal colitis; SA, small animals; UA, urinalysis; USG, urine specific gravity.

Rows: Dogs, Cats, Horses (RDC risk), Cattle/buffalo/small ruminants, CKD/geriatric, drug-interaction scenarios. Columns: Likely exposure and amplifiers (dehydration/heat, ACE-i/diuretic, steroid) | Immediate actions | GI protection | Renal watch (0–48 h) | Do-not-combine/washouts | One Health note.

RDC = right dorsal colitis; “triple-whammy” = NSAID + ACE-i + diuretic in hypovolemia; repeat charcoal for enterohepatic NSAIDs per protocol.

Source: Papich (2020); Kahn and Line (2020); Peterson and Talcott (2013).

Table 10.23 Corticosteroids – risk-mitigation checklist by species/context (pre-start screens, during-therapy monitoring, taper cues, and "avoid with …" flags).

Patient/context	Pre-start screen	On-treatment monitoring	Taper plan (if ≥7–10 d or high dose)	Avoid with …	Notes
Dog – healthy adult (short anti-inflammatory course ≤2–3 weeks)	Confirm indication; med list (no NSAIDs overlap). Baseline PCV/TP; ± chem/UA if >7–10 d planned.	Recheck at 7–10 d if continuing; watch PU/PD, appetite, stool/melena, behavior.	↓ 25–33% q3–7 d → q48 h → stop.	Recent GI bleed, uncontrolled infection, pancreatitis.	Dose AM with food; use lowest effective dose.
Dog – febrile in tick-endemic region	Infectious screen as indicated (e.g., *Ehrlichia*/*Anaplasma*/*Leishmania* by locale); CBC/chem/UA; thoracic/abdo focus as needed.	Temp curve; clinical status; labs per workup; start antimicrobials if indicated.	Begin only after infection addressed; taper slowly (↓ 10–25% q1–2 weeks).	Live vaccines at immunosuppressive doses; NSAIDs.	Consider steroid-sparing if prolonged therapy anticipated.
Dog – immune-mediated disease (high-dose/chronic)	CBC/chem/UA/UPC, BP, weight/BCS; baseline infectious screen; vaccine status (no live).	CBC/chem/UA q2–4 weeks, then q6–8 weeks; weight/BP monthly.	Once controlled: ↓ 10–25% q2–4 weeks to lowest effective; aim alternate-day.	NSAIDs, uncontrolled diabetes, active serious infection.	Add steroid-sparing early (e.g., azathioprine/cyclosporine) when indicated.
Cat – short course	Prefer prednisolone; renal panel if geriatric; med list (no NSAIDs).	Appetite, vomiting; PU/PD; weight/hydration.	↓ 25–33% q3–7 d → q48 h → stop.	Ibuprofen/naproxen exposure, recent GI bleed.	Keep courses brief; monitor for anorexia early.
Cat – diabetes risk/geriatric/CKD	Baseline glucose, UA (glucosuria/ketones), BP, renal panel.	BG at 1–2 weeks and with dose changes; UA if PU/PD; weight weekly.	Slow taper: ↓ 10–25% q2–3 weeks; avoid rapid swings.	Uncontrolled hyperglycemia/ketonuria; NSAIDs.	Higher risk for urinary tract infection (UTI); consider local/topical or budesonide (IBD).
Horse – laminitis-prone/EMS pony	Hoof history, digital pulses/hoof heat; metabolic screen if indicated.	Daily pulses/hoof heat; stance/lameness; colic signs.	↓ 10–20% q5–7 d to alternate-day; hold if laminitis signs.	NSAIDs overlap; active laminitis.	Soft footing; restrict NSC diet; avoid high stress/exertion during taper.
Horse – ulcer/colitis history	GI history; albumin/TP baseline; avoid NSAID stacking.	Feces/colic; TP/albumin trend.	As above; consider slower taper if GI signs.	NSAID combo; recent GI bleed.	Add omeprazole ± sucralfate prophylaxis if risk.
Ruminant (cattle/buffalo/sheep/goat) – late gestation	Confirm stage of pregnancy; withdrawal times/legal use.	Appetite/rumen motility; signs of parturition/abortion.	Usually no taper if ≤3–5 d; if longer, taper over 1–2 weeks.	Late-gestation use unless indicated; NSAIDs stacking.	Steroids may induce parturition/abortion; plan accordingly.

(*Continued*)

Table 10.23 (Continued)

Patient/context	Pre-start screen	On-treatment monitoring	Taper plan (if ≥7–10 d or high dose)	Avoid with ...	Notes
Camelid – heat/transport stress context	Hydration status; renal panel if prolonged course.	Appetite, feces, hydration; temp; "colic-like" signs.	If >5–7 d daily: taper over 1–2 weeks.	NSAIDs overlap; severe dehydration.	Provide cool/quiet environment during therapy.
Any species – cardiac/renal disease	BP, renal panel, electrolytes; review diuretics/ACE-i/NSAIDs.	BP, K^+/Na^+, edema, urine output.	Cautious: ↓ 10–25% q1–2 weeks with labs after each step.	Decompensated CHF/AKI; NSAID overlap.	Balance fluids carefully; coordinate with cardio/nephro plan.
Ocular steroid (topical) – any species	Fluorescein stain (no steroid with ulcer); IOP if glaucoma risk.	Re-stain as needed; watch keratomalacia; IOP if risk.	Step-down frequency (q6–8 h → q12 h → q24–48 h → stop).	Corneal ulcer, herpetic keratitis (cats).	Shield from self-trauma; add antimicrobials if infected.
Dermatologic use (SA)	Rule out deep pyoderma/demodicosis; secondary infections.	Pruritus score; skin culture response if used; weight.	Move to alternate-day quickly; introduce steroid-sparing (oclacitinib/lokivetmab/cyclosporine).	NSAIDs; uncontrolled infection.	Moisturize barrier; plan shortest effective course.
Any species – depot/long-acting preparations	Verify indication; ensure follow-up feasible.	Harder to adjust – monitor for GI bleed, infection, behavior changes.	Not adjustable once given – avoid depot when close monitoring/titration needed.	NSAID overlap; high infection risk.	Heat/dehydration/malnutrition increase adverse effects – opt for titratable oral where possible.

AKI, acute kidney injury; BCS, body condition score; BG, blood glucose; BP, blood pressure; CHF, congestive heart failure; EMS, equine metabolic syndrome; NSC, non-structural carbohydrates; PU/PD, polyuria/polydipsia; UA/UPC, urinalysis/urine protein-to-creatinine; SA, small animals; TP, total protein.
Source: Kahn and Line (2020) and Papich (2020).

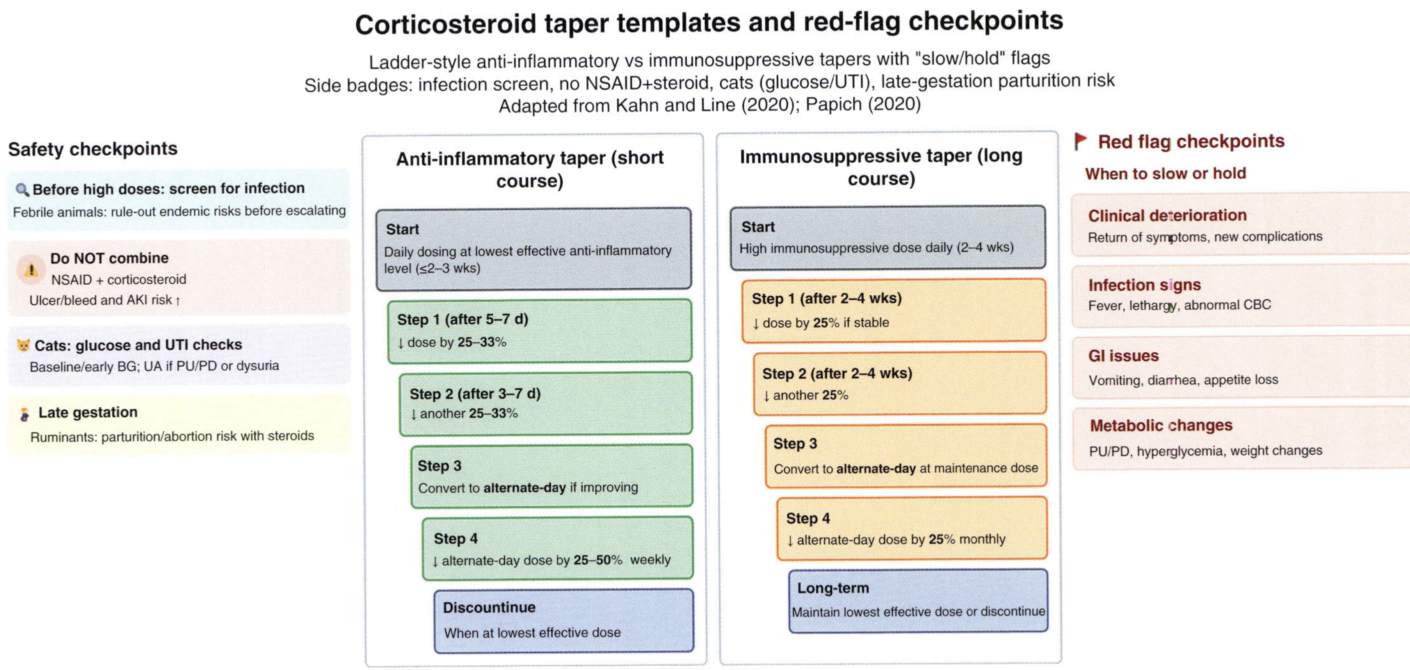

Figure 10.42 Corticosteroid taper templates and red-flag checkpoints. Ladder-style anti-inflammatory vs. immunosuppressive tapers with "slow/hold" flags (GI bleed, infection flare, hyperglycemia in cats, laminitis signs in horses). Side badges: screen for infection before high doses in febrile animals, no NSAID + steroid, cats – glucose/UTI checks, late gestation – parturition risk. *Source:* Kahn and Line (2020); Papich (2020).

severe, recent oral exposures alongside decontamination; for α_2-agonists, remove any residual topical source, reverse promptly with species-appropriate antagonists (yohimbine or atipamezole), and give IV fluids and thermal support while monitoring glucose and rhythm. These first-hour priorities are summarized in Figure 10.43, which pairs recognition cues with immediate actions to minimize secondary injury in hot, resource-limited settings (Kahn & Line, 2020; Papich, 2021; Peterson & Talcott, 2013). See Figure 10.43.

Barbiturates

Source

Barbiturates are derivatives of barbituric acid (malonylurea) in which C5 substitutions confer anesthetic potency and lipid solubility (see Figure 10.44). In veterinary contexts, pentobarbital, phenobarbital, and thiopental are most relevant. Exposures arise from anesthetic overdose, therapeutic phenobarbital misdosing, and scavenging of carcasses from barbiturate-euthanized livestock/equids – documented in dogs and zoo carnivores in tropical settings with variable carcass disposal practices (Kahn & Line, 2020; Papich, 2021).

Toxicity

Safety margins vary by agent and route; pentobarbital can be lethal at ~40–60 mg/kg IV or ~85 mg/kg PO in dogs (Kahn & Line, 2020). Tropical amplifiers include dehydration, heat stress (worsening hypoventilation), malnutrition, and delayed presentation after carcass ingestion (Bischoff, Jaeger and Ebel, 2011).

Mechanism of Action (Toxicity)

Barbiturates enhance GABA_A–mediated chloride currents and, at higher concentrations, can directly open the channel, producing dose-dependent CNS and medullary respiratory depression; cardiovascular depression follows with overdose (Papich, 2021; Peterson & Talcott, 2013).

Clinical Signs

Rapid progression from obtundation to coma; hypoventilation/apnea, loss of reflexes, hypotension, hypothermia. With chronic exposure/misdosing: ataxia, dull mentation. Post-euthanasia carcass ingestion may cause peracute respiratory failure in carnivores (Bischoff, Jaeger and Ebel, 2011).

Pathophysiology

Fatal cases may show brain/meningeal congestion and pulmonary edema; prolonged hypoxia leads to multi-organ congestion/edema (Kahn & Line, 2020).

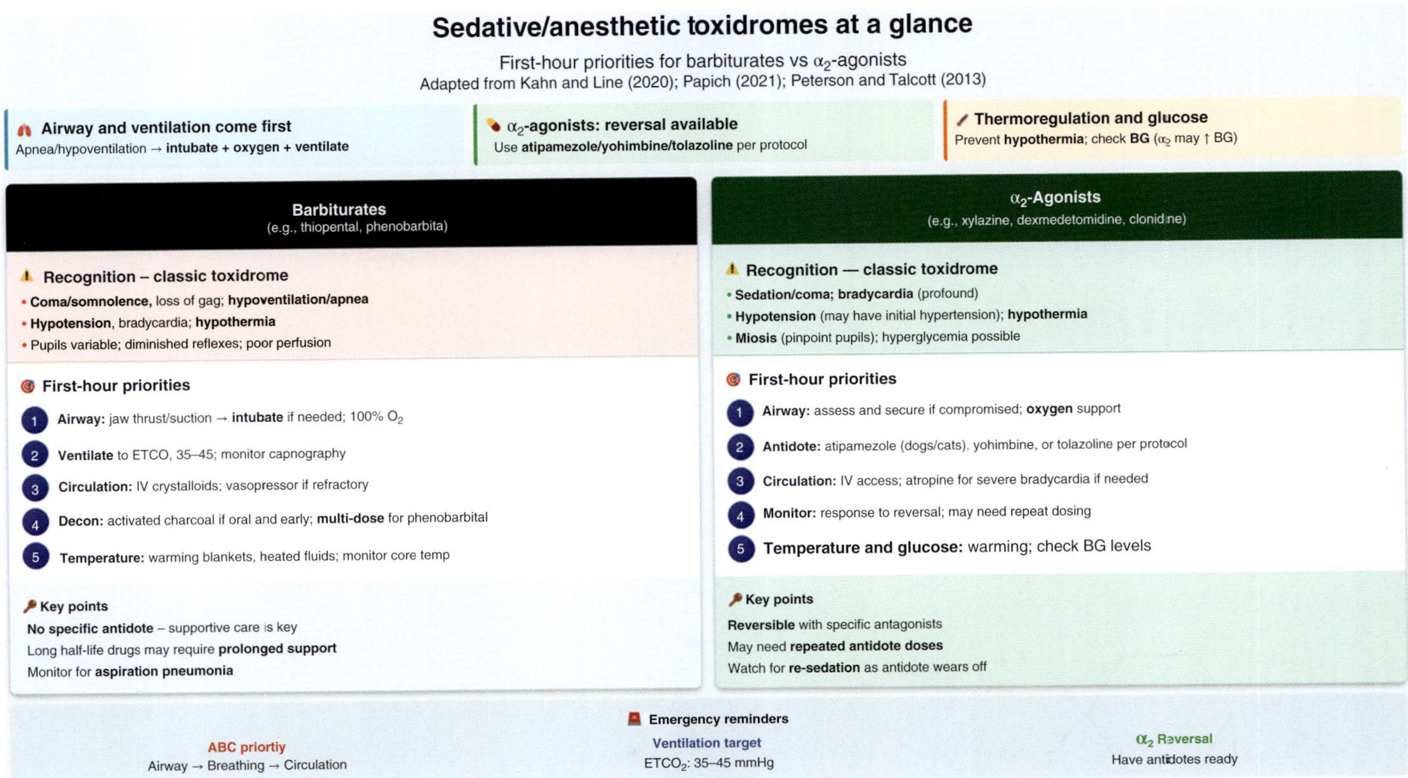

Figure 10.43 Sedative/anesthetic toxidromes at a glance – first-hour priorities for barbiturates vs. α_2-agonists (airway/ventilation vs. reversal/fluids/thermoregulation). *Source:* Kahn and Line (2020), Papich (2021), and Peterson and Talcott (2013).

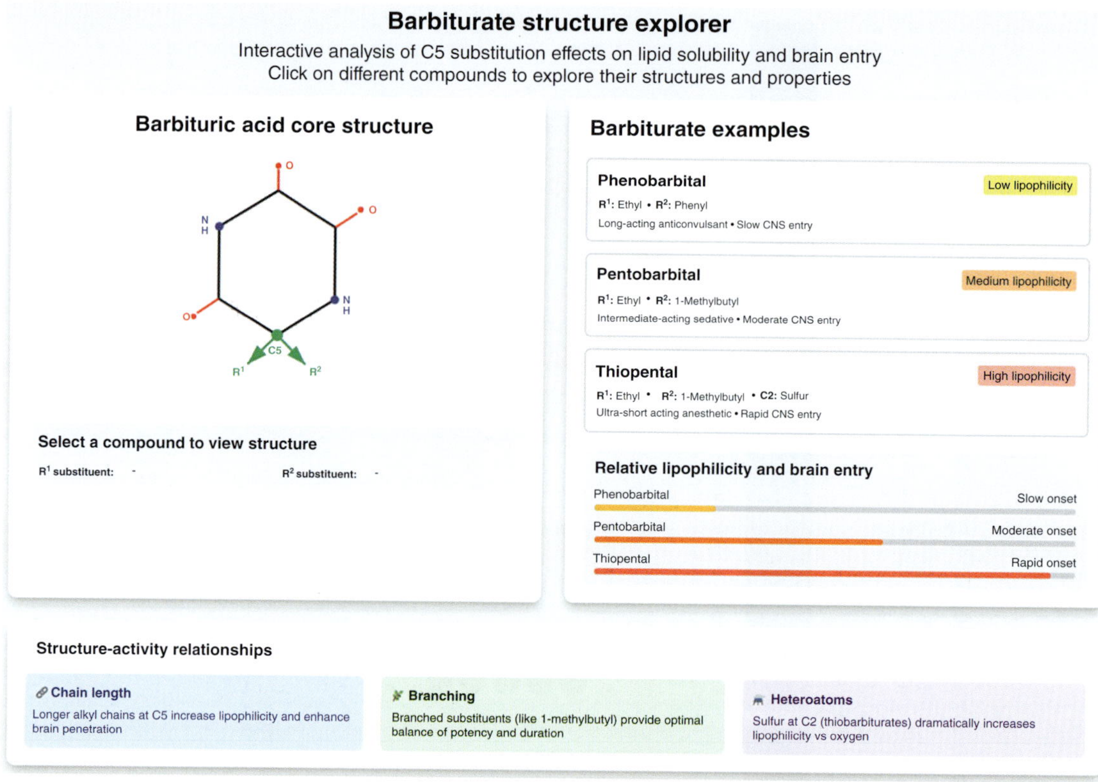

Figure 10.44 Barbituric acid core and C5 substitution sites; examples (phenobarbital, pentobarbital, thiopental) and relative lipid solubility/brain entry. *Source:* Papich (2021) and Kahn and Line (2020).

Diagnosis

History plus a "deep anesthesia" phenotype with respiratory and cardiovascular depression. Confirm with toxicology (serum/urine/gastric contents, liver). Phenobarbital may be detected on therapeutic drug assays; others typically require GC–MS/LC–MS (Peterson & Talcott, 2013) (Figure 10.45).

Treatment

First hour.

1) **Airway/ventilation first**: intubate early; oxygen and manual/mechanical ventilation to normocapnia.
2) **Decontamination**: if recent oral exposure and airway protected – gastric lavage + activated charcoal; for phenobarbital, begin multi-dose activated charcoal (MDAC) to interrupt enterohepatic recirculation (Papich, 2021; Peterson & Talcott, 2013).

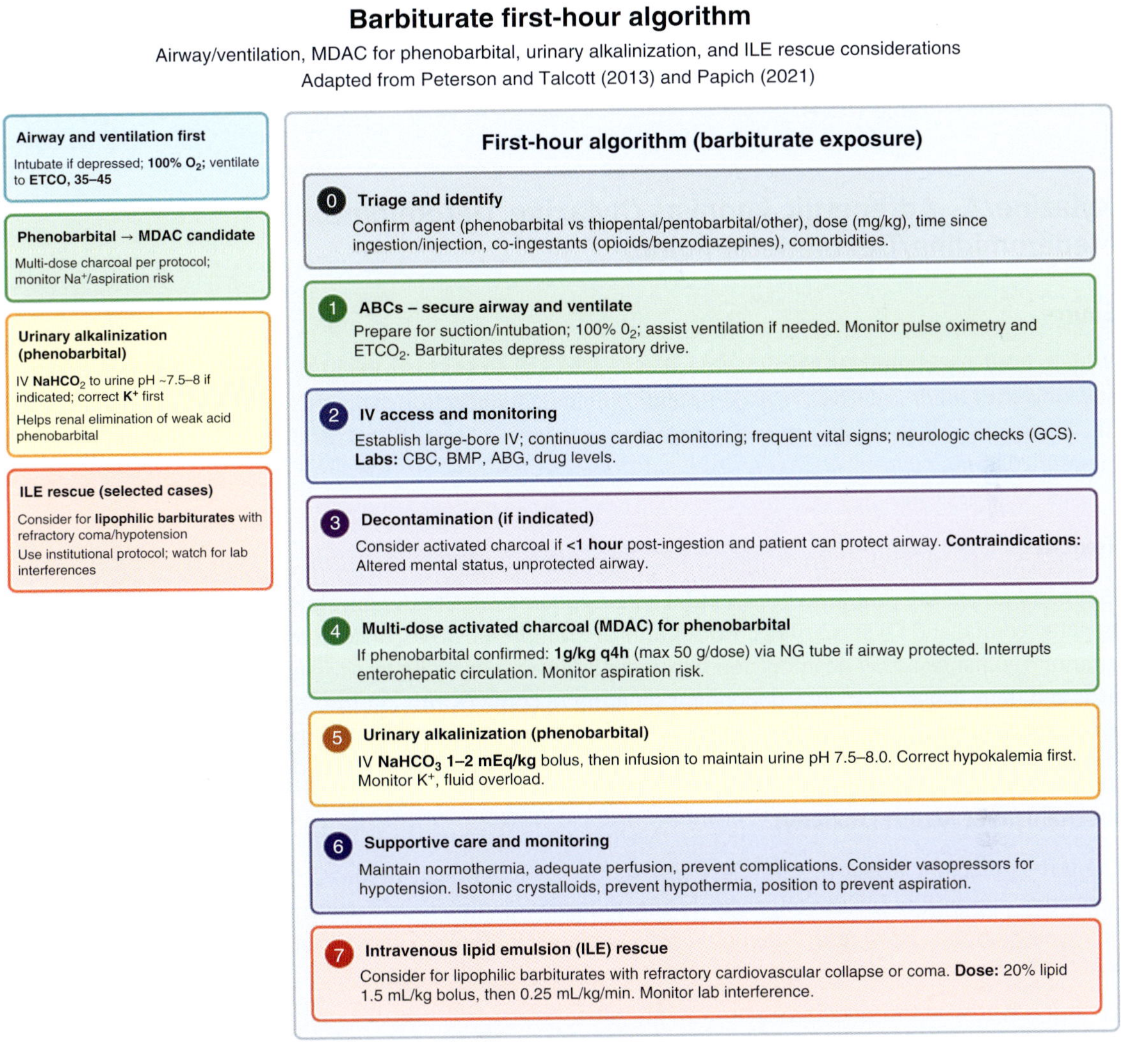

Figure 10.45 First-hour algorithm for suspected barbiturate toxicosis: recognition, airway/ventilation, decontamination, enhanced elimination, and escalation (dialysis/ILE). *Source:* Peterson and Talcott (2013); Kahn and Line (2020); Papich (2021).

3) **Enhanced elimination**: urinary alkalinization (IV $NaHCO_3$ with K^+ repletion) can increase phenobarbital clearance; hemodialysis/hemoperfusion is effective when available (Papich, 2021; Peterson & Talcott, 2013).
4) **Circulation/temperature**: isotonic crystalloids; vasopressors only if needed after ventilation; active rewarming.
5) **Rescue adjunct**: ILE may be considered after massive ingestion of highly lipophilic agents (e.g., thiopental) when conventional care fails (case-series level) (Kahn & Line, 2020; Peterson & Talcott, 2013).

Avoid. Older analeptics (e.g., nikethamide, bemegride) appear in legacy reports, but current references do not recommend CNS "stimulants" due to limited benefit and proconvulsant risk; management should prioritize airway/ventilation, decontamination, and enhanced elimination (Kahn & Line, 2020; Peterson & Talcott, 2013) (Table 10.24).

Xylazine/A₂-Adrenergic Agonists (Xylazine, Detomidine, Medetomidine/Dexmedetomidine)

Source

Widely used for chemical restraint/anesthesia across species; in tropical field conditions, overdosing, stacking with other sedatives (e.g., ketamine/opioids), dehydration/heat stress, and occasional accidental ingestions (dart waste, spilled concentrates) drive cases (Kahn & Line, 2020; Papich, 2021) (Figure 10.46).

Toxicity

Hallmark effects are profound bradycardia with hypotension, CNS/respiratory depression, hypothermia, hyperglycemia, and GI stasis/ileus. Ruminants are highly sensitive (dose in μg/kg) with bloat and regurgitation risk; sheep may develop non-cardiogenic pulmonary edema. Horses: ataxia/recumbency hazards and ileus. Dogs/cats: dose-dependent sedation to coma (Kahn & Line, 2020; Papich, 2021; Peterson & Talcott, 2013).

Mechanism of Action (Toxicity)

Central α_2-receptor agonism reduces sympathetic outflow (vagal predominance); pancreatic β-cell α_2 activation suppresses insulin (hyperglycemia/diuresis). A biphasic vascular response (early peripheral vasoconstriction → later central hypotension) explains monitor "swings" and why atropine alone can worsen hypertension/arrhythmias (Kahn & Line, 2020; Papich, 2021).

Clinical Signs

Sedation to unresponsiveness, small or variable pupils, bradycardia with weak pulses, cool extremities, hypothermia; shallow breathing/hypoventilation. Ruminants: tympany, salivation, regurgitation/aspiration risk. Horses: marked ataxia/recumbency; reduced gut sounds. Chemistry: stress hyperglycemia ± glucosuria (Kahn & Line, 2020; Peterson & Talcott, 2013).

Pathophysiology

Sympatholysis → decreased cardiac output and respiratory drive; GI smooth-muscle inhibition → stasis/tympany; β-cell inhibition → transient hyperglycemia/diuresis. In sheep, pulmonary edema likely reflects increased pulmonary capillary permeability (Kahn & Line, 2020; Papich, 2021).

Table 10.24 Barbiturates: toxidrome cues, bedside actions, "avoid" items, and escalation triggers (dialysis/ILE).

Agent/scenario	Toxidrome cues (bedside recognition)	Bedside actions (first hour)	Avoid (analeptics, pitfalls)	Escalate to dialysis/ILE when ...
Phenobarbital – acute oral overdose (dog/cat)	Progressive CNS depression → ataxia → coma; hypoventilation/apnea; bradycardia/hypotension; hypothermia; prolonged sedation	Airway/ventilation first (intubate/oxygen; assist-control to normocapnia); IV access, isotonic fluids; activated charcoal (if ≤~2 h and airway protected); begin multidose activated charcoal (MDAC) per protocol; active warming; glucose/electrolytes	Emesis in depressed patients; analeptics (e.g., doxapram, bemegride) → seizures/arrhythmias; flumazenil (not a barbiturate antidote); unprotected charcoal; routine forced diuresis	Dialysis/hemoperfusion if severe/refractory coma, very high level, or impaired clearance; urinary alkalinization (after correcting K^+) if pursuing enhanced renal clearance; ILE generally not primary (less lipophilic)
Pentobarbital (incl. euthanasia-solution ingestion)	Rapid deep coma; apnea; hypotension/bradycardia; hypothermia; possible ataxia/excitement before collapse	Secure airway and ventilate; oxygen; IV fluids ± vasopressor support per protocol; early activated charcoal if oral ingestion and safe; temperature control; glucose	Analeptics; unprotected gastric emptying; assuming flumazenil helps (it doesn't); delaying airway to pursue decon	ILE (intravenous lipid emulsion) may be considered for refractory hypotension/coma (high lipophilicity); dialysis usually low yield (large Vd, high lipophilicity) unless massive ingestion with prolonged coma and limited resources for ventilation
Thiopental (bolus or infusion mishap)	Immediate CNS/respiratory depression; apnea; hypotension; short context-sensitive half-time but prolonged effect if large dose/fat sequestration	Airway/ventilation; oxygen; IV fluids; treat hypothermia; consider repeat neurological checks as redistribution occurs	Analeptics; unnecessary flumazenil; aggressive atropine for hypertension-phase bradycardia	ILE can be considered in severe, refractory cases (lipophilic); dialysis minimal role
Mixed sedatives (barbiturate + opioid/benzodiazepine/ethanol)	Deeper than expected respiratory depression; pinpoint pupils (opioid), loss of gag; variable BP	Airway/ventilation; oxygen; naloxone trial if opioid co-ingestant suspected; charcoal if early and airway-safe; warming; glucose	Routine flumazenil use (may precipitate seizures, esp. mixed overdoses); analeptics; emesis	Dialysis as per dominant agent (phenobarbital > pento/thio); ILE if a strongly lipophilic co-ingestant contributes and shock/coma persists
Chronic/iatrogenic accumulation (phenobarbital)	Somnolence, ataxia, stupor; nystagmus; hepatopathy signs; often therapeutic miscalculation or drug interactions	Hold barbiturate; supportive care; check serum phenobarbital if available; consider MDAC if recent escalation; monitor glucose/electrolytes/temperature	Abrupt "antagonism" attempts; analeptics; skipping airway checks because exposure seems "chronic"	Dialysis if severe CNS depression with impaired clearance (hepatic/renal failure) or toxic level with deterioration; urinary alkalinization as adjunct if pursuing enhanced elimination

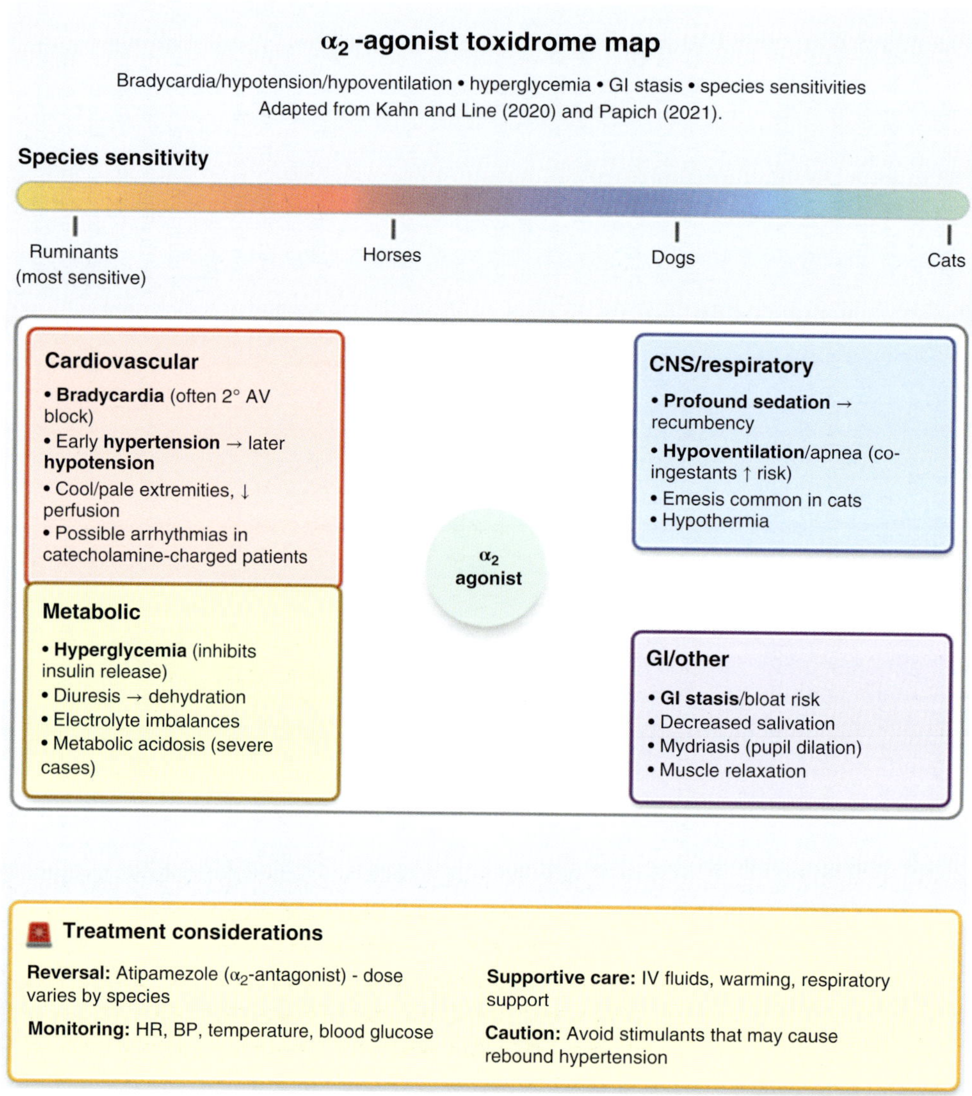

Figure 10.46 α_2-agonist toxidrome map – bradycardia/hypotension/hypoventilation, hyperglycemia, GI stasis, and species sensitivities (ruminants ≫ horses > dogs/cats). *Source:* Kahn and Line (2020) and Papich (2021).

Diagnosis

History of recent sedation/darting or access to concentrates/collars; exclude co-exposures (opioids, benzodiazepines, amitraz). Point-of-care glucose often elevated; ECG commonly shows sinus bradycardia or 2° AV block; ruminants – assess rumen gas and airway protection if recumbent (Kahn & Line, 2020).

Treatment

First-hour priorities

1) Reverse promptly (species-appropriate):
   - **Dogs/cats**: Atipamezole (preferred for dex/medetomidine; effective for xylazine), or yohimbine for xylazine.
   - **Horses/ruminants**: Yohimbine or tolazoline slow IV (monitor for hypotension/arrhythmias); atipamezole off-label with caution (Kahn & Line, 2020; Papich, 2021).
2) **Airway/oxygen/positioning**: O_2 supplementation; lateral/sternal positioning to protect airway; ruminants – decompress rumen if severe bloat and guard against aspiration.
3) **Perfusion and temperature**: isotonic crystalloids if hypotensive; avoid routine atropine – reserve for persistent, clinically significant bradycardia with hypotension after reversal (arrhythmia/hypertension risk). Active rewarming for hypothermia.
4) Decontamination if dermal/oral exposure and patient is stable (e.g., wipe spills, bathe; charcoal only with protected airway) (Peterson & Talcott, 2013) (Table 10.25).

Regional Considerations for Usage and Safety

Epidemiology of drug toxicity is not uniform across the tropics. Patterns reflect access pathways (OTC kiosks, communal dip vats), species mix (mixed farms with equids, small ruminants), climate (heat/humidity, drought), and regulatory posture (availability/restrictions, residue enforcement). Reading cases through this lens improves prevention and sharpens differentials (Gupta, 2018; Kahn & Line, 2020; Papich, 2020/2021; Peterson & Talcott, 2013).

Southeast Asia

- **Same-day combinations**: Levamisole followed within 24 hours by an organophosphate/carbamate dip or fogger in small ruminants → additive cholinergic/nicotinic signs. Safer: single-class deworming guided by FEC/FECRT; never stack within 72 hours; hydrate and weigh accurately.
- **Salicylanilides**: Closantel overdosing for *Haemonchus* in goats; malnutrition/hyperproteinemia increases free drug → delayed optic neuropathy. Weigh – don't estimate; avoid stacking salicylanilides.
- **Companion animals**: Doxycycline "dry-pilling" in cats (esophagitis/stricture); human ibuprofen/diclofenac given to dogs. Use client scripts and species icons to prevent.
- **Depot steroids**: Long-acting injections before transport/market → infection flares, wound-healing delay, and parturition risk near term.

Sub-Saharan Africa

- **Diminazene**: Neurotoxicity after high/repeat dosing or IM "top-ups" in dogs/small ruminants (onset 24–72 hours). Strict mg/kg dosing; never IV; observe 48–72 hours.
- **Ionophores**: Mill cross-contamination in mixed farms with equids → equine cardiotoxicity; institute mill QA and "NO HORSES" segregation; track CK/cTnI/ECG serials.
- **OP dip vats**: Community vats (small ruminants, dogs) → OP/carbamate crises. Sample before washing; atropine early; oxime for OPs.

Table 10.25 α_2-agonist overdoses: reversal options and monitoring by species (with "avoid/only-if" caveats).

Species	Common α_2 agonists/exposure	Preferred reversal and route	When to reverse vs. support only	First-hour bundle	Monitoring (0–6 h)	Avoid/only if
Dogs and cats	Xylazine (cats emesis), medetomidine/dexmedetomidine, accidental repeat sedation; amitraz collar/ingestion (α_2-like)	Atipamezole (dogs/cats) IM (label) or slow IV off-label per protocol; Yohimbine can reverse xylazine; Tolazoline alternative (esp. xylazine)	Reverse when airway/ventilation threatened, bradycardia with poor perfusion, hypothermia, or procedure finished. Support only (O_2, warmth, fluids) if mild, short-acting dose and monitoring feasible.	Airway/positioning; O_2; active warming; isotonic fluids if hypotensive; decontaminate amitraz (remove collar, bathe; charcoal if early and airway protected).	ECG (2° AV block), BP, temperature, glucose (hyperglycemia), urine output; watch for re-sedation, repeat reversal per protocol if needed.	Avoid atropine alone during hypertension-phase bradycardia; only reverse once painful stimuli managed (rebound agitation/arrhythmias risk); avoid emesis in depressed patients; with amitraz, avoid MAO-interacting drugs.
Horses (Equids)	Xylazine, detomidine, romifidine (field sedation overdoses or dose stacking)	Tolazoline IV slow or Yohimbine IV per protocol (xylazine); Atipamezole has limited equine use (consult protocol)	Reverse when marked bradycardia/poor perfusion, prolonged recumbency, or procedure complete and safe handling assured. Support if mild and standing with stable perfusion.	Large-bore IV access; O_2 if hypoxemic; cautious fluids if hypotension; controlled environment to prevent ataxia/falls after reversal.	ECG/BP, temp, ileus/colic watch (GI stasis); fecal output; re-sedation check 30–60 min after reversal.	Avoid rapid bolus reversal → acute hypertension/arrhythmias; only reverse when handlers ready for sudden arousal/ataxia; avoid atropine monotherapy; caution late gestation (uterine tone changes).
Ruminants	Xylazine (very sensitive; small doses), detomidine (less common), accidental topical/ingestion (e.g., cattle spray)	Tolazoline or yohimbine IV slow per protocol (xylazine); field use common	Reverse early with recumbency, bloat, severe bradycardia/poor perfusion, or respiratory compromise. Support if very mild and standing with good eructation.	Secure airway/position to prevent aspiration; decompress rumen if bloat; O_2 if available; warm, dry bedding; cautious fluids.	ECG/BP, temp, rumen motility/eructation, respiratory rate/SpO_2 if available; glucose (hyperglycemia possible).	Avoid atropine alone; only reverse once handling is safe (abrupt arousal); pregnancy: use with caution (uterine effects); avoid emesis attempts; monitor for re-sedation.

BP, blood pressure; ECG, electrocardiogram; IM, intramuscular; IV, intravenous; O_2, oxygen.
Practical notes

- Airway and temperature first. Hypoventilation, aspiration risk, and hypothermia commonly drive morbidity.
- Expect biphasic BP (early hypertension → later hypotension) and 2° AV block – treat the patient, not the monitor.
- Hyperglycemia and diuresis are common; check BG in cats and stressed patients.

Latin America

- **Pyrethroids**: Classic feline exposures from canine spot-ons and agricultural sprays; methocarbamol first, temperature control; consider ILE if refractory.
- **Aminoglycosides**: AKI in dehydrated calves treated empirically; hydrate first, use once-daily protocols where appropriate, monitor renal panel.
- **Macrocyclic lactones**: Environmental externalities (dung fauna); time treatments to pasture ecology.

Regulatory Notes

Bans/restrictions are common for nitrofurans, chloramphenicol, metronidazole in food animals; fipronil contraindicated in rabbits; observe withdrawal/residue intervals with documentation.

Resistance-Linked Toxicity and Combination Pitfalls

Selection pressure tempts higher doses, longer courses, and stacked drugs – each raises toxicity probability. Use these mini-scenarios to teach safer pathways.

Scenario 1 – Levamisole + Macrocyclic Lactone (Same Day) in Small Ruminants

Owner "double-covers" for *Haemonchus*: levamisole AM, ivermectin PM. Animal develops SLUD, abdominal pain, muscle fasciculations, ataxia. In farm dogs (MDR1-suspect) licking pour-ons, CNS depression may overlay.

Safer practice: Single class per day; weigh accurately; FEC/FECRT-guided rotation; rehydrate first; recheck FEC at 10–14 d.

First hour: Atropine for muscarinic signs; oxygen/suction; diazepam for seizures; oxime only if OP exposure is proven.

Scenario 2 – High-dose Moxidectin to "Blast" Encysted Cyathostomes (Horses)

Dose doubled "for larvae" → dullness, ataxia, reduced menace, bradycardia.

Safer practice: Staged larvicidal protocols (label moxidectin with monitoring; or fenbendazole multi-day where appropriate), hydration, stall rest; avoid P-gp inhibitors/sedative stacking.

Scenario 3 – Prolonged oxytetracycline for "resistant pneumonia"

Weeks of therapy under strong sun → photosensitivity and rising ALT/ALP.

Safer practice: Culture-guided de-escalation; UV avoidance; switch to targeted agent; monitor liver enzymes (Figure 10.47).

Diagnosis, Sampling and Immediate Management

Do not lose samples to the bathwater – collect first, decontaminate second. In hot, resource-limited settings, a disciplined first hour preserves diagnostics and improves outcome.

First 60 minutes (algorithm)

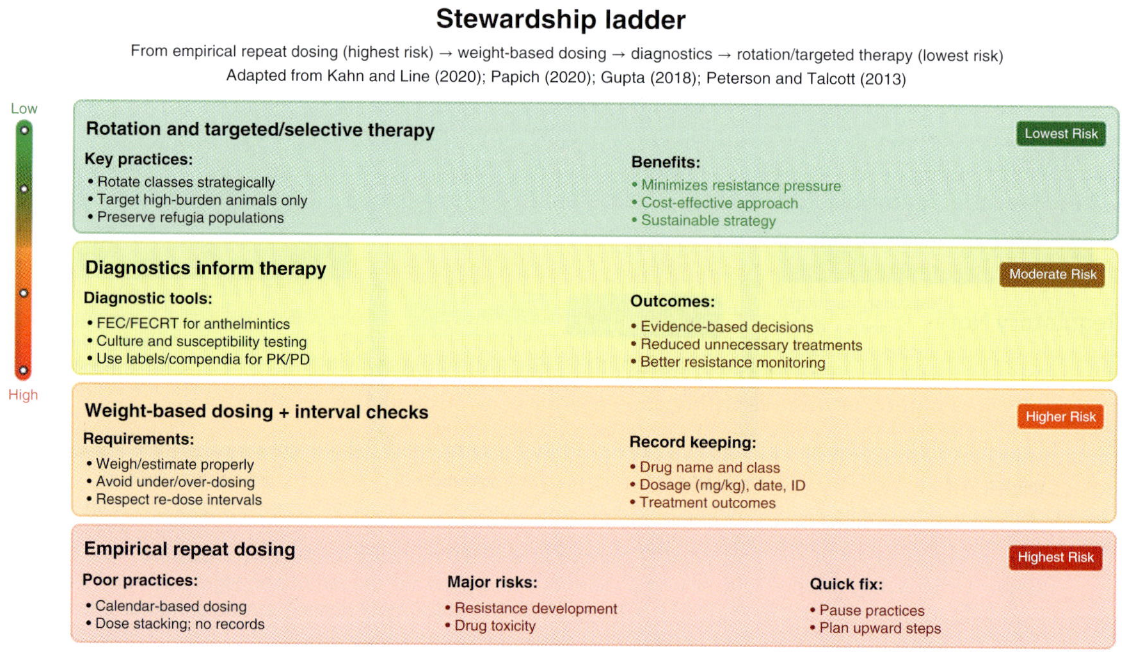

Figure 10.47 Stewardship ladder – from empirical repeat dosing (highest risk) → weight-based dosing with interval checks → diagnostics (FEC/culture), rotation/targeted therapy, and withdrawal compliance (lowest risk). *Source:* Kahn and Line (2020); Papich (2020); Gupta (2018); Peterson and Talcott (2013).

1) **Primary survey**: ABCs, oxygen, IV access; temperature; glucose.
2) **Sample before decon**:
   - Serum (chemistry); whole blood (AChE if OP/carbamate suspected).
   - Urine (aminoglycosides/NSAIDs); feed/spot-on vial; vomitus.
   - ECG/CK/cTnI for ionophores; ocular photos ± ERG pathway if closantel/enrofloxacin-cat risk.
3) **Decontamination**:
   - **Dermal**: mild detergent, clip mats; protect eyes/airway.
   - **GI**: emesis only if early and safe (no seizures/caustics/compromised airway); activated charcoal where indicated (repeat for enterohepatic drugs).
4) **Antidotes (give early by toxidrome)**:
   - Atropine ± oxime (OPs); atipamezole/yohimbine (amitraz/α_2s); NAC (feline paracetamol); methocarbamol (pyrethroid tremors); ILE in select massive lipophilic exposures.
5) **Control excitability**: Benzodiazepines; methocarbamol for tremors; propofol CRI if needed.
6) **Fluids/temperature**: Correct dehydration; active warming/cooling; monitor urine output.
7) **Monitoring cadence**: q6–8 h neuro checks (pyrethroids/amitraz); daily renal panel (aminoglycosides/NSAIDs); ECG/CK serials (ionophores); ocular recheck (closantel/enrofloxacin cats) (Table 10.26).

Table 10.26 First-hour playbooks by toxidrome (for quick bedside use).

Toxidrome	Likely culprits	Do now (0–15 min)	Next (15–60 min)	Labs/monitor	Avoid
Cholinergic crisis (muscarinic + nicotinic + CNS)	Organophosphates/carbamates (sprays, dips, baits)	Airway/oxygen; atropine for muscarinic signs; decon: wash/bathe, clip; if oral and safe → activated charcoal	Oxime (pralidoxime/obidoxime) if OP; fluids, control seizures (diazepam/midazolam); thermoregulation	HR, BP, temp; SpO_2; ECG; lactate; blood gas; ± cholinesterase where available	Delaying atropine; unnecessary oxime in pure carbamate exposure; emesis in depressed animals
Pyrethroid/permethrin tremor–seizure syndrome (cats ≫)	Spot-ons, shampoo/space sprays, dog products used on cats	Bathe with mild dish soap; control tremors/seizures (diazepam → methocarbamol; add phenobarbital if needed); oxygen; IV access	Repeat baths PRN; fluids; temperature control; consider ILE only for refractory cases	Temp q15–30 min; ECG; electrolytes (Ca, K, Mg); glucose	Phenytoin; lidocaine (cats); no emesis with neurological signs; hot water baths
Macrocyclic lactones – neurodepression (MDR1 dogs, dose stacking)	Ivermectin, moxidectin, doramectin, abamectin; high-dose or combos	Airway/oxygen; decon (charcoal if oral and protected airway); IV access; thermoregulate	Lipid emulsion consider for severe, lipophilic exposures; prolonged nursing care; treat aspiration risk	ECG; BP; glucose; temp; serial neurological checks	"Test doses"; repeated sedation; co-admin with P-gp inhibitors (ketoconazole, cyclosporine)
α_2-agonist toxidrome (bradycardia, hypotension, hypoventilation, GI stasis)	Xylazine, detomidine, romifidine, dex/medetomidine; amitraz	Position airway; O_2; active warming; if significant compromise → reversal by species (atipamezole dogs/cats; yohimbine/tolazoline xylazine in ruminants/equids)	Fluids if hypotensive after reversal; decon for amitraz (remove collar, bathe; charcoal if early/safe)	ECG (2° AV block), BP, temp, glucose; ruminant bloat/eructation; watch re-sedation	Atropine alone during hypertension phase; emesis in depressed patients; rapid IV reversal bolus in equids
Barbiturate overdose (respiratory depression/coma)	Phenobarbital, pentobarbital/thiopental	Airway/ventilate; 100% O_2; IV access; temperature support	Activated charcoal if ≤~2 h and airway protected; MDAC if phenobarbital; consider urinary alkalinization (after correcting K^+); ILE only for severe lipophilic cases	$ETCO_2$/ABG, ECG, BP, glucose, electrolytes; urine pH/output if alkalinizing	Emesis; analeptics (doxapram/bemegride); assuming flumazenil is helpful

(Continued)

Table 10.26 (Continued)

Toxidrome	Likely culprits	Do now (0–15 min)	Next (15–60 min)	Labs/monitor	Avoid
Paracetamol (acetaminophen)incats–methemoglobinemia ± hepatic injury	Human OTC tablets/liquids	O_2; IV access; start N-acetylcysteine ASAP; antiemetic; avoid stress; avoid methylene blue	Charcoal if ≤2 h and safe; SAMe/antioxidants per protocol; fluids; consider transfusion if severe	MetHb, SpO_2 (unreliable), venous color ("chocolate"), ALT/AST, bilirubin, PT/aPTT, glucose	Methylene blue (cats); delaying NAC; emesis with CNS depression
NSAID GI/renal toxidrome	Ibuprofen, naproxen, diclofenac, flunixin, phenylbutazone, carprofen, meloxicam	If oral & early → charcoal; start gastroprotection (PPI + sucralfate ± misoprostol); IV crystalloids if dehydrated	Continue PPI; antiemetics; pain control; remove co-nephrotoxins; horses: screen for RDC if on chronic therapy	BUN/Cr, UA (USG, casts), electrolytes; PCV/TP; fecal occult blood; in horses: albumin, US right dorsal colon	NSAID + steroid combo; NSAID redosing; aggressive fluids if CHF risk
Ionophore cardiomyopathy/ myonecrosis	Monensin, lasalocid, salinomycin; feed mix-ups – equids ≫	Remove feed immediately; quiet stall, O_2 PRN; single-dose charcoal if recent	Fluids (avoid overhydration if myocardial injury); antiarrhythmics as indicated; no exercise	CK/AST, troponin, ECG (arrhythmias), electrolytes; US or echo PRN	Forced exercise; Ca-rich supplements early; co-exposure with tetracyclines (potentiation)
Aminoglycoside nephrotoxicity (iatrogenic)	Gentamicin, amikacin, streptomycin (esp. dehydrated/CRI)	Stop drug; assess volume status; begin IV fluids if hypovolemic	Renal panel at 24–48 h; review dosing interval; consider alternative therapy	BUN/Cr, UA (casts, isosthenuria), urine output; FeNa if available	Continued dosing "to finish course"; other nephrotoxins (NSAIDs, amphotericin)
Tetracycline esophageal injury/ photosensitivity	Doxycycline dry-pilled cats; tetracyclines + sun on unpigmented skin	If pill stuck → water/food; antiemetic; sucralfate; pain control	Switch to liquid or give with water/food; counsel on sun avoidance	Oral exam; watch for dysphagia, hypersalivation; dermatologic checks	Dry-pilling cats; sun exposure after dose; co-admin with cation-rich feeds (↓ absorption)
Levamisole neurological/ respiratory stimulation + cholinergic features	Levamisole dewormers; mixing with OP/ carbamates	Airway/oxygen; do not combine with OP/ carbamates; benzodiazepines for seizures	Fluids; consider methocarbamol for tremors; symptomatic care	ECG, BP, temp; electrolytes; glucose	Additional cholinesterase inhibitors; repeated high dosing; using in late gestation without risk–benefit
Diminazene neurotoxicity	Overdose or repeated IM dosing	Airway, oxygen; benzodiazepines for seizures; IM-only if needed further; stop drug	Fluids; methocarbamol; nursing care; manage hyperthermia	Neurological checks; temp; CK; hydration status	IV dosing; combining with OP/carbamates; further dosing after neurological signs

ABG, arterial blood gas; BP, blood pressure; CK, creatine kinase; FECRT, fecal egg count reduction test; ILE, intravenous lipid emulsion; MDAC, multi-dose activated charcoal; MetHb, methemoglobin; OP, organophosphate; PPI, proton-pump inhibitor; RDC, right dorsal colitis; UA, urinalysis. *Source:* Kahn and Line (2020); Papich (2020, 2021); Gupta (2018); and Peterson and Talcott (2013).

One Health and Environmental Externalities (Concise)

- **Vultures – diclofenac**: Veterinary diclofenac residues in livestock carcasses were linked to vulture mortality in South Asia; meloxicam is a raptor-safer alternative where available.
- **Pyrethroids – fish/invertebrates**: High aquatic toxicity; bathe animals away from ponds/streams; dispose of rinse water per local guidance; keep wet animals away from aquaria.
- **Macrocyclic lactones – dung fauna**: Residual activity in dung alters pasture ecology; time treatments to minimize nontarget impacts; avoid unnecessary long-acting formulations.
- **Residues**: Adhere to withdrawal intervals; document lot, dose, date, and animal ID in all food animals.

Prevention Toolkit (Field-Ready)

Turn the chapter into practice with a compact set of guardrails.

A) Wallchart: Do-Not-Use/Use-With-Caution by Species
   - **Examples**: Cats – permethrin, paracetamol (high risk); rabbits – fipronil (contraindicated); chelonians – macrocyclic lactones (avoid); horses – ionophores (exquisitely sensitive); MDR1 herding breeds – high-dose macrocyclic lactones (avoid).

B) Weight-Based Dosing Cards
   - Species-specific quick cards (goats vs. sheep vs. cattle; foals vs. adults). Emphasize weigh – don't guess, calibrate drench guns/syringes, and avoid same-day "stacking."

C) Client Scripts (ready to hand out)
   - "Never use a dog flea spot-on on cats."
   - "Do not give human ibuprofen/diclofenac to pets."
   - "Always give doxycycline to cats with water/food; never dry-pill."
   - "Separate treated animals until topicals are fully dry; keep away from ponds/aquaria."

D) Discharge Checklist
   - Red-flag return signs; how to store/dispose pesticides/medications; sun-exposure advice for photosensitizers; residue/withdrawal reminders for food animals (Table 10.27).

Table 10.27 Prevention toolkit at a glance.

Tool	When to use	Key message	Handout/QR link (placeholder titles you can print/host)
Weight-tape and dose-by-weight card	Before prescribing any drug	Weigh or tape – don't guess. Dose mg/kg, record lot/date.	QR: "Weigh & Dose (mg/kg) – quick card"
Redose interval tracker	Any repeat/long course	Avoid dose stacking; respect drug- and species-specific intervals.	QR: "Redose Interval & Max Days – log sheet"
"No NSAID + Steroid" door sign	In all treatment areas	Never combine – ulcer/AKI risk; add gastroprotection if history unclear.	QR: "NSAID–Steroid Combo: Hard Stop" poster

(Continued)

Tool	When to use	Key message	Handout/QR link (placeholder titles you can print/host)
Heat/dehydration amplifier checklist	Hot season, working animals, diarrheic patients	Correct volume deficits before nephro/gastro-toxic drugs.	QR: "Hydration & Heat-Stress Pre-drug Checklist"
Anthelmintic FEC/ FECRT scheduler	Herd small ruminants/equids	Test, don't calendar-dose; treat high shedders; rotate on efficacy.	QR: "FEC & FECRT – When & How"
Antimicrobial culture and susceptibility prompt	Recurrent/deep infections or 2nd-line drugs	Obtain C&S early; match PK/PD targets; stop when cured.	QR: "Culture First" one-pager
Withdrawal-time and residue log	Food animals/ ELDU	Record drug, dose, route, WDT; confirm compliance before sale/slaughter.	QR: "Withdrawal-Time Log (Food Animal)"
Macrocyclic lactone genotype flag	Collies/related breeds, herding mixes	MDR1 status unknown ≠ high-dose ML; prefer labeled doses/alternatives.	QR: "MDR1 Safety – Owner Brief"
Cat OTC safety card	Any feline analgesia inquiry	No paracetamol/ acetaminophen; call clinic first; NAC window matters.	QR: "Cats & Human OTCs – Do Not Use"
Permethrin/ pyrethroid caution sticker	Households with cats	Use cat-safe products only; bathe/exam fast if exposure.	QR: "Pyrethroids & Cats – Emergency Steps"
Fipronil/ isoxazoline counseling	Seizure-prone pets, rabbits/fish households	Screen neurological history; avoid fipronil in rabbits; protect aquaria.	QR: "Ectoparasiticides: Species Cautions"
Ionophore feed-mill QA list	Equids, small ruminants near poultry feed	Segregate feeds; verify labels; pull suspect feed; check CK/troponin.	QR: "Ionophore Mix-Up – QA & Response"
Equine right dorsal colitis (RDC) screen	Horses on NSAIDs	Use minimum effective dose; monitor albumin/US right dorsal colon.	QR: "NSAIDs & RDC – Stable Checklist"
"First-hour toxidrome" pocket cards	Any suspected poisoning	ABCs first; early decon criteria; antidote sequence by syndrome.	QR: "First-Hour Toxidromes – Pocket Set"
α_2-agonist reversal quick guide	Oversedation or field mishaps	Choose atipamezole/ yohimbine/tolazoline by species; reverse safely.	QR: "α_2 Reversal by Species – Dose & Steps"
ILE (intravenous lipid) protocol	Refractory lipophilic tox cases	When, how, and labs affected; not first-line for most barbiturates.	QR: "ILE Protocol – Clinic SOP"
Owner discharge magnets	Households using pesticides/OTCs	Read labels; species-specific; storage; emergency phone/after-hours.	QR: "Safe Use & Storage – Home Checklist"

Replace the QR placeholders with your clinic's URLs or PDFs; keeping titles consistent makes printing QR labels easy.
Source: Kahn and Line (2020); Papich (2020, 2021); Gupta (2018); and Peterson and Talcott (2013).

References

Bischoff, K., Jaeger, R., & Ebel, J. G. (2011). An unusual case of relay pentobarbital toxicosis in a dog. *Journal of Medical Toxicology*, *7*(3), 236–239. https://doi.org/10.1007/s13181-011-0160-8

Carpenter, J. W., & Marion, C. J. (Eds.). (2018). *Exotic Animal Formulary* (5th ed.). Elsevier (Saunders). https://doi.org/10.1016/C2015-0-04281-2. ISBN 978-0-323-44450-7.

Constable, P. D., Hinchcliff, K. W., Done, S. H., & Grünberg, W. (2016). *Veterinary medicine: A textbook of the diseases of cattle, horses, sheep, pigs, and goats* (11th ed.). Elsevier.

Cornell University Animal Health Diagnostic Center (AHDC). (2023). *Sampling for toxicology screens*. https://www.vet.cornell.edu/animal-health-diagnostic-center/laboratories/toxicology

Dowling, P. M. (2020). Aspirin and salicylate toxicosis in cats. *Veterinary Clinics of North America: Small Animal Practice*, *50*(6), 1179–1191.

Fisher, B., & Thompson, L. (2021). Management of methemoglobinemia in cats. *Topics in Companion Animal Medicine*, *44*, 100541.

Gelatt, K. N. (Ed.). (2014). *Veterinary ophthalmology* (5th ed.). Wiley-Blackwell.

Giguère, S., Prescott, J. F., & Dowling, P. M. (Eds.). (2013). *Antimicrobial therapy in veterinary medicine* (5th ed.). Wiley-Blackwell.

Gupta, R. C. (Ed.). (2018). *Veterinary toxicology: Basic and clinical principles* (3rd ed.). Academic Press.

Hall, J. A., & Langston, C. E. (2020). Acetaminophen (paracetamol) poisoning in cats. *Journal of Veterinary Emergency and Critical Care*, *30*(1), 28–39.

Hugnet, C., Buronfosse, F., Pineau, X., Cadoré, J.-L., Lorgue, G., & Berny, P. J. (1996). Toxicity and kinetics of amitraz in dogs. *American Journal of Veterinary Research*, *57*(10), 1506–1510.

Jones, C. J., & Park, F. (2021). Gastrointestinal injury with NSAIDs in small animals. *Journal of Small Animal Practice*, *62*(4), 233–246.

Kahn, C. M., & Line, S. (Eds.). (2020). *The Merck veterinary manual* (11th ed.). Merck & Co., Inc.

Klaassen, C. D. (Ed.). (2019). *Casarett & Doull's toxicology: The basic science of poisons* (9th ed.). McGraw-Hill.

Ko, S., & Payton, M. E. (2022). Dialysis in veterinary toxicology: Indications and outcomes. *Journal of Veterinary Internal Medicine*, *36*(2), 456–468.

Michigan State University Veterinary Diagnostic Laboratory (MSU VDL). (2023). *Toxicology sample collection and handling*. https://cvm.msu.edu/vdl/laboratory-sections/toxicology

Papich, M. G. (2020). *Papich handbook of veterinary drugs* (5th ed.). Elsevier.

Papich, M. G. (2021). *Saunders handbook of veterinary drugs* (5th ed.). Elsevier.

Peterson, M. E., & Talcott, P. A. (Eds.). (2013). *Small animal toxicology* (3rd ed.). Elsevier.

Phillips, A., & Graham, J. (2019). Ibuprofen toxicosis in dogs and cats. *Veterinary Medicine and Science*, *5*(3), 315–324.

Plumb, D. C. (2018). *Plumb's veterinary drug handbook* (9th ed.). Wiley-Blackwell.

Serio, A. W., Keepers, T. R., Andrews, L., & Krause, K. M. (2018). Aminoglycoside adaptive resistance and toxicity. *Antimicrobial Agents and Chemotherapy*, *62*(4), e02360–e02317.

The Merck Veterinary Manual. (2024–2025). *Toxicology topics (online edition)*. https://www.merckvetmanual.com/

Wilson, R., & Sutton, D. (2022). N-acetylcysteine protocols for feline acetaminophen toxicity. *Veterinary Toxicology*, *16*(3), 145–152.

11

Case Studies and Practical Applications: Diagnostic Tools and Real-World Scenarios – Insights for Educators and Practitioners

Introduction: Why Case Studies Matter

Tropical veterinary toxicology is shaped by climate, agricultural practices, and socio-economic realities. High humidity and heat accelerate fungal growth in feed, while intense pest pressure drives pesticide use and, at times, misuse (Gupta, 2018; Kahn & Line, 2010). Informal supply chains and limited regulatory oversight further increase the likelihood of accidental or intentional exposures (Papich, 2021).

Real-world case studies illustrate how diagnostic frameworks and therapeutic playbooks from earlier chapters translate into field action. They also highlight the One Health dimensions of toxicology, where animal poisonings may foreshadow human and environmental consequences (Figure 11.1).

Case A – Acute Pesticide-Associated Mass Mortality in Cattle (Andhra Pradesh, India, 2018)

Background and Context

In tropical agricultural systems, pesticides are indispensable for controlling insect infestations and safeguarding crop yields. However, their indiscriminate or improper use creates significant risks for livestock health. In April 2018, one of the most dramatic examples of such misuse occurred in Andhra Pradesh, India, where 56 adult cattle died overnight after grazing on postharvest corn stubble that had been treated with a cyanide-based pesticide to manage armyworm infestations (The Times of India, 2018).

This tragedy illustrates the convergence of multiple risk factors unique to tropical regions:

- Climate drivers: High pest burdens after monsoon rains drive frequent pesticide applications.
- Management practices: Crop residues are commonly left accessible to wandering herds, as smallholders often graze animals on communal stubble.
- Regulatory gaps: Enforcement of pre-grazing intervals is limited; many farmers are unaware that residues persist in crop stubble for weeks.
- Socio-economic vulnerabilities: A single herder losing his entire herd, worth over USD 35,000, demonstrates how one mistake can devastate livelihoods.

This case is thus more than an isolated poisoning: It underscores the need for integrated crop–livestock safety planning and inter-sector communication between agricultural and veterinary services (Table 11.1).

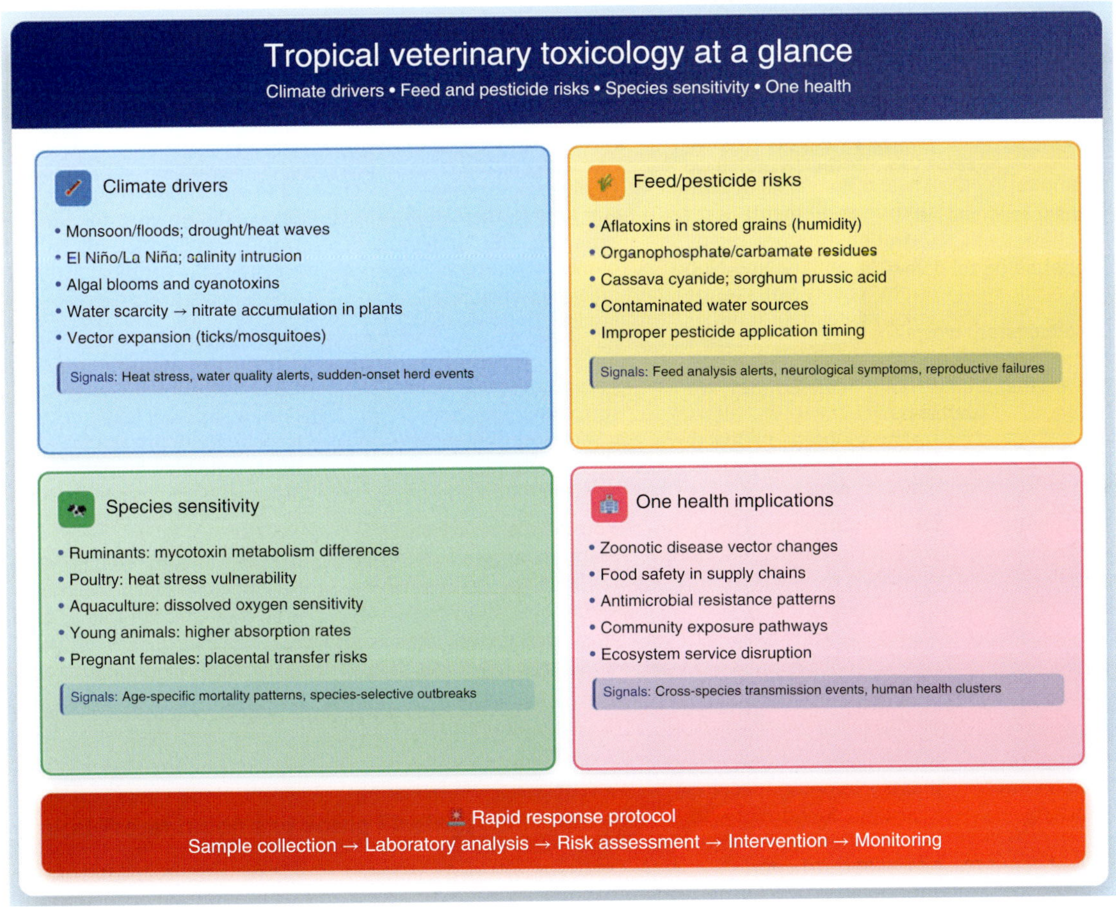

Figure 11.1 Tropical veterinary toxicology at a glance. Infographic: climate drivers; feed/pesticide risks; species sensitivity; One Health implications. *Source:* Adapted from Gupta (2018), and Kahn and Line (2010).

Table 11.1 Differential diagnosis of sudden herd collapse in grazing cattle: distinguishing features of cyanide, organophosphate/carbamate, and nitrate/nitrite toxicoses.

Feature	Cyanide (HCN; cyanogenic plants)	Organophosphates/carbamates (AChE inhibitors)	Nitrate/nitrite (methemoglobinemia)
Typical scene/ trigger	Access to wilted or stressed cyanogenic forage (sorghum, sudangrass, Johnsongrass), young cassava, cherry/ wild-rose hedge clippings; frost, drought, or trampling after rain; sudden ration change.	Recently sprayed pasture or spray drift; treated grain/ contaminated feed; recent pour-on/drench/dip; misuse of insecticide concentrates; dead insects present.	Drought then rain, heavy fertilization, cloudy weather; lush small-grain forages (oat, rye, millet, sorghum), pigweed; green-chop/silage not cured; high-nitrate water or lagoon seepage.

(*Continued*)

Table 11.1 (Continued)

Feature	Cyanide (HCN; cyanogenic plants)	Organophosphates/carbamates (AChE inhibitors)	Nitrate/nitrite (methemoglobinemia)
Time to onset after exposure	Seconds–minutes (often <1 h). Per-acute collapse of multiple animals.	Minutes–hours (rapid cluster of cases).	0.5–6 h after meal (peaks 3–8 h).
Dominant clinical signs	Acute dyspnea, tachycardia, anxiety/excitement, salivation, tremors, rapid collapse; mucosa and blood bright "cherry-red"; terminal seizures; death in minutes.	Cholinergic syndrome: SLUD (salivation, lacrimation, urination, defecation), miosis, bronchorrhea/bronchospasm, bradycardia; muscle fasciculations, weakness, recumbency, seizures.	Methemoglobinemia: chocolate-brown/cyanotic mucosa, tachypnea, ataxia, weakness, collapse; abortions with subacute exposure.
Field clues	Bright-red unclotted blood that fails to darken; chewed leaves of suspect plants; multiple animals down simultaneously.	Pinpoint pupils; copious secretions/diarrhea; responders may show cholinergic signs; animals improve with atropine.	Chocolate-brown blood/tissues; animals may transiently improve after methylene blue; brown aqueous humor postmortem.
Gross lesions (PM)	Often minimal; generalized congestion/edema; bright-red blood and tissues.	Nonspecific: pulmonary edema/congestion, watery GI contents; few distinguishing lesions.	Dark-brown blood and tissues; rumen with high-nitrate forage; fetal hypoxia if pregnant.
Rapid pen-side tests	Sodium picrate paper on rumen contents/plant; lab CN on whole blood/rumen; plant cyanogenic potential tests.	Field whole-blood cholinesterase (AChE/ChE) activity markedly depressed vs reference/herd-mates.	Griess/diphenylamine tests; nitrate test strips on water/forage; nitrite in ocular fluid.
Priority samples and handling	Rumen contents and suspect plants – freeze immediately in airtight containers with minimal headspace; whole blood (EDTA/heparin) chilled; liver. Cyanide is volatile – speed is critical.	Whole blood for AChE (refrigerate; avoid freezing); serum/plasma; rumen/gastric contents, liver, fat, feed; keep cold.	Aqueous humor (2–5 mL), serum/plasma; representative forage/water. Refrigerate plant/water; avoid freezing whole blood for nitrite assays.
First-hour treatment (individual)	Remove source; oxygen; antidote: nitrite–thiosulfate kit or hydroxocobalamin (per local protocols); consider rumen lavage with cold water + sodium thiosulfate.	Atropine for muscarinic signs; oxime (e.g., pralidoxime) for OPs where indicated; diazepam for seizures; decontaminate dermal/ingested sources.	Methylene blue IV (per local protocols); quiet handling; remove source; provide low-nitrate diet/fresh water.
Herd control actions	Immediate removal from suspect forage; test fields after stress; ensile/cure to reduce HCN potential; graze mature low-risk stands; avoid hungry turnout.	Respect reentry intervals; secure and label pesticides; correct mixing/application; enforce meat/milk withdrawals; PPE for staff.	Test and dilute high-nitrate feeds; adapt cattle gradually; harvest on sunny afternoons; avoid stacking NPN with high-nitrate forage; test water sources.
Distinguishing lab findings	Elevated blood/rumen cyanide; high lactate; plant cyanogenic capacity.	Markedly reduced ChE/AChE activity; OP/CB residues in feed/tissues.	High methemoglobin; nitrite in ocular fluid; nitrate in forage/water.

Use local dosing and laboratory protocols. Field tests guide triage but confirm with accredited laboratories.
Source: Adapted from Gupta (2018), Kahn and Line (2010), Peterson and Talcott (2013), and the Merck Veterinary Manual (online, updated 2024–2025).

Clinical Presentation and Scene Findings

At dawn, the herder found carcasses of 56 cows scattered across the stubble field, with another 40–50 animals nearby showing signs of distress (The Times of India, 2018). Surviving cattle exhibited tachypnea with open-mouth breathing, hypersalivation, generalized muscle tremors, ataxia with a staggering gait, and rapid collapse – with death in some animals within minutes of first signs.

The per-acute nature of the deaths, absence of prodromal illness, and simultaneous involvement of a large group are hallmarks of an acute toxic exposure rather than infectious disease. In tropical veterinary practice, primary differentials for sudden collapse of multiple grazing animals include cyanogenic plant toxicosis (e.g., sorghum, sudangrass, cassava leaves), chemical pesticide poisoning (cyanide-based fumigants, organophosphates, carbamates), nitrate/nitrite poisoning from fertilized forages, and anthrax (though carcasses here lacked hemorrhagic discharges or bloating). The strong association with a recently sprayed field and the bitter-almond odor detected from rumen contents pointed strongly to cyanide toxicosis (Gupta, 2018; Kahn & Line, 2010).

Diagnostic Workup

Field sampling. Rumen contents from several carcasses; blood samples from affected survivors; soil and stubble from the treated field.

Laboratory confirmation. Colorimetric assays and spectrophotometric analyses confirmed cyanide residues in rumen content and stubble (The Times of India, 2018). Reported concentrations exceeded lethal levels (>20 mg/kg body-weight equivalent for cattle).

Differentials. While organophosphate/carbamate poisoning can produce similar muscarinic signs (salivation, dyspnea), two key features pointed to cyanide: (i) extremely rapid progression from exposure to death and (ii) bright red blood and mucous membranes due to oxygen-saturated hemoglobin unable to release O_2, as noted postmortem (Gupta, 2018).

Pathology. Congested lungs with frothy airway exudate, bright cherry-red venous blood, and congested abomasal mucosa – findings consistent with per-acute cyanide poisoning (Gupta, 2018; Kahn & Line, 2010).

Toxicant and Pathophysiology

The culprit was a hydrogen cyanide (HCN)–releasing pesticide applied to corn stubble to suppress armyworms. Improper disposal of surplus pesticide in the field led to residues persisting for at least 3 weeks (The Times of India, 2018).

Mechanism of toxicity. Cyanide binds the ferric (Fe^{3+}) ion in cytochrome c oxidase (complex IV), blocking oxidative phosphorylation and preventing cellular oxygen utilization; the result is histotoxic hypoxia – oxygenated blood that tissues cannot use – leading to rapid neurological and cardiopulmonary collapse (Gupta, 2018; Kahn & Line, 2010) (Figure 11.2).

Tropical amplifiers. High ambient temperatures can accelerate volatilization and absorption of HCN from plant surfaces; thirsty cattle grazing aggressively after long treks ingest larger doses quickly; communal grazing increases simultaneous exposure, explaining catastrophic herd-level mortality.

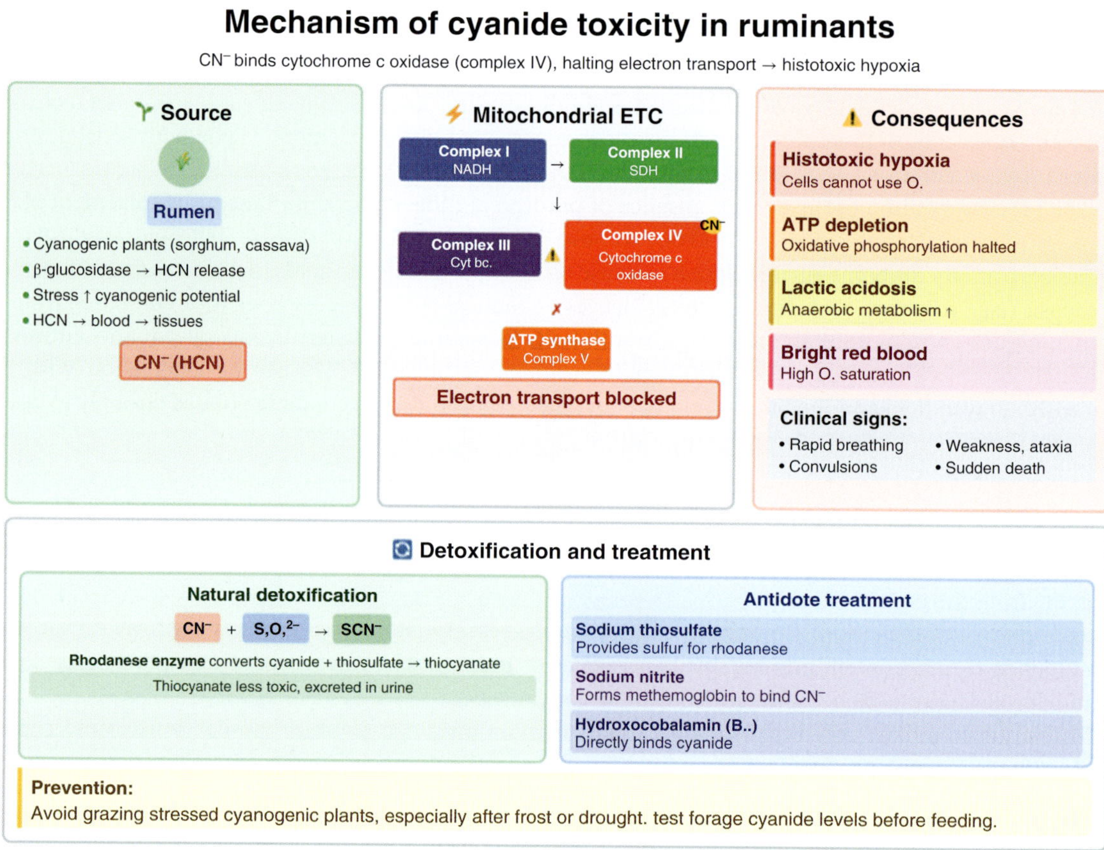

Figure 11.2 Mechanism of cyanide toxicity in ruminants. Cyanide binding to cytochrome oxidase blocks electron transport, causing histotoxic hypoxia and peracute collapse (Gupta, 2018; Kahn & Line, 2010).

Emergency Response and Treatment

Field priorities. (i) Immediate removal of surviving cattle from the contaminated field; (ii) on-site antidotes – intravenous sodium thiosulfate (enhances conversion of cyanide to thiocyanate, excreted in urine) and hydroxocobalamin (binds cyanide to form cyanocobalamin); and (iii) supportive oxygen where possible and IV fluids to support circulation (Gupta, 2018; Papich, 2021).

Outcomes. Reports indicated that ~20 cattle "revived from the brink of death," underscoring the effectiveness of early antidote deployment; however, once collapse progressed to seizures and coma, prognosis was grave (The Times of India, 2018) (Figure 11.3).

Outcome and Economic Impact

Animal loss. Fifty-six cattle died, representing catastrophic herd-level mortality.

Economic impact. Estimated direct losses exceeded USD 35,000 based on local cattle market values – near-total livelihood collapse for a single herder (The Times of India, 2018).

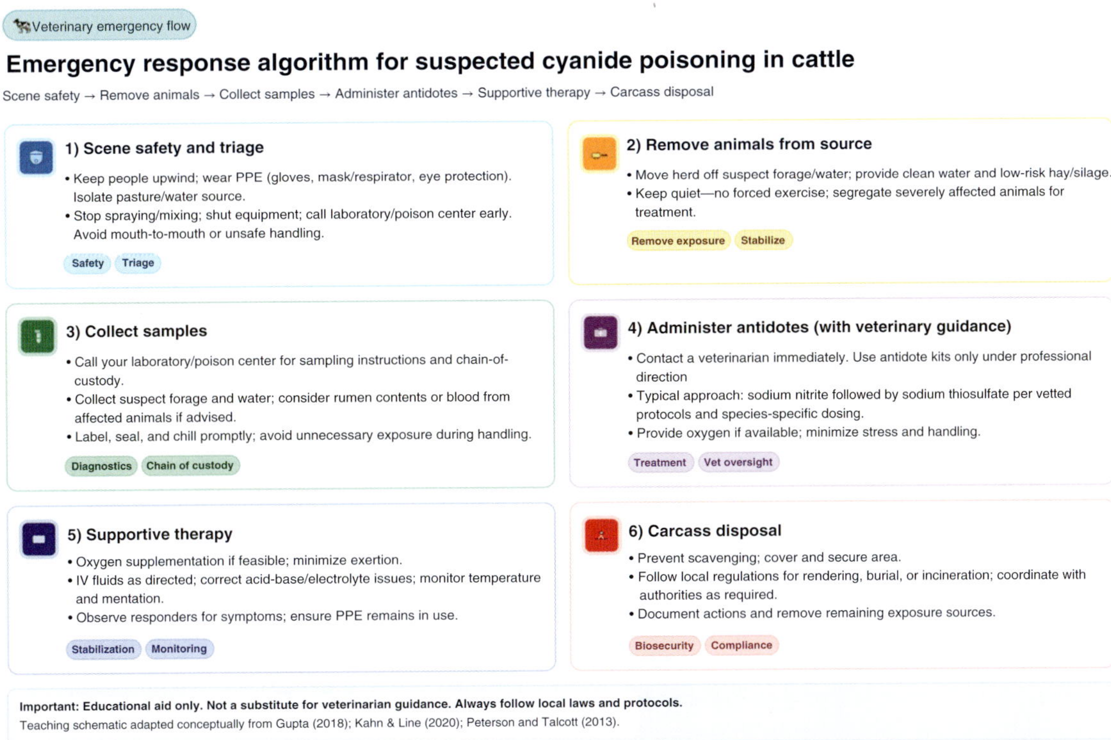

Figure 11.3 Emergency response algorithm for suspected cyanide poisoning in cattle. Scene safety → remove animals → collect priority samples → antidotes (nitrite–thiosulfate kit or hydroxocobalamin per local protocols) → oxygen and IV fluids → carcass control (Gupta, 2018; Kahn & Line, 2010; Papich, 2021).

Public health concern. Authorities warned villagers not to consume meat from carcasses due to risk of secondary poisoning; carcasses were buried under supervision (The Times of India, 2018).

Community impact. Local trust in pesticide safety declined; officials promised compensation and tighter oversight (Figure 11.4).

Lessons Learned and Implications for Practice

Education and stewardship. Train farmers on label instructions, pre-grazing intervals, and safe disposal.

Antidote preparedness. Regional clinics should stock sodium thiosulfate and hydroxocobalamin and maintain simple field kits for rapid deployment (Papich, 2021).

Cross-sector communication. Agricultural officers and applicators should proactively notify livestock owners after applications and during high-risk periods.

Policy implications. Enforce reentry/grazing intervals and container disposal in tropical mixed farming systems.

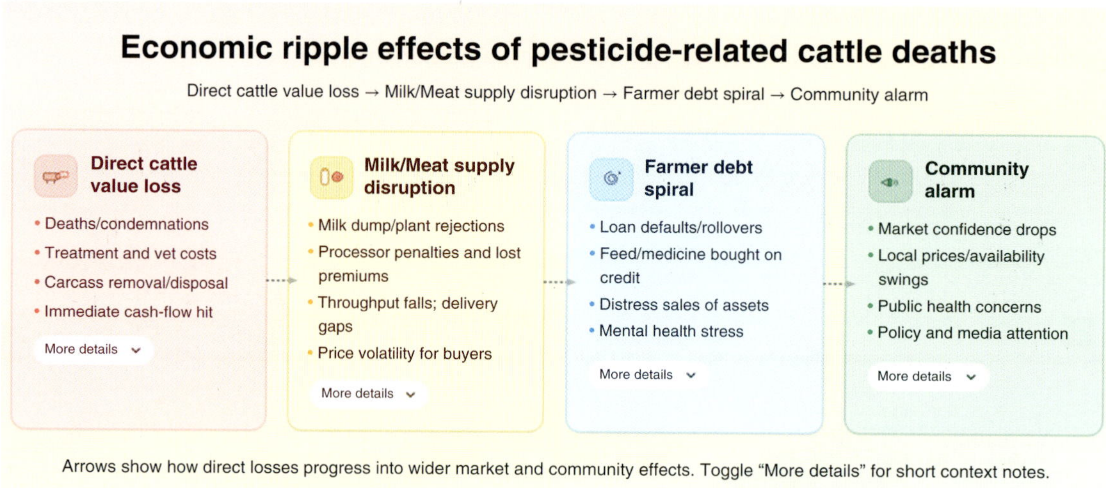

Figure 11.4 Economic ripple effects of pesticide-related cattle deaths. Direct animal value loss → supply disruption → farmer debt → community alarm/regulatory action. *Source:* Kahn & Line (2010)/with permission of Elsevier.

Teaching value. Classic case for veterinary curricula: sudden mass mortality in ruminants, rapid field diagnostics, and antidote-based emergency intervention (Gupta, 2018; Kahn & Line, 2010).

Case B – Aflatoxicosis: Abortion Storm in a Dairy Herd (Punjab, Pakistan, 2018)

Background and Context

Mycotoxins are an enduring problem in tropical and subtropical dairying, where high humidity and poor feed storage conditions create the perfect environment for fungal growth. Aflatoxins, produced mainly by *Aspergillus flavus* and *A. parasiticus*, are among the most potent hepatotoxic and carcinogenic compounds encountered in animal agriculture (Gupta, 2018).

In late 2018, a high-yield Holstein-Friesian dairy herd in Punjab, Pakistan experienced a severe reproductive crisis: 30 of 40 pregnant cows (75%) aborted within 5 weeks, and overall milk yield declined by nearly 19% (Penagos-Tabares et al., 2024). Investigations traced the outbreak to aflatoxin-contaminated concentrate feed, highlighting the economic and public health importance of mycotoxicosis in tropical dairy systems.

This case underscores:

- The vulnerability of large dairies to feed-borne toxins.
- The often-overlooked reproductive consequences of aflatoxin exposure.
- One Health implications. Aflatoxin B1 (AFB1) metabolizes to aflatoxin M1 (AFM1) in milk, posing a human health risk.

Clinical presentation:

- Reproductive losses: abortions between the 7th and 9th month of gestation.
- Production decline: ~19% drop in bulk-tank milk yield.
- Non-specific signs: transient anorexia, dullness, mild icterus in some cows.
- No infectious pattern: no fever spikes, uterine infections, or clustering suggestive of brucellosis or viral abortion storms.

The timing with a new batch of concentrate feed was the key epidemiological clue (Penagos-Tabares et al., 2024).

Diagnostic Workup

Field investigation. Feed samples (total mix ration [TMR] and concentrate); blood from aborting cows for biochemistry and serology to rule out infectious abortifacients; aborted fetuses for necropsy.

Laboratory findings. Feed enzyme linked immunosorbent assay (ELISA): aflatoxin B1 (AFB1) ≈ 60 µg/kg; total aflatoxins ≈ 100 µg/kg DM. Confirmatory liquid chromatography–tandem mass spectrometry (LC-MS/MS): total aflatoxins = 166 µg/kg (AFB1 = 134 µg/kg, aflatoxin B2 [AFB2] = 17.4 µg/kg, AFM1 = 14.9 µg/kg) (Penagos-Tabares et al., 2024). Histopathology: aborted fetuses with mild hepatic degeneration and centrilobular necrosis. Rule-outs: brucellosis, infectious bovine rhinotracheitis (IBR), leptospirosis negative.

Interpretation. AFB1 levels were >20-fold above EU limits (5–10 µg/kg for dairy feeds). With ~55% of the ration being contaminated concentrate, cows likely ingested >2 mg/day of AFB1 – sufficient to cause hepatic dysfunction and reproductive failure (Akbar et al., 2020) (Table 11.2).

Toxicant and Pathophysiology

Toxin. Aflatoxin B1 (AFB1), the most toxic and prevalent aflatoxin.

Metabolism. Ingested AFB1 is absorbed in the small intestine and transported to the liver. Hepatic cytochrome P450 enzymes convert AFB1 into the reactive AFB1-8,9-epoxide, which binds DNA and proteins, causing hepatocellular injury and carcinogenesis (Gupta, 2018). A fraction is hydroxylated to AFM1, excreted in milk; carry-over rates commonly range from 1% to 6% depending on dose, milk yield, and individual variation (Akbar et al., 2020).

Reproductive impact. Hepatic dysfunction reduces progesterone metabolism and can disrupt pregnancy maintenance; aflatoxins may directly impair placental and fetal development. The late-term abortions suggest cumulative hepatic and endocrine disruption rather than acute toxemia (Penagos-Tabares et al., 2024) (Figure 11.5).

Treatment and Management

Immediate actions. Withdraw contaminated feed and replace with verified toxin-free rations.

Supportive therapy. Hepatoprotectants (e.g., silymarin), vitamin E/selenium; toxin binders (e.g., bentonite) added to rations; B-complex vitamins to support hepatic metabolism.

Monitoring. Periodic milk testing for AFM1 before market release; reproductive monitoring for delayed fertility effects.

Table 11.2 Mycotoxin detection in tropical dairy practice: field and lab tools.

Tool/method	Targets (examples)	Matrix	Setting	Turnaround	Typical sensitivity/ LOD*	Strengths/use case	Limitations/caveats
Handheld UV "blacklight" (BGYF screen)	Aflatoxin risk indicator (toxigenic Aspergillus on grain/peanut kernels)	Corn/peanuts/ feeds (not milk)	Field	Minutes	Qualitative only (no LOD)	Very fast, zero consumables; flags hotspots for composite sampling	Not specific/ quantitative; many false results; screen only → confirm analytically
Lateral flow immunoassay (LFIA) strips ± reader	AFM1 (milk); AFB1, DON, Zearalenone (ZEN), T-2 toxin and HT-2 toxin (trichothecene mycotoxins) (T-2/ HT-2), fumonisins (FUM) (feed)	Raw milk/bulk tank; concentrates, grain, TMR, silage extracts	Field/parlor/ simple bench	5–10 min	Kit-dependent; AFM1 commonly ~0.025–0.10 μg/L; feed strips use screening cut-offs near action levels	Simple, fast, minimal equipment; semi-quant with reader – ideal for triage and supplier checks	Matrix effects; narrow dynamic range; toxin-class specific; positives require confirmatory lab testing
Portable fluorometric kits (e.g., Afla Test)	Aflatoxins (B_1+B_2+G_1+G_2); AFM1 variants available	Grain/feed; milk (kit-specific prep)	Field/basic lab	10–20 min	Low ppb (kit-specific)	Higher sensitivity than visual strips; portable reader; routine silo/lot screening	Consumable cost; single-class focus; calibration/controls needed
ELISA (microplate)	AFM1; AFB1; ZEN; DON; Ochratoxin A (OTA); FUM (single-analyte kits or small panels)	Milk, serum/urine (exposure), feed/ silage extracts	Basic lab	2–4 h (batch)	AFM1 often ~0.01–0.05 μg/L; feeds typically low μg/kg–mg/kg (analyte-dependent)	Cost-effective for batches; good sensitivity; widely available kits	Possible cross-reactivity; matrix validation/QC required; needs plate reader/washer/ pipettes
Thin-layer chromatography (TLC/HPTLC)	Aflatoxins, OTA, ZEN (method-dependent)	Feed, grain; milk after extraction	Lab	4–8 h	≈ μg/kg to tens μg/ kg	Low instrumentation cost;visualseparation– useful to confirm screens in resource-limited settings	Lower sensitivity/ throughput; solvent handling; semi-quant unless densitometry used
HPLC-FLD (often with post-column derivatization)	Aflatoxins; OTA (others with appropriate chemistry)	Feed/silage extracts; milk (AFM1)	Reference lab	4–24 h	Sub-ppb to low ppb (matrix & cleanup dependent)	Quantitative, specific; broadly accepted for regulatory decisions	Requires IAC or equivalent cleanup; trained staff; fewer analytes per run

LC-MS/MS (multi-mycotoxin)	Aflatoxins, ZEN, DON, T-2/HT-2, FUM, OTA, many others	Feed, TMR, silage, milk; urine/serum (biomonitoring)	Accredited lab	1–3 days (incl. logistics)	ng/kg to low µg/kg for many analytes	Gold-standard specificity; simultaneous multi-analyte quantification; confirmatory identification	Highest cost/complexity; rigorous QA/QC; matrix-matched calibration often needed
Immunoaffinity column (IAC) cleanup (prep step)	Class-specific (e.g., aflatoxins, ZEN, DON) – enables downstream detection	Milk and feed extracts	Lab (prep)	30–60 min	Not a detection method – improves LOD/SNR for HPLC/LC-MS	Removes matrix interferences; boosts sensitivity and accuracy	Per-sample cost; toxin-class specific; adds prep time
Near-infrared (spectroscopy) (NIR)/Fourier-transform infrared (spectroscopy) (FT-IR) spectroscopy (chemometric models)	Indirect screening correlated with contamination/risk	Ground feeds, grains, TMR (dry)	Field/mill/lab	Seconds–minutes	Model-dependent; no fixed LOD (screening classification)	Very rapid, nondestructive, high throughput for incoming QC	Requires robust local calibration; not confirmatory; sensitive to moisture/particle size
Biomarkers of exposure (lab)	AFM1 in milk; ZEN metabolites (α-zearalenol) in urine; DON-glucuronides (LC-MS/MS)	Milk, urine, serum	Lab	1–3 days	Low µg/L to ng/L (platform-dependent)	Assesses animal exposure/carry-over; evaluates interventions	Not directly equivalent to feed concentration; inter-animal variability; requires validated methods
Sampling plan (composite grabs; cold chain)	All classes (represents lot)	Grain, TMR, silage, milk	Field → lab	Add 10–20 composite increments; chill/ship same day	—	Reduces sampling error – the largest contributor to total test error	Requires discipline and documentation; improper handling can bias results

Screening and confirmatory methods for AFB1/AFM1 and other common mycotoxins, with typical turnaround times, LOD/sensitivity notes, and strengths/limitations across milk and feed matrices. (Adapted summary of strips/fluorometry/ELISA/TLC/HPLC-FLD/LC-MS/MS/IAC and sampling/biomarkers.)

LODs are indicative ranges – kits, matrices, and lab validation strongly influence performance. Screen-positive results should be **confirmed** using accredited methods.

Source: Adapted from Gupta (2018); Kahn and Line (2010); FAO/WHO guidance; AOAC/ISO method compendia; Merck Veterinary Manual (online, 2024–2025).

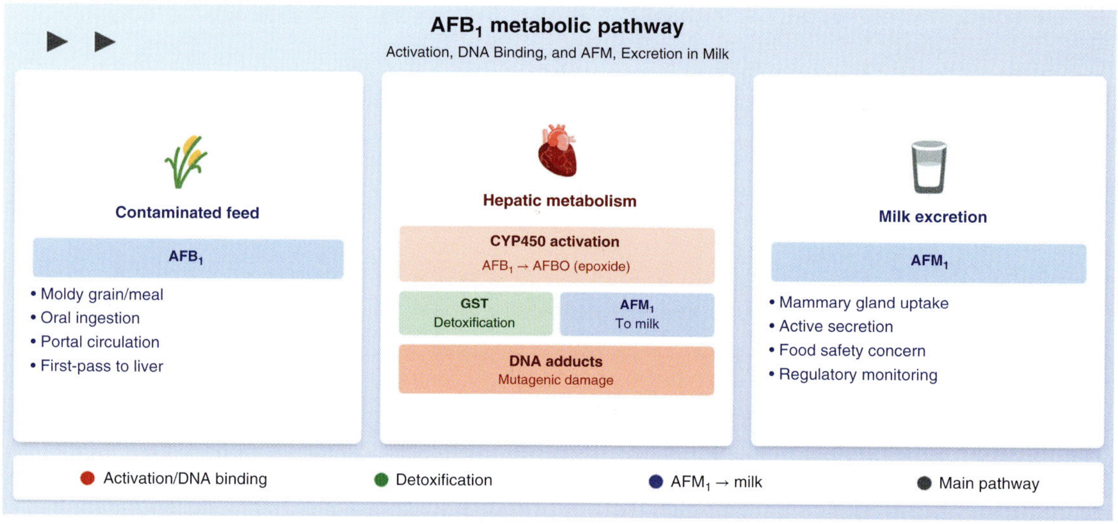

Figure 11.5 Metabolic pathway of aflatoxin B1: liver activation, DNA binding, and AFM1 excretion in milk. Pathway from feed ingestion to hepatic bioactivation and milk carry-over, highlighting typical AFM1 transfer ranges and sampling points. *Source:* After Gupta (2018), Akbar et al. (2020), Penagos-Tabares et al. (2024).

Outcome. Abortions ceased after feed replacement; milk yield recovered over weeks; some cows with severe liver damage showed prolonged reduced fertility (Penagos-Tabares et al., 2024).

Outcome and Economic Impact

Direct losses. Thirty calves lost (genetic/future productivity), ~19% herd milk reduction over 35 days (hundreds of liters) (Penagos-Tabares et al., 2024).

Indirect costs. Discarded milk due to AFM1; cost of replacement feed and binders; extended calving intervals.

Public health risk. AFM1-contaminated milk can enter the food chain if untested, increasing risk of hepatocellular carcinoma in humans (Akbar et al., 2020) (Figure 11.6).

Lessons Learned and Implications

Routine feed testing. Institutionalize rapid field screens (e.g., lateral-flow immunoassay [LFIA]) to triage lots and LC-MS/MS for confirmation and multi-mycotoxin profiling (Akbar et al., 2020).

Farmer awareness. In peri-urban Pakistan, ~95% of farmers had never heard of "aflatoxins" by name despite recognizing moldy feed as harmful; targeted training closes this prevention gap (Yunus et al., 2022).

Prevention. Proper drying (<15% moisture), aerated storage, mold inhibitors, supplier QA programs.

One Health. AFM1 in milk links animal health to human cancer risk; hold-and-test policies protect consumers and the dairy brand.

Teaching relevance. Include mycotoxins in differentials for abortion storms/production drops; know when to escalate from screening to confirmatory testing.

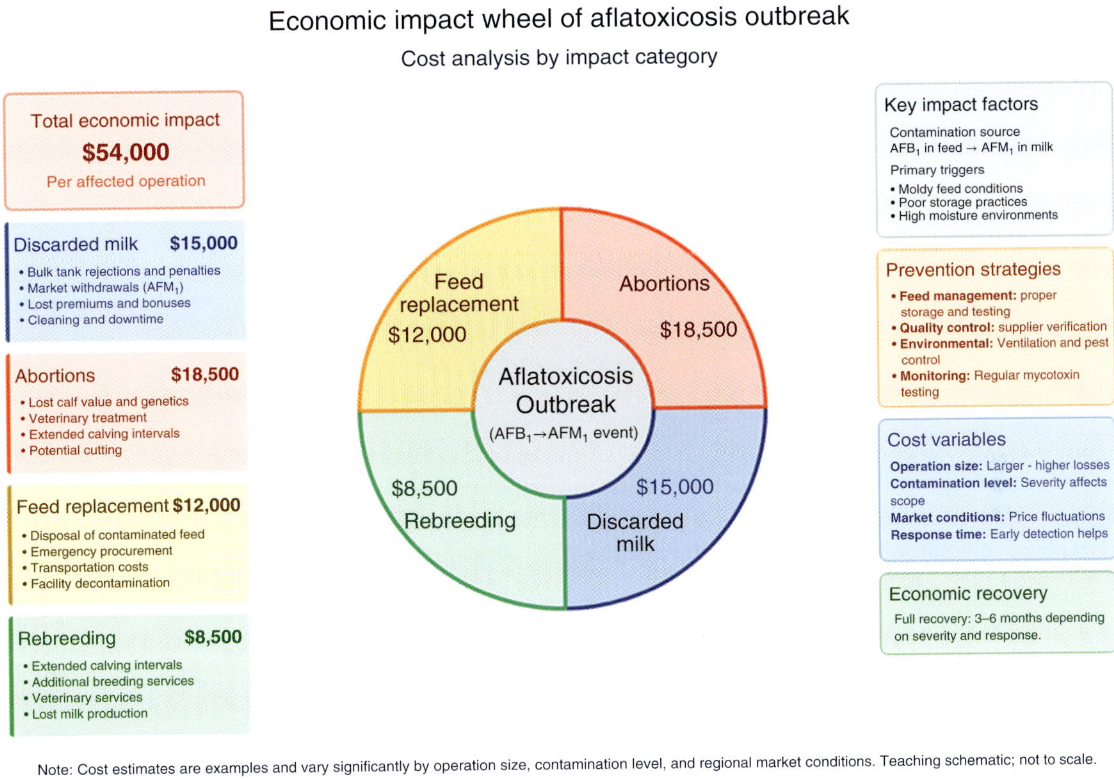

Figure 11.6 Economic impact wheel of an aflatoxicosis outbreak. Schematic allocation of losses across abortions, discarded milk, rebreeding, and feed replacement/binders for rapid stakeholder communication. *Source:* After Akbar et al. (2020), Penagos-Tabares et al. (2024).

Case C – Lead Poisoning in Livestock Near Artisanal Mining (Zamfara, Nigeria, 2010–2013)

Background and Context

In 2010, artisanal gold mining in Zamfara, Nigeria released extreme concentrations of lead (Pb) into the environment. Soil contamination in villages reached >10,000 ppm, far above safe levels (<85 ppm for livestock grazing) (Dooyema et al., 2012). Cattle, goats, poultry, and dogs grazing or scavenging in contaminated areas began dying in unusual numbers, often with neurological signs.

Livestock losses highlighted a One Health sentinel role: Animals were among the first to signal an environmental catastrophe that later claimed hundreds of human lives, especially children (Lo et al., 2012).

Clinical presentation and scene findings:

- Sudden deaths in goats and calves
- Neurological signs in surviving cattle: ataxia, blindness, head pressing
- Poultry with wing droop and depression

Postmortem findings included pale carcasses, swollen kidneys, and gastroenteritis in some goats (Blacksmith Institute, 2011). Differentiating Pb toxicosis from listeriosis or polioencephalomalacia was challenging.

Diagnostic Workup

Sampling. Blood from goats/cattle; soil, forage, water from village environments; liver and kidney from dead animals.

Laboratory results. Blood lead >100 μg/dL in goats/cattle (safe threshold <30 μg/dL). Soil lead up to 10,000 ppm (Dooyema et al., 2012). Kidney lead >50 ppm – diagnostic of chronic exposure (Gupta, 2018) (Table 11.3).

Toxicant and Pathophysiology

- Binds sulfhydryl groups → inhibits δ-aminolevulinic acid dehydratase and ferrochelatase.
- Disrupts heme synthesis → anemia with basophilic stippling.
- Competes with calcium at synapses → neurological dysfunction (ataxia, blindness, seizures).
- Deposits in bone → long-term reservoirs and chronic risk (Gupta, 2018; Kahn & Line, 2010).

Tropical amplifiers. Dry-season dust storms increase inhalational exposure; communal grazing intensifies simultaneous herd exposure; limited access to chelation prolongs disease impact (Figure 11.7).

Emergency Response and Treatment

Immediate removal of animals from contaminated sites; chelation (e.g., Ca-EDTA, DMSA) for high-value animals (cost/logistics often limiting); supportive care (B vitamins, thiamine), nutrition, and exposure control. In many herds, treatment was not feasible; control depended on relocation and soil remediation (Dooyema et al., 2012).

Outcome and Economic Impact

Livestock mortality. Hundreds of goats, cattle, and poultry lost (2010–2013).

Food-chain hazard. Contaminated milk/meat posed ongoing risks.

Economic devastation. Loss of draft animals and dairy cows worsened poverty; herd recovery lagged behind human remediation timelines (Lo et al., 2012) (Figure 11.8).

Lessons Learned and Implications

Livestock as sentinels. Unexplained animal deaths may foreshadow human epidemics; integrate veterinary findings into public health alerts.

Integrated surveillance. Veterinary, medical, and environmental agencies should codify joint sampling and action thresholds for mining regions.

Policy gaps. Enforce safer ore-processing practices and restrict in-village ore crushing; pair remediation with livelihood alternatives.

Teaching point. Connect clinical signs (blindness, anemia, behavior change) with field history (mining, tailings, windborne dust) when approaching herd cases.

Table 11.3 Diagnostic thresholds for lead exposure in livestock (cattle/goats). Safe/background, subclinical/exposed, and toxic/diagnostic ranges across blood, liver, kidney, and milk; common lab methods (GFAAS/ICP-MS/ICP-OES); collection and handling notes; unit conversions.

Specimen (matrix)	Species	Safe/background	Subclinical/ exposed (suspect)	Toxic/diagnostic	Common lab methods	Notes (collection and handling)
Blood (whole, EDTA)	Cattle/goats	<0.05 mg/L (<50 µg/L; <5 µg/dL)	0.05–0.35 mg/L (50–350 µg/L; 5–35 µg/dL)	>0.35 mg/L (>350 µg/L; >35 µg/dL); severe often >0.60 mg/L	Graphite-furnace AAS, ICP-MS (or ICP-OES at higher levels)	Use EDTA whole blood; avoid heparinized plasma for interpretation. Prevent contamination (no brass syringes/needles). Chill and ship promptly.
Liver (wet weight)	Cattle/goats	<1 mg/kg (ppm)	1–10 mg/kg	>10 mg/kg (often >30 mg/kg in clear poisoning)	ICP-MS, AAS after digestion	Collect fresh/frozen (~50–100 g). Rinse surface; place in trace-metal clean container.
Kidney (wet weight)	Cattle/goats	<1–2 mg/kg	2–10 mg/kg	>10–30 mg/kg (severe >30 mg/kg)	ICP-MS, AAS after digestion	Cortex preferred for chronic exposure. Store chilled/frozen; avoid cross-contamination.
Milk (raw)	Cattle/goats	Compliant/low: typically ≤0.02 mg/kg (jurisdiction-specific limit)	0.02–0.05 mg/kg (non-compliant; exposure likely)	>~0.05 mg/kg (public health concern; condemn)	ICP-MS, GFAAS (preconcentration), ICP-OES at higher levels	Collect into acid-washed plastic; chill. Milk reflects food-safety compliance rather than animal symptom severity.

Interpretation: Thresholds vary by laboratory validation and jurisdiction; interpret alongside clinical signs, exposure history (e.g., tailings/dust), and parallel tissues. Positive screens should be confirmed with accredited methods and QA/QC.

Source: Compiled from Gupta (2018); Kahn and Line (2010); Dooyema et al. (2012).Unit tips: 1 mg/L = 1,000 µg/L = 100 µg/dL.

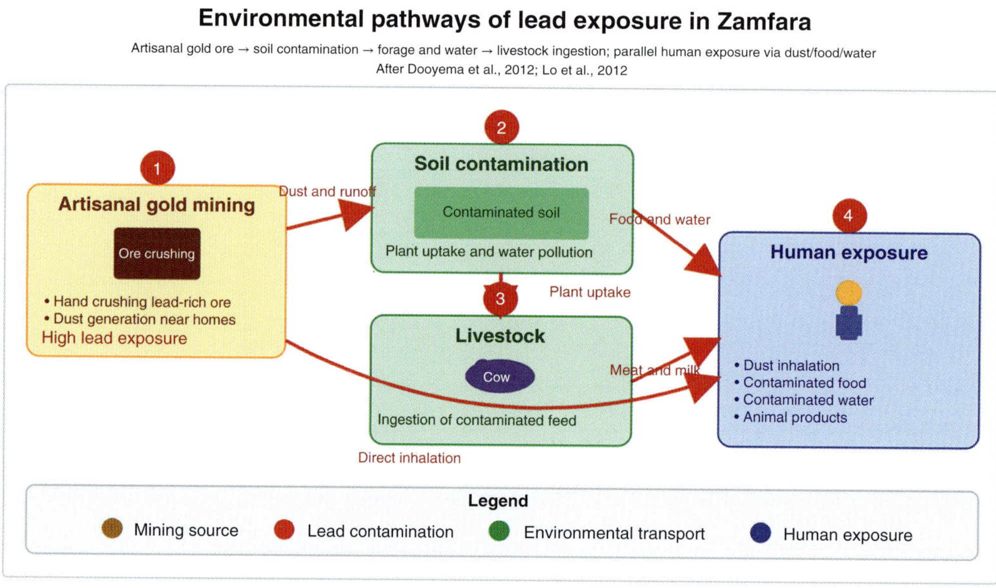

Figure 11.7 Environmental pathways of lead exposure in Zamfara. Diagram showing artisanal gold ore → soil contamination → forage and water → livestock ingestion; parallel human exposure via dust inhalation and contaminated food/water (Dooyema et al., 2012) and Lo et al. (2012).

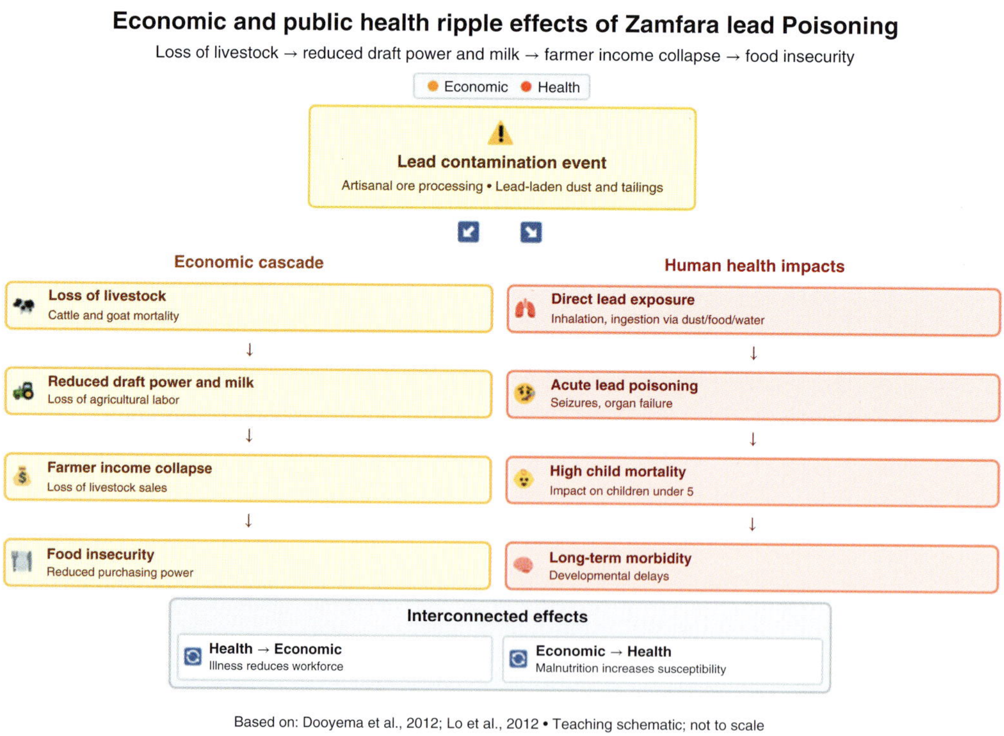

Figure 11.8 Economic and public health ripple effects of Zamfara lead poisoning. Livestock loss → reduced draft power/milk → debt and food insecurity → parallel human morbidity/mortality (Dooyema et al., 2012; Lo et al., 2012).

Case D – Ionophore (Monensin) Feed-Mixing Error in Water Buffaloes (Bahia, Brazil, 2022)

Background and Context

Ionophores are polyether antibiotics from *Streptomyces* spp. used widely in ruminant production (monensin, lasalocid, salinomycin, narasin). At label doses they improve feed efficiency and control coccidiosis; however, their therapeutic window is narrow, and mixing errors, cross-contamination, or species misapplication can lead to severe toxicosis (Gupta, 2018; Kahn & Line, 2010). Inter-species susceptibility is uneven: horses are highly sensitive; cattle tolerate moderate inclusion rates; field evidence suggests water buffaloes may be more vulnerable than cattle to monensin overexposure, likely due to differences in rumen metabolism and tissue handling (Gupta, 2018). Species-specific ionophore safety margins and approximate toxic exposure ranges for cattle, buffalo, horses, and poultry are summarized in Table 11.4.

In Bahia, Brazil (2022), a feed-mixing error placed excess monensin into a ration fed to a group of 21 adult buffaloes. Within days, 15 (71%) developed clinical signs, and all clinically affected animals died – one of the most detailed buffalo ionophore outbreaks reported regionally (Silva et al., 2022) (Figure 11.9).

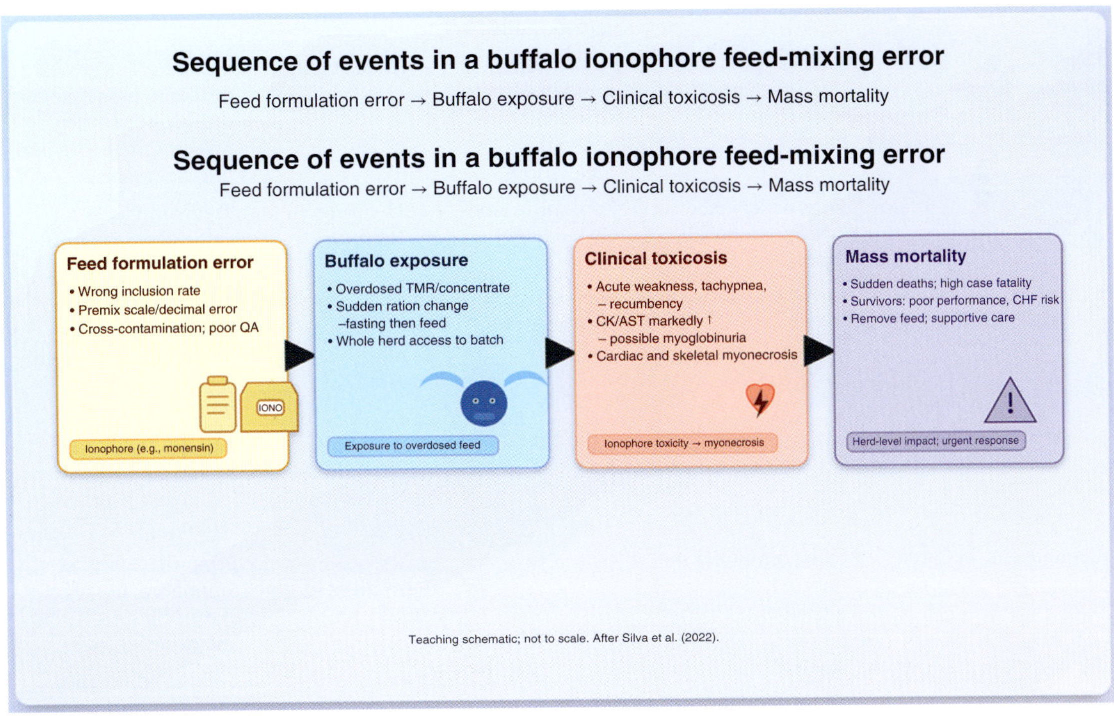

Figure 11.9 Sequence of events in a buffalo ionophore feed-mixing error. Flow: feed formulation error → buffalo exposure → cluster of myopathy cases → mass mortality. *Source:* Silva et al. (2022).

Table 11.4 Safe vs. toxic dose ranges of ionophores in major livestock species. Comparative label ranges, subclinical thresholds, and toxic/lethal exposures for cattle, buffalo, horses, and poultry; notes on mixing errors/cross-contamination. Compiled from Gupta (2018); Kahn & Line (2010); and Silva et al. (2022).

Ionophore (example brand)	Species	Typical label/safe use*	Subclinical/ suspect exposure (common red flags)	Toxic/lethal exposure (single-dose mg/kg bw unless noted)	Key notes
Monensin (Rumensin®)	Cattle	~10–40 ppm in feed (≈50–400 mg/head/ day, diet-dependent)	~≥2× label or sudden ration change; mix errors ≥100–200 ppm	~≥20–40 mg/kg bw (acute); severe outbreaks with high-ppm feed over hours–days	Cardiac/skeletal myonecrosis; ↑CK, ↑cTnI; drug interactions (macrolides) increase risk.
	Buffalo	Not widely labeled; if used off-label, keep ≤cattle ranges and introduce slowly	Similar triggers as cattle; case reports after high-ppm mixing errors	~≥15–30 mg/kg bw (approx., species likely ≥ cattle sensitivity)	Field outbreaks in Asia linked to premix decimal errors; high mortality clusters.
	Horses	None (contraindicated)	Any access to medicated feeds is unsafe	~≥1–3 mg/kg bw (often fatal)	Extremely sensitive; accidental access to cattle/poultry feed is a classic catastrophe.
	Poultry (broilers)	~100–125 ppm feed	≥150–200 ppm; feed mixing/ overlaps with other anticoccidials	LD_{50} roughly ~100–200 mg/kg bw (species/age dependent)	Growth depression before overt toxicosis; avoid combinations that potentiate effects.
Lasalocid (Bovatec®)	Cattle	~11–33 ppm feed (≈100–360 mg/ head/day)	≥60–80 ppm; rapid up-titration without adaptation	~≥30–60 mg/kg bw	Similar efficacy/risk profile to monensin but different chemistry; myocardium + skeletal muscle targets.
	Buffalo	Not widely labeled; use cautiously if considered	≥2× cattle label (by analogy)	~≥25–50 mg/kg bw (approx.)	Treat as at least cattle-sensitive until herd-level data are available.
	Horses	None (contraindicated)	Any exposure unsafe	~≥2–10 mg/kg bw (fatalities reported)	Horses sensitive, though usually slightly less than with monensin.
	Poultry	~75–125 ppm feed	≥150–200 ppm	LD_{50} on order of tens–hundreds mg/kg bw (strain/ age vary)	Performance drop, weakness; avoid ionophore overlaps in rations.
Salinomycin	Cattle	Not commonly labeled; avoid off-label use	—	— (use alternatives in cattle)	Primarily a poultry ionophore; horses extremely sensitive to any exposure.
	Horses	None (contraindicated)	Any exposure unsafe	Low mg/kg bw range (fatalities at small doses reported)	Treat as emergency exposure.
	Poultry	~50–70 ppm feed	≥80–120 ppm	LD_{50} typically tens of mg/kg bw	Neuromuscular weakness, recumbency at high feed ppm.

Table 11.4 (Continued)

Ionophore (example brand)	Species	Typical label/safe use*	Subclinical/ suspect exposure (common red flags)	Toxic/lethal exposure (single-dose mg/kg bw unless noted)	Key notes
Narasin	Poultry	~60–80 ppm feed	≥100–120 ppm	LD_{50} ≈ ~100 mg/kg bw (order-of-magnitude)	Often combined (e.g., narasin+nicarbazin); watch for potentiation.
Maduramicin	Poultry	~5–10 ppm feed	≥12–20 ppm	LD_{50} low single-digit mg/kg bw (very potent)	Narrow therapeutic index; rigorous QA in premix handling is essential.

* ppm feed ≈ mg of drug per kg of complete feed. "mg/kg bw" is milligrams per kilogram of body weight (single-dose acute reference).

Practical cautions

- Horses: any ionophore exposure is dangerous – treat as an emergency.
- Buffalo and cattle: most catastrophes stem from mixing/decimal errors or cross-contamination; abrupt ration changes can exacerbate toxicity.
- Poultry: usually managed safely at label ppm; toxicity arises from over-fortification, product overlap, or misfeed.
- Co-exposures (e.g., macrolide antibiotics), electrolyte disturbances, and poor hydration can worsen outcomes.

Source: Compiled from Gupta (2018); Kahn and Line (2010); and Silva et al. (2022).

Clinical Presentation and Scene Findings

Onset followed a 24–48 hours latency after the suspect ration was offered. Affected buffaloes showed muscular weakness and reluctance to move, tremors, staggering gait, tachycardia and dyspnea, and ruminal stasis, then recumbency with death 24–72 hours after first signs. Other species on the premises (cattle, horses) were unaffected, underscoring species-specific sensitivity (Silva et al., 2022). Differentials included clostridial myositis, selenium toxicosis, white muscle disease, toxic plant myopathies, and capture/overexertion myopathy. The tight temporal linkage to a new ration and herd-level clustering favored a feed-borne etiology.

Diagnostic Workup

Sampling. (i) Feed remnants from troughs/storage; (ii) serum from clinically affected buffaloes; (iii) cardiac and skeletal muscle at necropsy.

Laboratory results. Feed high-performance liquid chromatography (HPLC): monensin ≈ 461.7 mg/kg in the suspect material (Silva et al., 2022). Serum CK and aspartate transaminase (AST) were markedly elevated, consistent with myonecrosis. Necropsy: pale streaking of myocardium, pulmonary edema, diffuse skeletal muscle degeneration; histopathology: hyaline degeneration, segmental myofiber necrosis/lysis, early fibrosis in heart and locomotor muscles (Figure 11.10).

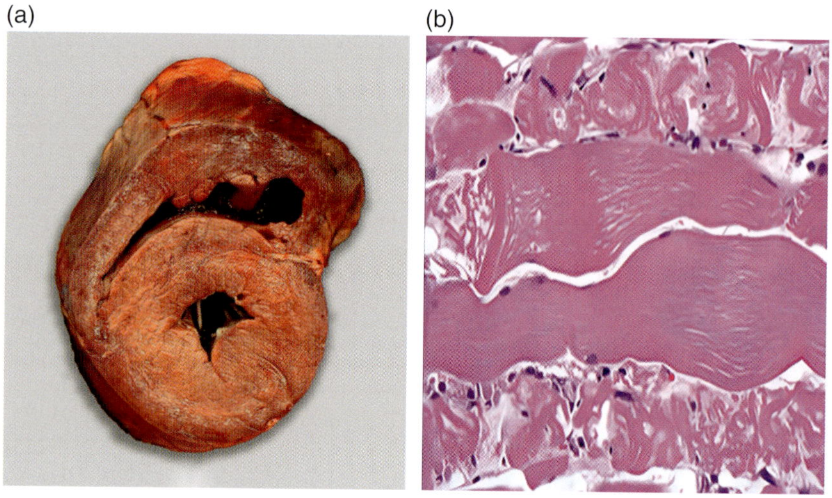

Figure 11.10 Gross and histologic lesions in ionophore toxicosis. (a) Severe concentric hypertrophy of the left ventricular wall, consistent with chronic pressure overload. (b) Myofiber degeneration and necrosis, with loss of the orderly myofibers appearance and replacement by clumped, amorphous material (H&E, 100×). *Source:* (a) UCDavis Comparative Pathology Laboratory. (n.d.). Specimen ID 6607 – Bovine heart, Case 17-198. Retrieved February 28, 2026, from https://www.ucvmpathology.ca/specimen.php?id=6607 and (b) National Hog Farmer. (n.d.). Diagnosis of ionophore intoxications in pigs. Retrieved February 28, 2026, from https://www.nationalhogfarmer.com/hog-nutrition/diagnosis-of-ionophore-intoxications-in-pigs.

Toxicant and Pathophysiology

Ionophores act as mobile ion carriers, collapsing transmembrane gradients. Monensin exchanges Na^+ for H^+, driving intracellular Na^+ accumulation; the Na^+ load triggers secondary Ca^{2+} influx, causing mitochondrial swelling, ATP depletion, and myofiber necrosis. Cardiac and skeletal muscle – high-energy tissues – are preferential targets (Gupta, 2018; Kahn & Line, 2010). Oxidative stress further amplifies injury, and sublethal exposures can leave survivors at risk of chronic cardiomyopathy and exercise intolerance.

Drug and diet interactions can potentiate toxicity (e.g., certain antimicrobials/ionophore co-exposures, severe electrolyte imbalances), and species-specific kinetics likely explain why buffaloes fare worse at similar exposures (Gupta, 2018) (Figure 11.11).

Emergency Response and Treatment

Immediate actions. Remove the suspect ration and isolate exposed buffaloes. Gastric/ruminal decontamination has limited utility once signs develop.

Supportive care. IV fluids, vitamin E/selenium, cautious non-steroidal anti-inflammatory drug (NSAID) use for pain, and rest; no specific antidote exists and response is often poor in fulminant cases (Gupta, 2018; Papich, 2021).

Herd management:

- Quarantine affected cohorts.
- Trace back and test all feed batches (HPLC/LC-MS/MS).
- Audit mill weighing/sequencing/flushing to prevent cross-contamination.
- Implement species-specific ration controls and staff retraining.

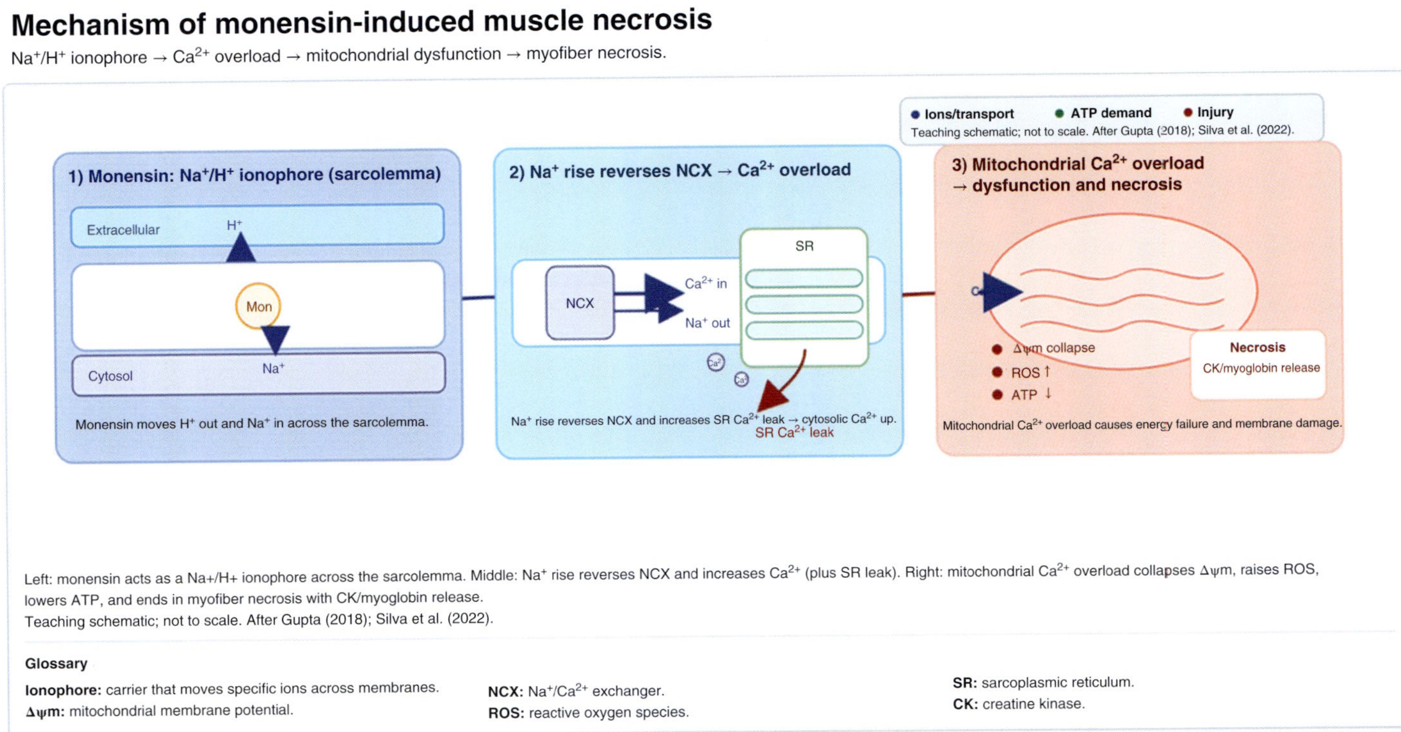

Figure 11.11 Mechanism of monensin-induced muscle necrosis. Ionophore-mediated Na^+/H^+ exchange → cytosolic Na^+ rise → Ca^{2+} overload → mitochondrial dysfunction → myofiber necrosis. Gupta (2018) and Kahn and Line (2010); informed by Silva et al. (2022).

Outcome and Economic Impact

In the Bahia incident, mortality among clinically affected buffaloes was 100%. Losses included animal value (breeding stock, milk, meat), draft power, veterinary/feed disposal costs, and opportunity costs (lost milk cycles, delayed breeding). At farm scale this equated to tens of thousands of USD; at regional scale, cases spur regulatory scrutiny of feed-mill QA/QC and traceability in multispecies supply chains (Silva et al., 2022) (Figure 11.12).

Lessons Learned and Implications

Narrow margins of safety. Ionophores demand disciplined weighing, batching, sequencing, and line flushing in mills.

Species sensitivity. Buffaloes may require extra caution vs. cattle; never cross-feed cattle premixes to other species.

Rapid confirmation. Keep HPLC/LC-MS/MS referral pathways ready for suspect feed; pair with serum CK/AST and necropsy to confirm myopathy.

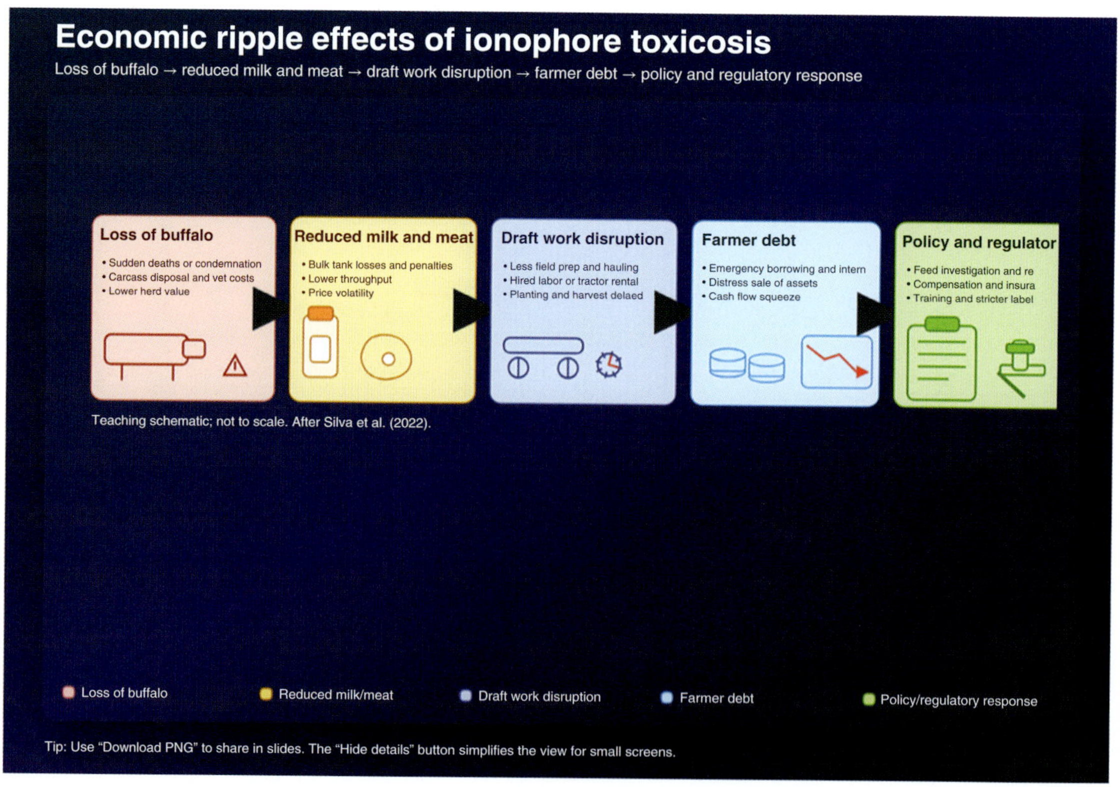

Figure 11.12 Economic ripple effects of ionophore toxicosis. Loss of buffalo → reduced milk/meat → draft work disruption → farmer debt → policy/regulatory response. *Source:* Silva et al. (2022).

Education and extension. Train staff to recognize the ionophore toxidrome and enact immediate feed holds.

Policy. Encourage labeling clarity, lot traceability, and routine proficiency checks for mills supplying mixed-species enterprises.

Teaching point. Use this case to integrate ration auditing, clinicopathologic interpretation, and One Health–aware economic analysis.

Case E – NSAID-Associated Vulture Collapse Linked to Diclofenac (South Asia, 1990s–Present)

Background and Context

From the early 1990s, three South Asian Gyps vultures – White-rumped (*Gyps bengalensis*), Long-billed (*G. indicus*), and Slender-billed (*G. tenuirostris*) – suffered catastrophic population crashes (>95–99%). Research traced the primary driver to veterinary diclofenac given to cattle and buffalo shortly before death; vultures feeding on those carcasses died of acute renal failure with visceral gout (Green et al., 2006; Oaks et al., 2004). Following the evidence, India, Nepal, and Pakistan banned veterinary diclofenac in 2006; India later capped human diclofenac vial sizes to deter diversion to livestock treatment (2015) and promoted meloxicam as a safe alternative (Cuthbert et al., 2011; SAVE, 2020). Despite policy gains, illegal/accidental exposure persists, and additional NSAIDs (e.g., ketoprofen, aceclofenac, nimesulide) have proven vulture-toxic or convert to toxic metabolites, keeping the conservation crisis active (Galligan et al., 2016, 2022; Naidoo et al., 2010) (Figure 11.13).

Clinical Presentation and Scene Findings

Carcasses of wild Gyps vultures are typically discovered near feeding areas with apparently good body condition but severe dehydration. Necropsy reveals white urate crystals on serosal surfaces (visceral gout), pale swollen kidneys, and minimal evidence of infectious disease – classic for NSAID-induced renal failure (Cuthbert et al., 2016; Oaks et al., 2004). In South Asia, epidemics clustered around carcass dumps and rural abattoirs where recently medicated livestock were disposed.

Diagnostic Workup

Field sampling. Dead vultures: kidney and liver for NSAID residue analysis; gross/histopathology for urate deposition. Carcasses/abattoirs: muscle/liver/kidney from livestock; pharmacy surveys to identify NSAIDs in circulation.

Analytical methods. HPLC/LC-MS/MS for residues; pathology to confirm urate nephrosis.

Results in South Asia. Diclofenac residues in vulture tissues and dosed carcasses reproduce renal failure and gout (Oaks et al., 2004). Ketoprofen is experimentally lethal to Gyps vultures at clinical dosing ranges (Naidoo et al., 2010). Aceclofenac rapidly biotransforms to diclofenac in cattle/buffalo, making it equivalently hazardous (Chandramohan et al., 2022; Galligan et al., 2016). Nimesulide at maximum likely exposure (MLE) killed Gyps vultures within ~30 hours with renal failure (Galligan et al., 2022) (Table 11.5).

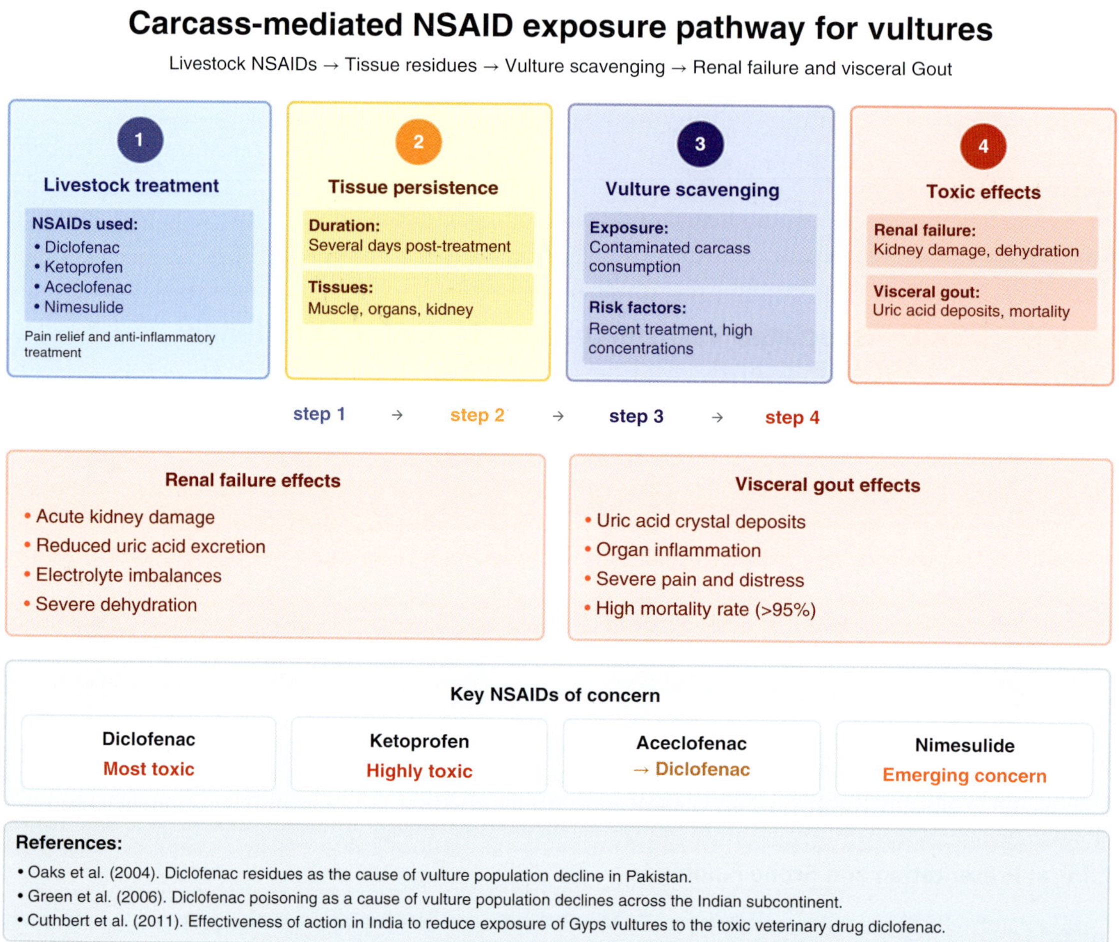

Figure 11.13 Carcass-mediated NSAID exposure pathway for vultures. Livestock treated with NSAIDs (diclofenac, ketoprofen, aceclofenac→diclofenac, nimesulide) → tissues retain residues for days → vulture scavenges carcass → renal failure and visceral gout (Cuthbert et al., 2011; Green et al., 2006; Oaks et al., 2004).

Table 11.5 Comparative NSAID risk to South Asian vultures (evidence synthesis). Diclofenac, ketoprofen, aceclofenac (→ diclofenac), and nimesulide: **toxic**; meloxicam: **safe** at likely exposure levels.

NSAID	Evidence in Gyps vultures	Population/field relevance	Overall risk (to Gyps)	Recommended action
Diclofenac	Experimentally lethal at ≤1 mg/kg body mass; classic lesions: acute renal failure with visceral gout. Residues from treated livestock carcasses sufficient to kill feeding vultures.	Mass declines in South Asia temporally linked to veterinary use; carcass surveys detected lethal residues; a single meal can be fatal.	Very high	Maintain/ strengthen bans; keep treated carcasses out of the scavenger food chain.

Table 11.5 (Continued)

NSAID	Evidence in Gyps vultures	Population/field relevance	Overall risk (to Gyps)	Recommended action
Ketoprofen	Lethal to Gyps at or near clinical (label) dosing levels (via contaminated tissues). Characteristic renal pathology/gout.	Carcass "hotspots" (e.g., injection-site muscle) can deliver lethal doses; field detections in the region.	High	Avoid in livestock where vultures scavenge; replace with vulture-safe alternatives.
Aceclofenac	Pro-drug rapidly biotransformed to diclofenac in cattle/buffalo; therefore inherits diclofenac's toxicity to Gyps.	Even if aceclofenac is used instead of diclofenac, carcasses pose the same lethal risk once converted.	Very high	Treat as diclofenac: avoid use; enforce substitution with meloxicam.
Nimesulide	Experimentally lethal to Gyps at MLE (maximum likely exposure) from a single contaminated meal; severe renal lesions and gout.	High residues documented at injection sites and in certain tissues for hours–days, creating carcass hotspots.	High–very high	Avoid use in vulture ranges; remove/secure carcasses from recently treated stock.
Meloxicam	Extensive experimental and field use shows no harm to Gyps at therapeutic exposures.	Scaled adoption associated with safe clinical outcomes and no vulture mortality signal.	Low/vulture-safe	Preferred alternative NSAID for livestock in South Asia.

MLE, *maximum likely exposure* (estimated dose to a vulture from a realistic meal of contaminated tissue). "Risk" reflects Gyps susceptibility and carcass-mediated exposure potential; other raptors may differ. Handling of treated-animal remains (especially **injection-site muscle**) is critical.
Source: Compiled from Oaks et al. (2004); Swan et al. (2006); Naidoo et al. (2010); Galligan et al. (2016, 2022).

Toxicant and Pathophysiology

Diclofenac and several other NSAIDs inhibit cyclooxygenase and disrupt renal prostaglandin-mediated autoregulation. In Gyps vultures, this causes acute tubulonephrosis, rapid hyperuricemia, and urate crystal precipitation (visceral gout) on serosae and in kidneys. Experimental dosing and feeding trials reproduced these lesions and mortality at doses consistent with field exposures (Green et al., 2006; Oaks et al., 2004). Nimesulide safety tests yielded similar pathophysiology with fatal renal failure (Galligan et al., 2022). By contrast, meloxicam safety trials at maximum likely exposure showed no renal injury, supporting policy substitution (Swan et al., 2006) (Figure 11.14).

Emergency Response and Management

Carcass management and exposure control. Rapid removal or burial/incineration of carcasses of NSAID-treated livestock prevents vulture exposure. Abattoir protocols and carcass-dump oversight are practical points of intervention – screen treated carcasses, improve disposal, and post clear signage/training.

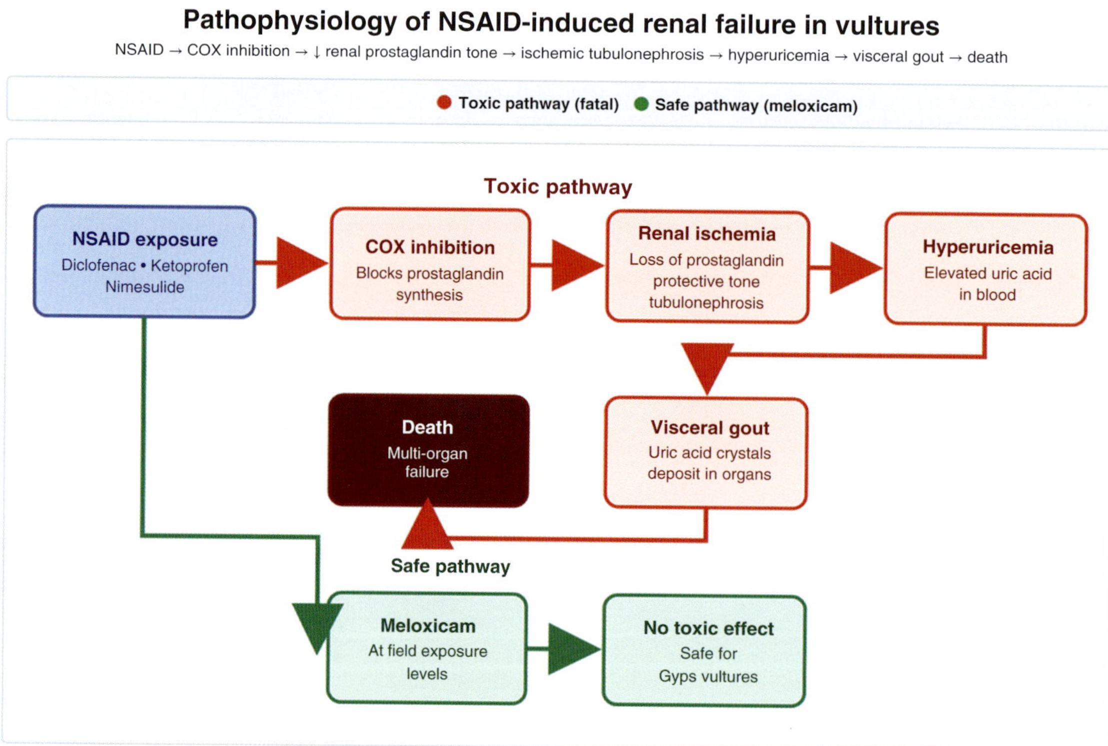

Figure 11.14 Pathophysiology of NSAID-induced renal failure in vultures. COX inhibition → loss of renal prostaglandins → tubulonephrosis → hyperuricemia → visceral gout → death; meloxicam pathway indicated as safe (Galligan et al., 2022; Oaks et al., 2004; Swan et al., 2006).

Drug policy and substitution. The 2006 veterinary diclofenac ban (India, Nepal, Pakistan) reduced carcass contamination and likely lowered annual vulture death rates; meloxicam (approved and widely available) is the recommended alternative (Cuthbert et al., 2011; SAVE, 2020). Ongoing action should address other vulture-toxic NSAIDs (ketoprofen, aceclofenac, nimesulide) through regulation and pharmacovigilance.

Clinical care for individual birds. Supportive therapy (fluids, thermal support, non-nephrotoxic analgesia) is possible in rehab settings, but prognosis is poor in advanced visceral gout.

Outcome and Economic/One Health Impact

Ecological function loss. With fewer vultures removing livestock carcasses, feral dog and rat populations increased, amplifying rabies and other zoonoses (Markandya et al., 2008).

Human health and economic costs. Modeling links vulture declines to substantial increases in rabies incidence and associated costs (post-exposure prophylaxis, mortality), with estimates in the billions of USD over multiple years (Markandya et al., 2008).

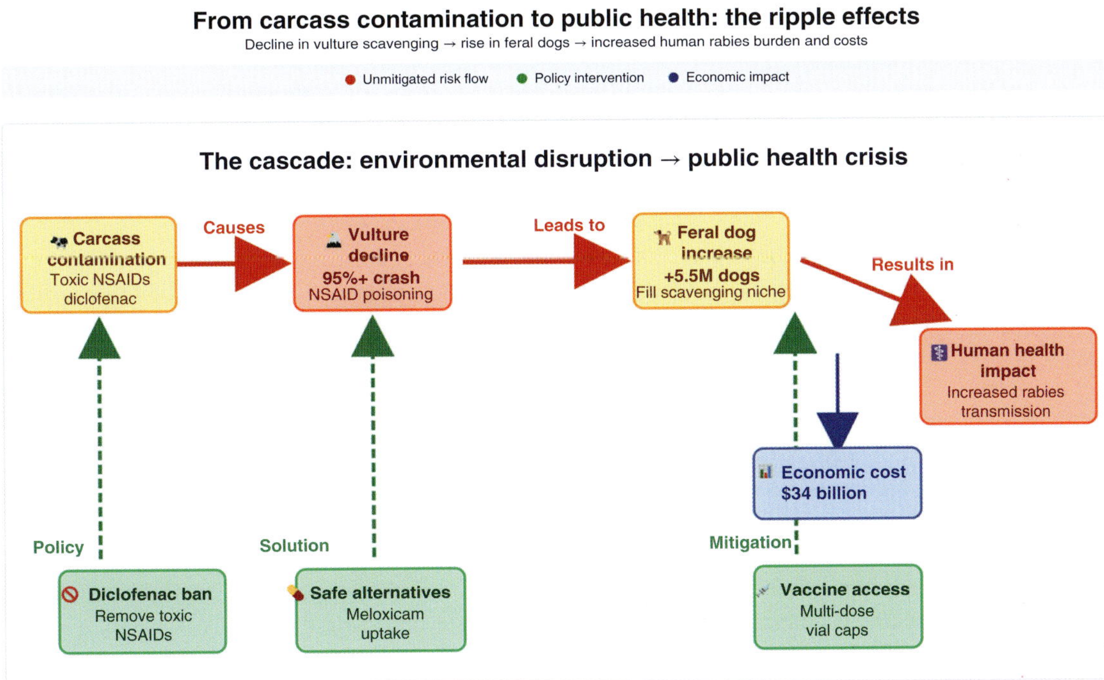

Figure 11.15 From carcass contamination to public health: the ripple effects. Vulture decline → dog population increase → higher human rabies burden; policy nodes show bans/substitutions (Cuthbert et al., 2011, 2016; Markandya et al., 2008).

Population trends after bans. Carcass surveys show declining diclofenac contamination post-ban, but continued illegal use and other toxic NSAIDs slow recovery; some colonies stabilize where enforcement and meloxicam uptake are strongest (Cuthbert et al., 2011, 2016) (Figure 11.15).

Lessons Learned and Implications

Evidence-based drug policy. Bans and restrictions work – but must extend beyond diclofenac to ketoprofen, aceclofenac (pro-drug → diclofenac), and nimesulide, all documented as vulture-toxic or hazardous via metabolism (Galligan et al., 2016, 2022; Naidoo et al., 2010).

Safer alternatives. Meloxicam is safe for Gyps vultures at field exposures and should be the default veterinary NSAID in vulture range states (Swan et al., 2006).

Carcass oversight. Dumps/abattoirs should implement screening and safe disposal protocols with staff training.

Surveillance. Incorporate routine residue testing (LC-MS/MS) of carcasses and necropsy-based NSAID screening for vultures into national action plans.

Teaching value. This case integrates toxicology, pharmacology, wildlife medicine, and One Health economics; it pairs well with problem-based learning on diagnostics plus policy.

Integrated Insights and Teaching Takeaways

These five case studies – (A) acute cyanide pesticide poisoning in cattle (India), (B) aflatoxicosis abortion storm in a dairy herd (Pakistan), (C) lead poisoning linked to artisanal mining (Zamfara, Nigeria), (D) ionophore (monensin) feed-mixing error in buffaloes (Brazil), and (E) NSAID-associated vulture collapse (South Asia) – illustrate recurring themes crucial for veterinary professionals and educators.

One Health and sentinel animals. Animals often serve as early warning signals for environmental toxicants. In Zamfara (Case C), unusual livestock deaths presaged a human lead-poisoning emergency investigated via a One Health team (Dooyema et al., 2012). In South Asia (Case E), cliff-edge Gyps declines revealed a veterinary-drug hazard in livestock systems (Green et al., 2006; Oaks et al., 2004). Teaching students to recognize unusual mortality patterns (e.g., multiple animals – sometimes across species – dying acutely) as potential toxin outbreaks can accelerate public health interventions. A One Health approach – deliberate collaboration among veterinarians, physicians, and environmental experts – is essential (Cuthbert et al., 2011; Dooyema et al., 2012) (Figure 11.16).

Importance of history and diagnostics. Each case underlines targeted history and fit-for-purpose testing. In the dairy aflatoxicosis (Case B), linking late-term abortions and a 19% milk drop to a new concentrate was decisive (Penagos-Tabares et al., 2024); in the cyanide mass mortality (Case A), a recent

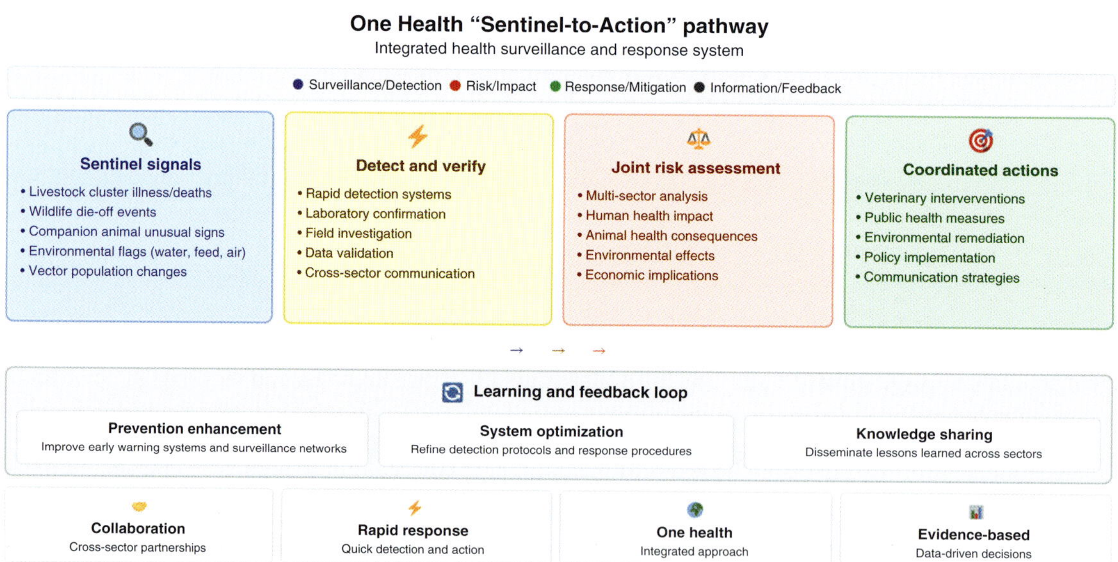

Figure 11.16 One Health escalation in toxicology: from sentinel animals to public health action. Unusual animal morbidity/mortality (e.g., Zamfara livestock; South Asian vultures) → field history & rapid tests → confirmatory analytics → risk communication → mitigation (carcass control, antidotes) → policy (e.g., diclofenac ban) (Cuthbert et al., 2011; Dooyema et al., 2012; Green et al., 2006; Oaks et al., 2004).

field spray and bitter-almond rumen odor rapidly narrowed the culprit (Gupta, 2018). Emphasize history domains (feed changes, pasture treatments, mining/industrial activity, recent medications) and align them to diagnostics: ELISA/LC-MS/MS for aflatoxins and AFM1 (Akbar et al., 2020; Penagos-Tabares et al., 2024), atomic absorption spectroscopy (AAS)/inductively coupled plasma mass spectrometry (ICP-MS) for lead (Dooyema et al., 2012), and field colorimetric tests for cyanide (Gupta, 2018). Context matters – e.g., ppb of aflatoxin in feed vs. AFM1 in milk, or blood-lead thresholds in cattle vs. goats (Table 11.6).

Clinical reasoning and differentials. The encountered syndromes – neurotoxicosis and per-acute collapse (Case A), reproductive failure (Case B), avian sudden deaths with visceral gout (Case E), and exertional weakness/myonecrosis (Case D) – compel practitioners to keep toxicological differentials in mind. These are ideal for problem-based learning: for tremors/sudden death in cattle, build and test a list (organophosphates/carbamates, cyanide from plants or pesticides, nitrate/nitrite, lightning); for abortion storms, include mycotoxins alongside infectious causes (Gupta, 2018; Kahn & Line, 2010) (Figure 11.17).

Emergency management and antidotes. Field action often precedes lab confirmation. Teams should know first-line measures and antidotes: atropine ± pralidoxime for organophosphates/carbamates; sodium thiosulfate ± hydroxocobalamin for suspected cyanide; chelators for lead where feasible (Gupta, 2018; Papich, 2021). Other syndromes (ionophore and aflatoxin toxicoses) lack specific antidotes, so supportive care and immediate exposure cessation are paramount (Akbar et al., 2020; Silva et al., 2022). Simulation of "sudden herd collapse" or "abortion-storm triage" improves readiness; clinics should maintain antidote kits and mass-care protocols (Table 11.7).

Prevention, education, and regulation. Most tragedies here were preventable: safe pesticide use and farmer training; feed QA/QC and medicated-feed stewardship; regulation/oversight of mining and vulture-toxic NSAIDs; and mycotoxin control (drying, aeration, storage, binders) (Akbar et al., 2020; Cuthbert et al., 2011; Dooyema et al., 2012; Silva et al., 2022). For educators, prevention deserves equal emphasis to treatment: integrated pest management, label-adherent drug use and carcass disposal, supplier quality systems, and practical checklists farmers can implement (Figure 11.18).

Economic and ethical implications. Beyond animal losses, toxicological events propagate ripple effects – discarded milk and market penalties (aflatoxin), loss of draft power (ionophores), and even national health costs (rabies burden after vulture declines) (Markandya et al., 2008). Framing these economics helps clinicians advocate for prevention and surveillance. Ethically, veterinarians have duties to prevent suffering: these cases (e.g., monensin-poisoned buffaloes, aflatoxin-affected fetuses) argue for proactive stewardship and chemical safety culture (Figure 11.19).

Cross-sector collaboration. Solving and preventing such incidents requires teamwork beyond the clinic. In Zamfara, a One Health investigation combined veterinary, medical, and environmental expertise to control lead exposure (Dooyema et al., 2012); in South Asia, conservation NGOs and vets helped translate toxicology into NSAID policy change (Cuthbert et al., 2011). Practical competencies include knowing who to call (public health, environment, wildlife, tox labs), how to ship samples with chain-of-custody, and how to communicate risk to farmers and the public (Table 11.8).

Table 11.6 Matching history cues to diagnostic samples and tests in tropical toxicology.

History/scene cue	Likely hazard(s)	Priority samples to collect (first 3)	Primary tests (screen → confirm)	Typical TAT* (field/lab)	Decision trigger/notes
New batch of concentrate/TMR; ration reformulated; sudden weakness/ recumbency	Ionophores (monensin, lasalocid, salinomycin, etc.)	1) Suspect feed/ premix (0.5–1 kg); 2) serum/EDTA blood (CK, cTnI); 3) heart + skeletal muscle (fresh + fixed)	Rapid CK/cTnI → LC-MS/ MS panel for ionophores (feed/rumen)	1–2 h/2–5 d	Pull feed immediately if CK ↑ or multiple animals affected; confirm dose in feed.
Moldy feed, hot/ humid storage; drop in milk; calves ill	Mycotoxins (AFB1, AFM1, ochratoxin, fumonisins)	1) Feed/TMR (composite); 2) milk (AFM1); 3) serum/liver (if sick)	ELISA screen (AFB1/ AFM1) → LC-MS/MS multi-mycotoxin	0.5 d/1–3 d	Dump milk if AFM1 over limit; segregate/ replace feed; binder only as adjunct.
Pasture or shed recently sprayed; SLUD signs	OP/carbamate insecticides	1) Whole blood (cholinesterase); 2) forage/surface swabs; 3) rumen content	AChE/BChE activity (colorimetry) → GC/ LC-MS compound ID	1–3 h/1–3 d	Treat as OP/Carb: atropine ± oxime; compare paired ChE to herd controls.
Sudden deaths after grazing wilted sorghum/cassava, chewing pits	Cyanogenic glycosides → HCN	1) Plant material; 2) rumen content; 3) liver	Picrate paper/spectro HCN → microdiffusion + spectro	15–60 min/1 d	If field HCN positive, give nitrite/thiosulfate per protocol; keep samples airtight & cold.
Drought-stressed, heavily fertilized forage; chocolate-brown blood	Nitrate/nitrite	1) Forage/water; 2) ocular fluid (postmortem); 3) rumen content	Dipstick/Griess spectro → Ion chromatography	15–30 min / 1–2 d	If methemoglobinemia suspected, give methylene blue (where permitted).
Mining/battery recycling nearby; neuro signs; abortions; wildlife deaths	Lead (Pb) (± other metals)	1) EDTA whole blood; 2) liver/kidney; 3) milk (dairy)	AAS/ICP-MS (blood/ tissues/milk); (soil: portable XRF for screening)	— / 1–3 d	Blood Pb >0.35 mg/L (35 µg/dL) strongly supportive; prevent further exposure, manage food-safety.
Warm pond/dam, scums; acute hepatic/neurologic cases	Cyanobacteria (microcystins, anatoxin-a, etc.)	1) Water (scum + subsurface); 2) stomach/rumen content; 3) liver	ELISA (microcystins) → LC-MS/ MS; histopath ± PP2A activity	0.5 d / 2–5 d	Remove access immediately; activated carbon if early; warn community.

Baleage/silage with carcass contamination; flaccid paralysis	Botulism (C/D)	1) Serum (paired); 2) GI/rumen content; 3) suspect feed/silage	ELISA/Endopep-MS (lab) ± PCR for C. botulinum genes	— / 1–3 d	Give antitoxin early if available; feed/source control; mouse bioassay where still used.
Access to rodenticide stores; bleeding, hematomas	Anticoagulants (brodifacoum, etc.)	1) Whole blood (PT/ ACT); 2) liver (if PM); 3) bait sample	PT/INR bedside → LC-MS/MS anticoagulant panel	<1 h / 2–7 d	Start vitamin K1 if coagulopathy; continue pending ID/half-life.
Urea lick/new NPN; rapid bloat, tremors	Urea–ammonia toxicosis	1) Rumen liquor; 2) ocular fluid; 3) feed/lick	Ammonia meter/ ISE → confirm enzymatic spectro	minutes/1 d	Give cold water + vinegar; treat promptly; collect rumen samples quickly.
Recent NSAID treatment in herd; concern for wildlife scavengers	Diclofenac/ketoprofen/ aceclofenac→diclofenac/ nimesulide	1) Injection-site muscle; 2) liver/kidney (PM); 3) drug vials/records	LC-MS/MS for NSAIDs (tissues)	—/2–5 d	Carcass management to protect vultures; substitute meloxicam going forward.
Salty well/ evaporation ponds; neurologic signs	Salt/water-deprivation	1) Serum/CSF Na; 2) brain (PM); 3) water sample	Electrolytes (Na, osmolality) → histo (eosinophilic meningoencephalitis)	<1 h/1–2 d	Gradual rehydration; avoid rapid shifts.

* TAT, **turnaround time** (approximate): field screens are same-day where equipment exists; confirmatory chemistry typically 1–5 business days depending on lab capacity and shipping.

Example cues (new feed, pasture spraying, mining nearby, recent medications) mapped to priority samples (feed, milk, blood, liver/kidney, rumen) and tests (ELISA/LC-MS/MS for aflatoxins; colorimetry for cyanide; AAS/ICP-MS for Pb), with decision-useful turnaround times.

General sampling and handling tips (fast decisions, fewer redraws)

- Collect duplicates of each matrix (one for screen, one for confirm); include a blank (unused container opened at site).
- Use EDTA whole blood for metals and cholinesterase; avoid brass needles for Pb.
- For volatile/reactive analytes (HCN, NH_3), keep airtight, cold, and analyze ASAP.
- For feed/TMR, submit a well-mixed composite; retain a split on farm.
- Maintain chain-of-custody, label with date/time, and ship chilled; freeze tissues if delayed.

Source: Compiled from Gupta (2018); Akbar et al. (2020); Dooyema et al. (2012); Penagos-Tabares et al. (2024).

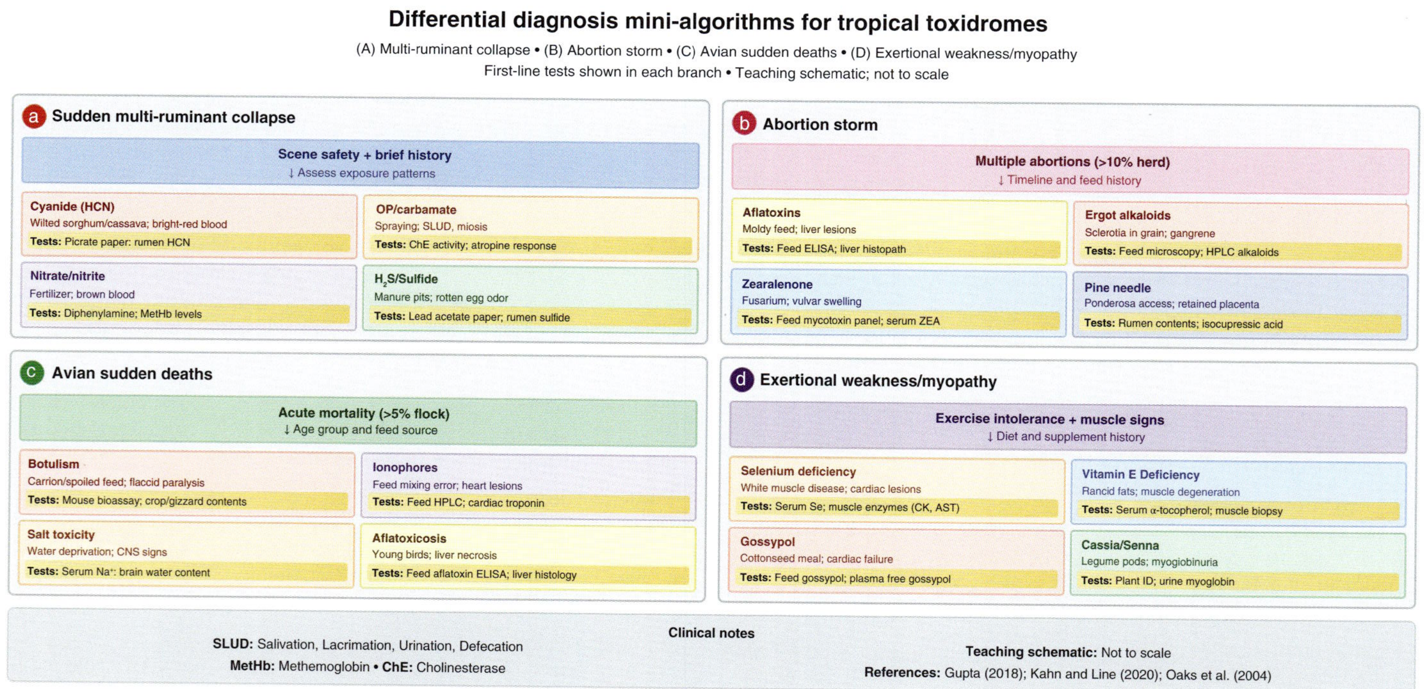

Figure 11.17 Differential diagnosis mini-algorithms for tropical toxidromes. Panels: (a) sudden multi-ruminant collapse; (b) abortion storm; (c) avian sudden deaths; (d) exertional weakness/myopathy. Each shows key differentials and "first tests." (Gupta, 2018; Kahn & Line, 2010; Oaks et al., 2004; Penagos-Tabares et al., 2024; Silva et al., 2022).

Table 11.7 Emergency actions and antidotes by syndrome.

Syndrome/scene cue	First actions (field)	Antidote/emergency drug(s)	Typical doses (adult cattle unless noted)	Monitoring and supportive care	Logistics/caveats
Organophosphate/carbamate insecticides (spraying, SLUD signs, miosis)	Remove from source; decontaminate skin (soap + water); minimize handling stress	Atropine sulfate (muscarinic blocker). Consider pralidoxime (2-PAM) for OPs with nicotinic signs (weakness, fasciculations).	Atropine: 0.6–1 mg/kg; give ~1/3 IV, remainder IM/SC; repeat to effect as signs recur. (MSD Veterinary Manual) 2-PAM (OPs): commonly 20 mg/kg IV slowly (30–120 min); may repeat (consult tox center/local protocol). (DVM 360)	Airway/oxygen as needed; fluids; control seizures if present. Expect tachycardia, decreased bronchial secretions as "endpoints" of atropinization.	Carbamates often respond to atropine alone; oxime benefit is less certain. Do not delay atropine while arranging oxime.
Suspected cyanide (wilted sorghum/cassava, cherry leaves; bright red blood; per-acute collapse)	Immediate removal from source; minimize exertion (↓ O_2 demand)	Sodium nitrite → sodium thiosulfate (sequential IV). Where available: hydroxocobalamin IV (alternative course).	Na nitrite: 20 mg/kg IV (10 g/100 mL); infuse over 3–4 min. Then Na thiosulfate 20%: ≥500 mg/kg slow IV. (MSD Veterinary Manual) (Field notes: amyl nitrite inhalation may be used as a bridge if on hand. (MSD Veterinary Manual)) Hydroxocobalamin: IV per product label; do not run in same line as nitrite/thiosulfate. (CHEMM)	Oxygen if available; handle quietly; consider repeat ½-dose of nitrite + thiosulfate if signs recur. (CHEMM)	Stock NITHIODOTE (nitrite+thiosulfate) or equivalent in ambulatory kits. Incompatibility: hydroxocobalamin + NITHIODOTE in same line. (CHEMM)
Lead (Pb) (battery dump/mining nearby; neuro signs; calves esp.)	Pull exposed animals; segregate high-risk classes (calves, dairy); prevent further ingestion	Chelation (where permitted): Calcium disodium EDTA (Ca-EDTA) ± thiamine	Ca-EDTA: 110 mg/kg/day IV or SC, divided BID for 3 d; repeat after 2-day rest. Thiamine: 2–4 mg/kg SC daily. (MSD Veterinary Manual)	Manage seizures; laxatives/rumenotomy in select cases; long withdrawals likely; monitor blood Pb serially. (MSD Veterinary Manual)	For food-producing animals, treatment often not recommended due to residues, poor prognosis, and regulatory issues; consult authorities before chelating. (MSD Veterinary Manual)

(*Continued*)

Table 11.7 (Continued)

Syndrome/scene cue	First actions (field)	Antidote/emergency drug(s)	Typical doses (adult cattle unless noted)	Monitoring and supportive care	Logistics/caveats
Aflatoxicosis (AFB1/AFM1) (moldy feed, hot/humid storage; drop in milk/ill calves)	Stop exposure immediately; switch to safe ration; discard contaminated milk as required	No specific antidote	—	Fluids; rumen support; vitamin/mineral repletion as needed; monitor liver enzymes; manage secondary infections; consider binders as adjunct (not curative).	Emphasize exposure control and regulatory milk/meat compliance; confirm by ELISA/LC-MS/MS as feasible. (Merck Veterinary Manual)
Ionophore toxicosis (monensin/lasalocid mix error; exertional weakness, myopathy, arrhythmias)	Pull feed immediately; strict rest; minimize stress/handling	No antidote	—	Aggressive supportive care: IV fluids, correct electrolytes/acid-base; manage arrhythmias; oxygen as needed; monitor CK and cTnI trends; prolonged convalescence for survivors. (Merck Veterinary Manual)	Prognosis guarded; cardiac/skeletal muscle injury can be permanent. Prevent with feed QA and label separation. (Merck Veterinary Manual)

Organophosphate/carbamate (atropine ± pralidoxime); suspected cyanide (sodium thiosulfate ± hydroxocobalamin); lead (chelation where available); aflatoxin and ionophores (no antidote: remove exposure + supportive care). Notes on dosing caveats and logistics.
Notes and reminders (field reality):

- Give antidotes while you're arranging confirmatory testing –don't wait when classic toxidromes are present. General treatment principles remain: remove exposure, supportive care, then specific antidotes when indicated.
- Cyanide kits: sequential nitrite → thiosulfate is standard in ruminants; some evidence supports IM routes when IV is impractical, but IV remains preferred when possible.
- Documentation: label every dose, route, and time; keep chain-of-custody for suspect feeds/waters and note carcass handling if wildlife risks exist.

Source: Compiled from Gupta (2018); Papich (2021); Dooyema et al. (2012); Silva et al. (2022).

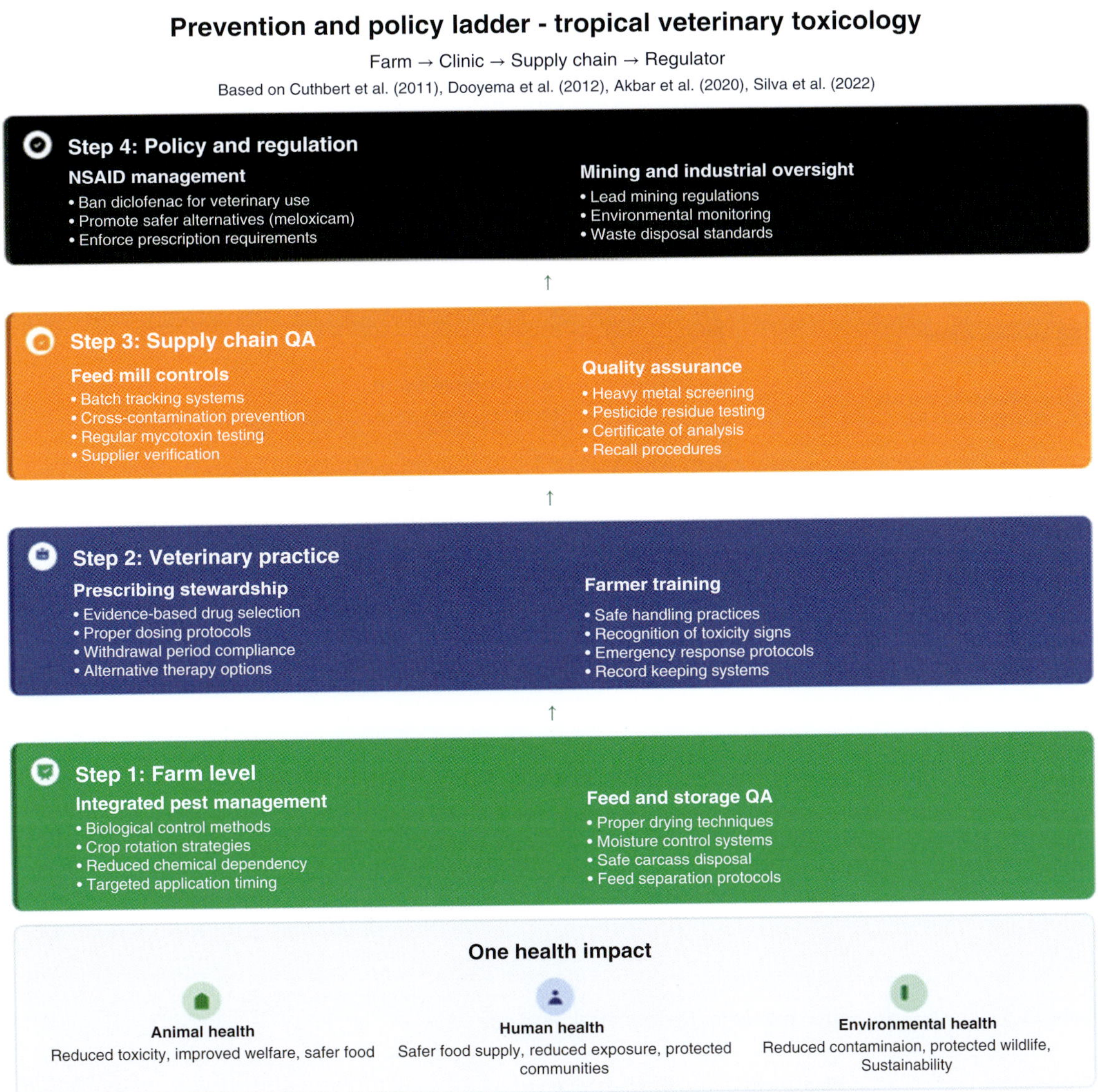

Figure 11.18 Prevention ladder for tropical veterinary toxicology. Farm-level (IPM, feed QA, storage/drying, carcass disposal) → veterinary practice (prescribing stewardship, farmer training) → supply chain (mill traceability, testing) → policy (NSAID bans/substitutions; mining oversight) (Akbar et al., 2020; Cuthbert et al., 2011; Dooyema et al., 2012; Silva et al., 2022).

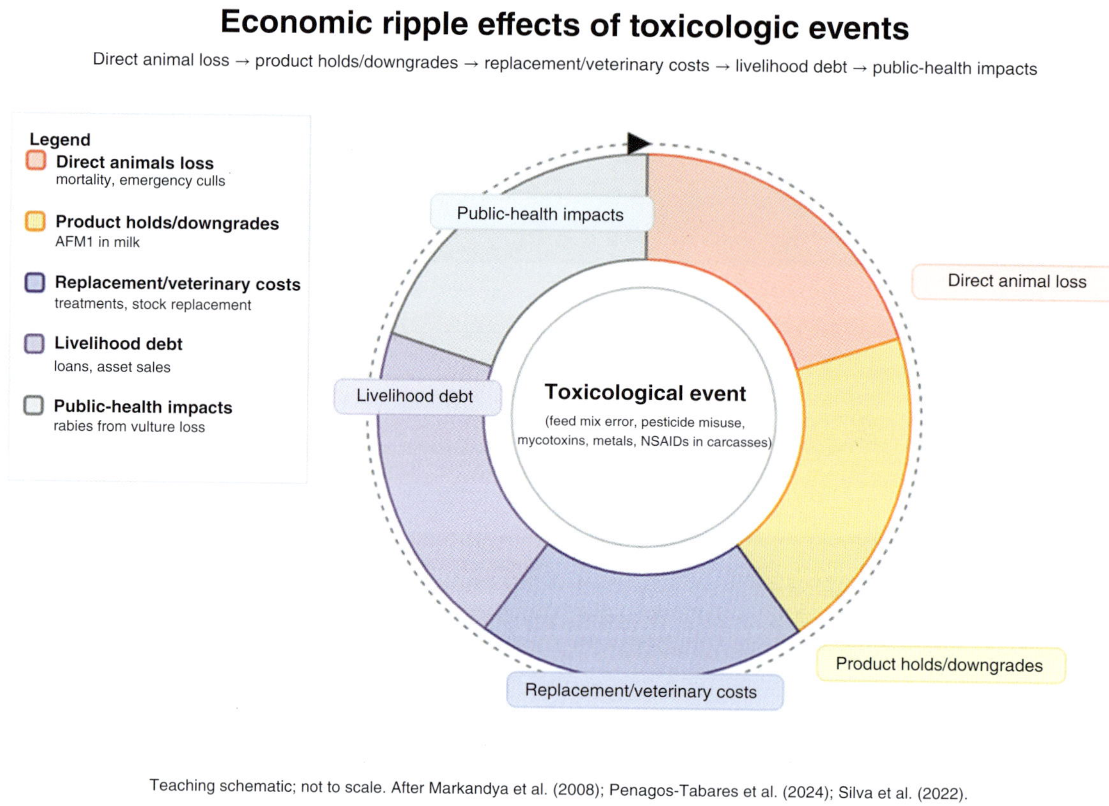

Figure 11.19 Economic ripple effects of toxicological events. Direct animal loss → product holds/downgrades (e.g., AFM1 in milk) → replacement/veterinary costs → livelihood debt → public health impacts (e.g., rabies from vulture loss) (Markandya et al., 2008; Penagos-Tabares et al., 2024; Silva et al., 2022).

Table 11.8 Cross-sector action matrix for toxicological incidents

Trigger/scenario (examples)	When to call	Who to call (primary → secondary)	What to send immediately (data packet)	Priority samples and target tests	Decision-useful TAT
Sudden multi-ruminant collapse (shared pasture/feed)	Now (≤1 h)	Vet authority/ animal health EOC → toxicology lab; poison center	Line list (IDs, signs, times), feed/water lot IDs, site photos, exposure map	Feed/TMR and premix (LC-MS/MS ionophores/ pesticides), rumen liquor (HCN colorimetry/ microdiffusion; nitrates), whole blood (ChE, metHb), heart/skeletal muscle (histo)	Field 15–60 min; lab 1–3 d

Table 11.8 (Continued)

Trigger/scenario (examples)	When to call	Who to call (primary → secondary)	What to send immediately (data packet)	Priority samples and target tests	Decision-useful TAT
Abortion storm/milk rejection (new or moldy feed)	Same day	Vet authority → dairy regulator/ food-safety lab	Bulk tank results, feed invoices, ration sheet, lot traceability	Feed composite (ELISA AFB1 → LC-MS/MS multi-mycotoxin), milk (AFM1 ELISA → confirm LC-MS/MS), liver if PM	Screen 0.5–1 d; confirm 1–3 d
Avian carcasses/ vulture deaths near carcasses	Now	Wildlife authority → environment ministry; tox lab	Carcass GPS, photos, livestock treatment records	Injection-site muscle, liver/kidney (LC-MS/MS NSAIDs); GI content (GC/LC-MS pesticides if baiting suspected)	2–5 d
Blue-green scums/stock deaths at water source	Now	Environment/ water resources → public health; vet authority	Waterbody location, bloom photos, recent weather	Scum + subsurface water (ELISA microcystins → LC-MS/ MS; anatoxin-a LC-MS/ MS), stomach/rumen content, liver (PP2A activity/histo)	Screen 0.5 d; confirm 2–5 d
OP/Carbamate spray drift; SLUD signs	Now	Vet authority → poison center; agriculture/ pesticide regulator	Spray records, product label, wind/ weather, map of drift	Whole blood (AChE/ BChE activity), forage swabs, GI/rumen (GC/ LC-MS compound ID)	ChE 1–3 h; confirm 1–3 d
Chocolate-brown blood; drought + fertilized forage (nitrate/nitrite)	Now	Vet authority → feed/forage lab	Field notes, pasture/ fertilizer history	Forage/water (dipstick/ Griess spectro), ocular fluid (PM nitrite), rumen content	Field 15–30 min; lab 1–2 d
Mining/battery recycling nearby; neuro signs; wildlife affected	Same day	Environment/ mines regulator → public health; tox lab	Site photos, GPS, list of exposed species/ ages, human co-exposures	EDTA blood (Pb by AAS/ ICP-MS), liver/kidney (Pb), milk (Pb), soil (portable XRF screen → lab confirm)	1–3 d
Flaccid paralysis in birds (ponds/ silage)	Same day	Wildlife authority → vet authority; reference lab	Carcass photos, feed/silage lot IDs, water source	Serum/GI/rumen content, suspect feed/ silage (Endopep-MS or ELISA; PCR adjunct; mouse bioassay where used)	1–3 d
Suspected malicious baiting/ criminal act	Now	Law enforcement → vet authority; wildlife and public health	Scene documentation, chain-of-custody forms, witness statements	Baits, GI content, liver/ kidney (GC/LC-MS wide screen), surface swabs	2–7 d (prioritize triage screens)

(Continued)

Table 11.8 (Continued)

Triggers (sudden cluster; multi-species; food-safety risk), contact tree (public health, environment, wildlife, labs), and sample/shipping checklists (chain-of-custody, cold chain, target analytes).

Contact tree (quick list)

- Animal health (lead): state/provincial veterinary authority / animal health EOC.
- Public health: zoonoses/food-safety unit; poison information center.
- Environment / water: environmental protection, water resources, fisheries.
- Wildlife: wildlife/veterinary services, conservation authority.
- Laboratories: nearest toxicology/chemistry lab (LC-MS/MS, ICP-MS), reference pathology lab, forage/water lab.
- Regulators / industry: pesticide regulator, feed mill QA, dairy/abattoir inspector.
- Law enforcement: if intentional poisoning or critical infrastructure risk.

Universal sample and shipping checklist (what to send)

- Sampling plan: duplicate samples per matrix (A = screen, B = confirm) + one blank; record date/time, GPS, collector.
- Matrices and volumes: feed/TMR (≥1 kg), water (2×250 mL), blood EDTA (≥3 mL), serum (≥3 mL), rumen (≥50 mL), liver/kidney (≥100 g each), milk (2×50 mL), plant material (≥200 g), injection-site muscle (≥50 g).
- Preservation: airtight for volatile/reactive (HCN, NH_3); cold chain (4°C) → freeze tissues if delay >24 h; protect from light for photolabile analytes.
- Packaging: leak-proof primary + absorbent + rigid secondary (triple packaging); label biohazard if appropriate; dry ice with UN1845 declaration when required.
- Chain-of-custody: numbered seals, signature trail; include request form with suspected hazards and target analytes.
- Documentation packet: case definition; line list; exposure timeline; site map/photos; product labels/SDS; treatment log; herd inventory; milk/feed lot IDs.

Turnaround and communication norms

- Field screens (HCN, nitrates, ChE, AFM1 ELISA): same day where kits exist.
- Confirmatory chemistry (LC-MS/MS, ICP-MS): 1–5 business days depending on lab capacity/shipping.
- Pathology/histology: preliminary 24–72 h; special stains/tests longer.
- Reporting cadence: initial notification <2 h for acute clusters; daily situation update until controlled; final report with corrective actions and prevention notes.

Escalation triggers

- Multi-species or wildlife + livestock affected; children/human co-exposures; food-chain entry (milk/meat).
- Geographically spreading events; suspected criminal intent; cross-border implications.

Source: Compiled from Dooyema et al. (2012); Gupta (2018); Kahn and Line (2010).

References

Akbar, N., Maqbool, A., Ashraf, M., Sultan, A., & Khan, S. (2020). Assessment of aflatoxin in milk and feed samples from dairy farms in Pakistan. *Food Science & Nutrition*, *8*(11), 6316–6324. https://doi.org/10.1002/fsn3.1557

Blacksmith Institute. (2011). *Lead poisoning crisis in Zamfara State, Nigeria: Report of the environmental remediation program*. Blacksmith Institute.

Chandramohan, S., Mathesh, K., Mallord, J. W., Naidoo, V., Mahendran, K., Kesavan, M., Gaur, G. K., Pawde, A. M., Prakash, N., Ranade, S., & Saikia, D. (2022). Metabolism of aceclofenac to diclofenac in the domestic water buffalo: Implications for vultures. *Environmental Toxicology and Pharmacology*, *92*, 103860. https://doi.org/10.1016/j.etap.2022.103984

Cuthbert, R., Taggart, M. A., Prakash, V., Saini, M., Swarup, D., Upreti, S., Mateo, R., Chakraborty, S. S., Deori, P., & Green, R. E. (2011). Effectiveness of action in India to reduce exposure of Gyps vultures to the toxic veterinary drug diclofenac. *PLoS One*, *6*(5), e19069. https://doi.org/10.1371/journal.pone.0019069

Cuthbert, R., Taggart, M., Saini, M., Sharma, A., Das, A., Kulkarni, M. D., ... Green, R. E. (2016). Continuing mortality of vultures in India associated with illegal veterinary use of diclofenac and a potential threat from nimesulide. *Oryx*, *50*(1), 104–112. https://doi.org/10.1017/S003060531500037X

Dooyema, C. A., Neri, A., Lo, Y.-C., Durant, J., Dargan, P. I., Swarthout, T., Biya, O., Gidado, S. O., Haladu, S., Sani-Gwarzo, N., Nguku, P. M., Akpan, H., Idris, S., Bashir, A. M., & Brown, M. J. (2012). Outbreak of fatal childhood lead poisoning related to artisanal gold mining in Northwestern Nigeria, 2010. *Environmental Health Perspectives*, *120*(4), 601–607. https://doi.org/10.1289/ehp.1103965

Galligan, T. H., Green, R. E., Wolter, K., Taggart, M. A., Duncan, N., Mallord, J. W., Alderson, D., Li, Y., & Naidoo, V. (2022). The non-steroidal anti-inflammatory drug nimesulide kills Gyps vultures at concentrations found in the muscle of treated cattle. *Science of the Total Environment*, *807*, 150788. https://doi.org/10.1016/j.scitotenv.2021.150788

Galligan, T. H., Taggart, M. A., Cuthbert, R. J., Svobodova, D., Chipangura, J., Alderson, D., Prakash, V. M., & Naidoo, V. (2016). Metabolism of aceclofenac in cattle to vulture-killing diclofenac. *Conservation Biology*, *30*(5), 1122–1127. Portico. https://doi.org/10.1111/cobi.12711

Green, R. E., Newton, I., Shultz, S., Cunningham, A. A., Gilbert, M., Pain, D. J., & Prakash, V. (2006). Collapse of Asian vulture populations: Risk of mortality from residues of the veterinary drug diclofenac. *Journal of Applied Ecology*, *43*(5), 949–956. https://doi.org/10.1111/j.1365-2664.2006.01225.x

Gupta, R. C. (Ed.). (2018). *Veterinary toxicology: Basic and clinical principles* (3rd ed.). Academic Press.

Kahn, C. M., & Line, S. (Eds.). (2010). *The Merck veterinary manual* (10th ed.). Merck & Co., Inc.

Lo, Y. C., Dooyema, C. A., Neri, A., Durant, J., Jefferies, T., Medina-Marino, A., ... Brown, M. J. (2012). Childhood lead poisoning associated with gold ore processing: A village-level investigation—Zamfara State, Nigeria, October–November 2010. *Environmental Health Perspectives*, *120*(10), 1450–1455. https://doi.org/10.1289/ehp.1104793

Markandya, A., Taylor, T., Longo, A., Murty, M. N., Murty, S., & Dhavala, K. (2008). Counting the cost of vulture decline—An appraisal of the human health and other benefits of vultures in India. *Ecological Economics*, *67*(2), 194–204. https://doi.org/10.1016/j.ecolecon.2008.04.020

Naidoo, V., Wolter, K., Cromarty, D., Diekmann, M., Duncan, N., Taggart, M., ... Cuthbert, R. (2010). Toxicity of non-steroidal anti-inflammatory drugs to Gyps vultures: A new threat from ketoprofen. *Biology Letters*, *6*(3), 339–341. https://doi.org/10.1098/rsbl.2009.0818

Oaks, J. L., Gilbert, M., Virani, M. Z., Watson, R. T., Meteyer, C. U., Rideout, B. A., ... Khan, A. A. (2004). Diclofenac residues as the cause of vulture population decline in Pakistan. *Nature*, *427*(6975), 630–633. https://doi.org/10.1038/nature02317

Papich, M. G. (2021). *Saunders handbook of veterinary drugs* (5th ed.). Elsevier.

Penagos-Tabares, F., Mahmood, M., Sulyok, M., Rafique, K., Khan, M. R., Zebeli, Q., Krska, R., & Metzler-Zebeli, B. (2024). Outbreak of aflatoxicosis in a dairy herd induced depletion in milk yield and high abortion rate in Pakistan. *Toxicon*, *246*, 107799. https://doi.org/10.1016/j.toxicon.2024.107799

Peterson, M. E., & Talcott, P. A. (Eds.). (2013). *Small Animal Toxicology* (3rd ed.). Elsevier/Saunders. https://doi.org/10.1016/C2010-0-67099-4

SAVE (Saving Asia's Vultures from Extinction). (2020). Saving Indian Vultures from Extinction: Policy Statement. https://save-vultures.org/wp-content/uploads/2020/02/Vulture-policy-brief-India-Feb-20-updated.pdf

Silva, A. W. O., Mendonça, M. F. F., Freitas, M. D., Ribeiro Filho, A. L., Silva, R. D. G., Leal, P. V., Pimentel, L. A., & Peixoto, T. C. (2022). Accidental monensin poisoning in buffaloes in Bahia, Brazil. *Pesquisa Veterinária Brasileira*, *42*. https://doi.org/10.1590/1678-5150-pvb-6937

Swan, G., Naidoo, V., Cuthbert, R., Green, R. E., Pain, D. J., Swarup, D., ... Prakash, V. (2006). Removing the threat of diclofenac to critically endangered Asian vultures. *PLoS Biology*, *4*(3), e66. https://doi.org/10.1371/journal.pbio.0040066

The Times of India. (2018, April 10). 56 cows die after feeding on pesticides in Andhra village. https://timesofindia.indiatimes.com/city/amaravati/56-cows-die-after-feeding-on-pesticides-in-andhra-village/articleshow/63689075.cms

Yunus, A. W., Lindahl, J. F., Anwar, Z., Ullah, A., & Ibrahim, M. N. M. (2022). Farmer's knowledge and suggested approaches for controlling aflatoxin contamination of raw milk in Pakistan. *Frontiers in Microbiology*, *13*. https://doi.org/10.3389/fmicb.2022.980105

Appendix – Reference Tables and Diagnostic Aids

This appendix summarizes key facts, tests, and sample-handling rules from Chapters 1–11 for rapid field and laboratory use. For context and case examples, see the parent chapters noted in each table.

A0. Systems of Weights and Measures

Toxicology literature has used several systems (metric/SI, imperial, apothecaries, avoirdupois). Use SI/metric for all calculations and prescribing. Older systems and household measures are listed here to interpret legacy texts and labels.

1) Metric system (SI)
   Base units: meter (m, length), liter (L, volume), gram (g, mass).
   Volume: 1 L = 1,000 milliliters (mL).
   Mass: 1 kilogram (kg) = 1,000 g; 1 g = 1,000 milligrams (mg); 1 mg = 1,000 micrograms (mcg).
   Prescription safety: Write microgram as mcg (not µg) to avoid misreading as mg.
   Length: 1 meter = 100 centimeters (cm) = 1,000 millimeters (mm); 1 mm = 1,000 micrometers (µm); 1 µm = 1,000 nanometers (nm).
   (Legacy terms: micron = µm; millimicron = nm.)
   Definition note: Historically, the gram was defined as the mass of 1 cm^3 of water at 4°C.
2) **Imperial System (Apothecaries and Avoirdupois)**
   Two weight systems coexisted under imperial.
   - **Apothecaries (pharmacy)** – archaic system using roman numerals/symbols.
     Weights: 20 grains (gr) = 1 scruple; 3 scruples (60 gr) = 1 dram (dr); 8 dr (480 gr) = 1 ounce (oz apoth.); 12 oz = 1 pound (lb apoth.) = 5,760 gr.
     Fluid measures (shared with Imperial): 60 minims = 1 fluid dram; 8 fluid drams (480 minims) = 1 fluid ounce (fl oz).
   - **Avoirdupois (commercial)** – official UK trade weights.
     Weights: 1 pound (lb avdp) = 7,000 gr; 1 ounce (oz avdp) = 437.5 gr.
     Style: Write numerals in Arabic with abbreviations, e.g., 50 gr; 2 oz; 2 lb; 1/20 gr.

Fluid measures:

Imperial: 1 fl oz (imp) = 28.41 mL; 1 pt (imp) = 568 mL; 1 gal (imp) = 4.546 L; 1 L ≈ 35.2 fl oz (imp) ≈ 1.76 pt (imp) ≈ 0.22 gal (imp).
US customary differs: 1 US fl oz = 29.57 mL; 1 US pt = 473 mL (US pints/quarts/gallons are 4/5 of imperial).

Approximate imperial–metric equivalents:

1 grain (gr) ≈ 64.8 mg (≈ 65 mg); 100 mg ≈ 1.54 gr.
1 oz (avdp) = 28.35 g (≈ 28 g); 1 oz (apoth.) = 31.10 g (≈ 31 g).
1 lb (avdp) = 453.59 g (≈ 454 g); 1 kg ≈ 2.205 lb (≈ 2.2 lb).

Household measures (legacy; avoid for dosing):

1 drop ≈ 1 minim ≈ 0.06 mL.
1 teaspoonful (tsp) ≈ 60 minims ≈ 3.55 mL (legacy); modern standard tsp = **5 mL.**
1 dessertspoonful ≈ 120 minims ≈ 7.1 mL.
1 tablespoonful (Tbsp) ≈ ½ fl oz ≈ 14.2 mL (legacy); modern standard Tbsp = **15 mL.**
1 cup (imp) = 8 fl oz (imp) ≈ 227 mL. (Modern metric cups vary: 240–250 mL.)

Safety note: For prescriptions, always use metric (mg, g, mL). Household spoons and cups vary; relying on them can cause dosing errors.

A1. One-look Blood/mucosa Color to Mechanism, Suspects, and First Aid (see Chapter 9)

Blood/mucosa color	Likely mechanism	Usual suspects	Immediate first aid priorities
Brown/ chocolate	Methemoglobinemia	Nitrate/nitrite; sodium chlorate	Oxygen if hypoxemic; methylene blue IV (see A7/A8 dosing notes); reduce ongoing rumen release (chilled water and mineral oil in ruminants).
Cherry red	Cytochrome oxidase block	Cyanide (prussic acid)	Secure airway and oxygen; nitrite + thiosulfate kit if available; strict sample handling (see A5).
Bright red	Carboxyhemoglobin	Carbon monoxide	Fresh air; oxygen; ventilatory support.
Dark/"air hunger"	Hypercapnia/asphyxia	CO_2 accumulation; confinement	Fresh air; oxygen.

"Cherry red" venous blood suggests cyanide; "bright red" arterial mucosa is typical for CO exposure.

A2. Field Spot Tests for Nitrate/Nitrite (see Chapter 9)

Nitrate field test (diphenylamine–sulfuric acid) – plant cut surfaces:

1) Dissolve 0.5 g diphenylamine in 20 mL distilled water; carefully add concentrated H_2SO_4 to a total volume of 100 mL. Cool; store in the dark.
2) Just before use, mix equal parts of this stock and **80% sulfuric acid**.
3) Place one drop on a freshly cut plant surface. Positive: green to blue shift (indicative of > ~2% nitrate in plant sap).

Nitrite field test (Griess reaction: sulfanilic acid + α-naphthylamine) – liquids/plant cuts
Prepare reagents:

a) 0.5 g sulfanilic acid in 150 mL 20% glacial acetic acid.
b) 0.2 g α-naphthylamine HCl in 20% acetic acid (warm gently to dissolve).
   Test: Combine 2 mL sample + 2 mL (a) + 2 mL (b) in a clean tube.
   Positive: pink to red (Griess reaction).

Field trigger (forage hazard): pasture > 10–15 mg/g nitrate is potentially lethal (see A7 for full workflow).

A3. Blood Cholinesterase (ChE) Reference Activity (Modified Michel Method; see Chapters 7 and 10)

Useful when confirming organophosphate (OP)/carbamate exposure; interpret trends vs. a known baseline where available.

Species	% total ChE in RBCs	Whole-blood ChE activity (ΔpH)
Cattle	90%	0.30–0.75
Sheep	90%	0.10–0.30
Goat	89%	0.04–0.24
Horse	90%	0.20–0.65
Dog	61%	~ 0.43
Pig	67–88%	—

Most activity is erythrocytic; whole-blood ChE is a surrogate for junctional AChE. Use species-appropriate ranges and the same method across serial tests.

A4. OP/Carbamate Toxidrome – Antidotes and Cautions (see Chapters 7 and 10)

Scenario	Antidote/priority	Practical dose cues (see parent chapter)	Key cautions
Muscarinic crisis (OP/carbamate)	Atropine sulfate	Ruminants ~ 0.5 mg/kg; horse ~ 65 mg total; dog ~ 2 mg total. Give ~ ¼ IV, remainder SC/IM; repeat every 3–4 h for 1–2 days based on response.	Atropine treats muscarinic signs only; titrate to dry bronchial sounds/↑HR.
OP confirmed/suspected (early)	Oxime (e.g., pralidoxime/2-PAM; regional alternatives)	Use early to reactivate AChE (aging limits benefit). In buffalo (where approved): diacetylmonoxime (DAM) 30 mg/kg IV, then 26 mg/kg q14 h as an alternative regimen.	Do not give oximes in pure carbamate poisoning.
All cases	Supportive care	Oxygen/ventilation; dermal decontamination; fluids; benzodiazepines for seizures (as needed); temperature/glucose/electrolyte management.	Collect prebath samples if feasible; monitor for pancreatitis risk.

A5. Specimen Collection and Handling – Quick Reference (see Chapters 6 and 9)

Suspected agent	What to collect	Container and preservative	Handling/shipping
Nitrate/nitrite	Ocular fluid, serum; suspect feed/ingesta; water	Leak-proof plastic or glass	Freeze all samples for nitrate/nitrite assays; ship cold.
Cyanide (prussic acid)	Rumen/gastric contents; liver; suspect plants/feed	Airtight containers, filled to the brim if possible	Immediate chilling/freezing; minimize headspace; rush to lab.
Chlorinated hydrocarbons (e.g., DDT, dieldrin)	Fat, liver, brain; suspect baits	No plastic; use glass or aluminum	Chill/freeze; protect from light; seal well.
Anticoagulant rodenticides	Liver, kidney, stomach contents, any bait; citrated blood (PT/INR)	Routine tox containers + sodium citrate tubes	Keep chilled; avoid hemolysis; include exposure history and coagulopathy timeline.
OP/carbamate insecticides	Whole blood (ChE), serum; liver; fat; stomach/rumen contents; any product	Standard tubes/containers	Refrigerate promptly; run ChE ASAP; note any decontamination already done.

A6. Ectoparasiticide Emergencies (see Chapter 10)

Class	Signature toxidrome	First-hour priorities
OPs/carbamates	Cholinergic crisis (SLUDGE-M; bronchorrhea/bronchospasm; fasciculations progressing to weakness)	Dermal wash (mild detergent), oxygen/ventilation, atropine; oxime early for OPs only; benzodiazepines as needed.

Class	Signature toxidrome	First-hour priorities
Pyrethroids	Neuroexcitation, tremor/seizure; sometimes hyperthermia	Mild detergent bath; methocarbamol/benzodiazepine; temperature control; consider intravenous lipid emulsion (ILE) if refractory.
Amitraz	alpha-2 agonist syndrome (bradycardia, CNS depression, hyperglycemia)	Remove product/wash; yohimbine/atipamezole; fluids/warmth.

A7. Nitrate/Nitrite – Diagnostic Triggers and Sampling Workflow (see Chapter 9)

- When to suspect: Per-acute onset; dyspnea/cyanosis; brown blood; recent fertilizer use; pasture regrowth after a drought-break or frost; herd cases.
- Field rapid test: Use A2 protocols on plants/water/ingesta.
- Forage trigger: > 10–15 mg/g nitrate = potentially lethal range.
- Samples: Ocular fluid (from deceased animals), serum, feed/ingesta, water. Freeze immediately; ship on ice/dry ice.
- Treatment anchor: Methylene blue 4 mg/kg IV (2–4% solution); may repeat if ongoing rumen release. In ruminants, add mineral oil PO and chilled water.

A8. Quick Preparation Facts (Common Antidotes/Tests)

- Methylene blue: 1% = 10 mg/mL. Treatment target 4 mg/kg IV (often supplied as 2–4% solutions; dilute to a manageable volume).
- Griess reagents: Keep in labeled dropper bottles; prepare fresh monthly; store cool/dark.
- Pralidoxime (2-PAM): Follow local product concentration/dose guidance; administer early when OP poisoning is suspected.

A9. Submission Checklist (Clip-and-go)

- Gather key case history details: timeline, herd/flock map, recent sprays/dips/feed changes/weather events, water sources.
- Collect samples before decontamination: whenever possible, obtain samples prior to washing the animal or starting therapy.
- Use appropriate containers: glass/aluminum for chlorinated hydrocarbons; **airtight and full** (then **freeze**) for cyanide; **freeze all** nitrate/nitrite samples.
- Label and document chain of custody: animal ID, matrix, date/time, preservative, collector; attach chain-of-custody form.

- Maintain temperature control: refrigerate/freeze immediately; use an **insulated shipper** with ice/dry ice as required.
- Run parallel clinical tests: **PT/INR** for suspected anticoagulants; **whole-blood ChE** for OP/carbamate exposure.
- Alert the lab for rush/unstable analytes: e.g., cyanide, nitrite.

Cross-references

- Chapter 7: Organophosphorus and carbamates – toxidrome, ChE testing, atropine/oximes.
- Chapter 9: Nitrates, cyanide, and other natural toxicants – color clues, field tests, methylene blue, sampling.
- Chapter 10: Ectoparasiticides – **first-hour** treatment map.
- Chapter 6: **Sample-handling** principles and matrices.

Use this appendix as a first-pass aid. Always confirm doses and protocols against the full chapter text before treating individual cases.

Index

a

d